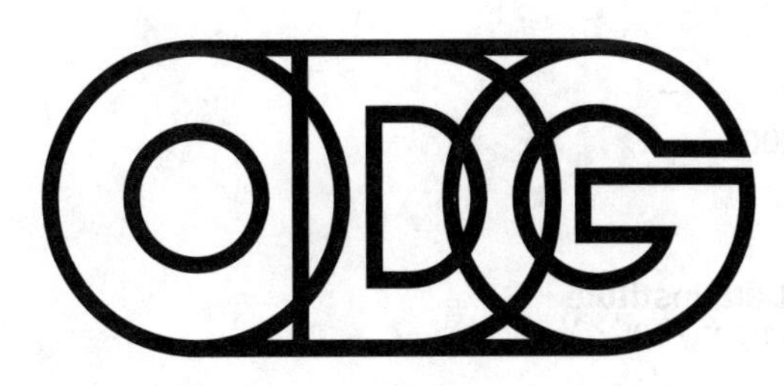

Official Disability Guidelines™

Special Edition
Top 200 Conditions

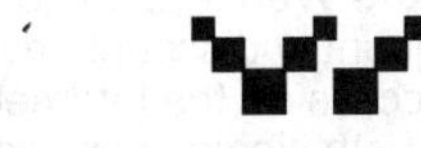

Work Loss Data Institute

Foureenth Edition
2009

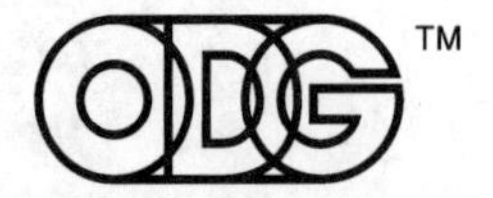

Official Disability Guidelines ™ 2009

FOURTEENTH EDITION

"The Evidence Based Guideline Company" ™
www.worklossdata.com

Printed and bound in the United States

ISBN 978-1-880891-50-6 **2009 *Official Disability Guidelines*** - January 2009, softbound, 2,112 pages, $195. *ODG's* return-to-work guidelines provide disability duration norms for every illness and injury, based on the largest experience database available. Thousands of employers are saving millions of dollars by using *ODG* to help employees recover and get back to work. Because the data is evidence based, it is fair to employees and defensible by employers. Includes a copy of *ODG Top 200.*

ISBN 978-1-880891-51-3 **2009 *ODG Top 200 Conditions*** - January 2009, softbound, 288 pages, $99. The Top 200 Conditions version of *ODG's* return-to-work guidelines covers those conditions that represent about 80% of total lost workdays, in a lightweight portable edition.

ISBN 978-1-880891-52-0 **2009 *ODG Treatment in Workers' Comp*** - January 2009, softbound, 4,224 pages, $325. *ODG's* treatment guidelines cover conditions likely to be seen in Workers' Comp, providing evidence based medical treatment recommendations. Includes a copy of *ODG Complete* and *ODG Top 200*, so this "ODG Treatment Library" contains a total of over 4,000 pages in 3 volumes.

ISBN 978-1-880891-53-7 **2009 *ODG on the Web*** - updated continuously, $195 per year. Access on the Internet via secure logon, using any standard Web browser. Available in both single user and network versions. Includes a copy of *ODG Top 200.*

ISBN 978-1-880891-55-1 **2009 *ODG Treatment on the Web*** - updated continuously, $325 per year (for single user access, quantity discounts available). Integrated treatment and return-to-work guidelines. Access on the Internet via secure logon, using any standard Web browser. Available in both single user and network versions. Includes access to *ODG on the Web* and a copy of *ODG Top 200.*

Work Loss Data Institute, LLC
169 Saxony Road, Suite 101
Encinitas, CA 92024

800-488-5548
760-753-9992
760-753-9995 (fax)

EDITORIAL ADVISORY BOARD
ODG/ODG TREATMENT

EDITORIAL ADVISORY BOARD
ODG/ODG TREATMENT
(continued)

EDITORIAL ADVISORY BOARD
ODG/ODG TREATMENT
(continued)

EDITORIAL ADVISORY BOARD
ODG/ODG TREATMENT
(continued)

FOREWORD

"Change" has been a real buzzword across the nation this past year. And, it appears there will be much of it before things settle down. Yet, we at Work Loss Data Institute (WLDI) are taking a different approach. Our intent as we update and enhance *Official Disability Guidelines* (*ODG*) is to continue to follow the steady course set 14 years ago by Phil Denniston, WLDI's president and co-founder. That is, to build upon one constant – the value of evidence-based medicine. As such, we continue to follow a strict, ongoing, and unwavering methodological approach for identifying and recommending timely care consistent with the least invasive, most effective treatment protocols today's science has to offer. States that have adopted *ODG* have found, in comparing pre and post implementation, that by following *ODG,* injured workers receive earlier access to quality care and return to functionality sooner. From that, all else follows: return-to-work durations decrease, indemnity and medical costs per claim decrease, productivity increases, and quality of life issues improve for the injured workers, their families and society in general; a win-win for all involved in the workers' comp system.

Working with a "constant" does not in any way imply being idle; on the contrary. When the "constant" is evidenced-based medicine, by definition a moving target, WLDI, our staff, and our Editorial Advisory Board, under the direction of Dr. Charles "Bud" Kennedy, must be diligent in uncovering and summarizing the outcomes from studies, trials and meta-analyses of the ever-changing advances, developments and applications of medical and pharmaceutical treatments. That's what makes our mission so exciting. Though our course never "changes", we are always in motion.

And, we are continually chartering new waters. Highlights of our developments this year include three major new additions to *ODG*, to answer the needs of many of our subscribers. First, we have provided a brand new Chapter to *ODG Treatment in Workers' Comp*, addressing pulmonary injuries and illnesses. Secondly, with drug costs becoming an increasingly significant portion of total workers' comp medical costs, and evidence that many injured workers are receiving inappropriate prescriptions, the need for a Drug Formulary emerged and has been added as an Appendix to the 2009 *ODG*. The Formulary provides easy-to-access status information for all the drugs covered throughout the ODG guidelines, including brand name and generic antidepressants, anti-epilepsy drugs, herbal medicines, muscle relaxants, nonprescription analgesics, NSAIDS, opioids, corticosteroids, topical analgesics and more. Lastly, we are including a section on "causality" to the

Procedure Summary in all the chapters of *ODG Treatment*, to help determine if, in fact, an injury is likely to have been caused by the workplace. Preliminary results of our causality findings are included in this edition, but the topic is complex and, it is a work-in-progress as we go to Press.

Any one of us who has attempted to set a steady course in our personal or professional lives, knows there are challenges along the way. A relationship – though committed – has its many ups and downs; a course of therapy which ultimately is destined for a good outcome, can have distressing side effects during treatment. A business, too, may experience unsettling winds which threaten its course, but, with a good captain, a strong sense of teamwork, a large dose of self-discipline and a clear vision of the ultimate goal or destination, the journey can be satisfying and the arrival victorious. Rest-assured, with our 14th edition of *Official Disability Guidelines* and our 7th edition of *ODG Treatment*, the journey continues. WLDI remains above board and outward bound.

Patricia Whelan
Publisher

CONTENTS
Special Edition
Top 200 Conditions

"At a Glance" Table of Contents to the Structure of ICD9-CM Codes
Level 1: to Major Categories

"At a Glance" Table of Contents to the Structure of ICD9-CM Codes
Level 2: to 3-digit ranges

Range of ICD9 Codes	Description
001-139	**1. INFECTIOUS AND PARASITIC DISEASES**
001-009	Intestinal Infectious Diseases
010-018	Tuberculosis
020-027	Zoonotic Bacterial Diseases
030-042	Other Bacterial Diseases
045-049	Poliomyelitis And Other Non-Arthropod-Borne Viral Diseases Of Central Nervous System
050-057	Viral Diseases Accompanied By Exanthem
060-066	Arthropod-Borne Viral Diseases
070-079	Other Diseases Due To Viruses And Chlamydiae
080-088	Rickettsioses And Other Arthropod-Borne Diseases
090-099	Syphilis And Other Venereal Diseases
100-104	Other Spirochetal Diseases
110-118	Mycoses
120-129	Helminthiases
130-136	Other Infectious And Parasitic Diseases
137-139	Late Effects Of Infectious And Parasitic Diseases
140-239	**2. NEOPLASMS**
140-149	Malignant Neoplasm Of Lip, Oral Cavity, And Pharynx
150-159	Malignant Neoplasm Of Digestive Organs And Peritoneum
160-165	Malignant Neoplasm Of Respiratory And Intrathoracic Organs
170-176	Malignant Neoplasm Of Bone, Connective Tissue, Skin, And Breast
179-189	Malignant Neoplasm Of Genitourinary Organs
190-199	Malignant Neoplasm Of Other And Unspecified Sites
200-208	Malignant Neoplasm Of Lymphatic And Hematopoietic Tissue
210-229	Benign Neoplasms
230-234	Carcinoma In Situ
235-238	Neoplasms Of Uncertain Behavior
240-279	**3. ENDOCRINE, NUTRITIONAL AND METABOLIC DISEASES, AND IMMUNITY DISORDERS**
240-246	Disorders Of Thyroid Gland
250-259	Diseases Of Other Endocrine Glands
260-269	Nutritional Deficiencies
270-279	Other Metabolic And Immunity Disorders
280-289	**4. DISEASES OF THE BLOOD AND BLOOD-FORMING ORGANS**
290-319	**MENTAL DISORDERS**
290-299	Psychoses
290-294	Organic Psychotic Conditions
295-299	Other Psychoses
300-316	Neurotic Disorders, Personality Disorders, And Other Nonpsychotic Mental Disorders

"At a Glance" Table of Contents to the Structure of ICD9-CM Codes
Level 2: to 3-digit ranges
[*continued* -page 2 of 4]

Range of ICD9 Codes	Description
290-319	**MENTAL DISORDERS** (*continued*)
317-319	Mental Retardation
320-389	**DISEASES OF THE NERVOUS SYSTEM AND SENSE ORGANS**
320-326	Inflammatory Diseases Of The Central Nervous System
330-337	Hereditary And Degenerative Diseases Of The Central Nervous System
340-349	Other Disorders Of The Central Nervous System
350-359	Disorders Of The Peripheral Nervous System
360-379	Disorders Of The Eye And Adnexa
380-389	Diseases Of The Ear And Mastoid Process
390-459	**DISEASES OF THE CIRCULATORY SYSTEM**
390-392	Acute Rheumatic Fever
393-398	Chronic Rheumatic Heart Disease
401-405	Hypertensive Disease
410-414	Ischemic Heart Disease
415-417	Diseases Of Pulmonary Circulation
420-429	Other Forms Of Heart Disease
430-438	Cerebrovascular Disease
440-448	Diseases Of Arteries, Arterioles, And Capillaries
451-459	Diseases Of Veins And Lymphatics, And Other Diseases Of Circulatory System
460-519	**DISEASES OF THE RESPIRATORY SYSTEM**
460-466	Acute Respiratory Infections
470-478	Other Diseases Of The Upper Respiratory Tract
480-487	Pneumonia And Influenza
490-496	Chronic Obstructive Pulmonary Disease And Allied Conditions
500-508	Pneumoconioses And Other Lung Diseases Due To External Agents
510-519	Other Diseases Of Respiratory System
520-579	**DISEASES OF THE DIGESTIVE SYSTEM**
520-529	Diseases Of Oral Cavity, Salivary Glands, And Jaws
530-537	Diseases Of Esophagus, Stomach, And Duodenum
540-543	Appendicitis
550-553	Hernia Of Abdominal Cavity
555-558	Noninfectious Enteritis And Colitis
560-569	Other Diseases Of Intestines And Peritoneum
570-579	Other Diseases Of Digestive System
580-629	**DISEASES OF THE GENITOURINARY SYSTEM**
580-589	Nephritis, Nephrotic Syndrome, And Nephrosis
590-599	Other Diseases Of Urinary System
600-608	Diseases Of Male Genital Organs
610-611	Disorders Of Breast
614-616	Inflammatory Disease Of Female Pelvic Organs

"At a Glance" Table of Contents to the Structure of ICD9-CM Codes

Level 2: to 3-digit ranges

[*continued* -page 3 of 4]

Range of ICD9 Codes	Description
580-629	**DISEASES OF THE GENITOURINARY SYSTEM** (*continued*)
617-629	Other Disorders Of Female Genital Tract
630-676	**COMPLICATIONS OF PREGNANCY, CHILDBIRTH, AND THE PUERPERIUM**
630-633	Ectopic And Molar Pregnancy
634-639	Other Pregnancy With Abortive Outcome
640-648	Complications Mainly Related To Pregnancy
650-659	Normal Delivery, And Other Indications For Care In Pregnancy, Labor, And Delivery
660-669	Complications Occurring Mainly In The Course Of Labor And Delivery
670-676	Complications Of The Puerperium
680-709	**DISEASES OF THE SKIN AND SUBCUTANEOUS TISSUE**
680-686	Infections Of Skin And Subcutaneous Tissue
690-698	Other Inflammatory Conditions Of Skin And Subcutaneous Tissue
700-709	Other Diseases Of Skin And Subcutaneous Tissue
710-739	**DISEASES OF THE MUSCULOSKELETAL SYSTEM AND CONNECTIVE TISSUE**
710-719	Arthropathies And Related Disorders
720-724	Dorsopathies
725-729	Rheumatism, Excluding The Back
730-739	Osteopathies, Chondropathies, And Acquired Musculoskeletal Deformities
740-759	**CONGENITAL ANOMALIES**
760-779	**CERTAIN CONDITIONS ORIGINATING IN THE PERINATAL PERIOD**
760-763	Maternal Causes Of Perinatal Morbidity And Mortality
764-779	Other Conditions Originating In The Perinatal Period
780-799	**SYMPTOMS, SIGNS, AND ILL-DEFINED CONDITIONS**
780-789	Symptoms
790-796	Nonspecific Abnormal Findings
797-799	Ill-Defined And Unknown Causes Of Morbidity And Mortality
800-999	**INJURY AND POISONING**
800-829	Fractures
800-804	Fracture Of Skull
805-809	Fracture Of Neck And Trunk
810-819	Fracture Of Upper Limb
820-829	Fracture Of Lower Limb
830-839	Dislocation
840-848	Sprains And Strains Of Joints And Adjacent Muscles
850-854	Intracranial Injury, Excluding Those With Skull Fracture

"At a Glance" Table of Contents to the Structure of ICD9-CM Codes
Level 2: to 3-digit ranges
[*continued* -page 4 of 4]

Range of ICD9 Codes	Description
800-999	**INJURY AND POISONING** (*continued*)
860-869	Internal Injury Of Thorax, Abdomen, And Pelvis
870-897	Open Wound
870-879	Open Wound Of Head, Neck, And Trunk
880-887	Open Wound Of Upper Limb
890-897	Open Wound Of Lower Limb
900-904	Injury To Blood Vessels
905-909	Late Effects Of Injuries, Poisonings, Toxic Effects, And Other External Causes
910-919	Superficial Injury
920-924	Contusion With Intact Skin Surface
925-929	Crushing Injury
930-939	Effects Of Foreign Body Entering Through Orifice
940-949	Burns
950-957	Injury To Nerves And Spinal Cord
958-959	Certain Traumatic Complications And Unspecified Injuries
960-979	Poisoning By Drugs, Medicinal And Biological Substances
980-989	Toxic Effects Of Substances Chiefly Nonmedicinal As To Source
990-995	Other And Unspecified Effects Of External Causes
996-999	Complications Of Surgical And Medical Care, Not Elsewhere Classified
V01-V82	**SUPPLEMENTARY CLASSIFICATION OF FACTORS INFLUENCING HEALTH STATUS AND CONTACT WITH HEALTH SERVICES**
V01-V09	Persons With Potential Health Hazards Related To Communicable Diseases
V10-V19	Persons With Potential Health Hazards Related To Personal And Family History
V20-V29	Persons Encountering Health Services In Circumstances Related To Reproduction And Development
V30-V39	Liveborn Infants According To Type Of Birth
V40-V49	Persons With A Condition Influencing Their Health Status
V50-V59	Persons Encountering Health Services For Specific Procedures And Aftercare
V60-V68	Persons Encountering Health Services In Other Circumstances
V70-V82	Persons Without Reported Diagnosis Encountered During Examination And Investigation Of Individuals And Populations

PREFACE

Official Disability Guidelines™ *(ODG)* links together four U.S. government databases to provide length-of-disability experience data that can be used to manage employee productivity. These four databases are the following:

ICD-9-CM — The International Classification of Diseases, 9th Revision, Clinical Modification. This is the principle coding system used worldwide for the diagnosis of any medical condition. The main section of *ODG* includes *verbatim* the complete "Volume 1, Diseases: Tabular List" of the current Official ICD-9-CM publication.

CDC NCHS NHIS — The National Health Interview Survey (NHIS) is conducted annually by the National Center for Health Statistics (NCHS) of the Centers for Disease Control and Prevention (CDC). *ODG* uses data from every year beginning in 1987 until the most current.

OSHA BLS OII — The Bureau of Labor Statistics (BLS) reports annually on Occupational Injuries and Illnesses (OII) from forms submitted by employers to the Occupational Safety and Health Administration (OSHA). *ODG* uses data from the latest available year.

HCUP — The Healthcare Cost and Utilization Project (HCUP) is a family of health care databases and related software tools and products developed through a Federal-State-Industry partnership and sponsored by the Agency for Healthcare Research and Quality (AHRQ) to create a national information resource of patient-level health care data. HCUP includes the largest collection of longitudinal medical care data in the United States. These databases enable research on a broad range of health policy issues, including cost and quality of health services, medical practice patterns, access to health care programs, and outcomes of treatments at the national, State, and local market levels. The latest available year is included in *ODG*.

From the beginning, the first edition of *Official Disability Guidelines* (ODG) in 1996 provided lost time guidelines using actual experience data from these federal government databases, specifically OSHA BLS (Occupational Safety and Health Administration – Bureau of Labor Statistics) and CDC NCHS NHIS (Centers for Disease Control and Prevention, National Center for Health Statistics, National Health Interview Survey). The raw data is presented graphically so users can compare it directly with their own experience, and it is designed to enhance a timely and appropriate return-to-work for workers suffering from illness or injury. From the beginning, ODG was based on actual experience, not "expert" opinion. This made ODG fair to employees and defensible by employers. With changes to the Federal Rules of Evidence, the ODG guidelines also became the most likely to stand up in court. As a result of recent U.S. Supreme Court decisions, the Federal Rules of Evidence were recently amended in December 2000. The new rules state that statistical studies will be admissible under the Federal Rules of Evidence, and that such methods generally satisfy important aspects of the "scientific knowledge" requirement articulated in the Daubert Decision.[1] Furthermore, it states that "courts have described surveys as the most direct form of evidence that can be offered, and several courts have drawn negative inferences from the absence of a survey."[2]

Official Disability Guidelines is based on actual reported data from the annual CDC National Health Interview Survey (NHIS), the BLS Survey of Occupational Injuries and Illnesses (SOII), and over 2 million medical records from actual workers' compensation claims. This includes actual observed case data - rather than government survey "patient recollection" data. All data is tracked by ICD-9-CM code and not just general body part. Since 2003 all of the ODG disability duration data has been validated and enhanced by actual client claims data, and this is reflected in the Return-To-Work Summary Guidelines (Claims data Midrange and At-Risk) as well as the Return-To-Work "Best Practice" Guidelines, the RTW Claims Data (Calendar-days away from work by decile), and the RTW Post Surgery (Calendar-days away from work by decile). *Official Disability Guidelines* also includes client data, based on over 2 million claims from WLDI's multi-year multi-state workers comp database, covering almost 50 million paid invoices on medical encounters for those claims. These medical costs represent a total of $10.0 billion dollars in actual incurred costs, and the indemnity costs represent a total of $7.2 billion dollars in actual incurred costs, for a total of over $17 billion of workers' compensation costs, and they are presented in the table, entitled "Workers' Comp Costs per Claim." A detailed Methodology Outline, covering both the Treatment Guidelines as well as the Return-to-Work Guidelines, has been posted on the Web at http://www.odg-disability.com/methodology_outline.pdf. There is also a detailed Methodology Description using the AGREE Instrument (Appraisal of Guidelines Research and Evaluation), posted online at http://www.odg-disability.com/ODG_AGREE.htm.

RETURN-TO-WORK "BEST PRACTICE" GUIDELINES

The next step in the evolution of ODG was the identification of pathways for each condition, based primarily on drilling down into the raw data in the NHIS, which has a wealth of detail on type of therapy, type of job, demographics, comorbidities and severity. These pathways provided the different treatment options with their resultant time out of work, including considerations for severity and type of job. When different types of jobs made a difference in disability duration, job considerations specific to that diagnosis are identified. For example, "light duty" is not the same for carpal tunnel as for back strain as for depression. With different return-to-work pathways for each type of job, modified duty opportunities can be identified, and the appropriate time frames determined. These treatment pathways are titled "Return-To-Work Best Practice Guidelines", and in effect, they brought *Official Disability Guidelines* halfway to offering treatment guidelines.

The term "Best Practice" describes the use of these pathways to manage disability. For example, for carpal tunnel syndrome (ICD9 354.0) the first entry in the "Best Practice" Guidelines is "Conservative treatment, modified work (no repetitive use of hand/wrist): 0 days". The "Best Practice" is to try to follow this initial treatment pathway, and, if it is followed, the actual data support a norm of 0 days. (Also under carpal tunnel syndrome, the CDC bar chart shows that in 43% of the cases reported to CDC, where a physician has diagnosed carpal tunnel syndrome, no time is missed. This is the data that supports that pathway.)

The "Best Practice" guidelines were first launched in the 1997 edition of ODG, but they

[1] *Reference Manual on Scientific Evidence*, Second Edition, Federal Judicial Center 2000, page 86.
[2] Above, page 236

have been expanded in each subsequent annual edition. Currently, *Official Disability Guidelines* has "Best Practice" guidelines for four times as many conditions as in 1997, and the average number of treatment options per condition is more than double what it was in 1997. With over 16,000 clients, the "Best Practice" guidelines in ODG are nationally recognized. Since they are based on actual experience data from the federal government, they are scientifically valid and outcome-based. New users of lost time guidelines have gravitated toward ODG because the "Best Practice" guidelines, the heart of ODG, identify what makes a difference in return-to-work. Rather than looking at an average or a median for all cases for a particular condition, ODG allows comparison among like cases. Within diagnoses, some cases should return earlier than others because they are on a different pathway. Trying to make them all adhere to an overall median will not only let some cases be out too long, but will also force some cases back to work too soon. As ODG became a focal point facilitating communication among all parties in the return-to-work process, including patients, it has been assisting all parties with regard to the appropriate treatment and management of work related injuries and illnesses. The framework of the "Best Practice" guidelines has established elements against which aspects of care can be compared, and allowed identification of treatments and services that are reasonable and medically necessary for treatment of a particular injury.

The "Best Practice" disability duration data is contained in boxed bold type under each diagnosis. These durations are what can be achieved through management of the disability case, based on analyzing the raw data and comparing findings with the experience of clients of Work Loss Data Institute. The "Best Practice" Guidelines also reflect the experience of the members of the *ODG* Editorial Advisory Board, comprised of about eighty medical professionals, typically medical directors at large corporations or other employers with significant disability experience, who review the "Best Practice" guidelines every year to identify new return-to-work pathways and compare the durations with their own experience.

Separate data is provided for whatever factors would significantly affect the disability duration. For example, choice of therapy may be identified, including different procedures, along with target disability durations for each of those. Each of these procedure names is also indexed in the Keyword Index for easy access to durations on procedures. In many cases there are significant differences between cases treated surgically versus medically (e.g., drug therapy). For diagnoses where co-morbidities are a significant factor, these may also be identified in the "Best Practice" Guidelines section. These "Best Practice" Guidelines focus on return-to-work, and are not as detailed as clinical best practice guidelines, but they should include the various paths of treatment suggested by clinical best practice guidelines.

Where type of job makes a difference, that is shown also. This may be clerical work versus manual work, but it may also be other factors such as sedentary versus standing, or use of a particular body part. Where clerical/modified work shows a shortened disability duration, the "modified" work may be an opportunity to return the worker to restricted duty, before he or she returns to their normal duties. Where other factors affect duration, such as non-dominant versus dominant arm, they are also identified. For each diagnosis, there may be specific job characteristics that affect length of disability. These characteristics may not correspond to the five job classifications in the Department of Labor's *Dictionary of Occupational Titles*. Where they do apply, "sedentary" corresponds to class 1 (sitting, up to 10 pounds of force), "clerical" is class 2 (up to 20 pounds), "manual" is class 3 (up to 50 pounds), and "heavy manual" covers class 4 or 5 (up to 100 pounds and over 100 pounds).

The graphs shown for each database of experience data may show different clusters of data. The "Best Practices" section helps explain what causes those clusters, e.g. medical treatment versus surgery, hospitalization versus non-hospitalization, light-duty versus heavy manual work, etc.

Throughout the "Best Practice" Guidelines there is consistency in the definition of days. Return-to-work durations are always in calendar days, as opposed to workdays, so they can be applied to workers on different shifts, full time versus part time, etc. Length of disability of 7 days is equal to one week. A partial day missed is treated as one day if the employee would be expected to be out for most of the day (e.g., for a colonoscopy). Time off for an hour or two, say for routine diagnostic examination, physical therapy, or limited chemotherapy, would be treated as zero days. Each of the treatment options under the "Best Practice" Guidelines generally has its own disability duration. For example, the time out of work for initial conservative treatment would be separate from time off for surgery, if the conservative treatment is chosen but it turns out to be unsuccessful, and then surgery is selected. On the other hand, a diagnostic procedure may be also part of a more extensive therapeutic procedure.

These guidelines are meant to be used to identify cases that are out of the norm, where questions may be asked, such as what makes them different. Especially where there is a great variation in severity, for example, for some cancers, additional information may be requested and the additional time out of work may be justified. If the patient has co-morbidities that are not specifically identified in the guidelines, application of the guidelines is more difficult. The final opinion regarding any medical condition and the ability of a patient to return to work should rest with the physician treating that patient. Where the "Best Practice" disability duration guidelines indicate "by report", variances in the data made it impossible to select a benchmark number of days, and the report by the evaluating physician should guide the amount of time off work.

It should also be noted that achieving the best practice guidelines disability durations typically requires appropriate job descriptions and availability of altered work. Depending on the type of work, some injuries will have a residual chronic pain syndrome that will require accommodation. It is recommended that these guidelines be achieved in a setting that includes modified duty work as well as case management. Some employers have found that with aggressive Return-To-Work modified duty programs, disability schedules can be considerably shortened compared to the "Best Practice" guidelines. On the other hand, modified duty policies are quite variable among employers, and the clinician needs to acknowledge that the level of RTW function they approve may not be accommodated by company policy.

Some physicians consider the return-to-work dates in the "Best Practice" guidelines to be aggressive, and there may be some cases that do not meet these guidelines. This may result in disagreement between case managers and physicians. The best practices take into account the best circumstances. Some patients can return to work earlier than the best practices suggest, and others later than suggested. Such variables as age, co-morbid conditions, severity, job type and other items can impact disability duration and <u>must always be taken into account</u>. When patients fall outside these values, most notably if the projected disability duration exceeds "Best Practice" estimates, the case manager should consult the treating physician as to why the case might not fit the "Best Practice" guidelines.

One of the challenges in disability management is what to do when a person has recurrent problems. For instance, when someone has headaches, rheumatoid arthritis, osteoarthritis, or cancer that has recurrent symptoms, it is very difficult to determine a "Best Practice" disability duration.

The Return-to-Work “Best Practice” Guidelines, comprising the most important feature in ODG, are now closer to the top within each condition, in the second box. These still show estimated days out of work (based on national norms) for typical cases within each condition depending on severity, type of treatment and type of job, including modified duty. They are indispensable to effective case management, by identifying up front what “pathway” a case is likely to follow. In addition, multipliers for many common comorbidities have been added, based on the raw experience data.

<u>Multiple incidences of disability duration</u>: When managing multiple incidences of disability duration for the same worker on a prospective basis, ODG users should consider each one separately when creating return-to-work expectations using the “Best Practice” Guidelines. The

disability duration data used to derive the pathways in the Return-to-Work "Best Practice" Guidelines is based on single incidences of missed work, because that is the only way to isolate the specific factors affecting return-to-work in each of the pathways. (On the other hand, when benchmarking claims on a retrospective basis, users should be aware that the RTW Summary Guidelines, as well as the ODG claims data by decile, include all instances of absence for each claim.) And, as with all disability durations in ODG, the length of disability is calculated by taking the return-to-work date minus the last day of work less one-day. When using durations in the "Best Practice" Guidelines to manage a specific worker's absence on a prospective basis, the expected disability duration should generally "reset to zero" if the worker has returned to work for a period, but then misses work again at a later time. Furthermore, because of the potential for abuse from multiple incidences of absence, users should probably "reset" the duration only for the second instance of absence for the same condition within a year (not the third, fourth, etc.), and only if the time during which the worker returned to work is significant, i.e., it exceeds the disability duration that preceded it. Specific absence situations that exceed these guidelines will need to be reviewed on a case-by-case basis. The return-to-work period need not be job specific, so it may be regular work that could have been impacted by the medical condition, or either regular work or modified duty where the condition should have a limited effect. In addition, please note that disability duration pathways in ODG that refer to surgery are calculated from the date of surgery, and not from the last day of work. These general principles should also apply to recommendations regarding number of treatment visits, for example, physical therapy, even though these visits may or may not be during an absence from work. In general, a second incidence of physical therapy visits after a substantial time back at work may represent a recurrence of the original condition that might allow another series of physical therapy visits. Without a disability-duration to trigger this, the "substantial time back at work" might be considered anything greater than the number of "At-Risk" days for that condition. And, physical therapy visits post surgery should be considered separately from visits used up in an attempt at conservative treatment that might have avoided surgery. Again with respect to retrospective benchmarking, as opposed to prospective claims management, disability duration data in ODG that is used for this benchmarking, for example, the Return-to-Work Summary Guidelines or the RTW Claims Data, includes all incidences of disability duration for a single claim with that primary diagnosis over the previous year.

Additional note on co-morbidities: With respect to co-morbidities, in most cases the expected disability duration will be driven by the most severe diagnosis. In fact, when disability durations are calculated in ODG from actual experience data, and a case has multiple ICD9 diagnosis codes, all of the lost workdays for that case are assigned to only one ICD9 code, the one with largest number in the ODG Return-To-Work Summary Guidelines (i.e., Midrange, All absences). Consequently, when using ODG to determine an expected return-to-work date, the disability durations should not generally be added together when the worker has multiple injuries or illnesses. Unless there are instructions that incorporate those specific co-morbidities, users should just take the longest duration and go with that. The healing time of the less serious condition should fall within that. For example, if a worker has a back sprain and a disc disorder, the return-to-work (RTW) date should be driven by the disc disorder diagnosis, and the healing time for the back sprain should fall within that. This is similar for RTW after surgery. For example, if someone has a spinal fusion and a discectomy, the return-to-work date would be driven by the fusion.

RETURN-TO-WORK SUMMARY GUIDELINES

Based on input from users, the 2003 edition of *Official Disability Guidelines* underwent a major re-design to facilitate finding the right information quickly. With the new format you can efficiently locate the number you need to reserve a claim, or you can get the in-depth backup information necessary for more extensive case management.

Return-to-Work Summary Guidelines show estimated days out of work (based on national norms) for each condition in summary, for those who just want to select a target, and you can now cost justify case management efforts by "beating the guideline" using the At-Risk date. These are followed by ODG's well-respected "Best Practice" Guidelines, which have proven indispensable to effective case management by identifying up front what "pathway" a case is likely to follow. This new "Summary Guideline" box brings to the front of each diagnosis, experience data that was previously contained in the ODG "decile table", using the 50% number for "Midrange" and the 90% number for "At-Risk".

Please note: An important distinction needs to be made between the Return-To-Work Summary Guidelines and the Return-To-Work "Best Practice" Guidelines. The Summary Guidelines were designed primarily for retrospective benchmarking of claims, requiring only a diagnosis, plus a disability duration. On the other hand, the "Best Practice" Guidelines were designed primarily for prospective case management, when more details about a case are known, for example type of therapy, type of job, severity, co-morbidities, etc. The At-Risk date in the Summary Guidelines should NOT be used for prospective case management – it may be too late to begin management at that point. This is the point when the case has already become an outlier and is at risk of never returning to work, no matter how effective additional case management may be. Instead, the At-Risk date may be used as a consistent measure across different operating units to determine how effective case management efforts have been against national norms in "beating the guideline", since unmanaged cases will tend to become outliers, and hit the At-Risk date.

Beginning with the 2005 edition, a new row was added to the Return-to-Work Summary Guidelines. This "Summary Guideline" box brought to the front of each diagnosis experience data that is contained in the ODG "decile table" (the *RTW Claims Data - Calendar-days away from work by decile*), using the 50% number for "Midrange" and the 90% number for "At-Risk", and this "decile table" includes only cases that were out more than 7 days, so that the data is consistent with and comparable to the claims data that most ODG clients use when benchmarking. Now these numbers continue to be shown in the Summary Guidelines in the first row, entitled "Claims data".

In recent years there has been increased focus on "incidental absence", those cases typically out for 7 days or less, that may never become claims under most workers' compensation rules or under the eligibility requirements of most disability benefit programs. Furthermore, many employers and their vendors have moved to early reporting of absence, in order to improve early return to work. Because of this, they are picking up cases in their case mix that never would have been in their database of reported absence in the past. In order to provide benchmarking data for these clients, a new row has been added, entitled "All absences". This row uses the 50% number for "Midrange" and the 90% number for "At-Risk", covering all absences, and not just cases that were out more than 7 days. Because this data includes the shorter duration cases, these "Midrange" and "At-Risk" numbers will generally be shorter than the previous numbers (which are still being displayed in the "Claims data" row).

When deciding which numbers to apply in benchmarking, users will need to ask themselves whether or not their own dataset generally includes cases out for 7 days or less. If so, to be consistent in their application of the national norms, they should use the row labeled "All absences". For some conditions, such as a broken leg, there will not be significant differences in the numbers in the two rows. For other conditions where a significant percentage of cases miss less than 8 days, such as colds or flu, the differences will be substantial.

As before, these Summary Guidelines are followed by ODG's well-respected "Best Practice" Guidelines, which have proven indispensable to effective case management by identifying up front what "pathway" a case is likely to follow

Some of the ways these upfront Summary Guidelines numbers (typically the At-Risk number) are used is as follows:

- Reserves: Estimating duration for purposes of setting conservative reserves.
- Targets: Selecting a duration as "the number to hit" or the "the number to beat".
- Pre-authorization rules: Some workers' compensation systems use the "At-Risk" date to trigger pre-authorization requirements, making providers submit approved treatment

plans prior to payment, for cases that have exceeded this limit.

- Budgeting: Making an initial prediction of disability duration, and keeping that prediction, unmodified, in a database in order to compare the eventual actual duration against that first estimate.
- Performance reviews: Using duration as a QA performance standard, as part of the qualitative evaluation of a few selected case manager files. A powerful way to evaluate the effectiveness of case managers or teams is to compare actual vs. estimated durations across whole caseloads or other large groups of claims.
- Organizational benchmarking: Using duration as an aggregate system benchmark for median duration of disability across the whole book of business, and providing top management a report every month tracking the actual performance of each operating unit against those benchmarks. In addition, innovations in claim and case management can be tracked for their effectiveness in reducing median durations.
- Client benchmarking: Claims organizations can measure overall performance, or individual performance, by adding up the actual durations for all cases and dividing that by the sum of the "at-risk" numbers. This can also indicate "total days saved".
- Grading performance: Sum up all internal claims durations, sum up corresponding At-Risk durations from ODG Summary Guidelines (with an ICD9 coded At-Risk date corresponding to each claim), divide the sum of the At-Risk dates minus the sum of your internal claims durations by the sum of the At-Risk dates, and multiply the result by 100 to get a percentage score. For more details on this technique, which is also described in a CE article in the February 2005 issue of the AAOHN Journal, request a copy of "Benchmarking Medical Absence" from Work Loss Data Institute, or find it on the Web at http://www.disabilitydurations.com/benchmarking_lost_time.htm.

OTHER KEY FEATURES

After the Summary Guidelines and Return-To-Work "Best Practice" guidelines are the following additional features, which appear under each condition where they apply and there is sufficient data available:

Capabilities & Activity Modifications

Activity Modifications shows condition-specific modifications for each level of job identified in the "Best Practice" Guidelines. These are meant to be used in conjunction with the "Best Practice" Guidelines to determine what level of job is appropriate and for how long. For example, if "Severe, clerical/modified work: 0-3 days" appears, then look at the definition of "*clerical/modified work*" for job modifications used to prevent re-injury. Then, "Severe, manual work: 14-17 days", about two weeks later the worker may transition to work defined under "*manual work*". Physicians can copy & paste these restrictions into a RTW form for use by employers, and all parties (doctors, patients, employers, and insurers) use them as a communication tool to create shared expectations. They can also facilitate return to modified duty, which is often a critical first step in the return-to-work process.

Description and Other Names

For most common injuries and illnesses there is a description of the diagnosis, along with common symptoms, causes, and complications, using terminology understandable to non-medical personnel. Common names for this diagnosis are also provided.

ICD-10 Codes

ICD-10 Codes are next, providing complete ICD-10 translations for each condition (Web version only).

Procedure Summary (from ODG Treatment)

This section lists procedures and other topics relevant to this diagnosis, as they appear in the Procedure Summary of *ODG Treatment in Workers' Comp*. (In the Web version each procedure is a hyperlink going directly to that entry.) The Procedure Summary is the most important section in *ODG Treatment*, and the first two sections, the Treatment Protocols and the Codes for Automated Approval, are based on the conclusions from the evidence in the Procedure Summary. The Procedure Summary lists all possible therapies and diagnostic methods, as well as other issues that apply for each condition, and provides a summary of the latest evidence from the highest quality medical studies. The studies providing this evidence are referenced so that they can be consulted directly, and if necessary, copied into a claims report. For each condition, there may be as many as 100 separate listings covered in this fashion. Many of these procedures are being performed regularly, but are not supported by the quality medical evidence as summarized in this guideline, and in some cases, are proven to be harmful. When patient selection is important to the success of a procedure, the criteria for patient selection is also outlined, and the appropriate study is referenced. In supporting decisions to approve or deny medical services, users of *ODG Treatment* can go beyond quoting a set of guidelines, and copy and paste the results of the actual study, taking "evidence based medicine" to its logical end point. Clicking on the hyperlinks (containing author name and study year) in the Web version of the Procedure Summary will take the user directly to the studies supporting that statement. These reference summaries, including an abstract, plus the WLDI evaluation and rating of the reference, are in alphabetical order for those who want to browse them all, and important points in the study are highlighted. WLDI uses a proprietary rating system to evaluate the quality of the studies, ranging from 1a to 11c. Within the Procedure Summary there are specialized guidelines for various topics that stand out because they are highlighted in light blue. For surgical procedures that may be supported by high quality medical studies, ODG Treatment presents a decision matrix called "ODG Indications for Surgery™" that itemizes the decision-making process and patient selection criteria for successful outcomes from the surgery. Also within the Procedure Summary there is another specialized guideline for various topics that stands out in light blue. Contained in this section, where appropriate under imaging procedures, such as Radiography, Magnetic resonance imaging (MRI), or Ultrasound, are the recommended criteria for those modalities.

Causality Likelihood

Based on the raw data, causality likelihood indicates what percentage of total lost workdays were occupational (Web version only). The data sets used for this calculation are OSHA lost workdays per 100 workers (for cases meeting the requirements as an OSHA recordable injury or illness), and CDC NHIS lost workdays per 100 workers (for all cases, including non-occupational illnesses and injuries) from these two ODG databases through the 2004 edition. (Methodology differences make this comparison difficult using data after 2004.) When the causality likelihood percentage is large, cases with that diagnosis are likely to be occupational in nature. This indicator may be used as an aid in evaluating causality, but any definitive determination of causality requires analysis of the specific details of each case.

Hospital Costs

Hospital Costs are next, showing average hospital costs for each condition, including total number of cases per sample (Web version only). Average costs are shown for each condition where there is sufficient data, and the number of cases is shown for the most recent year. These costs are from the Healthcare Cost & Utilization Project (HCUP), produced by the U.S. government Agency for Healthcare Research and Quality (AHRQ). The costs only cover cases that were hospitalized. For conditions where there are not enough cases of hospitalization to estimate average costs, no medical costs are shown.

Hospital Length Of Stay

Also from the Healthcare Cost & Utilization Project (HCUP), average Hospital Length Of Stay is shown for the most recent year (Web version only). Note: when using these numbers as benchmarks, it is important to use the most current edition of ODG, because there has been a continued decline in hospital length of stay, but a significant increase in average medical costs. For selected workers' comp conditions, average hospital length of stay will also be shown for surgical procedures done as an inpatient, along with the ICD9 procedure code for those procedures. (For hospital procedures, the ICD9 procedure coding system is used, whereas for physician office procedures, the CPT® coding system is used.)

Procedure Codes

Procedure Codes commonly performed for each condition are listed (Web version only).

Case Management Triage

Case Management Triage priority indicators are next (Web version only). Each condition has a heading, "CM Triage", which uses algorithms applied to the raw data to label each condition with priority indicators: Level 1 - "Low Touch", Level 2 - "Case Management", or Level 3 - "Long Term Planning". Level 1 conditions (66%) don't require initial management. If they reach their inflection point without resolution, they become Level 2 and require CM. Level 2 (17%) benefit immediately from CM, and Level 3 (17%) cases are anticipated to be long-term, with a large percentage out for a long period, allowing advance planning with respect to paperwork, reserves, SSDI, etc. Copies of the algorithms are available in electronic versions of ODG.

Physical Therapy Guidelines

Physical Therapy Guidelines, showing recommended frequency and duration of PT visits are next. Only appropriate conditions have physical therapy guidelines. These guidelines provide evidence-based benchmarks for the number of visits with a physical or occupational therapist and the period of time during which these visits take place. (Note: These guidelines do not include work hardening programs.) The physical therapy guidelines do not describe the type of therapy required, and the number of visits does not include physical therapy that the patient should perform in their own home or work site, after proper training from a clinician. Unless noted otherwise, the visits indicated are for outpatient physical therapy, and the physical therapist's judgment is always a consideration in the determination of the appropriate frequency and duration of treatment. Support for the physical therapy guidelines is relevant medical literature and actual experience data, combined with consensus review by experts. The most important data sources are the high quality medical studies that are referenced in the treatment guidelines, *ODG Treatment in Workers' Comp*, within the Procedure Summaries of each relevant chapter, summarized under the entry for "Physical Therapy." For clinical trials that show effectiveness for these therapies, the number of visits required to achieve this are isolated from each study and combined with the same information from other successful studies to arrive at the benchmark number of visits in ODG.

There are a number of overall physical therapy philosophies that may not be specifically mentioned within each guideline: (1) As time goes by, one should see an increase in the active regimen of care, a decrease in the passive regimen of care, and a fading of treatment frequency; (2) The exclusive use of "passive care" (e.g., palliative modalities) is not recommended; (3) Home programs should be initiated with the first therapy session and must include ongoing assessments of compliance as well as upgrades to the program; (4) Use of self-directed home therapy will facilitate the fading of treatment frequency, from several visits per week at the initiation of therapy to much less towards the end; (5) Patients should be formally assessed after a "six-visit clinical trial" to see if the patient is moving in a positive direction, no direction, or a negative direction (prior to continuing with the physical therapy); & (6) When treatment duration and/or number of visits exceeds the guideline, exceptional factors should be noted.

Generally there should be no more than 4 modalities/procedural units in total per visit, allowing the PT visit to focus on those treatments where there is evidence of functional improvement, and limiting the total length of each PT visit to 45-60 minutes unless additional circumstances exist requiring extended length of treatment. Treatment times per session may vary based upon the patient's medical presentation but typically may be 45-60 minutes in order to provide full, optimal care to the patient. Additional time may be required for the more complex and slow to respond patients. While an average of 3 or 4 modalities/ procedural units per visit reflect the typical number of units, this is not intended to limit or cap the number of units that are medically necessary for a particular patient, but documentation should support an average greater than 4 units per visit. These additional units should be reviewed for medical necessity, and authorized if determined to be medically appropriate for the individual injured worker.

As described above, for more detail users should refer to *ODG Treatment in Workers' Comp*, within the Procedure Summaries of each relevant chapter, for recommendations about specific treatments and modalities, along with supporting links to the highest quality relevant medical studies, which have been summarized, rated, and highlighted. In these Procedure Summaries ODG covers many different types of treatments that can be supported by the medical evidence, and it also identifies the maximum number of visits that can be justified by the evidence; however, this does not mean that a provider should do every possible treatment that may be recommended (actually, this would be highly unlikely since different specialties would be required), or always deliver the maximum number of visits, without taking into account what was needed to cure the patient in a particular case. Furthermore, duplication of services is not considered medically necessary. While the recommendations for number of visits are guidelines and are not meant to be absolute caps for every case, they are also not meant to be a minimum requirement on each case (i.e., they are not an "entitlement"). Any provider doing this is not using the guidelines correctly, and provider profiling would flag these providers as outliers. This applies to all types of treatment, and not just physical therapy. Furthermore, flexibility is especially important in the time frame recommendations. Generally, the number of weeks recommended should fall within a relatively cohesive time period, between date of first and last visit, but this time period should not restrict additional recommended treatments that come later, for example due to scheduling issues or necessary follow-up compliance with a home-based program. When there are co-morbidities, the same principles should apply as in the ODG guidelines for return-to-work. See Additional note on co-morbidities at the end of the description of the Return-To-Work "Best Practice" Guidelines. In estimating the maximum number of treatment visits for workers with multiple diagnoses, users should use the number from the diagnosis with the longest number of visits. This assumes that whatever separate therapy, if any, that the lesser diagnosis requires, it can be done during the same visits addressing the more serious problem. If there are reasons why these therapies cannot be concurrent, documentation should support medical necessity. Also see Multiple incidences of disability duration in the same section for recommendations regarding number of treatment visits, for example, physical therapy, in these situations. And physical therapy visits post surgery should be considered separately from visits used up in an attempt at conservative treatment that might have avoided surgery.

Physical medicine treatment (including PT, OT and chiropractic care) should be an option when there is evidence of a musculoskeletal or neurologic condition that is associated with functional limitations; the functional limitations are likely to respond to skilled physical medicine treatment (e.g., fusion of an ankle would result in loss of ROM but this loss would not respond to PT, though there may be PT needs for gait training, etc.); care is active and includes a home exercise program; & the patient is compliant with care and makes significant functional gains with treatment.

Chiropractic Guidelines

Chiropractic Guidelines are next, showing recommended frequency and duration of chiropractic care. These guidelines provide evidence-based benchmarks for the number of visits with a chiropractor and the period of time during which these visits take place. Support for the chiropractic guidelines is relevant medical literature and actual experience data, combined with consensus review by experts. The most important data sources are the high quality medical studies that are referenced in the treatment guidelines, *ODG Treatment in Workers' Comp*, within the Procedure Summaries of each relevant chapter, summarized under the entry for "Manipulation." For clinical trials that show effectiveness for manipulation, the number of visits required to achieve this are isolated from each study and combined with the same information from other successful studies to arrive at the benchmark number of visits in ODG. Another major source was the "Mercy Guidelines", the consensus document created by the American Chiropractic Association in conjunction with the Congress of State Chiropractic Associations, entitled *Guidelines for Chiropractic Quality Assurance and Practice Parameters, Proceedings of the Mercy Center Consensus Conference.* Many of the general philosophies described above under "Physical Therapy Guidelines" should also apply to the chiropractic guidelines. More specifically, in addition to a "six-visit clinical trial", every six visits thereafter the treating physical or occupational therapist/chiropractor should validate improvement in function as it relates to the patient's essential job functions, hours working, health related quality of life indicators (e.g. Oswestry) or a standard pain scale in order for treatment to continue. Pain reduction should be accompanied by improved function and/or reduced medication use. For other general guidelines that may apply to chiropractic care, also see Physical Therapy Guidelines.

Workers' Comp Costs per Claim

Indemnity costs, medical costs and total costs per claim for over 2000 ICD9 diagnosis codes seen in workers' comp are provided. Within each cost category ODG shows the cost distribution by quartile (25%, 50%, and 75%), the mean (or average) costs, and the percentage of claims with no costs in that category, plus total number of claims that the cost data is based. It includes almost 2 million claims from WLDI's multi-year multi-state workers' comp database, and it covers almost 50 million paid invoices on medical encounters for those claims. The medical costs cover multiple categories, including office visits, surgeries, PT, pharmaceuticals, hospital, durable medical equipment, etc. They are from medical provider bills that were approved and paid, but not bills from MCO's, so they do not include the cost of managed care services (bill review, case management, UR, etc). When there are multiple ICD9 diagnostic categories in a claim, all costs for that claim are assigned to the most severe ICD9 code, using the ODG disability duration database to identify the most severe ICD9 code. These medical costs represent a total of $10.0 billion dollars in actual incurred costs, and the indemnity costs represent a total of $7.2 billion dollars in actual incurred costs, for a total of over $17 billion of workers' compensation costs.

Age Adjustment Factors

Age Adjustment Factors are next, where there is sufficient raw data, in a boxed table providing condition-specific multipliers important for the aging workforce, plus the At-Risk date pre-adjusted by the multipliers. Most experts believe it is reasonable to modify return-to-work by multiplying the value from the appropriate category, ideally using the "Best Practice" Guidelines, by the value for the corresponding age of the patient.

RTW Claims Data

RTW Claims Data for benchmarking is the table formerly called "RTW Raw Data by Decile (with 7-day waiting period)", showing days away from work by decile (10 percent of claims back by tenth day, etc.), including mean. This boxed table displays the disability duration data by decile for only those cases with over 7 lost workdays. The 7-day cut-off was chosen so the data would be comparable to the most common reporting systems used for short-term disability, which have a 7-day waiting period. Showing calendar days off by percentile allows meaningful benchmarking of disability claims experience data, to identify opportunities for improvement. On the other hand, the bar chart for Integrated Disability Durations raw data shows all the disability duration data, starting at 1 day missed, and the footnote to that bar chart even identifies cases with no missed work.

RTW Post Surgery

This table is the same format as the RTW Claims Data above, but it shows disability duration data after selected surgical procedures that may be commonly done for this condition. These durations only include cases where the specific procedure was performed when the primary diagnosis was the ICD9 diagnosis code indicated above. Consequently, the post-surgical disability durations in ODG may vary for the same procedure when it appears under different ICD9 diagnosis codes.

Integrated Disability Durations Raw Data

Integrated Disability Durations raw data is next, including Length of Disability Data from CDC NCHS (Centers for Disease Control National Center for Health Statistics), charting disability duration data for all cases from the National Health Interview Survey. The "Impact on Total Absence", based on this data, is under this table showing impact on total absence for each condition (total incidence and prevalence data).

The two length-of-disability databases are each provided in a similar format, with summary information plus a graphical representation of the actual data using bar-chart format. The bar charts for each of the two different databases are of two different widths so they can be quickly distinguished from each other. Typographical differences are used to distinguish the disability databases from the ICD9 database, which serves as the organization of *ODG*, and the framework upon which the disability databases rely. Whereas the ICD9 data is in *serif* type, left-justified format with tabs denoting its hierarchical structure, the disability data is in smaller *san serif* type and centered.

The first database to appear is labeled Integrated Disability Durations. These include cases of calendar days away from work. Four data summaries are shown -- median (mid-point), mean (average), mode (most frequent), and calculated rec. This data is reflective only of those cases that report at least one day of lost work within the previous year (cases with no lost work have been excluded from calculations). The calculated recommendation data is a calculation that takes into account the other three summary data points, giving extra weight to the median. Following these summary calculations is a bar chart showing "Percent of Cases". The bar chart always has 14 bars. Depending on the data, there may be a bar for each length, e.g., "1 day", "2 days", etc., with the last bar showing "14 and more days". If 14 days is not long enough to show the detail, a different scale is used, saying "Range of Days (up to)". For example "3" means "1 to 3 days", then "6" means "4 to 6 days", etc. There may be a footnote to the bar chart if any cases were reported with no lost work, saying "cases with no lost workdays" with the percent of total cases, including the cases indicated graphically on the bar chart.

This data is also the basis for several other presentations of raw data. The heading "Impact on Total Absence" provides incidence and prevalence data for each diagnosis, as well as for higher-level groups of diagnoses. The prevalence data provides the frequency of a diagnosis in percent, by dividing the total lost workdays for that diagnosis by the total lost workdays for all diagnoses. The incidence data equates this prevalence rate to total lost days per year per 100 full time equivalent workers, using base absence data described below. With this data, users can easily target those conditions that have the largest impact on productivity and profitability. Total lost-work days, for any unscheduled absence due to illness or injury (including sick leave, short and long term disability, and workers' compensation), add up to 1,050 days per 100 workers (or 10.5 days per worker, equating to an absence rate of 4.2% assuming 250 work-days annually). This does not include scheduled absences (e.g., vacation, holidays, certain leave-of-absence) or unscheduled absences due to other causes (e.g., personal reasons, care of a family member, "no-shows", absences caused by an "entitlement" mentality). Other sources of absence data vary somewhat from this benchmark of 4.2% -- some are higher and some lower. A survey of very large employers by Mercer resulted in an estimate of 4.4%[3], and this estimate includes workers' comp medical costs and vendor administrative charges, plus the average employer size was over 5,000 employees. BNA's annual survey shows a much lower rate, 1.7%[4], but this is based only on absences reported to the human resources department, and it covers a cross section of U.S. employers, including smaller companies without a rich benefit structure. The results of CCH's annual survey were slightly higher than BNA's at 2.2%[5], with a similar methodology to the BNA survey. The highest rate of all was reported by the annual Watson Wyatt survey done in conjunction with the Washington Business Group on Health, showing 6.3%[6], but this survey is very much weighted toward the largest employers and those with the most generous benefit structures. It should be noted that, despite their widely differing estimates, the above studies are all based on surveying employers. On the other hand, *ODG* is based primarily on actual data reported to the federal government.

Occupational Disability Durations Raw Data

Occupational Disability Durations raw data is next, including OSHA DAW Data (Occupational Safety and Health Administration Days Away from Work), providing lost time statistics on work-related disabilities as reported to OSHA, and calculating estimated workers' compensation indemnity costs for each condition. The "Impact on Occupational Absence", based on this data, is under this table showing impact on occupational absence (occupational incidence and prevalence data).

This second database is based on reports by employers of missed workdays for occupational related injuries and illnesses. Only a median is provided for this data and the bar charts always have 7 columns. Beginning with the 2005 edition of ODG, OSHA now uses calendar days in its surveys. At the request of *ODG* users, a benchmark indemnity cost estimate is provided along with all OSHA tables. These costs are based on the State Average Weekly Wage (SAWW) used by the Texas Workers' Compensation Commission ($539). These costs do not include medical costs, but only the indemnity (lost work) portion of workers' comp costs. The total benchmark indemnity costs include both direct costs, the actual wages paid, as well as indirect costs, which include the costs of replacement, rehiring, retraining, overtime, down time, lost productivity, and infrastructure costs to manage current systems. Total costs including indirect costs have been estimated to be five times the direct costs, based on industry studies (Kalina, *AAOHN Journal*, August, 1998, page 385, and Guidotti, American Medical Association, *Occupational Health Services*, 1989). Of course, the percentage of indirect costs will vary

---

[3] *2001 Survey on Employers' Time-Off and Disability Programs*, April 2002, Mercer Human Resource Consulting and Marsh USA. "The total direct cost of unscheduled absence is 4.4 percent of payroll in direct expenses (that is, including salary continuation, benefit payments, and, in some cases, vendor administrative charges). Included in this category are incidental absence/sick days, salary continuation, STD benefits, LTD plans, and workers' compensation coverage (including work-related medical costs). A total of 476 US employers, in a wide range of industries, provided information for the survey. Almost two-thirds of the respondents have multi-state locations. The average number of employees covered in the plans described by respondents is 5,577."

[4] *BNA's Survey Of Job Absence*, March 20, 2001, Bureau of National Affairs. "Absenteeism in 2000 was little changed, on the whole, from a year earlier, signaling an apparent end to the upward trend in job absence observed in 1998 and 1999, according to a survey conducted by BNA, Inc. Median monthly rates of unscheduled absence averaged 1.7 percent of scheduled workdays last year. BNA's survey of job absence has been conducted quarterly since 1974. Absence rates for 2000 are based on responses from 170 human resource and employee relations executives representing a cross section of U.S. employers, both public and private. Job absence, for the purposes of the survey, excludes holidays, vacations, and other scheduled leave. "

[5] *2001 CCH Unscheduled Absence Survey*, October 23, 2001, CCH Incorporated "According to the latest CCH survey, conducted by Harris Interactive[sm], absenteeism rates rose slightly – increasing from 2.1 percent in 2000 to 2.2 percent in 2001 – while the average per-employee cost of absenteeism rose sharply from $610 per year in 2000 to $755. The survey, conducted May 31 through June 21, 2001, reflects experiences of HR executives in U.S. companies and organizations of all sizes and across various businesses and not-for-profit industry sectors."

[6] *The Staying @ Work Survey*, December 12, 2000, Watson Wyatt, "Average Direct Costs of Disability in Percentage of Payroll: 2.5% Workers' compensation, 1.7% Sick pay, 1.5% STD, 0.6% LTD, 6.3% Total for 1999/2000. 178 participating companies: 52% 1,000 to 4,999 employees, 18% 5,000 to 9,999, 30% 10,000+."

considerably from industry to industry. The OSHA data is the basis for the data following the heading "Impact on Occupational Absence". The prevalence rate is the total occupational lost workdays for that condition divided by the total occupational lost workdays for all conditions. The incidence rate is based on applying the incidence to total lost work-days for workers' comp cases based on data from NIOSH (the National Institute for Occupational Safety & Health).

FINDING THE RIGHT CONDITION

The framework for the main section of *ODG*, "Disability Guidelines", is the same as the ICD-9-CM, and each of the other three databases which provide disability durations are linked to the appropriate ICD9 for which they apply.

Official ICD9 data is organized by code number. These codes are hierarchical and may be three, four, or five digits, or may be at the group level, depending on the detail required, and they are grouped together for similar conditions. The "At a Glance" Tables of Contents indicate where each major section begins.

There are three ways to find the correct section of "Disability Guidelines" using ICD9 codes, as follows:

1) Medical Record Virtually all medical records and billing forms should have an ICD9 diagnostic code for the patient. These codes may not have a decimal point, and they may be padded out to 5 digits on the right with zeros. For example code "57200" would actually be "572.0" in the list of ICD9 codes, which are presented in numerical order by code.

2) Tables of Contents Using the "At a Glance" Table of Contents for Major Categories in *ODG*, it is possible to identify the major classification, e.g., "Diseases of the Digestive System". Then, the "At a Glance" Table of Contents for 3-digit Group Level Ranges will reveal the major sub-heads, such as "Appendicitis (540-543)". Reading the detail within the sub-head will help locate the correct code because inclusions and exclusions are spelled out.

3) Keyword Index At the end of *ODG* is an "ICD9 Keyword Index", which takes every word in the description plus the inclusions for an ICD9 code, and identifies that code along with its page number in the main section of *ODG*. The Keyword Index also contains procedures referred to in the "Best Practices" section of each diagnosis. Reviewing the information in the main section will confirm that the code is correct, as well as allowing access to the disability duration data for that code.

It should be noted that, whereas the main section of *ODG* includes ICD-9-CM "Volume 1, Tabular List" *verbatim*, the *ODG* "Keyword Index" is not the same as the ICD-9-CM, "Volume 2, Index to Diseases and Injuries". The *ODG* index allows more powerful searching; for example, the word "rotator" will help locate "rotator cuff tendonitis" in *ODG* and in Volume 1 of ICD9, but there is no such heading in Volume 2 of ICD9.

EVALUATING THE DATA

The ICD9 headings in *ODG* are complete -- every bit of detail in the official version is included. The raw data appears wherever there is collected data for that ICD9 code. This means some codes may have information from all three, from two, from only one, or not from any of the three databases. Of course, if no data appears that probably means that the diagnosis is very rare, it is unlikely that you would ever look up information for that diagnosis, and if you did, there is probably not enough experience to develop a reasonable estimate.

It is also possible that the data may not be available at the detailed diagnosis level, and a higher level, broader diagnosis should be checked. For example, HCUP hospital length-of-stay data are usually available at the 4-digit level, but the disability duration data may not be. It may be necessary to go up to the 3-digit level to find disability duration data. Sometimes the disability duration data is clustered at a 4-digit level ending in "9", for "unspecified". It may even be necessary to go back to a group level (a range of 3-digit codes) to find OSHA data, because the OSHA form is not always as specific in the diagnosis as ICD9 codes allow.

In evaluating the data that does appear, it is important to note the number of cases. Data is presented whenever it exists, so some sample sizes are large and some are small. The size of the sample is valuable for determining the relative frequency of a diagnosis. If it is very small, the diagnosis is rare. Perhaps that is not the best diagnosis to select, and there is a better, more common one not far away. The number of cases is also important in evaluating how well that data should predict disability durations in every case.

The bar charts showing detail are valuable in determining how to apply the data in your own situation. For example, the data may clump around several different points, indicating that there may be other variables, which could make the duration, be either "short" or "long". The most common point, the highest bar or the "mode", is also useful. For example, a disease may have a median duration of 2 days, but 1 day is the most likely duration for most cases.

Differences in the three databases for the same or similar conditions are also worth noting. For some diagnoses, for example Carpal Tunnel Syndrome, the OSHA days are longer than the self-reported days, possibly because incentives under Workers' Comp may delay how quickly workers return to work when their injury is related to their work, than if it might have been caused outside of work. Since the OSHA data is occupationally related, the incidences are much higher for injuries and illnesses that are "work-related".

The HCUP Hospital length of stay is provided as another benchmark for comparison with the two disability duration databases. For conditions in which hospitalization is the norm, the hospital length of stay may show how much of the total length of disability may be spent in the hospital. For many conditions this will not be true since the hospital data only shows cases where admission to hospital occurred, whereas the disability duration data shows all cases. In situations where the number of HCUP hospital cases is much smaller than the number of disability duration cases, it would appear that hospitalization is unlikely.

OTHER VERSIONS OF ODG

Official Disability Guidelines is also available in a "Top 200 Conditions" version. This book covers those diagnoses that represent about 75% of all lost workdays. With its smaller size, it is more portable than the complete edition, and it is easier to find the more common conditions. Of course, information on the vast majority of conditions is missing. Raw data from *ODG* is also available for licensing on computer tape or CD-ROM. With electronic versions of *Official Disability Guidelines*, users can link into the *ODG* disability duration data as they bring up each of their computerized cases. Of course, a Web-based version is available, so that users can access *ODG* from any location using a secure login and password. *ODG* is also available as an integrated treatment disability duration guideline, *ODG Treatment in Workers' Comp (ODG – TWC)*.

For assistance in using this publication, or information on other services, please call 1-800-488-5548.

COPYRIGHT PAGE

Printed and bound in the United States

1. INFECTIOUS AND PARASITIC DISEASES (001-139)

Impact on Total Absence: Prevalence 0.7091% of total lost workdays; Incidence 7.45 days per 100 workers

RTW Claims Data (Calendar-days away from work by decile)										
10%	20%	30%	40%	**50%**	60%	70%	80%	**90%**	100%	Mean
8	10	11	13	**14**	15	16	18	**35**	365	23.13

Note: Categories for "late effects" of infectious and parasitic diseases are to be found at 137-139.

Includes: diseases generally recognized as communicable or transmissible as well as a few diseases of unknown but possibly infectious origin

Excludes:

acute respiratory infections (460-466)
carrier or suspected carrier of infectious organism (V02.0-V02.9)
certain localized infections
influenza (487.0-487.8)

INTESTINAL INFECTIOUS DISEASES (001-009)

Excludes:
helminthiases (120.0-129)

RTW Claims Data (Calendar-days away from work by decile)										
10%	20%	30%	40%	**50%**	60%	70%	80%	**90%**	100%	Mean
8	8	9	10	**11**	12	14	17	**34**	365	20.44

Impact on Total Absence: Prevalence 0.1901% of total lost workdays; Incidence 2.00 days per 100 workers

Occupational Disability Durations, in days
Median (mid-point) 7 - Benchmark Indemnity Costs $5,250
(80 cases)
Impact on Occupational Absence: Prevalence 0.0063% of occupational lost workdays

008 Intestinal infections due to other organisms

Return-To-Work Summary Guidelines		
Dataset	**Midrange**	**At-Risk**
Claims data	11 days	59 days
All absences	2 days	10 days

Return-To-Work "Best Practice" Guidelines
1-2 days
Food handling work (possible disease transmission): 7 days

Description: Intestinal infection, usually caused by ingesting bacteria or parasites through food, water, or direct contact with infested feces. Symptoms may include diarrhea, gas, abdominal cramps, nausea, vomiting, and/or blood or mucous in the stool.

Includes: any condition classifiable to 009.0-009.3 with mention of the responsible organisms

Excludes:
food poisoning by these organisms (005.0-005.9)

Disability Duration Adjustment Factors by Age						
Age Group	18-24	25-34	35-44	45-54	55-64	65-74
Adjustment Factor	0.63	0.79	1.04	1.17	1.89	NA

RTW Claims Data (Calendar-days away from work by decile)										
10%	20%	30%	40%	**50%**	60%	70%	80%	**90%**	100%	Mean
8	8	9	10	**11**	12	15	25	**59**	365	24.50

008 Intestinal infections due to other organisms *(cont'd)*

Integrated Disability Durations, in days*
Median (mid-point) 2.0 Mean (average) 6.11
Mode (most frequent) 1 Calculated rec. 3

Percent of Cases
(8714 cases)

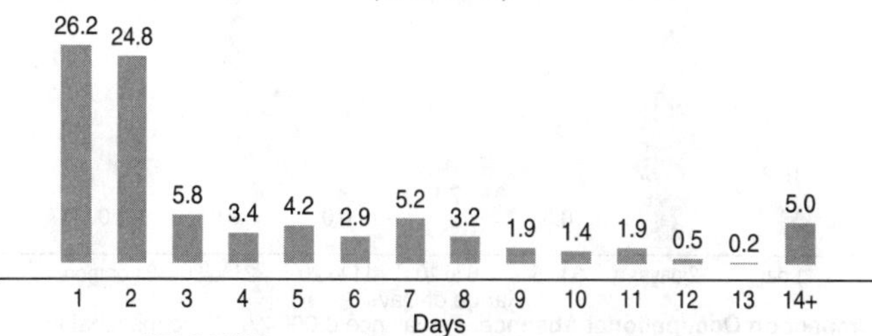

*CDC NHIS cases with no lost workdays: 1149 (13.2%)

Impact on Total Absence: Prevalence 0.1365% of total lost workdays; Incidence 1.43 days per 100 workers

OTHER BACTERIAL DISEASES (030-042)

Excludes:
bacterial venereal diseases (098.0-099.9)
bartonellosis (088.0)

RTW Claims Data (Calendar-days away from work by decile)										
10%	20%	30%	40%	**50%**	60%	70%	80%	**90%**	100%	Mean
9	10	10	12	**13**	14	15	27	**42**	365	29.96

Impact on Total Absence: Prevalence 0.1281% of total lost workdays; Incidence 1.35 days per 100 workers

Occupational Disability Durations, in days
Median (mid-point) 6 - Benchmark Indemnity Costs $4,500
(250 cases)
Impact on Occupational Absence: Prevalence 0.0170% of occupational lost workdays

034 Streptococcal sore throat and scarlet fever

Return-To-Work Summary Guidelines		
Dataset	**Midrange**	**At-Risk**
Claims data	12 days	15 days
All absences	3 days	5 days

Return-To-Work "Best Practice" Guidelines
See 034.0

RTW Claims Data (Calendar-days away from work by decile)										
10%	20%	30%	40%	**50%**	60%	70%	80%	**90%**	100%	Mean
8	9	10	11	**12**	12	14	15	**15**	36	11.94

Integrated Disability Durations, in days*
Median (mid-point) 3.0 Mean (average) 3.27
Mode (most frequent) 2 Calculated rec. 3

Percent of Cases
(4518 cases)

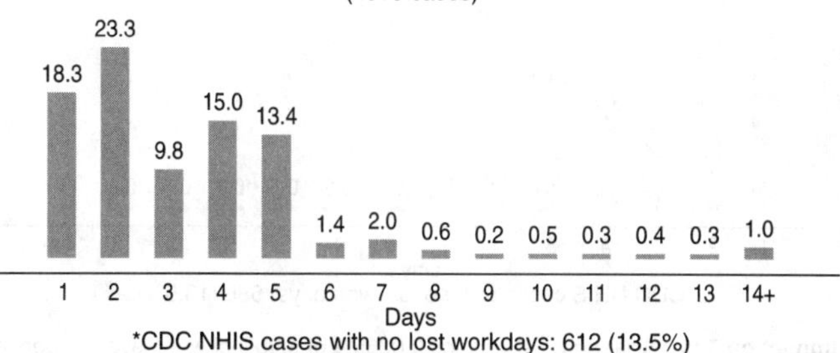

*CDC NHIS cases with no lost workdays: 612 (13.5%)

Impact on Total Absence: Prevalence 0.0377% of total lost workdays; Incidence 0.40 days per 100 workers

034 Streptococcal sore throat and scarlet fever

Occupational Disability Durations, in days
Median (mid-point) 2 - Benchmark Indemnity Costs $1,500

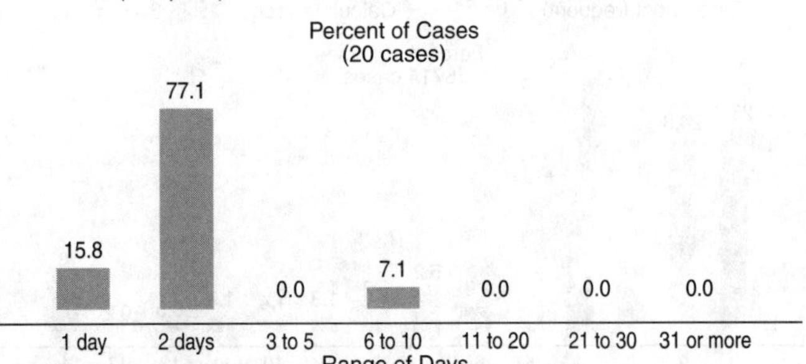

Impact on Occupational Absence: Prevalence 0.0004% of occupational lost workdays

034.0 Streptococcal sore throat

Return-To-Work Summary Guidelines		
Dataset	**Midrange**	**At-Risk**
Claims data	11 days	15 days
All absences	2 days	5 days

Return-To-Work "Best Practice" Guidelines
Without temperature: 0-2 days
With temperature, antibiotic treatment: 4-5 days
Severe complications: see rheumatic fever

Description: Bacterial infection most common in the throat. Symptoms may include sore throat, fever, nausea, vomiting, chills, and swollen lymph nodes in the neck.

Other names: Strep throat

Septic:
- sore throat

Streptococcal:
- angina
- laryngitis
- pharyngitis
- tonsillitis

Disability Duration Adjustment Factors by Age						
Age Group	18-24	25-34	35-44	45-54	55-64	65-74
Adjustment Factor	0.63	0.79	1.04	1.17	1.89	NA

RTW Claims Data (Calendar-days away from work by decile)										
10%	20%	30%	40%	**50%**	60%	70%	80%	**90%**	100%	Mean
8	9	10	10	**11**	12	13	14	**15**	30	11.61

Integrated Disability Durations, in days*

Median (mid-point)	2.0	Mean (average)	3.20
Mode (most frequent)	2	Calculated rec.	2

Percent of Cases
(4353 cases)

Days	1	2	3	4	5	6	7	8	9	10	11	12	13	14+
Percent	18.5	25.2	8.5	14.7	13.4	1.4	1.8	0.6	0.3	0.5	0.3	0.3	0.3	0.9

*CDC NHIS cases with no lost workdays: 586 (13.5%)

Impact on Total Absence: Prevalence 0.0355% of total lost workdays; Incidence 0.37 days per 100 workers

2. NEOPLASMS (140-239)

Impact on Total Absence: Prevalence 2.5860% of total lost workdays; Incidence 27.15 days per 100 workers

RTW Claims Data (Calendar-days away from work by decile)										
10%	20%	30%	40%	**50%**	60%	70%	80%	**90%**	100%	Mean
13	15	20	28	**34**	40	44	53	**77**	365	45.80

Notes:

1. Content:
   This chapter contains the following broad groups:
   140-195 Malignant neoplasms, stated or presumed to be primary, of specified sites, except of lymphatic and hematopoietic tissue
   196-198 Malignant neoplasms, stated or presumed to be secondary, of specified sites
   199 Malignant neoplasms, without specification of site
   200-208 Malignant neoplasms, stated or presumed to be primary, of lymphatic and hematopoietic tissue
   210-229 Benign neoplasms
   230-234 Carcinoma in situ
   235-238 Neoplasms of uncertain behavior [see Note, at beginning of section 235-238]
   239 Neoplasms of unspecified nature
2. Functional activity
   All neoplasms are classified in this chapter, whether or not functionally active. An additional code from Chapter 3 may be used to identify such functional activity associated with any neoplasm, e.g.:
   catecholamine-producing malignant pheochromocytoma of adrenal:
   code 194.0, additional code 255.6
   basophil adenoma of pituitary with Cushing's syndrome:
   code 227.3, additional code 255.0
3. Morphology [Histology]
   For those wishing to identify the histological type of neoplasms, a comprehensive coded nomenclature, which comprises the morphology rubrics of the ICD-Oncology, is given after the E-code chapter.
4. Malignant neoplasms overlapping site boundaries
   Categories 140-195 are for the classification of primary malignant neoplasms according to their point of origin. A malignant neoplasm that overlaps two or more subcategories within a three-digit rubric and whose point of origin cannot be determined should be classified to the subcategory .8 "Other." For example, "carcinoma involving tip and ventral surface of tongue" should be assigned to 141.8. On the other hand, "carcinoma of tip of tongue, extending to involve the ventral surface" should be coded to 141.2, as the point of origin, the tip, is known. Three subcategories (149.8, 159.8, 165.8) have been provided for malignant neoplasms that overlap the boundaries of three-digit rubrics within certain systems. Overlapping malignant neoplasms that cannot be classified as indicated above should be assigned to the appropriate subdivision of category 195 (Malignant neoplasm of other and ill-defined sites).

MALIGNANT NEOPLASM OF RESPIRATORY AND INTRATHORACIC ORGANS (160-165)

Excludes:
carcinoma in situ (231.0-231.9)

RTW Claims Data (Calendar-days away from work by decile)										
10%	20%	30%	40%	**50%**	60%	70%	80%	**90%**	100%	Mean
15	27	30	35	**40**	43	48	53	**60**	365	45.96

Impact on Total Absence: Prevalence 0.4180% of total lost workdays; Incidence 4.39 days per 100 workers

162 Malignant neoplasm of trachea, bronchus, and lung

Return-To-Work Summary Guidelines		
Dataset	**Midrange**	**At-Risk**
Claims data	39 days	59 days
All absences	32 days	59 days

Return-To-Work "Best Practice" Guidelines
Asymptomatic: 0 days
Bronchoscopy, local anesthesia: 1 day
Bronchoscopy, general anesthesia: 1-2 days
Lung biopsy, percutaneous: 3-5 days
Lung biopsy, thoracotomy, clerical/modified work: 35 days
Lung biopsy, thoracotomy, manual work: 42 days
Chemotherapy, clerical/modified work: 28 days
Chemotherapy, manual work: 42 days
Radiation therapy, clerical/modified work: 28 days
Radiation therapy, manual work: 42 days
Lobectomy, clerical/modified work: 35 days
Lobectomy, manual work: 49 days
Pneumonectomy, clerical/modified work: 42 days
Pneumonectomy, manual work: 59 days

Description: Cancerous cell growth usually originating from cells within the lung, although it is also possible that the cancer spread to the respiratory tract from other parts of the body. Symptoms usually include a persistent cough, as well as coughing up blood and chest pain. Late symptoms include weight loss and weakness. This is the most common cancer and most common cause of cancer-related death.

Other names: Lung cancer, Cancer of the bronchus, Cancer of the trachea

Workers' Comp Costs per Claim (based on 59 claims)					
Quartile	25%	50%	75%	Mean	% no cost
Indemnity	$18,039	$68,775	$88,001	$61,018	16%
Medical	$263	$441	$704	$3,644	10%
Total	$9,860	$60,218	$87,182	$54,467	0%

Disability Duration Adjustment Factors by Age						
Age Group	18-24	25-34	35-44	45-54	55-64	65-74
Adjustment Factor	0.61	0.92	0.98	0.75	1.14	1.38

RTW Claims Data (Calendar-days away from work by decile)										
10%	20%	30%	40%	**50%**	60%	70%	80%	**90%**	100%	Mean
14	26	29	35	**39**	42	46	50	**59**	365	41.42

Integrated Disability Durations, in days*
Median (mid-point) 32.0 Mean (average) 32.65
Mode (most frequent) 3 Calculated rec. 25

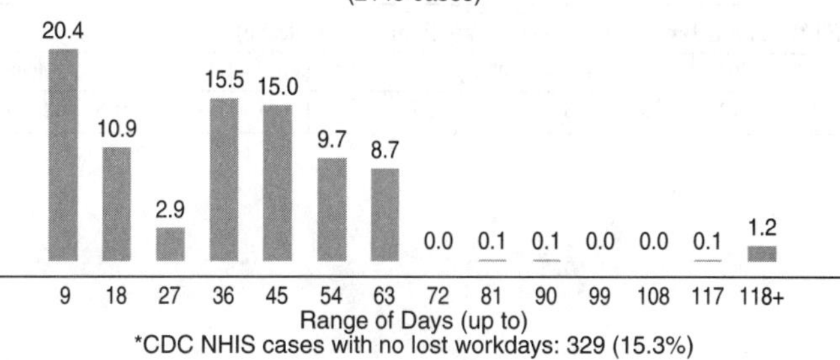

*CDC NHIS cases with no lost workdays: 329 (15.3%)

Impact on Total Absence: Prevalence 0.1752% of total lost workdays; Incidence 1.84 days per 100 workers

MALIGNANT NEOPLASM OF BONE, CONNECTIVE TISSUE, SKIN, AND BREAST (170-176)

Excludes:
carcinoma in situ:
breast (233.0)
skin (232.0-232.9)

RTW Claims Data (Calendar-days away from work by decile)										
10%	20%	30%	40%	**50%**	60%	70%	80%	**90%**	100%	Mean
12	14	15	17	**21**	30	36	42	**44**	365	33.02

Impact on Total Absence: Prevalence 0.4042% of total lost workdays; Incidence 4.24 days per 100 workers

174 Malignant neoplasm of female breast

Return-To-Work Summary Guidelines		
Dataset	**Midrange**	**At-Risk**
Claims data	22 days	43 days
All absences	16 days	42 days

Return-To-Work "Best Practice" Guidelines
Mammogram: 0 days
Breast biopsy, core needle: 0 days
Breast biopsy, incisional: 1 day
Radiation therapy/chemotherapy: 1-7 days
Lumpectomy, clerical/modified work: 7 days
Lumpectomy, manual work: 14 days
Simple mastectomy, clerical/modified work: 14 days
Simple mastectomy, manual work: 35 days
Modified radical mastectomy, clerical/modified work: 21 days
Modified radical mastectomy, manual work: 42 days

Description: Cancerous growth in the breast tissues indicated by a lump in the breast or armpit. There could be dimpled or leathery skin over the lump. Other symptoms may include discharge from the nipple and a change in breast shape or size.
Other names: Breast cancer

Includes: breast (female)
connective tissue
soft parts
Paget's disease of:
breast
nipple

Excludes:
skin of breast (172.5, 173.5)

Disability Duration Adjustment Factors by Age						
Age Group	18-24	25-34	35-44	45-54	55-64	65-74
Adjustment Factor	NA	NA	NA	1.01	0.81	NA

RTW Claims Data (Calendar-days away from work by decile)										
10%	20%	30%	40%	**50%**	60%	70%	80%	**90%**	100%	Mean
12	14	15	18	**22**	31	36	41	**43**	365	29.71

174 Malignant neoplasm of female breast *(cont'd)*

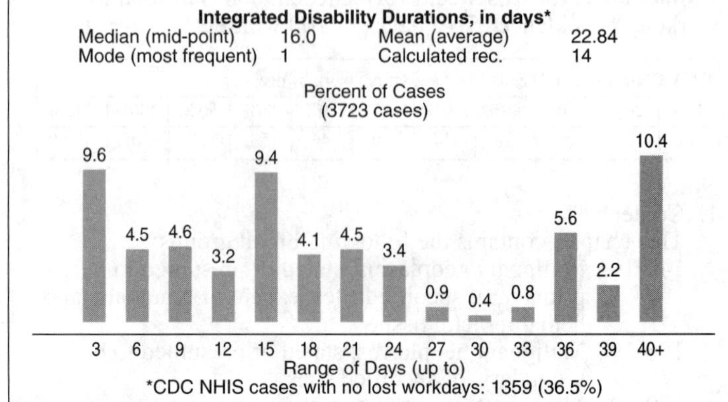

Impact on Total Absence: Prevalence 0.1596% of total lost workdays; Incidence 1.68 days per 100 workers

BENIGN NEOPLASMS (210-229)

RTW Claims Data (Calendar-days away from work by decile)										
10%	20%	30%	40%	**50%**	60%	70%	80%	**90%**	100%	Mean
10	13	15	20	**28**	35	43	54	**62**	365	38.15

Impact on Total Absence: Prevalence 0.2427% of total lost workdays; Incidence 2.55 days per 100 workers

218 Uterine leiomyoma

Return-To-Work Summary Guidelines		
Dataset	**Midrange**	**At-Risk**
Claims data	35 days	59 days
All absences	27 days	57 days

Return-To-Work "Best Practice" Guidelines
Without surgery: 0-1 days
Hysteroscopy, diagnostic: 2 days
Dilation & curettage/D&C: 3 days
Uterine artery embolization, clerical/modified work: 10 days
Uterine artery embolization, manual work: 28 days
Vaginal hysterectomy, clerical/modified work: 14-42 days
Vaginal hysterectomy, manual work: 35-42 days
Laparoscopically assisted vaginal hysterectomy/LAVH, clerical/modified work: 14-42 days
Laparoscopically assisted vaginal hysterectomy/LAVH, manual work: 35-42 days
Abdominal hysterectomy, clerical/modified work: 21-42 days
Abdominal hysterectomy, manual work: 56 days
Myomectomy, clerical/modified work: 28-42 days
Myomectomy, manual work: 56 days

Description: Non-cancerous tumors made of fibrous connective tissue found in the uterus. The fibrous tissue begins as smooth muscle, gradually becoming firm and round. If symptoms are present, which they often aren't in non-pregnant women, they include constipation, painful menstruation with excessive bleeding, and frequent urination.
Other names: Uterine Myoma, Fibroid tumor of the uterus

Includes: fibroid (bleeding) (uterine)
uterine:
fibromyoma
myoma

RTW Claims Data (Calendar-days away from work by decile)										
10%	20%	30%	40%	**50%**	60%	70%	80%	**90%**	100%	Mean
12	15	21	28	**35**	41	44	55	**59**	365	37.76

218 Uterine leiomyoma *(cont'd)*

Integrated Disability Durations, in days*

Median (mid-point)	27.0	Mean (average)	30.77
Mode (most frequent)	2	Calculated rec.	22

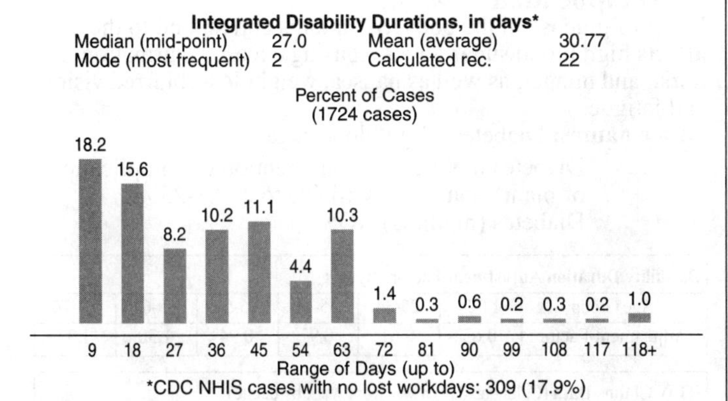

*CDC NHIS cases with no lost workdays: 309 (17.9%)

Impact on Total Absence: Prevalence 0.1287% of total lost workdays; Incidence 1.35 days per 100 workers

Occupational Disability Durations, in days

Median (mid-point) 1 - Benchmark Indemnity Costs $750 (20 cases)

Impact on Occupational Absence: Prevalence 0.0002% of occupational lost workdays

3. ENDOCRINE, NUTRITIONAL AND METABOLIC DISEASES, AND IMMUNITY DISORDERS (240-279)

Impact on Total Absence: Prevalence 1.3642% of total lost workdays; Incidence 14.32 days per 100 workers

RTW Claims Data (Calendar-days away from work by decile)										
10%	20%	30%	40%	**50%**	60%	70%	80%	**90%**	100%	Mean
10	11	13	14	**15**	18	23	31	**45**	365	26.10

Excludes:
endocrine and metabolic disturbances specific to the fetus and newborn (775.0-775.9)
Note: All neoplasms, whether functionally active or not, are classified in Chapter 2. Codes in Chapter 3 (i.e., 242.8, 246.0, 251-253, 255-259) may be used to identify such functional activity associated with any neoplasm, or by ectopic endocrine tissue.

250 Diabetes mellitus

Return-To-Work Summary Guidelines		
Dataset	**Midrange**	**At-Risk**
Claims data	42 days	115 days
All absences	40 days	115 days

Return-To-Work "Best Practice" Guidelines
See 250.0

Excludes:
gestational diabetes (648.8)
hyperglycemia NOS (790.6)
neonatal diabetes mellitus (775.1)
nonclinical diabetes (790.2)
that complicating pregnancy, childbirth, or the puerperium (648.0)

The following fifth-digit subclassification is for use with category 250:

0 type II [non-insulin dependent type] [NIDDM type] [adult-onset type] or unspecified type, not stated as uncontrolled
1 type I [insulin dependent type] [IDDM] [juvenile type], not stated as uncontrolled
2 type II [non-insulin dependent type] [NIDDM type] [adult-onset type] or unspecified type, uncontrolled
3 type I [insulin dependent type] [IDDM] [juvenile type], uncontrolled

250.0 Diabetes mellitus without mention of complication

Return-To-Work Summary Guidelines		
Dataset	**Midrange**	**At-Risk**
Claims data	14 days	18 days
All absences	10 days	17 days

Return-To-Work "Best Practice" Guidelines
Symptoms under control: 0 days
Medical treatment without hospitalization: 0-2 days
With hospitalization, clerical/modified work: 5-7 days
With hospitalization, manual work: 10-14 days
Depression comorbidity, multiply by: 2
Hypertension comorbidity, multiply by: 2
Obesity comorbidity (BMI >= 30), multiply by: 2.4

Description: A chronic endocrine syndrome in which the body is unable to metabolize carbohydrates, proteins, and fats, and unable to use or release insulin adequately, thereby causing high levels of glucose in the body. Symptoms correspond to the affects high blood sugar levels, causing excessive urination, thirst, and hunger, as well as nausea, weight loss, blurred vision and fatigue.

Other names: Diabetes, High blood sugar

Diabetes mellitus without mention of complication or manifestation classifiable to 250.1-250.9
Diabetes (mellitus) NOS

Disability Duration Adjustment Factors by Age						
Age Group	18-24	25-34	35-44	45-54	55-64	65-74
Adjustment Factor	0.63	0.61	0.97	0.94	1.30	1.33

RTW Claims Data (Calendar-days away from work by decile)										
10%	20%	30%	40%	**50%**	60%	70%	80%	**90%**	100%	Mean
10	11	12	13	**14**	15	15	16	**18**	365	21.02

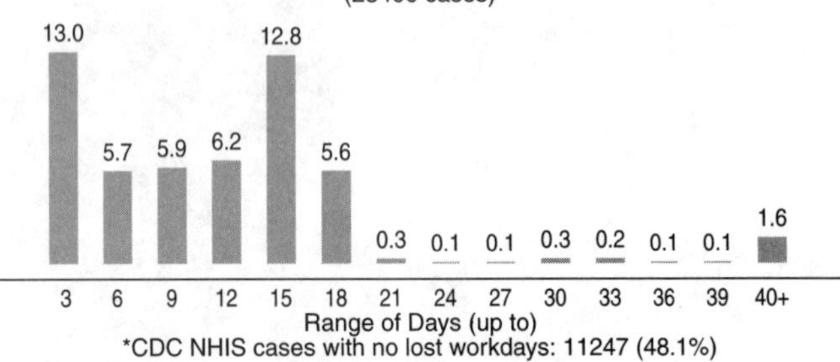

Impact on Total Absence: Prevalence 0.4908% of total lost workdays; Incidence 5.15 days per 100 workers

OTHER METABOLIC AND IMMUNITY DISORDERS (270-279)

Use additional code to identify any associated mental retardation

RTW Claims Data (Calendar-days away from work by decile)										
10%	20%	30%	40%	**50%**	60%	70%	80%	**90%**	100%	Mean
10	12	15	20	**23**	29	32	43	**46**	365	30.96

Impact on Total Absence: Prevalence 0.8764% of total lost workdays; Incidence 9.20 days per 100 workers

278 Overweight, obesity and other hyperalimentation

Return-To-Work Summary Guidelines		
Dataset	**Midrange**	**At-Risk**
Claims data	31 days	47 days
All absences	8 days	45 days

Return-To-Work "Best Practice" Guidelines
See 278.0

Excludes:
hyperalimentation NOS (783.6)
poisoning by vitamins NOS (963.5)
polyphagia (783.6)

RTW Claims Data (Calendar-days away from work by decile)										
10%	20%	30%	40%	**50%**	60%	70%	80%	**90%**	100%	Mean
11	20	23	29	**31**	35	43	45	**47**	315	35.01

278 Overweight, obesity and other hyperalimentation *(cont'd)*

Integrated Disability Durations, in days*

Median (mid-point)	8.0	Mean (average)	19.38
Mode (most frequent)	3	Calculated rec.	10

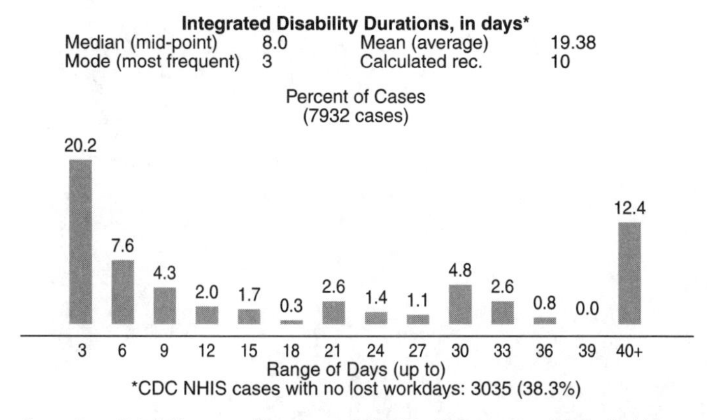

Impact on Total Absence: Prevalence 0.2804% of total lost workdays; Incidence 2.94 days per 100 workers

278.0 Overweight and obesity

Return-To-Work Summary Guidelines		
Dataset	**Midrange**	**At-Risk**
Claims data	31 days	47 days
All absences	8 days	45 days

Return-To-Work "Best Practice" Guidelines
Medical treatment (diet & exercise): 0 days
Liposuction (lipectomy), clerical/modified work: 3 days
Liposuction (lipectomy), manual work: 21 days
Abdominoplasty (tummy-tuck), clerical/modified work: 7 days
Abdominoplasty (tummy-tuck), manual work: 28 days
Gastric bypass (bariatric surgery), clerical/modified work: 30 days
Gastric bypass, manual work: 42-45 days

Description: An excess of body fat, most commonly occurring when energy intake exceeds energy use, though obesity could be a result of a genetic condition or a disturbance in body hormones. Other problems that occur as a result of obesity often include difficulty breathing, including sleep apnea, low back pain, excessive sweating, and skin disorders.
Other names: Overweight

Excludes:
adiposogenital dystrophy (253.8)
obesity of endocrine origin NOS (259.9)

Disability Duration Adjustment Factors by Age						
Age Group	18-24	25-34	35-44	45-54	55-64	65-74
Adjustment Factor	0.70	0.78	0.94	1.20	1.32	1.54

RTW Claims Data (Calendar-days away from work by decile)										
10%	20%	30%	40%	**50%**	60%	70%	80%	**90%**	100%	Mean
11	20	23	29	**31**	34	42	45	**47**	315	34.77

278.0 Overweight and obesity *(cont'd)*

Integrated Disability Durations, in days*

Median (mid-point)	8.0	Mean (average)	19.13
Mode (most frequent)	3	Calculated rec.	10

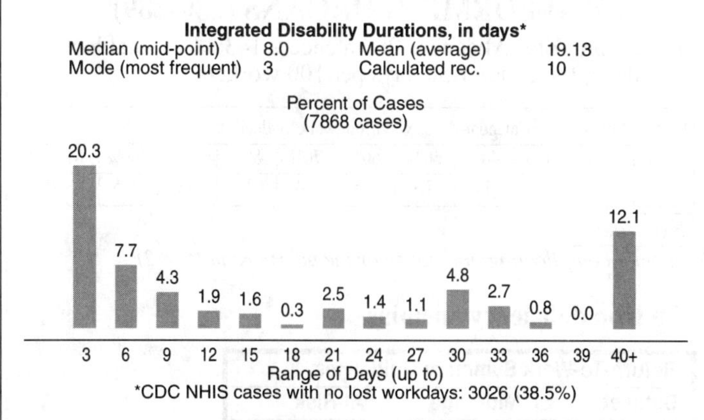

Impact on Total Absence: Prevalence 0.2737% of total lost workdays; Incidence 2.87 days per 100 workers

4. DISEASES OF THE BLOOD AND BLOOD-FORMING ORGANS (280-289)

Impact on Total Absence: Prevalence 0.1430% of total lost workdays; Incidence 1.50 days per 100 workers

RTW Claims Data (Calendar-days away from work by decile)										
10%	20%	30%	40%	**50%**	60%	70%	80%	**90%**	100%	Mean
10	12	13	14	**15**	16	24	38	**71**	365	33.26

Excludes:
anemia complicating pregnancy or the puerperium (648.2)

280 Iron deficiency anemias

Return-To-Work Summary Guidelines		
Dataset	**Midrange**	**At-Risk**
Claims data	13 days	47 days
All absences	6 days	16 days

Return-To-Work "Best Practice" Guidelines
Clerical/modified work, without acute blood loss, iron therapy: 0 day
Manual work, with blood loss: 3 days
With blood transfusion: 7 days

Description: The most common form of anemia, characterized by a low number of red blood cells circulating throughout the body, usually caused by excessive bleeding. Other symptoms may include fatigue, shortness of breath, and a craving for non-foods such as ice, dirt, or starch.
Other names: Anemia, Iron deficiency

Includes: anemia:
asiderotic
hypochromic-microcytic
sideropenic

Excludes:
familial microcytic anemia (282.4)

RTW Claims Data (Calendar-days away from work by decile)										
10%	20%	30%	40%	**50%**	60%	70%	80%	**90%**	100%	Mean
8	9	10	12	**13**	14	15	17	**47**	365	24.58

Integrated Disability Durations, in days*

Median (mid-point)	6.0	Mean (average)	11.79
Mode (most frequent)	3	Calculated rec.	7

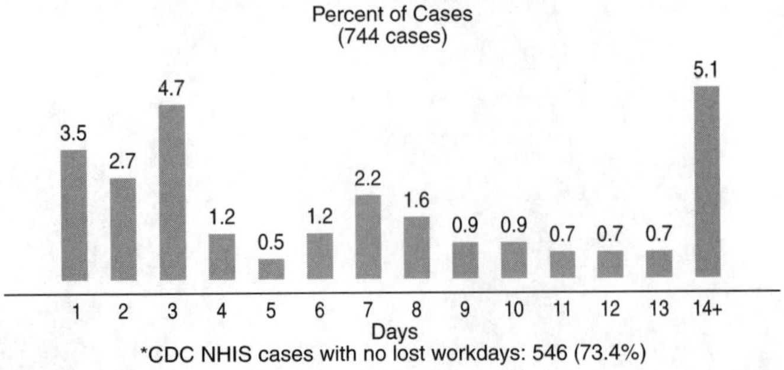

Percent of Cases
(744 cases)

Days	1	2	3	4	5	6	7	8	9	10	11	12	13	14+
Percent	3.5	2.7	4.7	1.2	0.5	1.2	2.2	1.6	0.9	0.9	0.7	0.7	0.7	5.1

*CDC NHIS cases with no lost workdays: 546 (73.4%)

Impact on Total Absence: Prevalence 0.0069% of total lost workdays; Incidence 0.07 days per 100 workers

5. MENTAL DISORDERS (290-319)

Impact on Total Absence: Prevalence 8.4896% of total lost workdays; Incidence 89.14 days per 100 workers

RTW Claims Data (Calendar-days away from work by decile)										
10%	20%	30%	40%	**50%**	60%	70%	80%	**90%**	100%	Mean
10	13	14	18	**21**	25	30	42	**56**	365	37.28

In the International Classification of Diseases, 9th Revision (ICD-9), the corresponding Chapter V, "Mental Disorders," includes a glossary which defines the contents of each category. The introduction to Chapter V in ICD-9 indicates that the glossary is intended so that psychiatrists can make the diagnosis based on the descriptions provided rather than from the category titles. Lay coders are instructed to code whatever diagnosis the physician records.

Chapter 5, "Mental Disorders," in ICD-9-CM uses the standard classification format with inclusion and exclusion terms, omitting the glossary as part of the main text.

The mental disorders section of ICD-9-CM has been expanded to incorporate additional psychiatric disorders not listed in ICD-9. The glossary from ICD-9 does not contain all these terms. It now appears in Appendix B, which also contains descriptions and definitions for the terms added in ICD-9-CM. Some of these were provided by the American Psychiatric Association's Task Force on Nomenclature and Statistics who are preparing the Diagnostic and Statistical Manual, Fourth Edition (DSM-IV), and others from A Psychiatric Glossary.

The American Psychiatric Association provided invaluable assistance in modifying Chapter 5 of ICD-9-CM to incorporate detail useful to American clinicians and gave permission to use material from the aforementioned sources.

1. Manual of the International Statistical Classification of Diseases, Injuries, and Causes of Death, 9th Revision, World Health Organization, Geneva, Switzerland, 1975.
2. American Psychiatric Association, Task Force on Nomenclature and Statistics, Robert L. Spitzer, M.D., Chairman.
3. A Psychiatric Glossary, Fourth Edition, American Psychiatric Association, Washington, D.C., 1975.

PSYCHOSES (290-299)

Excludes:
mental retardation (317-319)

OTHER PSYCHOSES (295-299)

Use additional code to identify any associated physical disease, injury, or condition affecting the brain with psychoses classifiable to 295-298

RTW Claims Data (Calendar-days away from work by decile)										
10%	20%	30%	40%	**50%**	60%	70%	80%	**90%**	100%	Mean
11	14	18	21	**24**	30	41	43	**55**	365	34.26

Impact on Total Absence: Prevalence 3.1868% of total lost workdays; Incidence 33.46 days per 100 workers

Occupational Disability Durations, in days
Median (mid-point) 30 - Benchmark Indemnity Costs $22,500 (80 cases)
Impact on Occupational Absence: Prevalence 0.0272% of occupational lost workdays

296 Episodic mood disorders

Return-To-Work Summary Guidelines		
Dataset	**Midrange**	**At-Risk**
Claims data	14 days	52 days
All absences	10 days	31 days

Includes: episodic affective disorders

Excludes:
neurotic depression (300.4)
reactive depressive psychosis (298.0)
reactive excitation (298.1)

The following fifth-digit subclassification is for use with categories 296.0-296.6:
0 unspecified
1 mild
2 moderate
3 severe, without mention of psychotic behavior
4 severe, specified as with psychotic behavior
5 in partial or unspecified remission
6 in full remission

Workers' Comp Costs per Claim (based on 1,759 claims)					
Quartile	25%	50%	75%	Mean	% no cost
Indemnity	$36,047	$56,259	$84,861	$64,290	1%
Medical	$28,781	$46,457	$75,033	$58,710	0%
Total	$73,364	$107,525	$160,556	$122,514	0%

RTW Claims Data (Calendar-days away from work by decile)										
10%	20%	30%	40%	**50%**	60%	70%	80%	**90%**	100%	Mean
9	10	12	13	**14**	15	16	27	**52**	365	25.89

Integrated Disability Durations, in days*
Median (mid-point) 10.0 Mean (average) 16.91
Mode (most frequent) 14 Calculated rec. 13

Percent of Cases
(1925 cases)

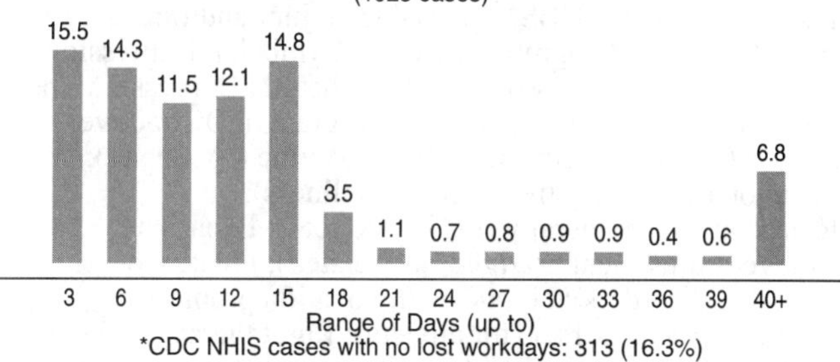

*CDC NHIS cases with no lost workdays: 313 (16.3%)

Impact on Total Absence: Prevalence 0.0805% of total lost workdays; Incidence 0.85 days per 100 workers

296.2 Major depressive disorder, single episode

Return-To-Work Summary Guidelines		
Dataset	**Midrange**	**At-Risk**
Claims data	26 days	58 days
All absences	20 days	48 days

Return-To-Work "Best Practice" Guidelines
Rule out impaired mood/personality disorder: 0 days
Outpatient therapy, without symptoms affecting work: 0-7 days
Outpatient therapy, with symptoms interfering with work: 21-42 days
With hospitalization, non-cognitive/modified work: 21 days
With hospitalization, cognitive work: 42 days

Capabilities & Activity Modifications:

296.2 Major depressive disorder, single episode

Avoid eliciting symptoms affecting work/other job issues: Limit to low project responsibility and minimal supervision of others; avoid situations of conflict and stress; minimal interaction with the public; personal driving only; minimal handling of heavy machinery (if not limited by medication).
Non-cognitive/modified work: Limit to moderate project responsibility and moderate supervision of others; personal driving only; minimal handling of heavy machinery (if not limited by medication).
Description: A single episode of excessively long or intense sadness or extreme apathy. Other symptoms may include irritability, poor concentration, decreased appetite, social withdrawal, and an inability to experience pleasure.
Other names: Depression

Depressive psychosis, single episode or unspecified
Endogenous depression, single episode or unspecified
Involutional melancholia, single episode or unspecified
Manic-depressive psychosis or reaction, depressed type, single episode or unspecified
Monopolar depression, single episode or unspecified
Psychotic depression, single episode or unspecified

Excludes:
circular type, if previous attack was of manic type (296.5)
depression NOS (311)
reactive depression (neurotic) (300.4)
psychotic (298.0)

Procedure Summary (from ODG Treatment): Acceptance and commitment therapy (ACT); Activity restrictions; Acupressure; Acupuncture; Antidepressants (therapy); Antidepressants - SSRI's versus tricyclics (class); Aromatherapy; Brain wave synchronizers (for stress reduction); Cognitive therapy for depression; Cognitive therapy for panic disorder; Cognitive therapy for stress; Cognitive behavioral stress management (CBSM) to reduce injury and illness; Computer-assisted cognitive therapy; Cymbalta; Depression screening; Depression: effect on heart health; Depression: the gene factor; Disease management (programs); Distractive methods (to reduce acute stress); Duloxetine (Cymbalta); Education (to reduce stress related to illness); Electroconvulsive therapy (ECT); Exercise; Expatriate employee adjustment; Fatigue (job related); Folate (for depressive disorders); Hypnosis; Innovation promotion (program); Kava extract (for anxiety); Light therapy; Massage therapy (MT); Mind/body interventions (for stress relief); Music (for relaxation/stress management); Opioid antagonists (especially naltrexone) for alcohol dependence; Optimism (and its effect on schema-focused therapy); Peer support (for postpartum depression); Psychological debriefing (for preventing post-traumatic stress disorder); Psychosocial/pharmacological treatments (for deliberate self harm); Psychosocial empowerment (programs); Psychotherapy; Return to work; SAMe (S-adenosylmethionine); St. John's wort (for depression); Stress & atherosclerosis (effect); Stress & blood pressure (effect); Stress & depression (effect); Stress & physiology/mental performance (effect); Stress & post-myocardial infarction (effect); Stress & myocardial ischemia (effect); Stress inoculation training ; Stress management, behavioral/cognitive (interventions); Stress management, physical (interventions); Tension headaches (pharmaceuticals vs. behavioral therapy); Technological stress; Vitamin B6; Vitamin use (for stress reduction); Work; Yoga

296.2 Major depressive disorder, single episode

Workers' Comp Costs per Claim (based on 1,444 claims)					
Quartile	25%	50%	75%	Mean	% no cost
Indemnity	$36,656	$55,939	$85,586	$64,738	1%
Medical	$29,673	$46,694	$75,054	$58,478	0%
Total	$74,435	$107,804	$162,446	$122,875	0%

RTW Claims Data (Calendar-days away from work by decile)										
10%	20%	30%	40%	**50%**	60%	70%	80%	**90%**	100%	Mean
10	15	21	22	**26**	39	42	44	**58**	365	38.34

Integrated Disability Durations, in days*

Median (mid-point)	20.0	Mean (average)	27.49
Mode (most frequent)	1	Calculated rec.	17

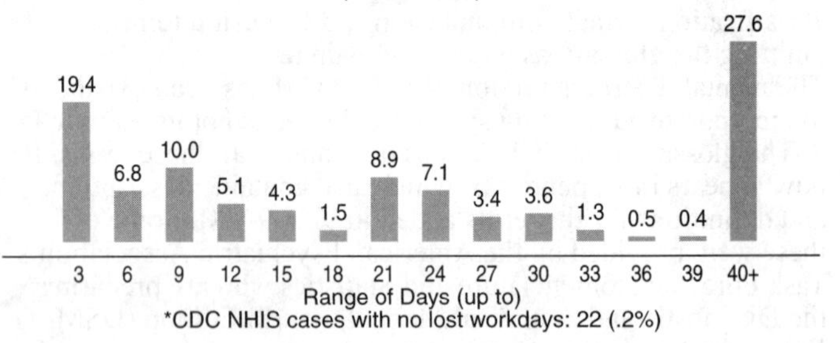

*CDC NHIS cases with no lost workdays: 22 (.2%)

Impact on Total Absence: Prevalence 1.1571% of total lost workdays; Incidence 12.15 days per 100 workers

296.5 Bipolar I disorder, most recent episode (or current) depressed

Return-To-Work Summary Guidelines		
Dataset	**Midrange**	**At-Risk**
Claims data	23 days	45 days
All absences	20 days	44 days

Return-To-Work "Best Practice" Guidelines
Rule out impaired mood/personality disorder: 0 days
Without hospitalization: 0-21 days
With hospitalization: 21-42 days

Capabilities & Activity Modifications:
Avoid eliciting symptoms affecting work/other job issues: Limit to low project responsibility and minimal supervision of others; avoid situations of conflict and stress; minimal interaction with the public; personal driving only; minimal handling of heavy machinery (if not limited by medication).
Non-cognitive/modified work: Limit to moderate project responsibility and moderate supervision of others; personal driving only; minimal handling of heavy machinery (if not limited by medication).
Description: A psychiatric illness in which extreme mood swings alternate between depression and mania. The depressed phase is often indistinguishable from major depression (See 296.2) or it could be a mixed stage of depression and mania, which usually marks the end of a manic phase and the start of a depressive stage.

Bipolar disorder, now depressed
Manic-depressive psychosis, circular type but currently depressed

Excludes:
brief compensatory or rebound mood swings (296.99)

Procedure Summary (from ODG Treatment): Acceptance and commitment therapy (ACT); Activity restrictions; Acupressure; Acupuncture; Antidepressants (therapy);

296.5 Bipolar I disorder, most recent episode (or current) depressed *(cont'd)*

Antidepressants - SSRI's versus tricyclics (class); Aromatherapy; Brain wave synchronizers (for stress reduction); Cognitive therapy for depression; Cognitive therapy for panic disorder; Cognitive therapy for stress; Cognitive behavioral stress management (CBSM) to reduce injury and illness; Computer-assisted cognitive therapy; Cymbalta; Depression screening; Depression: effect on heart health; Depression: the gene factor; Disease management (programs); Distractive methods (to reduce acute stress); Duloxetine (Cymbalta); Education (to reduce stress related to illness); Electroconvulsive therapy (ECT); Exercise; Expatriate employee adjustment; Fatigue (job related); Folate (for depressive disorders); Hypnosis; Innovation promotion (program); Kava extract (for anxiety); Light therapy; Massage therapy (MT); Mind/body interventions (for stress relief); Music (for relaxation/stress management); Opioid antagonists (especially naltrexone) for alcohol dependence; Optimism (and its effect on schema-focused therapy); Peer support (for postpartum depression); Psychological debriefing (for preventing post-traumatic stress disorder); Psychosocial/ pharmacological treatments (for deliberate self harm); Psychosocial empowerment (programs); Psychotherapy; Return to work; SAMe (S-adenosylmethionine); St. John's wort (for depression); Stress & atherosclerosis (effect); Stress & blood pressure (effect); Stress & depression (effect); Stress & physiology/mental performance (effect); Stress & post-myocardial infarction (effect); Stress & myocardial ischemia (effect); Stress inoculation training ; Stress management, behavioral/cognitive (interventions); Stress management, physical (interventions); Tension headaches (pharmaceuticals vs. behavioral therapy); Technological stress; Vitamin B6; Vitamin use (for stress reduction); Work; Yoga

RTW Claims Data (Calendar-days away from work by decile)

10%	20%	30%	40%	**50%**	60%	70%	80%	**90%**	100%	Mean
12	17	21	21	**23**	25	42	43	**45**	365	35.27

Integrated Disability Durations, in days*

Median (mid-point)	20.0	Mean (average)	25.55
Mode (most frequent)	1	Calculated rec.	17

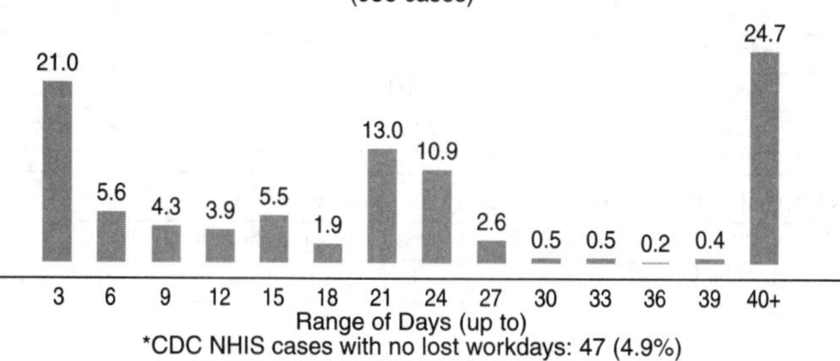

*CDC NHIS cases with no lost workdays: 47 (4.9%)

Impact on Total Absence: Prevalence 0.0686% of total lost workdays; Incidence 0.72 days per 100 workers

296.6 Bipolar I disorder, most recent episode (or current) mixed

Return-To-Work Summary Guidelines		
Dataset	**Midrange**	**At-Risk**
Claims data	21 days	44 days
All absences	19 days	43 days

296.6 Bipolar I disorder, most recent episode (or current) mixed *(cont'd)*

Return-To-Work "Best Practice" Guidelines
Without hospitalization: 0-14 days
With hospitalization: 21-42 days

Capabilities & Activity Modifications:
Avoid eliciting symptoms affecting work/other job issues: Limit to low project responsibility and minimal supervision of others; avoid situations of conflict and stress; minimal interaction with the public; personal driving only; minimal handling of heavy machinery (if not limited by medication).
Non-cognitive/modified work: Limit to moderate project responsibility and moderate supervision of others; personal driving only; minimal handling of heavy machinery (if not limited by medication).
Description: A form of bipolar disorder in which the person experiences both manic and depressive symptoms simultaneously. Symptoms could include crying, sadness, or suicidal thoughts as well as intense and sometimes unpleasant feelings of excitement, anger, agitation, and confusion.
Manic-depressive psychosis, circular type, mixed
Procedure Summary (from ODG Treatment): Acceptance and commitment therapy (ACT); Activity restrictions; Acupressure; Acupuncture; Antidepressants (therapy); Antidepressants - SSRI's versus tricyclics (class); Aromatherapy; Brain wave synchronizers (for stress reduction); Cognitive therapy for depression; Cognitive therapy for panic disorder; Cognitive therapy for stress; Cognitive behavioral stress management (CBSM) to reduce injury and illness; Computer-assisted cognitive therapy; Cymbalta; Depression screening; Depression: effect on heart health; Depression: the gene factor; Disease management (programs); Distractive methods (to reduce acute stress); Duloxetine (Cymbalta); Education (to reduce stress related to illness); Electroconvulsive therapy (ECT); Exercise; Expatriate employee adjustment; Fatigue (job related); Folate (for depressive disorders); Hypnosis; Innovation promotion (program); Kava extract (for anxiety); Light therapy; Massage therapy (MT); Mind/body interventions (for stress relief); Music (for relaxation/stress management); Opioid antagonists (especially naltrexone) for alcohol dependence; Optimism (and its effect on schema-focused therapy); Peer support (for postpartum depression); Psychological debriefing (for preventing post-traumatic stress disorder); Psychosocial/ pharmacological treatments (for deliberate self harm); Psychosocial empowerment (programs); Psychotherapy; Return to work; SAMe (S-adenosylmethionine); St. John's wort (for depression); Stress & atherosclerosis (effect); Stress & blood pressure (effect); Stress & depression (effect); Stress & physiology/mental performance (effect); Stress & post-myocardial infarction (effect); Stress & myocardial ischemia (effect); Stress inoculation training ; Stress management, behavioral/cognitive (interventions); Stress management, physical (interventions); Tension headaches (pharmaceuticals vs. behavioral therapy); Technological stress; Vitamin B6; Vitamin use (for stress reduction); Work; Yoga

RTW Claims Data (Calendar-days away from work by decile)

10%	20%	30%	40%	**50%**	60%	70%	80%	**90%**	100%	Mean
14	15	16	20	**21**	23	25	42	**44**	365	28.16

296.6 Bipolar I disorder, most recent episode (or current) mixed *(cont'd)*

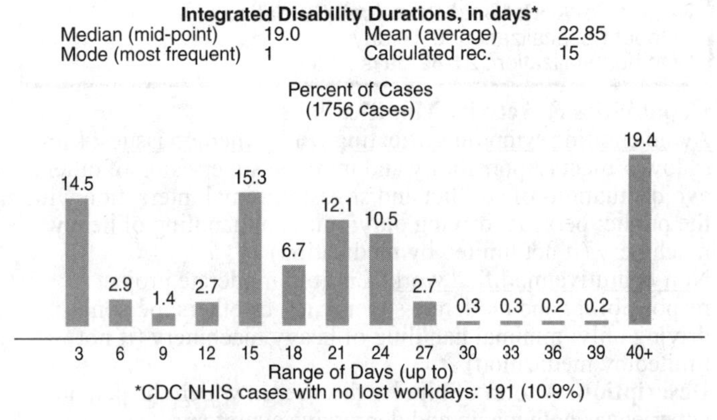

Impact on Total Absence: Prevalence 0.1056% of total lost workdays; Incidence 1.11 days per 100 workers

NEUROTIC DISORDERS, PERSONALITY DISORDERS, AND OTHER NONPSYCHOTIC MENTAL DISORDERS (300-316)

RTW Claims Data (Calendar-days away from work by decile)

10%	20%	30%	40%	**50%**	60%	70%	80%	**90%**	100%	Mean
10	12	14	15	**20**	22	28	32	**57**	365	38.67

Impact on Total Absence: Prevalence 5.1796% of total lost workdays; Incidence 54.39 days per 100 workers

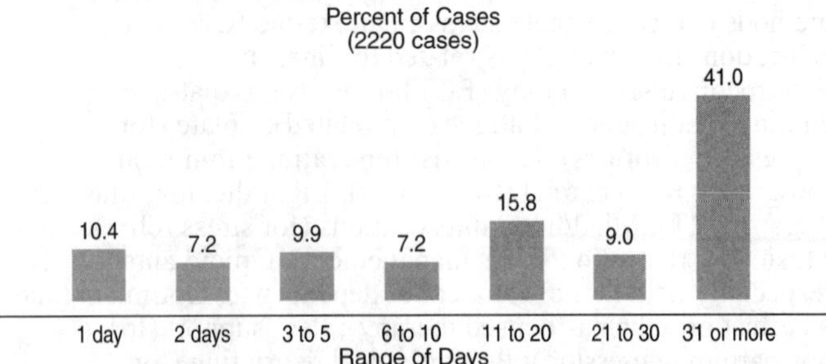

Impact on Occupational Absence: Prevalence 0.5036% of occupational lost workdays; Incidence 0.08 days per 100 workers

300 Anxiety, dissociative and somatoform disorders

Return-To-Work Summary Guidelines		
Dataset	**Midrange**	**At-Risk**
Claims data	19 days	25 days
All absences	10 days	23 days

Return-To-Work "Best Practice" Guidelines
Rule out impaired mood/personality disorder: 0 days
Without hospitalization: 0-7 days
With hospitalization: 7-21 days

Capabilities & Activity Modifications:
Avoid eliciting symptoms affecting work/other job issues: Limit to low project responsibility and minimal supervision of others; avoid situations of conflict and stress; minimal interaction with the public; personal driving only; minimal handling of heavy machinery (if not limited by medication).

300 Anxiety, dissociative and somatoform disorders *(cont'd)*

Non-cognitive/modified work: Limit to moderate project responsibility and moderate supervision of others; personal driving only; minimal handling of heavy machinery (if not limited by medication).

Procedure Summary (from ODG Treatment): Acceptance and commitment therapy (ACT); Activity restrictions; Acupressure; Acupuncture; Antidepressants (therapy); Antidepressants - SSRI's versus tricyclics (class); Aromatherapy; Brain wave synchronizers (for stress reduction); Cognitive therapy for depression; Cognitive therapy for panic disorder; Cognitive therapy for stress; Cognitive behavioral stress management (CBSM) to reduce injury and illness; Computer-assisted cognitive therapy; Cymbalta; Depression screening; Depression: effect on heart health; Depression: the gene factor; Disease management (programs); Distractive methods (to reduce acute stress); Duloxetine (Cymbalta); Education (to reduce stress related to illness); Electroconvulsive therapy (ECT); Exercise; Expatriate employee adjustment; Fatigue (job related); Folate (for depressive disorders); Hypnosis; Innovation promotion (program); Kava extract (for anxiety); Light therapy; Massage therapy (MT); Mind/body interventions (for stress relief); Music (for relaxation/stress management); Opioid antagonists (especially naltrexone) for alcohol dependence; Optimism (and its effect on schema-focused therapy); Peer support (for postpartum depression); Psychological debriefing (for preventing post-traumatic stress disorder); Psychosocial/ pharmacological treatments (for deliberate self harm); Psychosocial empowerment (programs); Psychotherapy; Return to work; SAMe (S-adenosylmethionine); St. John's wort (for depression); Stress & atherosclerosis (effect); Stress & blood pressure (effect); Stress & depression (effect); Stress & physiology/mental performance (effect); Stress & post-myocardial infarction (effect); Stress & myocardial ischemia (effect); Stress inoculation training ; Stress management, behavioral/cognitive (interventions); Stress management, physical (interventions); Tension headaches (pharmaceuticals vs. behavioral therapy); Technological stress; Vitamin B6; Vitamin use (for stress reduction); Work; Yoga

Workers' Comp Costs per Claim (based on 654 claims)

Quartile	25%	50%	75%	Mean	% no cost
Indemnity	$23,720	$46,163	$73,185	$56,573	2%
Medical	$20,811	$36,881	$60,018	$49,380	0%
Total	$49,550	$92,552	$130,673	$104,967	0%

RTW Claims Data (Calendar-days away from work by decile)

10%	20%	30%	40%	**50%**	60%	70%	80%	**90%**	100%	Mean
9	11	14	15	**19**	21	22	23	**25**	365	24.05

300 Anxiety, dissociative and somatoform disorders *(cont'd)*

Integrated Disability Durations, in days*

Median (mid-point)	10.0	Mean (average)	15.17
Mode (most frequent)	1	Calculated rec.	9

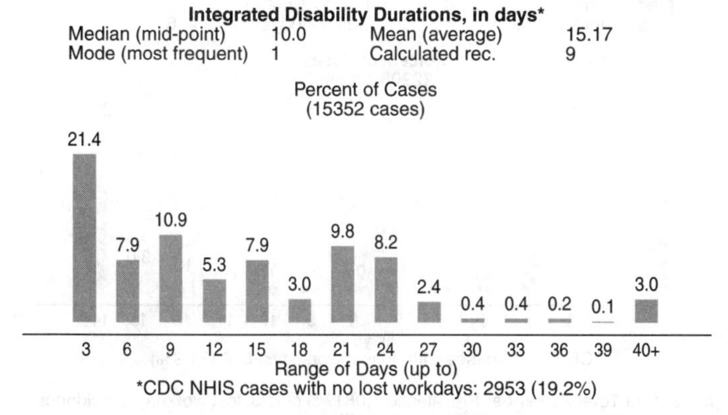

*CDC NHIS cases with no lost workdays: 2953 (19.2%)

Impact on Total Absence: Prevalence 0.5558% of total lost workdays; Incidence 5.84 days per 100 workers

Occupational Disability Durations, in days
Median (mid-point) 22 - Benchmark Indemnity Costs $16,500

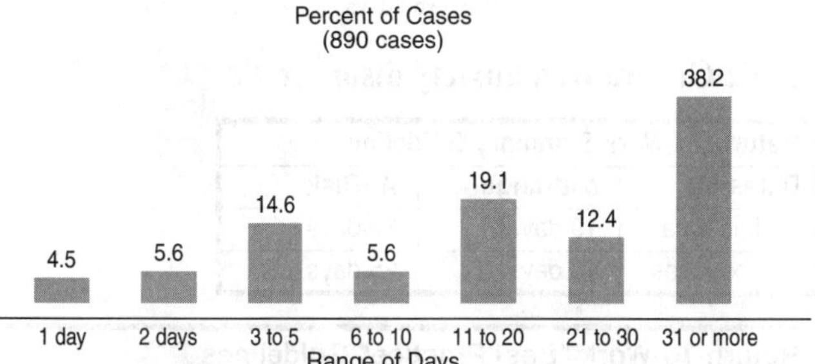

Impact on Occupational Absence: Prevalence 0.2221% of occupational lost workdays; Incidence 0.04 days per 100 workers

300.0 Anxiety states

Return-To-Work Summary Guidelines		
Dataset	**Midrange**	**At-Risk**
Claims data	17 days	42 days
All absences	11 days	25 days

Return-To-Work "Best Practice" Guidelines
Rule out impaired mood/personality disorder: 0 days
Without hospitalization: 0-7 days
With hospitalization: 14-21 days

Capabilities & Activity Modifications:
Avoid eliciting symptoms affecting work/other job issues: Limit to low project responsibility and minimal supervision of others; avoid situations of conflict and stress; minimal interaction with the public; personal driving only; minimal handling of heavy machinery (if not limited by medication).
Non-cognitive/modified work: Limit to moderate project responsibility and moderate supervision of others; personal driving only; minimal handling of heavy machinery (if not limited by medication).

Description: The most common type of psychiatric disorder consisting of excessive anxiety and worry about a variety of events or activities, usually lasting six months or longer. Resulting symptoms may include restlessness, trouble concentrating, irritability, sore muscles, and disturbed sleep.

Other names: Neurosis, Anxiety disorders

300.0 Anxiety states *(cont'd)*

Excludes:
anxiety in:
acute stress reaction (308.0)
transient adjustment reaction (309.24)
neurasthenia (300.5)
psychophysiological disorders (306.0-306.9)
separation anxiety (309.21)

Procedure Summary (from ODG Treatment): Acceptance and commitment therapy (ACT); Activity restrictions; Acupressure; Acupuncture; Antidepressants (therapy); Antidepressants - SSRI's versus tricyclics (class); Aromatherapy; Brain wave synchronizers (for stress reduction); Cognitive therapy for depression; Cognitive therapy for panic disorder; Cognitive therapy for stress; Cognitive behavioral stress management (CBSM) to reduce injury and illness; Computer-assisted cognitive therapy; Cymbalta; Depression screening; Depression: effect on heart health; Depression: the gene factor; Disease management (programs); Distractive methods (to reduce acute stress); Duloxetine (Cymbalta); Education (to reduce stress related to illness); Electroconvulsive therapy (ECT); Exercise; Expatriate employee adjustment; Fatigue (job related); Folate (for depressive disorders); Hypnosis; Innovation promotion (program); Kava extract (for anxiety); Light therapy; Massage therapy (MT); Mind/body interventions (for stress relief); Music (for relaxation/stress management); Opioid antagonists (especially naltrexone) for alcohol dependence; Optimism (and its effect on schema-focused therapy); Peer support (for postpartum depression); Psychological debriefing (for preventing post-traumatic stress disorder); Psychosocial/ pharmacological treatments (for deliberate self harm); Psychosocial empowerment (programs); Psychotherapy; Return to work; SAMe (S-adenosylmethionine); St. John's wort (for depression); Stress & atherosclerosis (effect); Stress & blood pressure (effect); Stress & depression (effect); Stress & physiology/mental performance (effect); Stress & post-myocardial infarction (effect); Stress & myocardial ischemia (effect); Stress inoculation training ; Stress management, behavioral/cognitive (interventions); Stress management, physical (interventions); Tension headaches (pharmaceuticals vs. behavioral therapy); Technological stress; Vitamin B6; Vitamin use (for stress reduction); Work; Yoga

Workers' Comp Costs per Claim (based on 222 claims)

Quartile	25%	50%	75%	Mean	% no cost
Indemnity	$21,588	$37,601	$62,507	$54,267	3%
Medical	$19,152	$35,564	$59,903	$49,238	0%
Total	$43,187	$86,447	$115,637	$102,114	0%

RTW Claims Data (Calendar-days away from work by decile)

10%	20%	30%	40%	**50%**	60%	70%	80%	**90%**	100%	Mean
10	13	14	15	**17**	20	22	24	**42**	365	26.92

300.0 Anxiety states *(cont'd)*

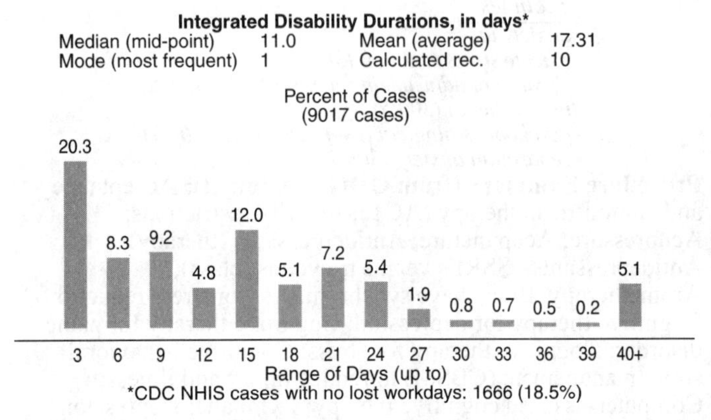

Impact on Total Absence: Prevalence 0.3761% of total lost workdays; Incidence 3.95 days per 100 workers

300.01 Panic disorder without agoraphobia

Return-To-Work Summary Guidelines		
Dataset	**Midrange**	**At-Risk**
Claims data	15 days	39 days
All absences	5 days	18 days

Return-To-Work "Best Practice" Guidelines
1-14 days

Description: A condition consisting of sudden, brief, and unpredictable episodes of acute anxiety with feelings intense fear and apprehension. Bodily symptoms include a racing heart, breathlessness, dizziness, sweating, trembling, palpitations, and chest pain, all of which usually lasts less than one hour.

Panic:
- attack
- state

Workers' Comp Costs per Claim (based on 93 claims)					
Quartile	25%	50%	75%	Mean	% no cost
Indemnity	$25,736	$48,799	$77,826	$70,749	2%
Medical	$14,039	$37,979	$61,184	$60,148	0%
Total	$49,938	$97,199	$143,525	$129,453	0%

Disability Duration Adjustment Factors by Age						
Age Group	18-24	25-34	35-44	45-54	55-64	65-74
Adjustment Factor	0.77	0.78	0.96	1.16	1.76	1.81

RTW Claims Data (Calendar-days away from work by decile)										
10%	20%	30%	40%	**50%**	60%	70%	80%	**90%**	100%	Mean
12	13	14	14	**15**	15	17	18	**39**	365	25.37

300.01 Panic disorder without agoraphobia *(cont'd)*

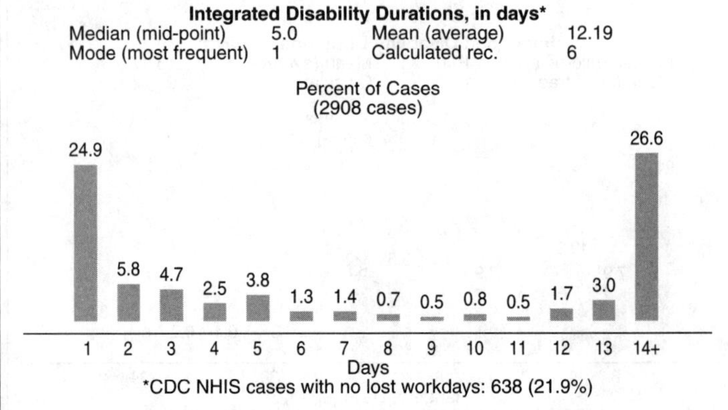

Impact on Total Absence: Prevalence 0.0817% of total lost workdays; Incidence 0.86 days per 100 workers

Occupational Disability Durations, in days
Median (mid-point) 1 - Benchmark Indemnity Costs $750
(90 cases)
Impact on Occupational Absence: Prevalence 0.0010% of occupational lost workdays

300.02 Generalized anxiety disorder

Return-To-Work Summary Guidelines		
Dataset	**Midrange**	**At-Risk**
Claims data	19 days	30 days
All absences	15 days	25 days

Return-To-Work "Best Practice" Guidelines
14-21 days

Description: A chronic state of anxiety characterized by excessive worry and fear which is noticed immediately upon waking and disturbs the person's ability to function socially and otherwise. Restlessness, disturbed sleep, fatigue, difficulty concentrating, muscle tension, and irritability are also possible symptoms.

Workers' Comp Costs per Claim (based on 36 claims)					
Quartile	25%	50%	75%	Mean	% no cost
Indemnity	$27,332	$54,989	$73,070	$52,579	5%
Medical	$20,507	$39,134	$52,206	$42,072	0%
Total	$46,095	$104,570	$125,297	$91,884	0%

Disability Duration Adjustment Factors by Age						
Age Group	18-24	25-34	35-44	45-54	55-64	65-74
Adjustment Factor	0.73	0.70	0.99	1.21	1.45	1.94

RTW Claims Data (Calendar-days away from work by decile)										
10%	20%	30%	40%	**50%**	60%	70%	80%	**90%**	100%	Mean
13	14	15	16	**19**	21	22	23	**30**	365	25.33

300.02 Generalized anxiety disorder *(cont'd)*

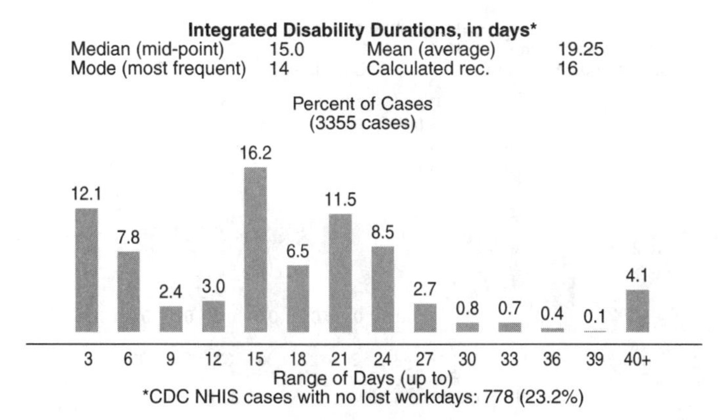

Impact on Total Absence: Prevalence 0.1466% of total lost workdays; Incidence 1.54 days per 100 workers

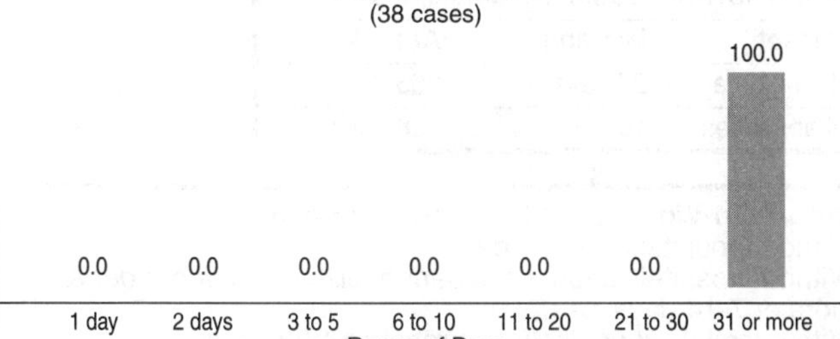

Impact on Occupational Absence: Prevalence 0.0159% of occupational lost workdays

300.4 Dysthymic disorder

Return-To-Work Summary Guidelines		
Dataset	**Midrange**	**At-Risk**
Claims data	28 days	44 days
All absences	26 days	44 days

Return-To-Work "Best Practice" Guidelines
Outpatient therapy, without symptoms affecting work: 0 days
Outpatient therapy, with symptoms interfering with work: 21 days
With hospitalization, non-cognitive/modified work: 28 days
With hospitalization, cognitive work: 42 days

Capabilities & Activity Modifications:
Avoid eliciting symptoms affecting work/other job issues: Limit to low project responsibility and minimal supervision of others; avoid situations of conflict and stress; minimal interaction with the public; personal driving only; minimal handling of heavy machinery (if not limited by medication).
Non-cognitive/modified work: Limit to moderate project responsibility and moderate supervision of others; personal driving only; minimal handling of heavy machinery (if not limited by medication).
Description: A milder form of depression with longer-lasting symptoms of two or more years. Symptoms usually include persistent sadness, pessimism, withdrawal, preoccupation with one's own failure or inadequacy, and gloominess. Often there are physical complaints such as aches and pains, over or under-eating, and oversleeping or inability to sleep.
Other names: Dysthymia

300.4 Dysthymic disorder *(cont'd)*

Anxiety depression
Depression with anxiety
Depressive reaction
Dysthymic disorder
Neurotic depressive state
Reactive depression

Excludes:
adjustment reaction with depressive symptoms (309.0-309.1)
depression NOS (311)
manic-depressive psychosis, depressed type (296.2-296.3)
reactive depressive psychosis (298.0)

Procedure Summary (from ODG Treatment): Acceptance and commitment therapy (ACT); Activity restrictions; Acupressure; Acupuncture; Antidepressants (therapy); Antidepressants - SSRI's versus tricyclics (class); Aromatherapy; Brain wave synchronizers (for stress reduction); Cognitive therapy for depression; Cognitive therapy for panic disorder; Cognitive therapy for stress; Cognitive behavioral stress management (CBSM) to reduce injury and illness; Computer-assisted cognitive therapy; Cymbalta; Depression screening; Depression: effect on heart health; Depression: the gene factor; Disease management (programs); Distractive methods (to reduce acute stress); Duloxetine (Cymbalta); Education (to reduce stress related to illness); Electroconvulsive therapy (ECT); Exercise; Expatriate employee adjustment; Fatigue (job related); Folate (for depressive disorders); Hypnosis; Innovation promotion (program); Kava extract (for anxiety); Light therapy; Massage therapy (MT); Mind/body interventions (for stress relief); Music (for relaxation/stress management); Opioid antagonists (especially naltrexone) for alcohol dependence; Optimism (and its effect on schema-focused therapy); Peer support (for postpartum depression); Psychological debriefing (for preventing post-traumatic stress disorder); Psychosocial/pharmacological treatments (for deliberate self harm); Psychosocial empowerment (programs); Psychotherapy; Return to work; SAMe (S-adenosylmethionine); St. John's wort (for depression); Stress & atherosclerosis (effect); Stress & blood pressure (effect); Stress & depression (effect); Stress & physiology/mental performance (effect); Stress & post-myocardial infarction (effect); Stress & myocardial ischemia (effect); Stress inoculation training ; Stress management, behavioral/cognitive (interventions); Stress management, physical (interventions); Tension headaches (pharmaceuticals vs. behavioral therapy); Technological stress; Vitamin B6; Vitamin use (for stress reduction); Work; Yoga

Workers' Comp Costs per Claim (based on 374 claims)					
Quartile	25%	50%	75%	Mean	% no cost
Indemnity	$27,867	$50,547	$77,732	$57,236	2%
Medical	$23,352	$39,176	$59,556	$49,149	0%
Total	$58,076	$95,603	$134,379	$105,513	0%

RTW Claims Data (Calendar-days away from work by decile)										
10%	20%	30%	40%	**50%**	60%	70%	80%	**90%**	100%	Mean
16	21	22	25	**28**	30	40	42	**44**	365	33.32

300.4 Dysthymic disorder *(cont'd)*

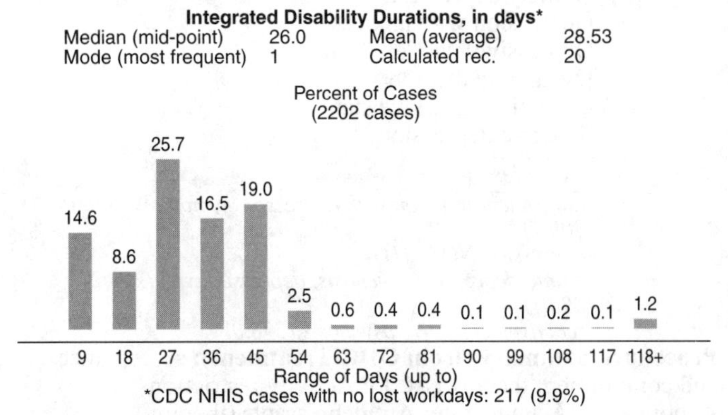

Impact on Total Absence: Prevalence 0.1673% of total lost workdays; Incidence 1.76 days per 100 workers

300.5 Neurasthenia

Return-To-Work Summary Guidelines		
Dataset	**Midrange**	**At-Risk**
Claims data	11 days	14 days
All absences	10 days	14 days

Return-To-Work "Best Practice" Guidelines
Without hospitalization: 0 days
With hospitalization: 10 days

Description: Overwhelming fatigue and exhaustion caused by psychological factors, mainly nervousness, anxiety, frustration, or boredom. Physical symptoms may include pains, dizziness, digestive disorders, palpitations, sexual malfunction, and complaints of being unusually cold or hot. Mental changes may include disturbing dreams, dissatisfaction, envy, and lack of concentration.

Other names: Nervous exhaustion
Fatigue neurosis
Nervous debility
Psychogenic:
asthenia
general fatigue
Use additional code to identify any associated physical disorder

Excludes:
anxiety state (300.00-300.09)
neurotic depression (300.4)
psychophysiological disorders (306.0-306.9)
specific nonpsychotic mental disorders following organic brain damage (310.0-310.9)

RTW Claims Data (Calendar-days away from work by decile)										
10%	20%	30%	40%	**50%**	60%	70%	80%	**90%**	100%	Mean
9	10	10	10	**11**	11	12	13	**14**	100	11.66

300.5 Neurasthenia *(cont'd)*

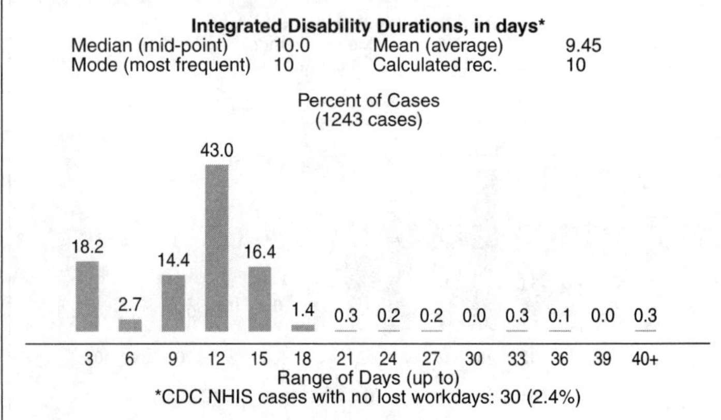

Impact on Total Absence: Prevalence 0.0338% of total lost workdays; Incidence 0.36 days per 100 workers

303 Alcohol dependence syndrome

Return-To-Work Summary Guidelines		
Dataset	**Midrange**	**At-Risk**
Claims data	27 days	365 days
All absences	15 days	228 days

Return-To-Work "Best Practice" Guidelines
Without hospitalization: 1 day
Without hospitalization, considering fellow worker danger & morale: 7-14 days
With hospitalization, including rehab: 14-28 days
Safety sensitive position: as determined by the SAP

Capabilities & Activity Modifications:
Avoid eliciting symptoms affecting work/other job issues: Limit to low project responsibility and minimal supervision of others; avoid situations of conflict and stress; minimal interaction with the public; personal driving only; minimal handling of heavy machinery (if not limited by medication).
Non-cognitive/modified work: Limit to moderate project responsibility and moderate supervision of others; personal driving only; minimal handling of heavy machinery (if not limited by medication).

Description: Chronic disease of excessive alcohol consumption despite adverse social, physical, and occupational consequences, defined by an inability to stop or limit drinking. As the brain becomes tolerant to more alcohol, the amount needed to attain the same level of intoxication must be increased, leading to withdrawal symptoms of tremor, vomiting, weakness, sweating, headache, depression, and anxiety if more alcohol is not consumed. Patterns could include excessive daily drinking or short or long periods of sobriety followed by intense binges. Long-term effects could include gastrointestinal deterioration or cancer, cardiovascular problems, anemia, and reduced brain and nerve function.

Other names: Alcoholism
Use additional code to identify any associated condition, as:
alcoholic psychoses (291.0-291.9)
drug dependence (304.0-304.9)
physical complications of alcohol, such as:
cerebral degeneration (331.7)
cirrhosis of liver (571.2)
epilepsy (345.0-345.9)
gastritis (535.3)
hepatitis (571.1)
liver damage NOS (571.3)

303 Alcohol dependence syndrome *(cont'd)*

Excludes:
drunkenness NOS (305.0)

The following fifth-digit subclassification is for use with category 303:
0 unspecified
1 continuous
2 episodic
3 in remission

Procedure Summary (from ODG Treatment): Acceptance and commitment therapy (ACT); Activity restrictions; Acupressure; Acupuncture; Antidepressants (therapy); Antidepressants - SSRI's versus tricyclics (class); Aromatherapy; Brain wave synchronizers (for stress reduction); Cognitive therapy for depression; Cognitive therapy for panic disorder; Cognitive therapy for stress; Cognitive behavioral stress management (CBSM) to reduce injury and illness; Computer-assisted cognitive therapy; Cymbalta; Depression screening; Depression: effect on heart health; Depression: the gene factor; Disease management (programs); Distractive methods (to reduce acute stress); Duloxetine (Cymbalta); Education (to reduce stress related to illness); Electroconvulsive therapy (ECT); Exercise; Expatriate employee adjustment; Fatigue (job related); Folate (for depressive disorders); Hypnosis; Innovation promotion (program); Kava extract (for anxiety); Light therapy; Massage therapy (MT); Mind/body interventions (for stress relief); Music (for relaxation/stress management); Opioid antagonists (especially naltrexone) for alcohol dependence; Optimism (and its effect on schema-focused therapy); Peer support (for postpartum depression); Psychological debriefing (for preventing post-traumatic stress disorder); Psychosocial/ pharmacological treatments (for deliberate self harm); Psychosocial empowerment (programs); Psychotherapy; Return to work; SAMe (S-adenosylmethionine); St. John's wort (for depression); Stress & atherosclerosis (effect); Stress & blood pressure (effect); Stress & depression (effect); Stress & physiology/mental performance (effect); Stress & post-myocardial infarction (effect); Stress & myocardial ischemia (effect); Stress inoculation training ; Stress management, behavioral/cognitive (interventions); Stress management, physical (interventions); Tension headaches (pharmaceuticals vs. behavioral therapy); Technological stress; Vitamin B6; Vitamin use (for stress reduction); Work; Yoga

Disability Duration Adjustment Factors by Age						
Age Group	18-24	25-34	35-44	45-54	55-64	65-74
Adjustment Factor	0.50	0.97	1.06	1.42	NA	NA

RTW Claims Data (Calendar-days away from work by decile)										
10%	20%	30%	40%	**50%**	60%	70%	80%	**90%**	100%	Mean
10	13	15	18	**27**	29	30	50	**365**	365	72.52

303 Alcohol dependence syndrome *(cont'd)*

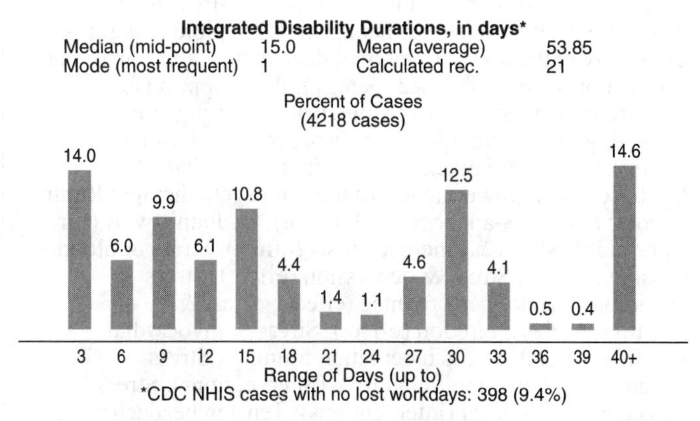

Impact on Total Absence: Prevalence 0.6079% of total lost workdays; Incidence 6.38 days per 100 workers

308 Acute reaction to stress

Return-To-Work Summary Guidelines		
Dataset	**Midrange**	**At-Risk**
Claims data	11 days	15 days
All absences	8 days	14 days

Return-To-Work "Best Practice" Guidelines
Without hospitalization (on-going counseling/drug therapy): 1 day
With hospitalization: 10 days

Capabilities & Activity Modifications:
Avoid eliciting symptoms affecting work/other job issues: Limit to low project responsibility and minimal supervision of others; avoid situations of conflict and stress; minimal interaction with the public; personal driving only; minimal handling of heavy machinery (if not limited by medication).
Non-cognitive/modified work: Limit to moderate project responsibility and moderate supervision of others; personal driving only; minimal handling of heavy machinery (if not limited by medication).

Includes: catastrophic stress
combat fatigue
gross stress reaction (acute)
transient disorders in response to exceptional physical or mental stress which usually subside within hours or days

Excludes:
adjustment reaction or disorder (309.0-309.9)
chronic stress reaction (309.1-309.9)

Procedure Summary (from ODG Treatment): Acceptance and commitment therapy (ACT); Activity restrictions; Acupressure; Acupuncture; Antidepressants (therapy); Antidepressants - SSRI's versus tricyclics (class); Aromatherapy; Brain wave synchronizers (for stress reduction); Cognitive therapy for depression; Cognitive therapy for panic disorder; Cognitive therapy for stress; Cognitive behavioral stress management (CBSM) to reduce injury and illness; Computer-assisted cognitive therapy; Cymbalta; Depression screening; Depression: effect on heart health; Depression: the gene factor; Disease management (programs); Distractive methods (to reduce acute stress); Duloxetine (Cymbalta); Education (to reduce stress related to illness); Electroconvulsive therapy (ECT); Exercise; Expatriate employee adjustment; Fatigue (job related); Folate (for depressive disorders); Hypnosis; Innovation promotion (program); Kava extract (for anxiety); Light therapy; Massage

308 Acute reaction to stress *(cont'd)*

therapy (MT); Mind/body interventions (for stress relief); Music (for relaxation/stress management); Opioid antagonists (especially naltrexone) for alcohol dependence; Optimism (and its effect on schema-focused therapy); Peer support (for postpartum depression); Psychological debriefing (for preventing post-traumatic stress disorder); Psychosocial/pharmacological treatments (for deliberate self harm); Psychosocial empowerment (programs); Psychotherapy; Return to work; SAMe (S-adenosylmethionine); St. John's wort (for depression); Stress & atherosclerosis (effect); Stress & blood pressure (effect); Stress & depression (effect); Stress & physiology/mental performance (effect); Stress & post-myocardial infarction (effect); Stress & myocardial ischemia (effect); Stress inoculation training ; Stress management, behavioral/cognitive (interventions); Stress management, physical (interventions); Tension headaches (pharmaceuticals vs. behavioral therapy); Technological stress; Vitamin B6; Vitamin use (for stress reduction); Work; Yoga

Workers' Comp Costs per Claim (based on 222 claims)

Quartile	25%	50%	75%	Mean	% no cost
Indemnity	$11,319	$20,029	$41,381	$34,019	9%
Medical	$4,211	$11,036	$24,192	$17,585	0%
Total	$14,438	$30,387	$67,400	$48,406	0%

RTW Claims Data (Calendar-days away from work by decile)

10%	20%	30%	40%	**50%**	60%	70%	80%	**90%**	100%	Mean
9	10	10	10	**11**	12	13	14	**15**	365	18.61

Integrated Disability Durations, in days*

Median (mid-point) 8.5 Mean (average) 10.86
Mode (most frequent) 1 Calculated rec. 7

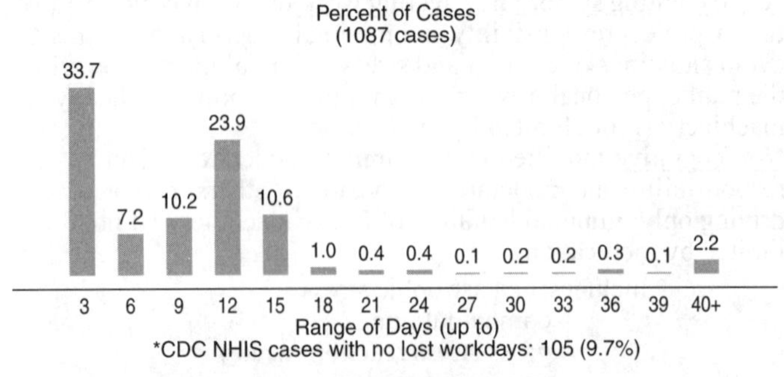

*CDC NHIS cases with no lost workdays: 105 (9.7%)

Impact on Total Absence: Prevalence 0.0315% of total lost workdays; Incidence 0.33 days per 100 workers

Occupational Disability Durations, in days

Median (mid-point) 15 - Benchmark Indemnity Costs $11,250

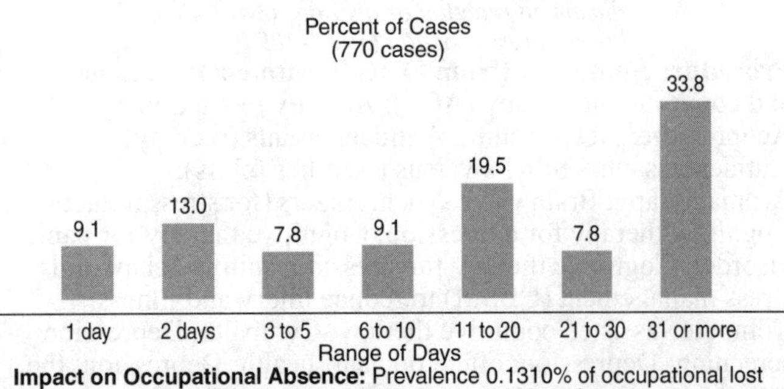

Impact on Occupational Absence: Prevalence 0.1310% of occupational lost workdays; Incidence 0.02 days per 100 workers

308.9 Unspecified acute reaction to stress

Return-To-Work Summary Guidelines

Dataset	Midrange	At-Risk
Claims data	14 days	37 days
All absences	11 days	31 days

Return-To-Work "Best Practice" Guidelines
Without hospitalization (on-going counseling): 1 day
With hospitalization: 10 days
Chemical dependence comorbidity: 28 days

Capabilities & Activity Modifications:
Avoid eliciting symptoms affecting work/other job issues: Limit to low project responsibility and minimal supervision of others; avoid situations of conflict and stress; minimal interaction with the public; personal driving only; minimal handling of heavy machinery (if not limited by medication).
Non-cognitive/modified work: Limit to moderate project responsibility and moderate supervision of others; personal driving only; minimal handling of heavy machinery (if not limited by medication).

Description: An anxiety disorder brought on by exposure to an extraordinarily traumatic event. Symptoms could include numbed emotional responsiveness, feelings of fear, helplessness, and/or guilt, depression, amnesia about the event, or repeated feelings of re-experiencing the event.

Other names: Acute/brief post-traumatic stress disorder, Acute stress disorder

Procedure Summary (from ODG Treatment): Acceptance and commitment therapy (ACT); Activity restrictions; Acupressure; Acupuncture; Antidepressants (therapy); Antidepressants - SSRI's versus tricyclics (class); Aromatherapy; Brain wave synchronizers (for stress reduction); Cognitive therapy for depression; Cognitive therapy for panic disorder; Cognitive therapy for stress; Cognitive behavioral stress management (CBSM) to reduce injury and illness; Computer-assisted cognitive therapy; Cymbalta; Depression screening; Depression: effect on heart health; Depression: the gene factor; Disease management (programs); Distractive methods (to reduce acute stress); Duloxetine (Cymbalta); Education (to reduce stress related to illness); Electroconvulsive therapy (ECT); Exercise; Expatriate employee adjustment; Fatigue (job related); Folate (for depressive disorders); Hypnosis; Innovation promotion (program); Kava extract (for anxiety); Light therapy; Massage therapy (MT); Mind/body interventions (for stress relief); Music (for relaxation/stress management); Opioid antagonists (especially naltrexone) for alcohol dependence; Optimism (and its effect on schema-focused therapy); Peer support (for postpartum depression); Psychological debriefing (for preventing post-traumatic stress disorder); Psychosocial/pharmacological treatments (for deliberate self harm); Psychosocial empowerment (programs); Psychotherapy; Return to work; SAMe (S-adenosylmethionine); St. John's wort (for depression); Stress & atherosclerosis (effect); Stress & blood pressure (effect); Stress & depression (effect); Stress & physiology/mental performance (effect); Stress & post-myocardial infarction (effect); Stress & myocardial ischemia (effect); Stress inoculation training ; Stress management, behavioral/cognitive (interventions); Stress management, physical (interventions); Tension headaches (pharmaceuticals vs. behavioral therapy); Technological stress; Vitamin B6; Vitamin use (for stress reduction); Work; Yoga

RTW Claims Data (Calendar-days away from work by decile)

10%	20%	30%	40%	**50%**	60%	70%	80%	**90%**	100%	Mean
9	10	11	12	**14**	21	28	30	**37**	365	27.34

308.9 Unspecified acute reaction to stress *(cont'd)*

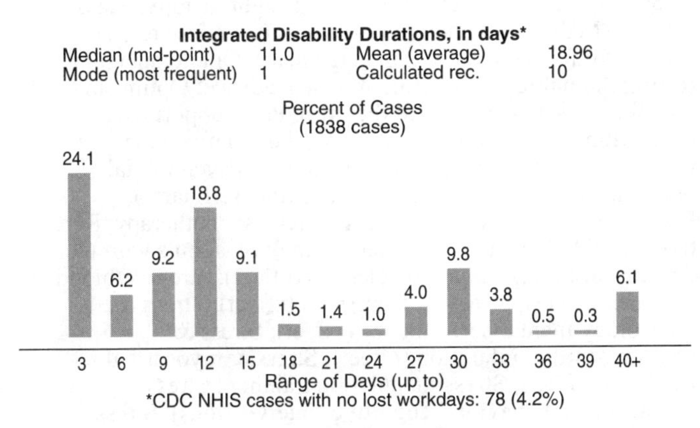

Impact on Total Absence: Prevalence 0.0986% of total lost workdays; Incidence 1.04 days per 100 workers

309 Adjustment reaction

Return-To-Work Summary Guidelines		
Dataset	**Midrange**	**At-Risk**
Claims data	16 days	35 days
All absences	13 days	30 days

Return-To-Work "Best Practice" Guidelines
Without hospitalization: 1-6 day
Outpatient care: 1-6 days
With inpatient hospitalization: 14-28 days

Capabilities & Activity Modifications:
Avoid eliciting symptoms affecting work/other job issues: Limit to low project responsibility and minimal supervision of others; avoid situations of conflict and stress; minimal interaction with the public; personal driving only; minimal handling of heavy machinery (if not limited by medication).
Non-cognitive/modified work: Limit to moderate project responsibility and moderate supervision of others; personal driving only; minimal handling of heavy machinery (if not limited by medication).

Description: Response to environmental stress or change causing symptoms which could include maladjustment, anxiety, crying, conduct problems, recklessness, or impaired social or occupational functioning.

Includes: adjustment disorders
reaction (adjustment) to chronic stress

Excludes:
acute reaction to major stress (308.0-308.9)
neurotic disorders (300.0-300.9)

Procedure Summary (from ODG Treatment): Acceptance and commitment therapy (ACT); Activity restrictions; Acupressure; Acupuncture; Antidepressants (therapy); Antidepressants - SSRI's versus tricyclics (class); Aromatherapy; Brain wave synchronizers (for stress reduction); Cognitive therapy for depression; Cognitive therapy for panic disorder; Cognitive therapy for stress; Cognitive behavioral stress management (CBSM) to reduce injury and illness; Computer-assisted cognitive therapy; Cymbalta; Depression screening; Depression: effect on heart health; Depression: the gene factor; Disease management (programs); Distractive methods (to reduce acute stress); Duloxetine (Cymbalta); Education (to reduce stress related to illness); Electroconvulsive therapy (ECT); Exercise; Expatriate employee adjustment; Fatigue (job related); Folate (for depressive disorders); Hypnosis; Innovation promotion (program); Kava extract (for anxiety); Light therapy; Massage

309 Adjustment reaction *(cont'd)*

therapy (MT); Mind/body interventions (for stress relief); Music (for relaxation/stress management); Opioid antagonists (especially naltrexone) for alcohol dependence; Optimism (and its effect on schema-focused therapy); Peer support (for postpartum depression); Psychological debriefing (for preventing post-traumatic stress disorder); Psychosocial/pharmacological treatments (for deliberate self harm); Psychosocial empowerment (programs); Psychotherapy; Return to work; SAMe (S-adenosylmethionine); St. John's wort (for depression); Stress & atherosclerosis (effect); Stress & blood pressure (effect); Stress & depression (effect); Stress & physiology/mental performance (effect); Stress & post-myocardial infarction (effect); Stress & myocardial ischemia (effect); Stress inoculation training ; Stress management, behavioral/cognitive (interventions); Stress management, physical (interventions); Tension headaches (pharmaceuticals vs. behavioral therapy); Technological stress; Vitamin B6; Vitamin use (for stress reduction); Work; Yoga

Workers' Comp Costs per Claim (based on 1,387 claims)					
Quartile	25%	50%	75%	Mean	% no cost
Indemnity	$24,717	$43,922	$76,755	$57,392	5%
Medical	$16,076	$31,925	$58,874	$46,217	0%
Total	$42,074	$80,882	$137,078	$100,622	0%

RTW Claims Data (Calendar-days away from work by decile)										
10%	20%	30%	40%	**50%**	60%	70%	80%	**90%**	100%	Mean
12	13	14	15	**16**	26	28	30	**35**	365	26.47

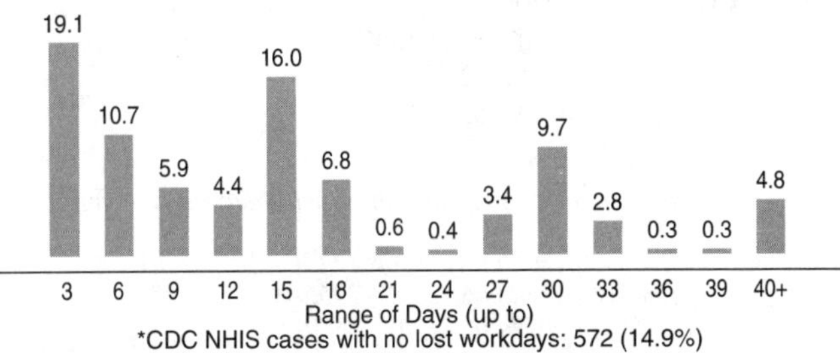

Impact on Total Absence: Prevalence 0.1688% of total lost workdays; Incidence 1.77 days per 100 workers

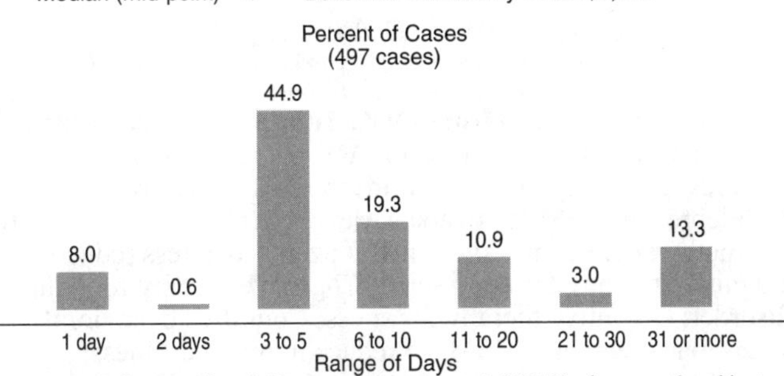

Impact on Occupational Absence: Prevalence 0.0225% of occupational lost workdays

311 Depressive disorder, not elsewhere classified

Return-To-Work Summary Guidelines		
Dataset	**Midrange**	**At-Risk**
Claims data	29 days	57 days
All absences	22 days	56 days

Return-To-Work "Best Practice" Guidelines
Rule out impaired mood/personality disorder: 0 days
Outpatient therapy, without symptoms affecting work or other job issues: 0-7 days
Outpatient therapy, with symptoms interfering with work: 21 days
Outpatient therapy, with serious job satisfaction issues: 28-42 days
With hospitalization, non-cognitive/modified work: 28 days
With hospitalization, cognitive work: 42-56 days

Capabilities & Activity Modifications:
Avoid eliciting symptoms affecting work/other job issues: Limit to low project responsibility and minimal supervision of others; avoid situations of conflict and stress; minimal interaction with the public; personal driving only; minimal handling of heavy machinery (if not limited by medication).
Non-cognitive/modified work: Limit to moderate project responsibility and moderate supervision of others; personal driving only; minimal handling of heavy machinery (if not limited by medication).
Description: An excessively long or intense period of deep sadness or extreme apathy. Depression varies in length from recurring bouts of several hours to a sustained depression lasting two years or more, with recurring episodes throughout a lifetime, sometimes resulting in suicide. Other symptoms may include irritability, poor concentration, decreased appetite, social withdrawal, and an inability to experience pleasure.
Other names: Depression

Depressive disorder NOS
Depressive state NOS
Depression NOS

Excludes:

acute reaction to major stress with depressive symptoms (308.0)
affective personality disorder (301.10-301.13)
affective psychoses (296.0-296.9)
brief depressive reaction (309.0)
depressive states associated with stressful events (309.0-309.1)
disturbance of emotions specific to childhood and adolescence, with misery and unhappiness (313.1)
mixed adjustment reaction with depressive symptoms (309.4)
neurotic depression (300.4)
prolonged depressive adjustment reaction (309.1)
psychogenic depressive psychosis (298.0)

Procedure Summary (from ODG Treatment): Acceptance and commitment therapy (ACT); Activity restrictions; Acupressure; Acupuncture; Antidepressants (therapy); Antidepressants - SSRI's versus tricyclics (class); Aromatherapy; Brain wave synchronizers (for stress reduction); Cognitive therapy for depression; Cognitive therapy for panic disorder; Cognitive therapy for stress; Cognitive behavioral stress management (CBSM) to reduce injury and illness; Computer-assisted cognitive therapy; Cymbalta; Depression screening; Depression: effect on heart health; Depression: the gene factor; Disease management (programs); Distractive methods (to reduce acute stress); Duloxetine (Cymbalta); Education (to reduce stress related to illness); Electroconvulsive therapy (ECT); Exercise; Expatriate employee adjustment; Fatigue (job related); Folate (for depressive disorders); Hypnosis; Innovation promotion (program); Kava extract (for anxiety); Light therapy; Massage therapy (MT); Mind/body interventions (for stress relief); Music (for relaxation/stress management); Opioid antagonists (especially naltrexone) for alcohol dependence; Optimism (and its effect on schema-focused therapy); Peer support (for postpartum depression); Psychological debriefing (for preventing post-traumatic stress disorder); Psychosocial/pharmacological treatments (for deliberate self harm); Psychosocial empowerment (programs); Psychotherapy; Return to work; SAMe (S-adenosylmethionine); St. John's wort (for depression); Stress & atherosclerosis (effect); Stress & blood pressure (effect); Stress & depression (effect); Stress & physiology/mental performance (effect); Stress & post-myocardial infarction (effect); Stress & myocardial ischemia (effect); Stress inoculation training ; Stress management, behavioral/cognitive (interventions); Stress management, physical (interventions); Tension headaches (pharmaceuticals vs. behavioral therapy); Technological stress; Vitamin B6; Vitamin use (for stress reduction); Work; Yoga

Workers' Comp Costs per Claim (based on 1,522 claims)					
Quartile	25%	50%	75%	Mean	% no cost
Indemnity	$35,532	$54,999	$82,541	$62,593	1%
Medical	$29,516	$48,426	$79,233	$60,678	0%
Total	$73,973	$111,468	$158,498	$122,724	0%

Disability Duration Adjustment Factors by Age						
Age Group	18-24	25-34	35-44	45-54	55-64	65-74
Adjustment Factor	0.58	0.91	0.95	1.19	1.38	1.66

RTW Claims Data (Calendar-days away from work by decile)										
10%	20%	30%	40%	**50%**	60%	70%	80%	**90%**	100%	Mean
11	17	21	26	**29**	37	43	54	**57**	365	36.97

Integrated Disability Durations, in days*

Median (mid-point)	22.0	Mean (average)	27.70
Mode (most frequent)	1	Calculated rec.	18

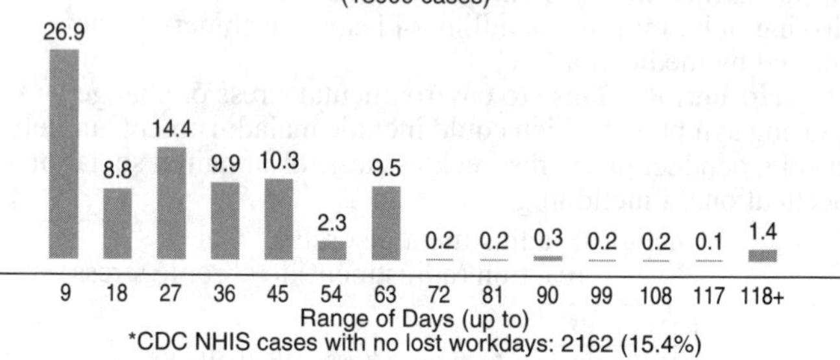

*CDC NHIS cases with no lost workdays: 2162 (15.4%)

Impact on Total Absence: Prevalence 0.9692% of total lost workdays; Incidence 10.18 days per 100 workers

6. DISEASES OF THE NERVOUS SYSTEM AND SENSE ORGANS (320-389)

Impact on Total Absence: Prevalence 6.3741% of total lost workdays; Incidence 66.93 days per 100 workers

RTW Claims Data (Calendar-days away from work by decile)										
10%	20%	30%	40%	**50%**	60%	70%	80%	**90%**	100%	Mean
10	13	14	16	**20**	24	29	38	**84**	365	45.22

This section covers diagnoses involving the nervous system and sense organs.

PAIN (338-339)

RTW Claims Data (Calendar-days away from work by decile)										
10%	20%	30%	40%	**50%**	60%	70%	80%	**90%**	100%	Mean
14	17	22	28	**32**	63	87	209	**216**	365	92.57

Impact on Total Absence: Prevalence 0.2801% of total lost workdays; Incidence 2.94 days per 100 workers

338 Pain, not elsewhere classified

Return-To-Work Summary Guidelines		
Dataset	**Midrange**	**At-Risk**
Claims data	28 days	211 days
All absences	23 days	211 days

Return-To-Work "Best Practice" Guidelines
Medical treatment, clerical/modified work: 14 days
Medical treatment, manual work: 63 days

Use additional code to identify:
pain associated with psychological factors (307.89)

Excludes: generalized pain (780.96)
localized pain, unspecified type - code to pain by site
pain disorder exclusively attributed to psychological factors (307.80)

Procedure Summary (from ODG Treatment): Actiq®; Acupuncture; Antidepressants (therapy); Antidepressants - SSRI's versus tricyclics (class); Anti-inflammatory medications; Autonomic test battery; Barbituate-containing analgesic agents (BCAs); Behavioral interventions; Biofeedback; Botulinum toxin (Botox); Capsaicin; Celebrex®; Cod liver oil; Cold lasers; CRPS (complex regional pain syndrome); Cyclobenzaprine; Cymbalta; Diagnostic criteria for CRPS; Education; Electrical stimulators (E-stim); Electroceutical therapy (bioelectric nerve block); Electrodiagnostic testing (EMG/NCS); Epidural steroid injections (ESI's); Exercise; Facet blocks; Fibromyalgia syndrome (FMS); Gabapentin; Glucosamine (and Chondroitin Sulfate); H-wave stimulation (devices); Ibuprofen; Implantable pumps for narcotics; Implantable spinal cord stimulators; Injection with anaesthetics and/or steroids; Interdisciplinary rehabilitation programs; Interferential current stimulation (ICS); Intrathecal pumps; Intravenous regional sympathetic blocks (for RSD, nerve blocks); Ketamine; Low level laser therapy (LLLT); Lumbar sympathetic block; Magnet therapy; Manual therapy & manipulation; Massage therapy; Medications; Microcurrent electrical stimulation (MENS devices); Morphine pumps; Multi-disciplinary treatment; Muscle relaxants; Myofascial pain; Naproxen; Neuroreflexotherapy; Neuromodulation devices; Neuromuscular electrical stimulation (NMES devices); Neurontin®; Nonprescription medications; NSAIDs (non steroidal anti-inflammatory drugs); Nucleoplasty; Occupational therapy (OT); Oral morphine; Opioids; Oxycontin®; Pain management programs; Percutaneous electrical nerve stimulation (PENS); Percutaneous neuromodulation therapy (PNT); Phentolamine infusion test; Physical therapy (PT); Prolotherapy; Psychological evaluations; Return to work; RSD (reflex sympathetic dystrophy); Salicylate topicals; Sclerotherapy (prolotherapy); Spinal cord stimulators (SCS); Stellate ganglion block; Stress infrared telethermography; Sympathectomy; Sympathetic therapy; Thermography (infrared stress thermography); Transcutaneous electrical nerve stimulation (TENS); Treatment for CRPS; Trigger point injections; Vicodin®; Vioxx®; Yoga

RTW Claims Data (Calendar-days away from work by decile)										
10%	20%	30%	40%	**50%**	60%	70%	80%	**90%**	100%	Mean
14	15	20	23	**28**	31	64	180	**211**	365	75.89

Integrated Disability Durations, in days*

Median (mid-point)	23.0	Mean (average)	63.71
Mode (most frequent)	3	Calculated rec.	28

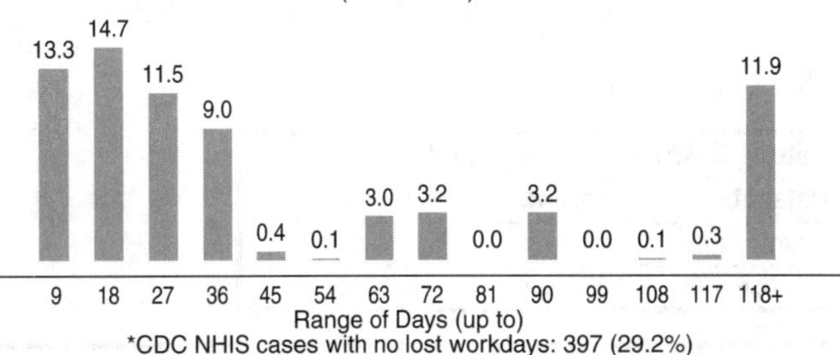

*CDC NHIS cases with no lost workdays: 397 (29.2%)

Impact on Total Absence: Prevalence 0.1811% of total lost workdays; Incidence 1.90 days per 100 workers

338.0 Central pain syndrome

Return-To-Work Summary Guidelines		
Dataset	**Midrange**	**At-Risk**
Claims data	28 days	211 days
All absences	23 days	211 days

Déjérine-Roussy syndrome
Myelopathic pain syndrome
Thalamic pain syndrome (hyperesthetic)

338.1 Acute pain

Return-To-Work Summary Guidelines		
Dataset	**Midrange**	**At-Risk**
Claims data	28 days	211 days
All absences	23 days	211 days

338.11 Acute pain due to trauma

Return-To-Work Summary Guidelines		
Dataset	**Midrange**	**At-Risk**
Claims data	28 days	211 days
All absences	23 days	211 days

338.12 Acute post-thoracotomy pain

Return-To-Work Summary Guidelines		
Dataset	**Midrange**	**At-Risk**
Claims data	28 days	211 days
All absences	23 days	211 days

338.12 Acute post-thoracotomy pain *(cont'd)*

Post-thoracotomy pain NOS

338.18 Other acute postoperative pain

Return-To-Work Summary Guidelines		
Dataset	Midrange	At-Risk
Claims data	28 days	211 days
All absences	23 days	211 days

Postoperative pain NOS

338.19 Other acute pain

Return-To-Work Summary Guidelines		
Dataset	Midrange	At-Risk
Claims data	28 days	211 days
All absences	23 days	211 days

Excludes: neoplasm related acute pain (338.3)

338.2 Chronic pain

Return-To-Work Summary Guidelines		
Dataset	Midrange	At-Risk
Claims data	124 days	364 days
All absences	103 days	355 days

Return-To-Work "Best Practice" Guidelines
60 days to indefinite
See the Pain Chapter in ODG Treatment

Excludes: causalgia (355.9)
lower limb (355.71)
upper limb (354.4)
chronic pain syndrome (338.4)
myofascial pain syndrome (729.1)
neoplasm related chronic pain (338.3)
reflex sympathetic dystrophy (337.20-337.29)

Procedure Summary (from ODG Treatment): Actiq®; Acupuncture; Antidepressants (therapy); Antidepressants - SSRI's versus tricyclics (class); Anti-inflammatory medications; Autonomic test battery; Barbituate-containing analgesic agents (BCAs); Behavioral interventions; Biofeedback; Botulinum toxin (Botox); Capsaicin; Celebrex®; Cod liver oil; Cold lasers; CRPS (complex regional pain syndrome); Cyclobenzaprine; Cymbalta; Diagnostic criteria for CRPS; Education; Electrical stimulators (E-stim); Electroceutical therapy (bioelectric nerve block); Electrodiagnostic testing (EMG/NCS); Epidural steroid injections (ESI's); Exercise; Facet blocks; Fibromyalgia syndrome (FMS); Gabapentin; Glucosamine (and Chondroitin Sulfate); H-wave stimulation (devices); Ibuprofen; Implantable pumps for narcotics; Implantable spinal cord stimulators; Injection with anaesthetics and/or steroids; Interdisciplinary rehabilitation programs; Interferential current stimulation (ICS); Intrathecal pumps; Intravenous regional sympathetic blocks (for RSD, nerve blocks); Ketamine; Low level laser therapy (LLLT); Lumbar sympathetic block; Magnet therapy; Manual therapy & manipulation; Massage therapy; Medications; Microcurrent electrical stimulation (MENS devices); Morphine pumps; Multi-disciplinary treatment; Muscle relaxants; Myofascial pain; Naproxen; Neuroreflexotherapy; Neuromodulation devices; Neuromuscular electrical stimulation (NMES devices); Neurontin®; Nonprescription medications; NSAIDs (non steroidal anti-inflammatory drugs); Nucleoplasty; Occupational

338.2 Chronic pain *(cont'd)*

therapy (OT); Oral morphine; Opioids; Oxycontin®; Pain management programs; Percutaneous electrical nerve stimulation (PENS); Percutaneous neuromodulation therapy (PNT); Phentolamine infusion test; Physical therapy (PT); Prolotherapy; Psychological evaluations; Return to work; RSD (reflex sympathetic dystrophy); Salicylate topicals; Sclerotherapy (prolotherapy); Spinal cord stimulators (SCS); Stellate ganglion block; Stress infrared telethermography; Sympathectomy; Sympathetic therapy; Thermography (infrared stress thermography); Transcutaneous electrical nerve stimulation (TENS); Treatment for CRPS; Trigger point injections; Vicodin®; Vioxx®; Yoga

RTW Claims Data (Calendar-days away from work by decile)										
10%	20%	30%	40%	**50%**	60%	70%	80%	**90%**	100%	Mean
28	52	62	95	**124**	156	196	278	**364**	365	154.39

Integrated Disability Durations, in days*

Median (mid-point)	103.0	Mean (average)	136.12
Mode (most frequent)	6	Calculated rec.	87

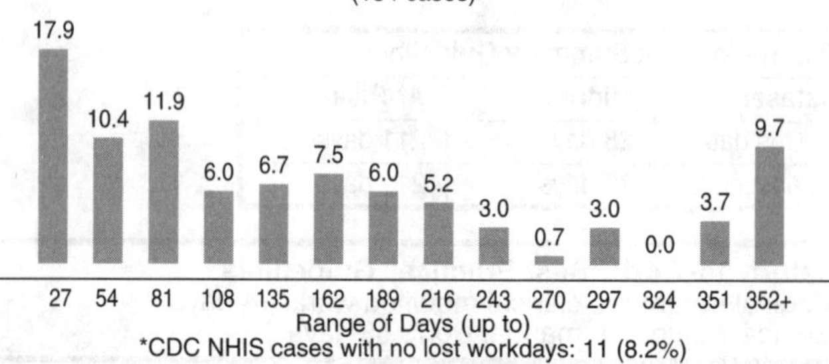

*CDC NHIS cases with no lost workdays: 11 (8.2%)

Impact on Total Absence: Prevalence 0.0494% of total lost workdays; Incidence 0.52 days per 100 workers

338.21 Chronic pain due to trauma

Return-To-Work Summary Guidelines		
Dataset	Midrange	At-Risk
Claims data	124 days	364 days
All absences	103 days	355 days

338.22 Chronic post-thoracotomy pain

Return-To-Work Summary Guidelines		
Dataset	Midrange	At-Risk
Claims data	124 days	364 days
All absences	103 days	355 days

338.28 Other chronic postoperative pain

Return-To-Work Summary Guidelines		
Dataset	Midrange	At-Risk
Claims data	124 days	364 days
All absences	103 days	355 days

338.29 Other chronic pain

Return-To-Work Summary Guidelines		
Dataset	Midrange	At-Risk
Claims data	124 days	364 days
All absences	103 days	355 days

338.3 Neoplasm related pain (acute) (chronic)

Return-To-Work Summary Guidelines		
Dataset	**Midrange**	**At-Risk**
Claims data	28 days	211 days
All absences	23 days	211 days

Cancer associated pain
Pain due to malignancy (primary) (secondary)
Tumor associated pain

338.4 Chronic pain syndrome

Return-To-Work Summary Guidelines		
Dataset	**Midrange**	**At-Risk**
Claims data	124 days	364 days
All absences	103 days	355 days

Return-To-Work "Best Practice" Guidelines
Note: this is a controversial diagnosis
60 days to indefinite
See the Pain Chapter in ODG Treatment

Chronic pain associated with significant psychosocial dysfunction

Procedure Summary (from ODG Treatment): Actiq®; Acupuncture; Antidepressants (therapy); Antidepressants - SSRI's versus tricyclics (class); Anti-inflammatory medications; Autonomic test battery; Barbituate-containing analgesic agents (BCAs); Behavioral interventions; Biofeedback; Botulinum toxin (Botox); Capsaicin; Celebrex®; Cod liver oil; Cold lasers; CRPS (complex regional pain syndrome); Cyclobenzaprine; Cymbalta; Diagnostic criteria for CRPS; Education; Electrical stimulators (E-stim); Electroceutical therapy (bioelectric nerve block); Electrodiagnostic testing (EMG/NCS); Epidural steroid injections (ESI's); Exercise; Facet blocks; Fibromyalgia syndrome (FMS); Gabapentin; Glucosamine (and Chondroitin Sulfate); H-wave stimulation (devices); Ibuprofen; Implantable pumps for narcotics; Implantable spinal cord stimulators; Injection with anaesthetics and/or steroids; Interdisciplinary rehabilitation programs; Interferential current stimulation (ICS); Intrathecal pumps; Intravenous regional sympathetic blocks (for RSD, nerve blocks); Ketamine; Low level laser therapy (LLLT); Lumbar sympathetic block; Magnet therapy; Manual therapy & manipulation; Massage therapy; Medications; Microcurrent electrical stimulation (MENS devices); Morphine pumps; Multi-disciplinary treatment; Muscle relaxants; Myofascial pain; Naproxen; Neuroreflexotherapy; Neuromodulation devices; Neuromuscular electrical stimulation (NMES devices); Neurontin®; Nonprescription medications; NSAIDs (non steroidal anti-inflammatory drugs); Nucleoplasty; Occupational therapy (OT); Oral morphine; Opioids; Oxycontin®; Pain management programs; Percutaneous electrical nerve stimulation (PENS); Percutaneous neuromodulation therapy (PNT); Phentolamine infusion test; Physical therapy (PT); Prolotherapy; Psychological evaluations; Return to work; RSD (reflex sympathetic dystrophy); Salicylate topicals; Sclerotherapy (prolotherapy); Spinal cord stimulators (SCS); Stellate ganglion block; Stress infrared telethermography; Sympathectomy; Sympathetic therapy; Thermography (infrared stress thermography); Transcutaneous electrical nerve stimulation (TENS); Treatment for CRPS; Trigger point injections; Vicodin®; Vioxx®; Yoga

338.4 Chronic pain syndrome *(cont'd)*

RTW Claims Data (Calendar-days away from work by decile)

10%	20%	30%	40%	**50%**	60%	70%	80%	**90%**	100%	Mean
28	52	62	95	**124**	156	196	278	**364**	365	154.39

Integrated Disability Durations, in days*

Median (mid-point)	103.0	Mean (average)	136.12
Mode (most frequent)	6	Calculated rec.	87

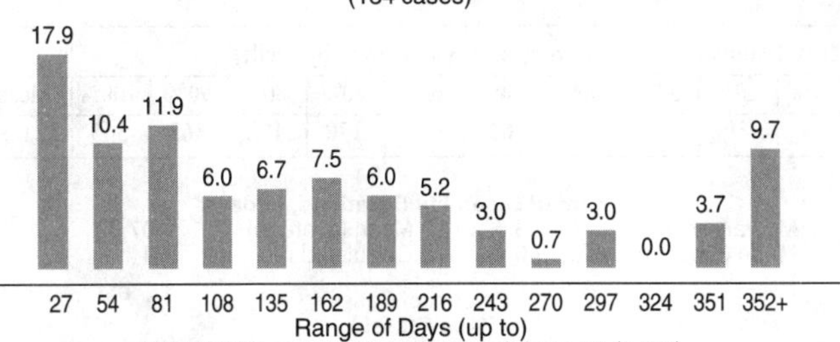

*CDC NHIS cases with no lost workdays: 11 (8.2%)

Impact on Total Absence: Prevalence 0.0494% of total lost workdays; Incidence 0.52 days per 100 workers

OTHER DISORDERS OF THE CENTRAL NERVOUS SYSTEM (340-349)

RTW Claims Data (Calendar-days away from work by decile)

10%	20%	30%	40%	**50%**	60%	70%	80%	**90%**	100%	Mean
11	14	14	16	**20**	22	27	30	**60**	365	39.91

Impact on Total Absence: Prevalence 2.4082% of total lost workdays; Incidence 25.29 days per 100 workers

Occupational Disability Durations, in days
Median (mid-point) 50 - Benchmark Indemnity Costs $37,500

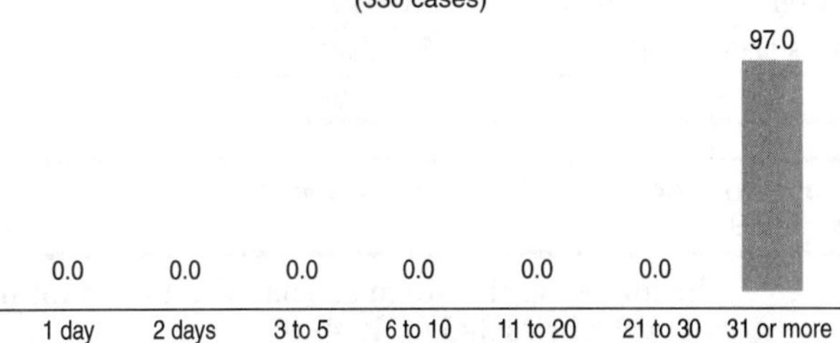

Impact on Occupational Absence: Prevalence 0.1871% of occupational lost workdays; Incidence 0.03 days per 100 workers

340 Multiple sclerosis

Return-To-Work Summary Guidelines		
Dataset	**Midrange**	**At-Risk**
Claims data	61 days	365 days
All absences	53 days	364 days

Return-To-Work "Best Practice" Guidelines
In remission: 0 days
With hospitalization: 40-60 days
With hospitalization, severe episode: 170 days to indefinite

Description: Slow progressive disease of the central nervous system occurring when the fatty substance that surrounds nerve processes (myelin) is lost, leading to slow or blocked nerve impulse conduction in the brain or spinal cord. Symptoms vary,

340 Multiple sclerosis *(cont'd)*

but common early symptoms could include tingling or numbness in the arms, legs, trunk or face, as well as vision problems or impaired dexterity.

Other names: MS

Disseminated or multiple sclerosis:
- NOS
- brain stem
- cord
- generalized

RTW Claims Data (Calendar-days away from work by decile)

10%	20%	30%	40%	**50%**	60%	70%	80%	**90%**	100%	Mean
16	39	41	43	**61**	169	170	172	**365**	365	121.55

Integrated Disability Durations, in days*

Median (mid-point)	53.5	Mean (average)	107.62
Mode (most frequent)	40	Calculated rec.	64

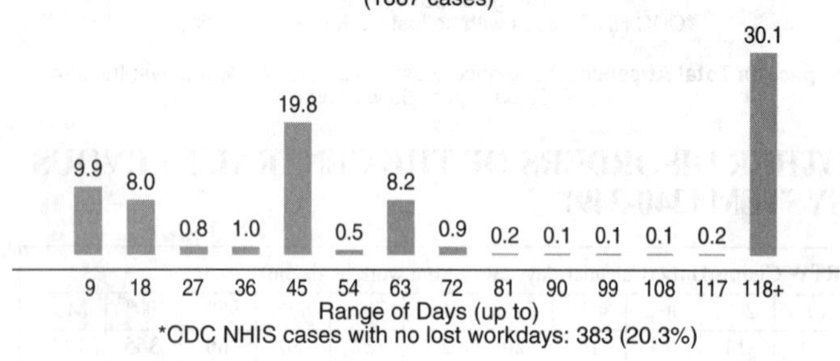

*CDC NHIS cases with no lost workdays: 383 (20.3%)

Impact on Total Absence: Prevalence 0.4784% of total lost workdays; Incidence 5.02 days per 100 workers

345 Epilepsy and recurrent seizures

Return-To-Work Summary Guidelines

Dataset	Midrange	At-Risk
Claims data	41 days	365 days
All absences	24 days	365 days

Return-To-Work "Best Practice" Guidelines
See 345.9

The following fifth-digit subclassification is for use with categories 345.0, .1, .4-.9:
- 0 without mention of intractable epilepsy
- 1 with intractable epilepsy

Excludes:
progressive myoclonic epilepsy (333.2)

345.1 Generalized convulsive epilepsy

Return-To-Work Summary Guidelines

Dataset	Midrange	At-Risk
Claims data	34 days	365 days
All absences	21 days	365 days

Return-To-Work "Best Practice" Guidelines
Controlled by medication: 0 days
Seizure, clerical/modified work: 1 day
Seizure, dangerous work, with written restrictions: 21 days to indefinite (driving based on state law)
Seizure, dangerous work: 365 days to indefinite
Rhizotomy, clerical/modified work: 21 days
Rhizotomy, manual work: 35 days

345.1 Generalized convulsive epilepsy *(cont'd)*

Description: Seizure caused by abnormal electrical activity of the brain which usually lasts one to two minutes and leaves the person in a disoriented mental state for the next few hours. Grand mal seizures are usually characterized by the tonic phase (15-30 seconds) where the body becomes rigid and collapses, followed by the clonic phase, consisting of violent muscular contractions and abnormal breathing. Following the seizure, the person usually falls asleep for a few minutes and wakes up disoriented.

Other names: Grand mal seizure

Epileptic seizures:
- clonic
- myoclonic
- tonic
- tonic-clonic

Grand mal
Major epilepsy

Excludes:
convulsions:
- *NOS (780.3)*
- *infantile (780.3)*
- *newborn (779.0)*

infantile spasms (345.6)

RTW Claims Data (Calendar-days away from work by decile)

10%	20%	30%	40%	**50%**	60%	70%	80%	**90%**	100%	Mean
13	20	21	22	**34**	35	38	364	**365**	365	114.80

Integrated Disability Durations, in days*

Median (mid-point)	21.0	Mean (average)	84.96
Mode (most frequent)	1	Calculated rec.	32

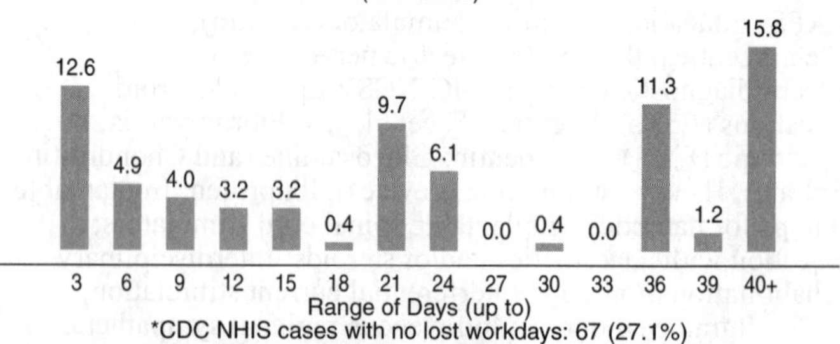

*CDC NHIS cases with no lost workdays: 67 (27.1%)

Impact on Total Absence: Prevalence 0.0452% of total lost workdays; Incidence 0.47 days per 100 workers

345.9 Epilepsy, unspecified

Return-To-Work Summary Guidelines

Dataset	Midrange	At-Risk
Claims data	41 days	365 days
All absences	24 days	365 days

Return-To-Work "Best Practice" Guidelines
Controlled by medication: 0 days
Seizure, clerical/modified work: 1 day
Seizure, dangerous work, with precautions: 28-42 days
Seizure, dangerous work: 365 days to indefinite

Description: Disorder of the brain's electrical activity characterized by the tendency to have recurring seizures that may or may not cause loss of consciousness.

Epileptic convulsions, fits, or seizures NOS

Excludes:
convulsive seizure or fit NOS (780.3)

345.9 Epilepsy, unspecified *(cont'd)*

RTW Claims Data (Calendar-days away from work by decile)										
10%	20%	30%	40%	**50%**	60%	70%	80%	**90%**	100%	Mean
15	21	27	29	**41**	44	364	365	**365**	365	141.83

Integrated Disability Durations, in days*

Median (mid-point) 24.0 Mean (average) 97.69

Mode (most frequent) 1 Calculated rec. 37

Percent of Cases
(3534 cases)

17.3 4.0 7.2 5.5 5.6 0.8 0.2 0.0 0.0 0.0 0.0 0.0 0.0 12.4

9 18 27 36 45 54 63 72 81 90 99 108 117 118+

Range of Days (up to)

*CDC NHIS cases with no lost workdays: 1659 (46.9%)

Impact on Total Absence: Prevalence 0.5414% of total lost workdays; Incidence 5.68 days per 100 workers

346 Migraine

Return-To-Work Summary Guidelines		
Dataset	**Midrange**	**At-Risk**
Claims data	19 days	31 days
All absences	6 days	28 days

Return-To-Work "Best Practice" Guidelines
1-3 days
Intractable (new diagnosis): 7-21 days
Depression/stress comorbidity: 14-28 days

Description: Severe, throbbing, recurring headaches that usually, but not always, affect only one side of the head and last from a few hours to three days. There could be an onset of symptoms such as nausea, restlessness, depression, blurred vision, and irritability 10-30 minutes before the headache begins.

The following fifth-digit subclassification is for use with category 346:
0 without mention of intractable migraine
1 with intractable migraine, so stated

Procedure Summary (from ODG Treatment): Activity restrictions; Acupuncture; Anticonvulsants; Antidepressants; Antiepilectics; Bed rest; Behavioral therapy; Botulinum toxin type A; Branched-chain amino acids (BCAAs); Cell transplantation therapy ; Complementary and alternative medicine (CAM); Corticosteroids (for acute traumatic brain injury); Cognitive therapy; Craniectomy; Craniotomy; CT (computed tomography); Decompressive surgery; EEG (Electroencephalography); Field of vision testing; Fluid resuscitation; Glasgow Coma Scale (GCS); Greater occipital nerve block (GONB); Hyperventilation; Hypothermia; Imaging; Interdisciplinary rehabilitation programs; Lumbar puncture; Mannitol; Melatonin; Methylphenidate; Modified Ashworth Scale (MAS); MRI (magnetic resonance imaging); Nutrition; Occupational therapy (OT); Oxygen therapy; PET (positron emission tomography); Physical therapy (PT); QEEG (Quantified Electroencephalography); Relaxation treatment (for migraines); Return to work; Sedation; Skull x-rays; Sleep aids; SPECT (single photon emission computed tomography); Steroids; Triptans; Vision evaluation; Wilsonii injecta; Work

346 Migraine *(cont'd)*

Disability Duration Adjustment Factors by Age						
Age Group	18-24	25-34	35-44	45-54	55-64	65-74
Adjustment Factor	0.63	0.82	1.10	1.15	1.90	0.89

RTW Claims Data (Calendar-days away from work by decile)										
10%	20%	30%	40%	**50%**	60%	70%	80%	**90%**	100%	Mean
10	13	14	15	**19**	21	24	28	**31**	365	24.17

Integrated Disability Durations, in days*

Median (mid-point) 6.0 Mean (average) 12.42

Mode (most frequent) 1 Calculated rec. 6

Percent of Cases
(33518 cases)

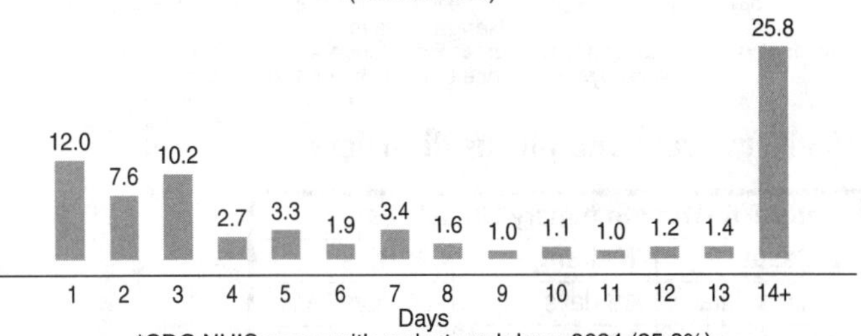

*CDC NHIS cases with no lost workdays: 8634 (25.8%)

Impact on Total Absence: Prevalence 0.9133% of total lost workdays; Incidence 9.59 days per 100 workers

Occupational Disability Durations, in days

Median (mid-point) 50 - Benchmark Indemnity Costs $37,500

Percent of Cases
(310 cases)

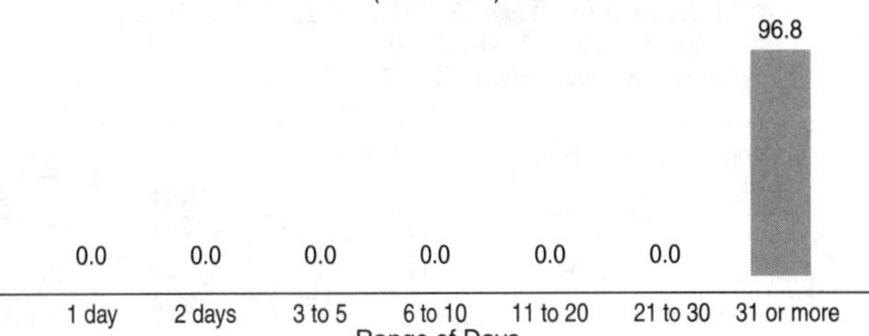

Impact on Occupational Absence: Prevalence 0.1758% of occupational lost workdays; Incidence 0.03 days per 100 workers

DISORDERS OF THE PERIPHERAL NERVOUS SYSTEM (350-359)

Excludes:
diseases of:
acoustic [8th] nerve (388.5)
oculomotor [3rd, 4th, 6th] nerves (378.0-378.9)
optic [2nd] nerve (377.0-377.9)
peripheral autonomic nerves (337.0-337.9)
neuralgia NOS or "rheumatic" (729.2)
neuritis NOS or "rheumatic" (729.2)
radiculitis NOS or "rheumatic" (729.2)
peripheral neuritis in pregnancy (646.4)

RTW Claims Data (Calendar-days away from work by decile)										
10%	20%	30%	40%	**50%**	60%	70%	80%	**90%**	100%	Mean
13	14	16	22	**29**	42	50	82	**145**	365	59.58

Impact on Total Absence: Prevalence 1.0251% of total lost workdays; Incidence 10.76 days per 100 workers

DISORDERS OF THE PERIPHERAL NERVOUS SYSTEM (350-359) *(cont'd)*

Occupational Disability Durations, in days
Median (mid-point) 27 - Benchmark Indemnity Costs $20,250

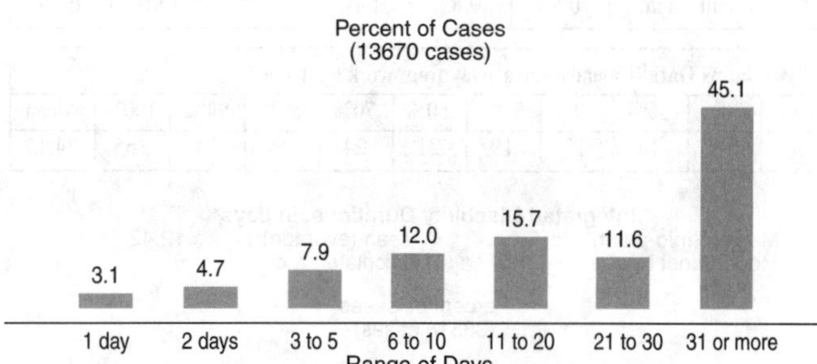

Impact on Occupational Absence: Prevalence 4.1870% of occupational lost workdays; Incidence 0.67 days per 100 workers

353 Nerve root and plexus disorders

Return-To-Work Summary Guidelines		
Dataset	**Midrange**	**At-Risk**
Claims data	16 days	84 days
All absences	13 days	43 days

Return-To-Work "Best Practice" Guidelines
See 353.0

Excludes:
conditions due to:
intervertebral disc disorders (722.0-722.9)
spondylosis (720.0-721.9)
vertebrogenic disorders (723.0-724.9)

Workers' Comp Costs per Claim (based on 410 claims)

Quartile	25%	50%	75%	Mean	% no cost
Indemnity	$6,101	$15,477	$41,013	$26,437	25%
Medical	$4,757	$11,513	$29,621	$21,938	1%
Total	$6,962	$21,305	$62,444	$41,827	1%

353.0 Brachial plexus lesions

Return-To-Work Summary Guidelines		
Dataset	**Midrange**	**At-Risk**
Claims data	42 days	131 days
All absences	32 days	115 days

Return-To-Work "Best Practice" Guidelines
Diagnostic testing: 0-1 days
Medical treatment, clerical/modified work: 7-14 days
Medical treatment, manual work: 42 days
Scalenectomy, clerical/modified work: 14 days
Scalenectomy, manual work: 42 days
Rib resection, clerical/modified work: 21 days
Rib resection, manual work: 84 days

Description: Pain and unusual sensations in the hand, neck, shoulder or arm caused by compression of the surrounding nerves. There could be a tingling or numbness in the arm and hands, sensitivity to cold, or a swelling of the arms, hands, and shoulders, as well as a bluish tint in those areas.

Cervical rib syndrome
Costoclavicular syndrome
Scalenus anticus syndrome
Thoracic outlet syndrome

353.0 Brachial plexus lesions *(cont'd)*

Excludes:
brachial neuritis or radiculitis NOS (723.4)
that in newborn (767.6)

Procedure Summary (from ODG Treatment):
Acromioplasty; Activity restrictions; Acupuncture; Adson's test (AT); Anterior scalene block; Arthrography; Arthroplasty (shoulder); Arthroscopy; Arthroscopic release of adhesions; Bipolar interferential electrotherapy; Biofeedback; Biopsychosocial rehab; Cardiovascular functional testing; Chiropractic; Cold lasers; Continuous-flow cryotherapy; Continuous passive motion (CPM); Corticosteroid injections; Costoclavicular maneuver (CCM); Cutaneous laser treatment; Deep friction massage; Diagnostic arthroscopy; Diathermy; Distension arthrography; Electrical stimulation; Electrodiagnostic testing for TOS (thoracic outlet syndrome); Elevated arm stress test (EAST); Ergonomic interventions; Exercises; Extracorporeal shock wave therapy (ESWT); Hydroplasty/ hydrodilation; Imaging; Immobilization; Impingement test; Injections; Interferential therapy; Laser therapy; Low level laser therapy (LLLT); Magnetic resonance imaging (MRI); Manipulation; Manipulation under anesthesia (MUA); Massage; Mechanical traction; Modified duty; Multidisciplinary biopsychosocial rehab; Nerve blocks; Osteochondral autologous transplantation (OATS); Physical therapy; Porcine small intestinal submucosa (SIS); Pulsed electromagnetic field; Radiography; Return to work; Rotator cuff repair; Rotator cuff porcine graft repair; Shock wave therapy; Shoulder repair; Steroid injections; Supraclavicular pressure (SCP); Surgery for AC joint separation; Surgery for adhesive capsulitis; Surgery for impingement syndrome; Surgery for rotator cuff repair; Surgery for ruptured biceps tendon; Surgery for shoulder dislocation; Surgery for Thoracic Outlet Syndrome; Thermal capsulorrhaphy; Thermotherapy; Transcutaneous electrical neurostimulation (TENS); Transdermal nitroglycerin; Ultrasound, diagnostic; Ultrasound, therapeutic; Work

Physical Therapy Guidelines:
Allow for fading of treatment frequency (from up to 3 visits per week to 1 or less), plus active self-directed home PT
Medical treatment: 14 visits over 6 weeks
Post-surgical treatment: 20 visits over 10 weeks

Workers' Comp Costs per Claim (based on 228 claims)

Quartile	25%	50%	75%	Mean	% no cost
Indemnity	$6,059	$15,367	$46,200	$29,784	23%
Medical	$4,757	$12,773	$31,868	$23,154	0%
Total	$6,836	$23,578	$65,646	$45,988	0%

RTW Claims Data (Calendar-days away from work by decile)

10%	20%	30%	40%	**50%**	60%	70%	80%	**90%**	100%	Mean
14	16	21	32	**42**	51	84	96	**131**	365	62.46

353.0 Brachial plexus lesions *(cont'd)*

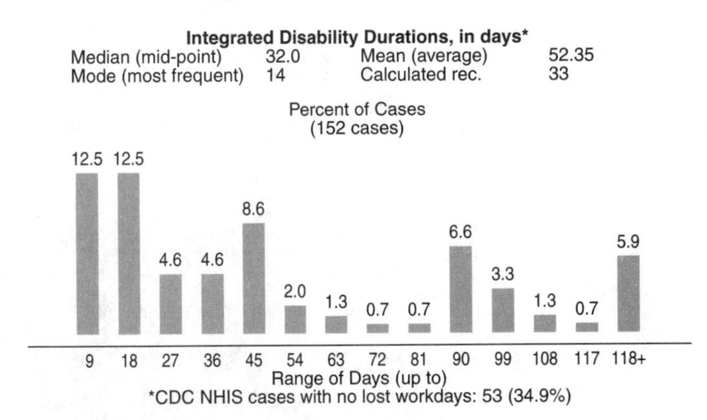

Impact on Total Absence: Prevalence 0.0153% of total lost workdays; Incidence 0.16 days per 100 workers

353.2 Cervical root lesions, not elsewhere classified

Return-To-Work Summary Guidelines		
Dataset	**Midrange**	**At-Risk**
Claims data	16 days	44 days
All absences	15 days	43 days

Return-To-Work "Best Practice" Guidelines
Diagnostic testing: 0 days
Treatment, clerical/modified work: 14 days
Treatment, manual work: 42 days

Description: Compression at the roots of the cervical nerves (the eight pairs of spinal nerves that arise from the neck area and supply the head, neck, back, upper limbs, and scalp). Symptoms include pain that may increase with sharp movement, headache, blurred vision, muscular weakness, decreased reflexes, and sensory abnormalities.

RTW Claims Data (Calendar-days away from work by decile)										
10%	20%	30%	40%	**50%**	60%	70%	80%	**90%**	100%	Mean
13	14	14	15	**16**	40	42	43	**44**	365	28.42

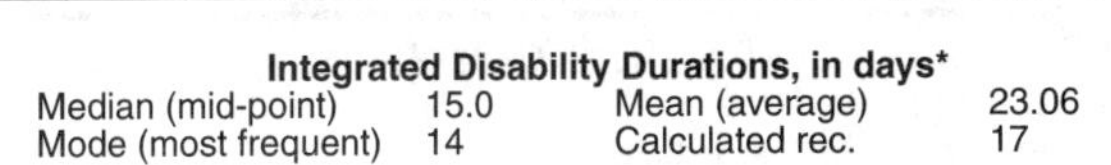

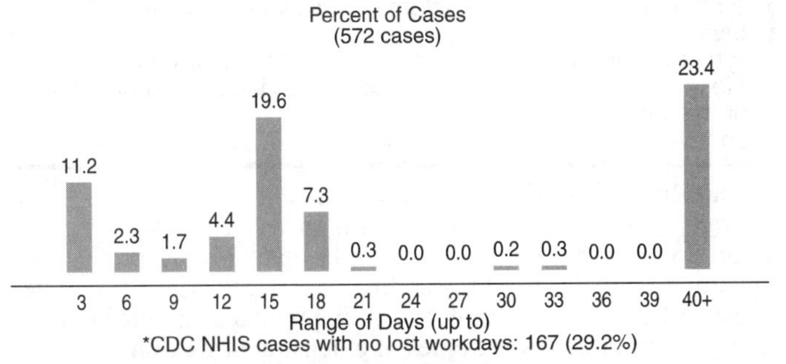

Impact on Total Absence: Prevalence 0.0276% of total lost workdays; Incidence 0.29 days per 100 workers

354 Mononeuritis of upper limb and mononeuritis multiplex

Return-To-Work Summary Guidelines		
Dataset	**Midrange**	**At-Risk**
Claims data	15 days	84 days
All absences	13 days	32 days

354 Mononeuritis of upper limb and mononeuritis multiplex *(cont'd)*

Return-To-Work "Best Practice" Guidelines
See 354.0

Workers' Comp Costs per Claim (based on 12,861 claims)					
Quartile	25%	50%	75%	Mean	% no cost
Indemnity	$3,287	$6,395	$13,619	$12,096	30%
Medical	$2,384	$4,820	$9,251	$8,019	1%
Total	$4,053	$9,083	$18,480	$16,517	1%

354.0 Carpal tunnel syndrome

Return-To-Work Summary Guidelines		
Dataset	**Midrange**	**At-Risk**
Claims data	41 days	134 days
All absences	24 days	91 days

Return-To-Work "Best Practice" Guidelines
Conservative treatment, modified work (limit repetitive use of hand/wrist): 0 days
Conservative treatment, regular work (if not aggravating to disability/use of splint): 0-5 days
Conservative treatment, regular work (if work related & electrodiagnostically confirmed): 28 days
Conservative treatment, regular work (with severe nerve impairment): indefinite
Endoscopic/mini-palm surgery, modified work: 3-5 days
Endoscopic/mini-palm surgery, regular work, non-dominant arm: 28 days
Endoscopic/mini-palm surgery, regular/repetitive/heavy manual work, dominant arm: 42 days to indefinite
Open surgery (median nerve neurolysis), modified work: 10-14 days
Open surgery, regular work, non-dominant arm: 42 days
Open surgery, regular/repetitive/heavy manual work, dominant arm: 56 days to indefinite
Open surgery, regular/repetitive/heavy manual work, bilateral: 84 days to indefinite
Pregnancy comorbidity, modified work until 28 days after delivery

Capabilities & Activity Modifications:
Modified work: Repetitive motion activities (w or w/o splint) not more than 4 times/hr; repetitive keying up to 15 keystrokes/min not more than 2 hrs/day; gripping and using light tools (pens, scissors, etc.) with 5-minute break at least every 20 min; no pinching; driving car up to 2 hrs/day; light work up to 5 lbs 3 times/hr; avoidance of prolonged periods in wrist flexion or extension.
Regular work (if not cause or aggravating to disability) : Repetitive motion activities not more than 25 times/hr; repetitive keying up to 45 keystrokes/min 8 hrs/day; gripping and using moderate tools (pliers, screwdrivers, etc.) fulltime; pinching up to 5 times/min; driving car or light truck up to 6 hrs/day or heavy truck up to 3 hrs/day; moderate to heavy work up to 35 lbs not more than 7 times/hr.

Description: Compression of the nerve that travels through the wrist to the thumb side of the hand causing pain, tingling, or numbness along the wrist, palm, and fingers. Pain may also be felt in the arm or shoulder, and is often worse while sleeping.
Median nerve entrapment
Partial thenar atrophy

Procedure Summary (from ODG Treatment): Activity restrictions; Acupuncture; Aerobic exercise; Arnica; Biofeedback; Brace; Breaks (microbreaks); Carpal tunnel release surgery (CTR); Chiropractic; Closed fist sign; Cold packs; Comorbidities; Corticosteroid injections;

354.0 Carpal tunnel syndrome *(cont'd)*

Corticosteroids, oral; Depression (comorbidity); Diabetes (comorbidity); Differential diagnosis; Diuretics; Durkan's compression test; Electrodiagnostic studies; Electromyography (EMG); Endoscopic surgery; Ergonomic interventions; Exercises; Flick sign (shaking hand); Gel-padded glove ; Heat therapy; Hypalgesia (in the median nerve territory); Hypnosis; Hypothyroidism (comorbidity); Imaging; Injections; Insulin; Iontophoresis; Katz hand diagram scores; Laser acupuncture; Low-level laser therapy (LLLT); Magnet therapy; Manipulation; Mobilization; Modified duty; Mouse use; MRI's (magnetic resonance imaging); Nerve conduction studies (NCS); Nerve gliding exercises; Night pain symptoms; Nocturnal paresthesias; Nonprescription medications; NSAIDs; Obesity (comorbidity); Occupational therapy (OT); Paresthesia; Phalen's test; Phonophoresis; Physical therapy (PT); Polarized polychromatic light (Bioptron light); Portable nerve conduction devices; Pregnancy (comorbidity); Psychosocial management; Pyridoxine; Return to work; Semmes-Weinstein monofilament test; Splinting; Square wrist sign; Static 2-point discrimination (>6mm); Surgery; Tendon gliding exercises; TENS (transcutaneous electrical neurostimulation); Tests (CTS diagnosis); Thenar atrophy; Therapeutic touch; Tinel's sign; Tourniquet test; Traumatic CTS; Ultrasound, therapeutic; Ultrasound, diagnostic; Vitamin B6 (pyridoxine); Weak thumb abduction strength; Work ; Wrist pain; Yoga

Physical Therapy Guidelines:
Allow for fading of treatment frequency (from up to 3 visits per week to 1 or less), plus active self-directed home PT
Medical treatment: 1-3 visits over 3-5 weeks
Post-surgical treatment (endoscopic): 3-8 visits over 3-5 weeks
Post-surgical treatment (open): 3-8 visits over 3-5 weeks

Chiropractic Guidelines:
Allow for fading of treatment frequency (from up to 3 visits per week to 1 or less), plus active self-directed home therapy
3-6 visits over 3 weeks
Note: this is not a recommended treatment for this condition

Workers' Comp Costs per Claim (based on 10,642 claims)

Quartile	25%	50%	75%	Mean	% no cost
Indemnity	$3,087	$5,849	$11,382	$10,009	31%
Medical	$2,300	$4,547	$8,127	$6,713	2%
Total	$3,938	$8,411	$15,981	$13,682	1%

Disability Duration Adjustment Factors by Age

Age Group	18-24	25-34	35-44	45-54	55-64	65-74
Adjustment Factor	0.34	0.75	1.08	1.15	1.10	NA

RTW Claims Data (Calendar-days away from work by decile)

10%	20%	30%	40%	**50%**	60%	70%	80%	**90%**	100%	Mean
12	15	22	29	**41**	45	57	83	**134**	365	66.78

RTW Post Surgery (Calendar-days away from work by decile)

	10%	20%	30%	40%	**50%**	60%	70%	80%	**90%**	100%	Mean
Remove wrist/forearm lesion	18	33	47	55	**62**	69	90	118	**218**	365	85.60
Wrist endoscopy/surgery	16	26	32	40	**46**	57	68	83	**130**	365	65.88
Carpal tunnel surgery	18	30	39	46	**54**	65	81	107	**185**	365	81.96

354.0 Carpal tunnel syndrome *(cont'd)*

Integrated Disability Durations, in days*
Median (mid-point) 24.0 Mean (average) 49.12
Mode (most frequent) 1 Calculated rec. 25

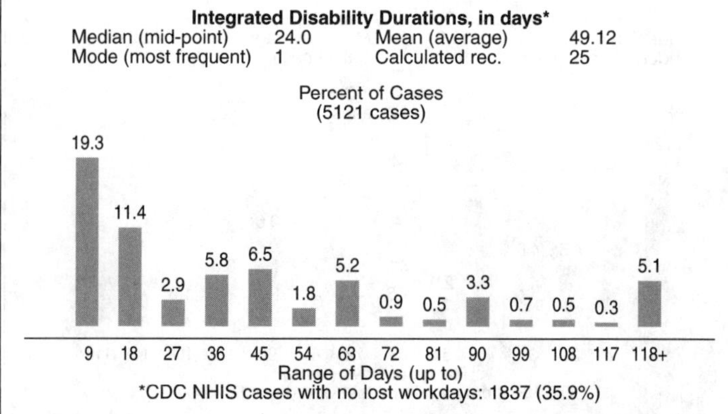

*CDC NHIS cases with no lost workdays: 1837 (35.9%)

Impact on Total Absence: Prevalence 0.4767% of total lost workdays; Incidence 5.01 days per 100 workers

Occupational Disability Durations, in days
Median (mid-point) 27 - Benchmark Indemnity Costs $20,250

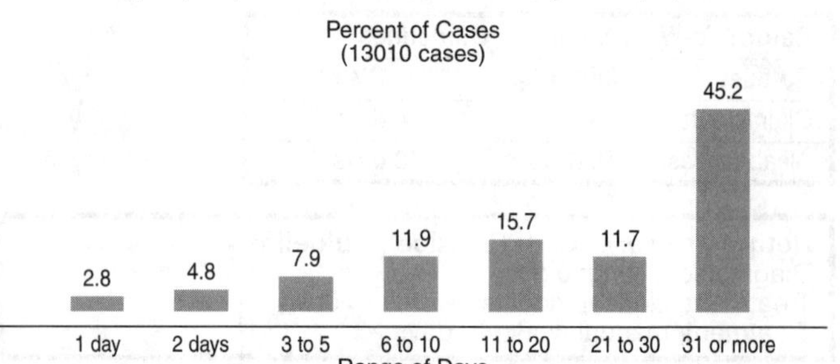

Impact on Occupational Absence: Prevalence 3.9849% of occupational lost workdays; Incidence 0.64 days per 100 workers

354.4 Causalgia of upper limb

Return-To-Work Summary Guidelines

Dataset	Midrange	At-Risk
Claims data	15 days	84 days
All absences	13 days	32 days

Return-To-Work "Best Practice" Guidelines
Medical treatment: 0 days
Sympathetic nerve block: 2 day
Sympathectomy/ganglionectomy, clerical/modified work: 21 days
Sympathectomy/ganglionectomy, manual work: 28 days
(Note: sympathectomy is not a recommended treatment option for this diagnosis)
Complex regional pain syndrome (CRPS-II): 28-84 days

Capabilities & Activity Modifications:
Clerical/modified work: Lifting with knees (with a straight back, no stooping) not more than 5 lbs up to 3 times/hr; squatting up to 4 times/hr; standing or walking with a 5-minute break at least every 20 minutes; sitting with a 5-minute break every 30 minutes; no extremes of extension or flexion; no extremes of twisting; no climbing ladders; driving car only up to 2 hrs/day.
Manual work: Lifting with knees (with a straight back) not more than 25 lbs up to 15 times/hr; squatting up to 16 times/hr; standing or walking with a 10-minute break at least every 1-2 hours; sitting with a 10-minute break every 1-2 hours; extremes of flexion or extension allowed up to 12 times/hr; extremes of twisting allowed up to 16 times/hr; climbing ladders allowed up to 25 rungs 6 times/hr; driving car or light truck up to a full work day; driving heavy truck up to 4 hrs/day.

354.4 Causalgia of upper limb *(cont'd)*

Description: Chronic pain occurring after a major injury to the nerves in an upper limb, most commonly seen when a nerve has been completely or partially severed. Pain is constant, burning, and easily aggravated, and there could be tingling or numbness.
Other names: Causalgia, Complex regional pain syndrome (CRPS II)

Excludes:
causalgia:
NOS (355.9)
lower limb (355.71)

Procedure Summary (from ODG Treatment): Actiq®; Acupuncture; Antidepressants (therapy); Antidepressants - SSRI's versus tricyclics (class); Anti-inflammatory medications; Autonomic test battery; Barbituate-containing analgesic agents (BCAs); Behavioral interventions; Biofeedback; Botulinum toxin (Botox); Capsaicin; Celebrex®; Cod liver oil; Cold lasers; CRPS (complex regional pain syndrome); Cyclobenzaprine; Cymbalta; Diagnostic criteria for CRPS; Education; Electrical stimulators (E-stim); Electroceutical therapy (bioelectric nerve block); Electrodiagnostic testing (EMG/NCS); Epidural steroid injections (ESI's); Exercise; Facet blocks; Fibromyalgia syndrome (FMS); Gabapentin; Glucosamine (and Chondroitin Sulfate); H-wave stimulation (devices); Ibuprofen; Implantable pumps for narcotics; Implantable spinal cord stimulators; Injection with anaesthetics and/or steroids; Interdisciplinary rehabilitation programs; Interferential current stimulation (ICS); Intrathecal pumps; Intravenous regional sympathetic blocks (for RSD, nerve blocks); Ketamine; Low level laser therapy (LLLT); Lumbar sympathetic block; Magnet therapy; Manual therapy & manipulation; Massage therapy; Medications; Microcurrent electrical stimulation (MENS devices); Morphine pumps; Multi-disciplinary treatment; Muscle relaxants; Myofascial pain; Naproxen; Neuroreflexotherapy; Neuromodulation devices; Neuromuscular electrical stimulation (NMES devices); Neurontin®; Nonprescription medications; NSAIDs (non steroidal anti-inflammatory drugs); Nucleoplasty; Occupational therapy (OT); Oral morphine; Opioids; Oxycontin®; Pain management programs; Percutaneous electrical nerve stimulation (PENS); Percutaneous neuromodulation therapy (PNT); Phentolamine infusion test; Physical therapy (PT); Prolotherapy; Psychological evaluations; Return to work; RSD (reflex sympathetic dystrophy); Salicylate topicals; Sclerotherapy (prolotherapy); Spinal cord stimulators (SCS); Stellate ganglion block; Stress infrared telethermography; Sympathectomy; Sympathetic therapy; Thermography (infrared stress thermography); Transcutaneous electrical nerve stimulation (TENS); Treatment for CRPS; Trigger point injections; Vicodin®; Vioxx®; Yoga

Impact on Total Absence: Prevalence 0.0003% of total lost workdays

Occupational Disability Durations, in days
Median (mid-point) 27 - Benchmark Indemnity Costs $20,250

Percent of Cases (310 cases)

Range of Days	1 day	2 days	3 to 5	6 to 10	11 to 20	21 to 30	31 or more
Percent	9.7	0.0	6.5	12.9	6.5	16.1	48.4

Impact on Occupational Absence: Prevalence 0.0949% of occupational lost workdays; Incidence 0.02 days per 100 workers

355 Mononeuritis of lower limb

Return-To-Work Summary Guidelines		
Dataset	**Midrange**	**At-Risk**
Claims data	29 days	214 days
All absences	24 days	212 days

Return-To-Work "Best Practice" Guidelines
See 355.9

Workers' Comp Costs per Claim (based on 557 claims)					
Quartile	25%	50%	75%	Mean	% no cost
Indemnity	$4,536	$12,532	$34,104	$23,851	19%
Medical	$3,749	$11,603	$26,891	$23,171	0%
Total	$6,962	$21,672	$55,545	$42,545	0%

355.0 Lesion of sciatic nerve

Return-To-Work Summary Guidelines		
Dataset	**Midrange**	**At-Risk**
Claims data	25 days	51 days
All absences	22 days	51 days

Return-To-Work "Best Practice" Guidelines
Clerical/modified work: 5 days
Manual work: 21 days
Heavy manual work: 49 days

Description: Damage to the sciatic nerve, which runs along the buttocks, thigh, calf, and foot, resulting in pain in those areas.

Excludes:
sciatica NOS (724.3)

Workers' Comp Costs per Claim (based on 32 claims)					
Quartile	25%	50%	75%	Mean	% no cost
Medical	$1,155	$11,687	$24,896	$17,357	0%
Total	$2,174	$16,674	$39,701	$33,773	0%

RTW Claims Data (Calendar-days away from work by decile)										
10%	20%	30%	40%	**50%**	60%	70%	80%	**90%**	100%	Mean
14	20	21	22	**25**	48	49	50	**51**	365	39.23

Integrated Disability Durations, in days*
Median (mid-point) 22.0 Mean (average) 32.34
Mode (most frequent) 21 Calculated rec. 24

Percent of Cases (398 cases)

Range of Days (up to)	9	18	27	36	45	54	63	72	81	90	99	108	117	118+
Percent	18.3	6.3	24.9	2.5	0.5	23.9	0.5	0.3	0.0	0.5	0.0	0.0	0.3	1.5

*CDC NHIS cases with no lost workdays: 82 (20.6%)

Impact on Total Absence: Prevalence 0.0302% of total lost workdays; Incidence 0.32 days per 100 workers

355.9 Mononeuritis of unspecified site

Return-To-Work Summary Guidelines		
Dataset	**Midrange**	**At-Risk**
Claims data	29 days	214 days
All absences	24 days	212 days

Return-To-Work "Best Practice" Guidelines
Note: this is a controversial diagnosis
Sympathetic nerve block: 3-7 days
Sympathectomy/ganglionectomy, clerical/modified work: 21 days
Sympathectomy/ganglionectomy, manual work: 28 days
(Note: sympathectomy is not a recommended treatment option for this diagnosis)
Complex regional pain syndrome (CRPS-II), early stage: 28-84 days
Complex regional pain syndrome (CRPS-II), late stage: 210 days to indefinite

Capabilities & Activity Modifications:
Clerical/modified work: Lifting with knees (with a straight back, no stooping) not more than 5 lbs up to 3 times/hr; squatting up to 4 times/hr; standing or walking with a 5-minute break at least every 20 minutes; sitting with a 5-minute break every 30 minutes; no extremes of extension or flexion; no extremes of twisting; no climbing ladders; driving car only up to 2 hrs/day.
Manual work: Lifting with knees (with a straight back) not more than 25 lbs up to 15 times/hr; squatting up to 16 times/hr; standing or walking with a 10-minute break at least every 1-2 hours; sitting with a 10-minute break every 1-2 hours; extremes of flexion or extension allowed up to 12 times/hr; extremes of twisting allowed up to 16 times/hr; climbing ladders allowed up to 25 rungs 6 times/hr; driving car or light truck up to a full work day; driving heavy truck up to 4 hrs/day.
Description: Chronic pain experienced after major nerve surgery.

Causalgia NOS

Excludes:
causalgia:
lower limb (355.71)
upper limb (354.4)

Procedure Summary (from ODG Treatment): Actiq®; Acupuncture; Antidepressants (therapy); Antidepressants - SSRI's versus tricyclics (class); Anti-inflammatory medications; Autonomic test battery; Barbituate-containing analgesic agents (BCAs); Behavioral interventions; Biofeedback; Botulinum toxin (Botox); Capsaicin; Celebrex®; Cod liver oil; Cold lasers; CRPS (complex regional pain syndrome); Cyclobenzaprine; Cymbalta; Diagnostic criteria for CRPS; Education; Electrical stimulators (E-stim); Electroceutical therapy (bioelectric nerve block); Electrodiagnostic testing (EMG/NCS); Epidural steroid injections (ESI's); Exercise; Facet blocks; Fibromyalgia syndrome (FMS); Gabapentin; Glucosamine (and Chondroitin Sulfate); H-wave stimulation (devices); Ibuprofen; Implantable pumps for narcotics; Implantable spinal cord stimulators; Injection with anaesthetics and/or steroids; Interdisciplinary rehabilitation programs; Interferential current stimulation (ICS); Intrathecal pumps; Intravenous regional sympathetic blocks (for RSD, nerve blocks); Ketamine; Low level laser therapy (LLLT); Lumbar sympathetic block; Magnet therapy; Manual therapy & manipulation; Massage therapy; Medications; Microcurrent electrical stimulation (MENS devices); Morphine pumps; Multi-disciplinary treatment; Muscle relaxants; Myofascial pain; Naproxen; Neuroreflexotherapy; Neuromodulation devices; Neuromuscular electrical stimulation (NMES devices);

355.9 Mononeuritis of unspecified site *(cont'd)*

Neurontin®; Nonprescription medications; NSAIDs (non steroidal anti-inflammatory drugs); Nucleoplasty; Occupational therapy (OT); Oral morphine; Opioids; Oxycontin®; Pain management programs; Percutaneous electrical nerve stimulation (PENS); Percutaneous neuromodulation therapy (PNT); Phentolamine infusion test; Physical therapy (PT); Prolotherapy; Psychological evaluations; Return to work; RSD (reflex sympathetic dystrophy); Salicylate topicals; Sclerotherapy (prolotherapy); Spinal cord stimulators (SCS); Stellate ganglion block; Stress infrared telethermography; Sympathectomy; Sympathetic therapy; Thermography (infrared stress thermography); Transcutaneous electrical nerve stimulation (TENS); Treatment for CRPS; Trigger point injections; Vicodin®; Vioxx®; Yoga

Workers' Comp Costs per Claim (based on 59 claims)					
Quartile	25%	50%	75%	Mean	% no cost
Indemnity	$5,408	$13,671	$41,517	$26,154	32%
Medical	$903	$5,954	$23,972	$16,823	0%
Total	$1,218	$14,333	$50,820	$34,541	0%

RTW Claims Data (Calendar-days away from work by decile)										
10%	20%	30%	40%	**50%**	60%	70%	80%	**90%**	100%	Mean
14	19	22	27	**29**	32	86	210	**214**	365	93.12

Integrated Disability Durations, in days*
Median (mid-point) 24.0 Mean (average) 74.50
Mode (most frequent) 3 Calculated rec. 31

Percent of Cases
(1356 cases)

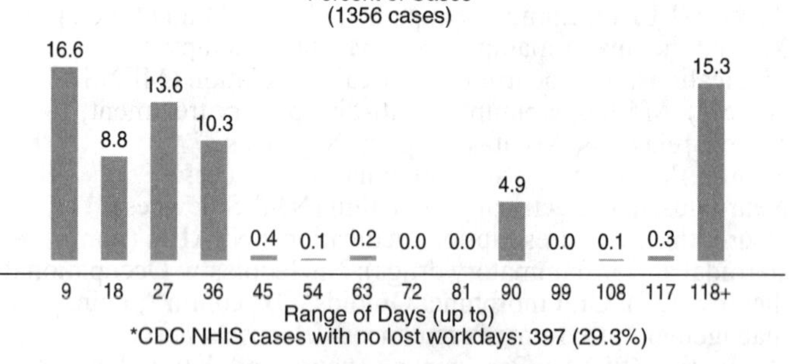

*CDC NHIS cases with no lost workdays: 397 (29.3%)

Impact on Total Absence: Prevalence 0.2111% of total lost workdays; Incidence 2.22 days per 100 workers

DISORDERS OF THE EYE AND ADNEXA (360-379)

RTW Claims Data (Calendar-days away from work by decile)										
10%	20%	30%	40%	**50%**	60%	70%	80%	**90%**	100%	Mean
10	13	14	14	**15**	18	27	29	**47**	365	27.33

Impact on Total Absence: Prevalence 0.5874% of total lost workdays; Incidence 6.17 days per 100 workers

Occupational Disability Durations, in days
Median (mid-point) 2 - Benchmark Indemnity Costs $1,500

Percent of Cases
(4490 cases)

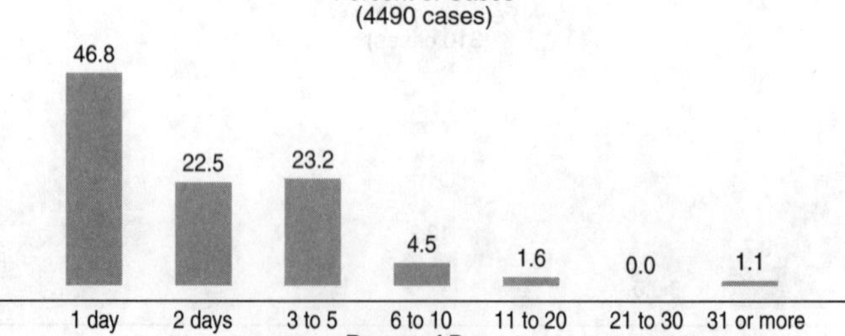

Impact on Occupational Absence: Prevalence 0.1018% of occupational lost workdays; Incidence 0.02 days per 100 workers

365 Glaucoma

Return-To-Work Summary Guidelines		
Dataset	**Midrange**	**At-Risk**
Claims data	15 days	64 days
All absences	13 days	41 days

Description: Increased pressure in the eye (usually affecting both eyes) caused by an obstruction in the channel in which fluid flows out of the eye, causing optic nerve damage and progressive vision loss. Except for slow, gradual loss of vision, leading to tunnel vision or blindness, symptoms are usually undetectable and regular eye examinations are recommended in order for the pressure inside the eye to be measured.

Excludes:
blind hypertensive eye [absolute glaucoma] (360.42)
congenital glaucoma (743.20-743.22)

RTW Claims Data (Calendar-days away from work by decile)

10%	20%	30%	40%	**50%**	60%	70%	80%	**90%**	100%	Mean
12	13	14	14	**15**	16	18	36	**64**	365	34.50

Integrated Disability Durations, in days*
Median (mid-point) 13.0 Mean (average) 22.99
Mode (most frequent) 14 Calculated rec. 16

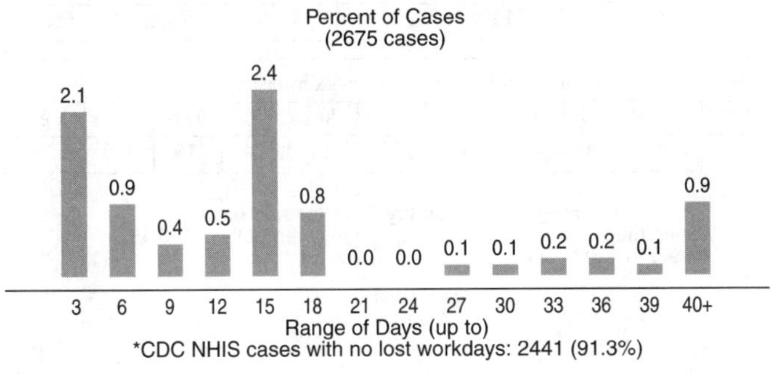

*CDC NHIS cases with no lost workdays: 2441 (91.3%)

Impact on Total Absence: Prevalence 0.0158% of total lost workdays; Incidence 0.17 days per 100 workers

365.1 Open-angle glaucoma

Return-To-Work Summary Guidelines		
Dataset	**Midrange**	**At-Risk**
Claims data	15 days	30 days
All absences	14 days	29 days

Return-To-Work "Best Practice" Guidelines
Medical treatment: 0 days
Trabeculoplasty by laser: 1 day
Trabeculectomy, clerical/modified work: 7 days
Trabeculectomy, manual work: 14-28 days

Description: Increased pressure in the eye which initially causes a gradual loss of peripheral vision and, if untreated, eventual loss of central vision and ultimate blindness. See 365 for more information.

RTW Claims Data (Calendar-days away from work by decile)

10%	20%	30%	40%	**50%**	60%	70%	80%	**90%**	100%	Mean
12	13	14	14	**15**	16	17	27	**30**	365	21.51

365.1 Open-angle glaucoma *(cont'd)*

Integrated Disability Durations, in days*
Median (mid-point) 14.0 Mean (average) 16.63
Mode (most frequent) 14 Calculated rec. 15

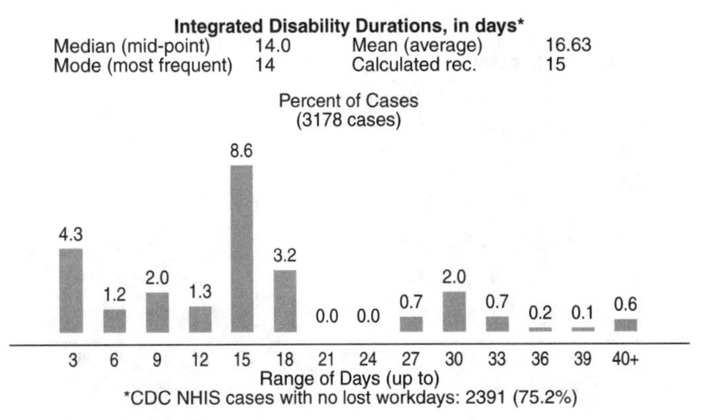

*CDC NHIS cases with no lost workdays: 2391 (75.2%)

Impact on Total Absence: Prevalence 0.0386% of total lost workdays; Incidence 0.41 days per 100 workers

366 Cataract

Return-To-Work Summary Guidelines		
Dataset	**Midrange**	**At-Risk**
Claims data	16 days	30 days
All absences	14 days	30 days

Return-To-Work "Best Practice" Guidelines
Without treatment: 0 days
Laser discission of cataract: 2 days
Extracapsular cataract extraction w/IOL, clerical/modified work: 14 days
Extracapsular cataract extraction w/IOL, manual work: 28 days

Description: Cloudiness in the eye's lens that may either cover the entire lens or form as scattered cloudy areas causing painless, progressive vision loss. Although cataracts can stop developing within the early stages, causing only minor vision loss, those that don't stop growing could eventually lead to blindness unless they are surgically removed. Decreased or cloudy vision is the most detectable symptom.

Excludes:
congenital cataract (743.30-743.34)

Workers' Comp Costs per Claim (based on 105 claims)

Quartile	25%	50%	75%	Mean	% no cost
Indemnity	$5,975	$47,933	$82,436	$53,057	27%
Medical	$5,376	$9,807	$19,383	$24,271	0%
Total	$8,894	$27,573	$92,232	$62,857	0%

RTW Claims Data (Calendar-days away from work by decile)

10%	20%	30%	40%	**50%**	60%	70%	80%	**90%**	100%	Mean
12	14	14	15	**16**	24	28	29	**30**	365	22.93

366 Cataract *(cont'd)*

Integrated Disability Durations, in days*

Median (mid-point) 14.0 Mean (average) 16.76
Mode (most frequent) 2 Calculated rec. 12

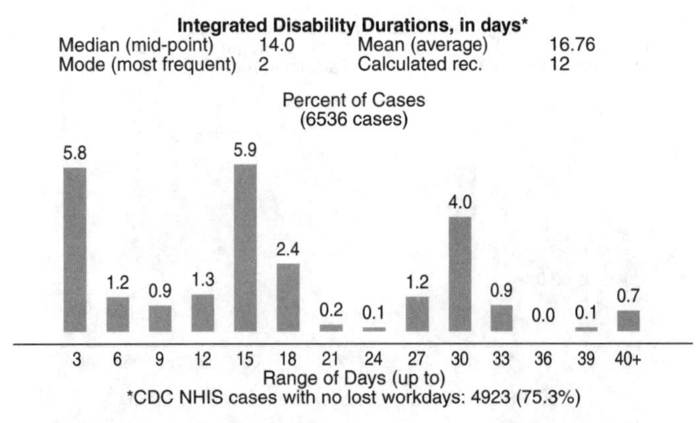

*CDC NHIS cases with no lost workdays: 4923 (75.3%)

Impact on Total Absence: Prevalence 0.0798% of total lost workdays; Incidence 0.84 days per 100 workers

372 Disorders of conjunctiva

Return-To-Work Summary Guidelines		
Dataset	**Midrange**	**At-Risk**
Claims data	11 days	15 days
All absences	2 days	7 days

Return-To-Work "Best Practice" Guidelines
See 372.0

Excludes:
keratoconjunctivitis (370.3-370.4)

Workers' Comp Costs per Claim (based on 17,138 claims)					
Quartile	25%	50%	75%	Mean	% no cost
Indemnity	$242	$536	$1,113	$948	99%
Medical	$126	$221	$336	$261	6%
Total	$126	$221	$336	$276	6%

Occupational Disability Durations, in days

Median (mid-point) 1 - Benchmark Indemnity Costs $750

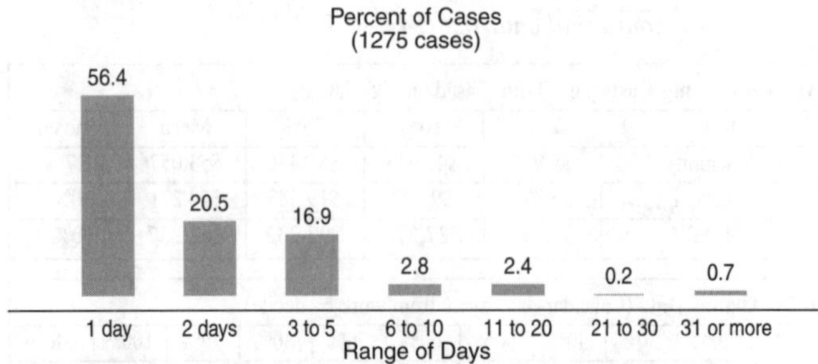

Impact on Occupational Absence: Prevalence 0.0144% of occupational lost workdays

372.0 Acute conjunctivitis

Return-To-Work Summary Guidelines		
Dataset	**Midrange**	**At-Risk**
Claims data	11 days	15 days
All absences	2 days	7 days

Return-To-Work "Best Practice" Guidelines
Modified work: 0 days
Regular work: 1-2 days

Capabilities & Activity Modifications:

372.0 Acute conjunctivitis *(cont'd)*

Modified work: In injuries occurring to one eye no binocular vision requirements, e.g., as required in the operation of high speed or mobile equipment (bilateral eye injuries such as welding flash burns, chemical burns, and allergic reactions, need to be off any work until the vision in one eye has returned to a functional level); limited stereopsis/fields of vision requirements; no exposure to significant vibration (e.g., affecting intra-ocular foreign bodies or retinal detachment); limit exposure to allergic substances (e.g., allergic conjuctivitis requiring removal of the substance from the workplace) and provision for hygiene to prevent spread of infection by direct contact or shared articles; wearing protective eyewear to prevent recurrent injury; possible workstation adjustment.

Description: Inflammation of the eyeball and inner eyelids caused by bacteria, viruses, or allergies, which usually doesn't cause vision problems, but could cause redness, unusual discharge, a swollen or itchy eye, or a burning in the eye, spreading from one eye to both eyes within a few days.

Other names: Pink eye

Workers' Comp Costs per Claim (based on 9,757 claims)					
Quartile	25%	50%	75%	Mean	% no cost
Indemnity	$242	$494	$882	$737	98%
Medical	$137	$231	$357	$274	6%
Total	$137	$231	$368	$286	6%

RTW Claims Data (Calendar-days away from work by decile)										
10%	20%	30%	40%	**50%**	60%	70%	80%	**90%**	100%	Mean
8	9	10	10	**11**	12	13	14	**15**	133	12.69

Integrated Disability Durations, in days*

Median (mid-point) 2.0 Mean (average) 3.19
Mode (most frequent) 1 Calculated rec. 2

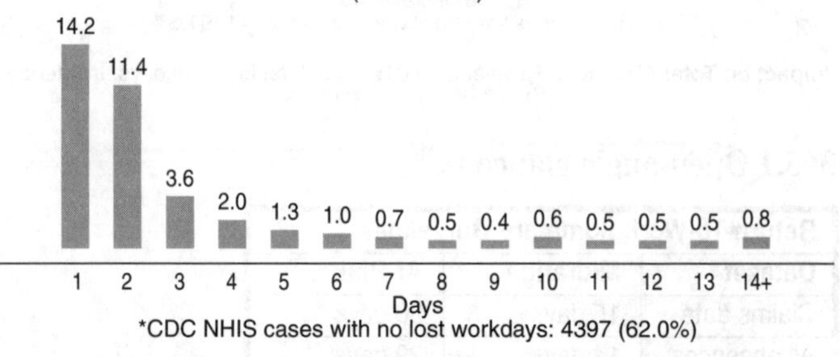

*CDC NHIS cases with no lost workdays: 4397 (62.0%)

Impact on Total Absence: Prevalence 0.0254% of total lost workdays; Incidence 0.27 days per 100 workers

Occupational Disability Durations, in days

Median (mid-point) 2 - Benchmark Indemnity Costs $1,500

Percent of Cases
(1540 cases)

1 day	2 days	3 to 5	6 to 10	11 to 20	21 to 30	31 or more
43.5	22.7	21.4	8.4	1.3	0.0	1.9

Range of Days

Impact on Occupational Absence: Prevalence 0.0349% of occupational lost workdays; Incidence 0.01 days per 100 workers

DISEASES OF THE EAR AND MASTOID PROCESS (380-389)

RTW Claims Data (Calendar-days away from work by decile)										
10%	20%	30%	40%	**50%**	60%	70%	80%	**90%**	100%	Mean
9	10	11	13	**16**	21	24	29	**35**	365	20.31

Impact on Total Absence: Prevalence 0.6338% of total lost workdays; Incidence 6.66 days per 100 workers

Occupational Disability Durations, in days
Median (mid-point) 5 - Benchmark Indemnity Costs $3,750 (180 cases)
Impact on Occupational Absence: Prevalence 0.0102% of occupational lost workdays

382 Suppurative and unspecified otitis media

Return-To-Work Summary Guidelines		
Dataset	**Midrange**	**At-Risk**
Claims data	13 days	17 days
All absences	2 days	5 days

Return-To-Work "Best Practice" Guidelines
Medical treatment: 0-1 days
Tympanostomy/myringotomy, unilateral: 1 day
Tympanostomy/myringotomy, bilateral: 2 days

Description: Inflammation of the middle ear, including the eardrum, small bones of the ear, and the tube that connects the ear to the throat, from a bacterial or viral infection, often as a complication of the common cold. Symptoms include severe earache, temporary hearing loss, and sometimes fever, chills, a full feeling in the ear, nausea, and diarrhea.
Other names: Middle ear infection

Workers' Comp Costs per Claim (based on 67 claims)					
Quartile	25%	50%	75%	Mean	% no cost
Medical	$137	$168	$305	$329	9%
Total	$137	$168	$305	$521	9%

RTW Claims Data (Calendar-days away from work by decile)										
10%	20%	30%	40%	**50%**	60%	70%	80%	**90%**	100%	Mean
9	10	10	12	**13**	14	15	16	**17**	365	16.48

Integrated Disability Durations, in days*
Median (mid-point) 2.0 Mean (average) 2.99
Mode (most frequent) 2 Calculated rec. 2

Percent of Cases (3328 cases)

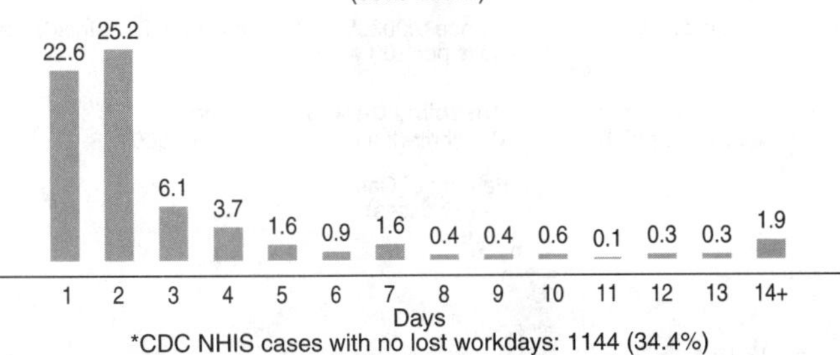

*CDC NHIS cases with no lost workdays: 1144 (34.4%)

Impact on Total Absence: Prevalence 0.0193% of total lost workdays; Incidence 0.20 days per 100 workers

386 Vertiginous syndromes and other disorders of vestibular system

Return-To-Work Summary Guidelines		
Dataset	**Midrange**	**At-Risk**
Claims data	21 days	36 days
All absences	6 days	34 days

Return-To-Work "Best Practice" Guidelines
See 386.0

Excludes:
vertigo NOS (780.4)

Workers' Comp Costs per Claim (based on 95 claims)					
Quartile	25%	50%	75%	Mean	% no cost
Indemnity	$4,053	$16,191	$39,375	$30,183	24%
Medical	$2,699	$7,854	$22,575	$16,426	0%
Total	$4,473	$16,711	$62,181	$39,366	0%

RTW Claims Data (Calendar-days away from work by decile)										
10%	20%	30%	40%	**50%**	60%	70%	80%	**90%**	100%	Mean
10	12	14	20	**21**	23	26	34	**36**	365	22.92

Integrated Disability Durations, in days*
Median (mid-point) 6.0 Mean (average) 11.98
Mode (most frequent) 1 Calculated rec. 6

Percent of Cases (6536 cases)

14.8 9.8 4.9 2.8 1.9 0.8 1.4 0.8 1.3 2.3 1.6 1.3 0.8 23.9
1 2 3 4 5 6 7 8 9 10 11 12 13 14+
Days

*CDC NHIS cases with no lost workdays: 2065 (31.6%)

Impact on Total Absence: Prevalence 0.1583% of total lost workdays; Incidence 1.66 days per 100 workers

386.0 Meniere's disease

Return-To-Work Summary Guidelines		
Dataset	**Midrange**	**At-Risk**
Claims data	21 days	35 days
All absences	12 days	34 days

Return-To-Work "Best Practice" Guidelines
Medical treatment, depending on job safety issues: 1-10 days
Labyrinthectomy: 21-35 days

Description: Chronic disorder of the inner ear characterized by recurring attacks of vertigo (spinning or moving sensations which often cause vomiting and loss of balance), hearing loss, ringing in the ears, and sometimes pressure in the ear.

Endolymphatic hydrops
Lermoyez's syndrome
Meniere's syndrome or vertigo

RTW Claims Data (Calendar-days away from work by decile)										
10%	20%	30%	40%	**50%**	60%	70%	80%	**90%**	100%	Mean
10	12	15	20	**21**	22	24	29	**35**	152	23.26

386.0 Meniere's disease *(cont'd)*

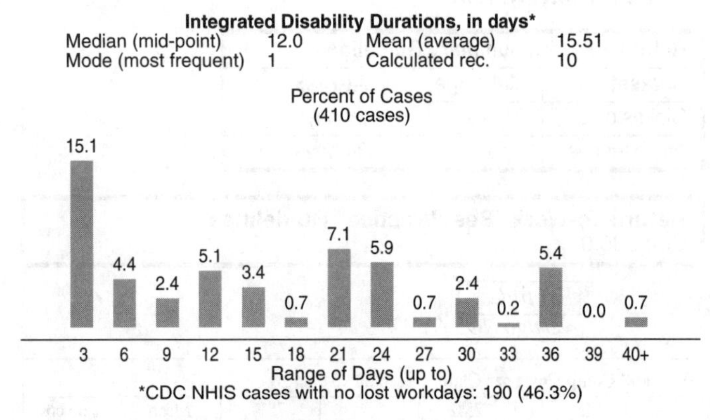

Impact on Total Absence: Prevalence 0.0100% of total lost workdays; Incidence 0.11 days per 100 workers

386.3 Labyrinthitis

Return-To-Work Summary Guidelines		
Dataset	**Midrange**	**At-Risk**
Claims data	14 days	30 days
All absences	4 days	28 days

Return-To-Work "Best Practice" Guidelines
Medical treatment, depending on job safety issues: 1-10 days
Labyrinthectomy: 7-28 days

Description: Viral infection in the inner ear affecting the fluid-filled chamber that controls balance and hearing. Symptoms include vertigo (spinning or moving sensation usually causing nausea and loss of balance) and hearing loss.
Other names: Inner ear infection, Otitis interna

RTW Claims Data (Calendar-days away from work by decile)										
10%	20%	30%	40%	**50%**	60%	70%	80%	**90%**	100%	Mean
9	10	10	11	**14**	27	28	29	**30**	365	19.51

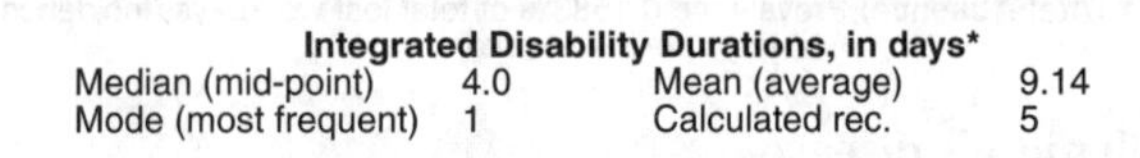

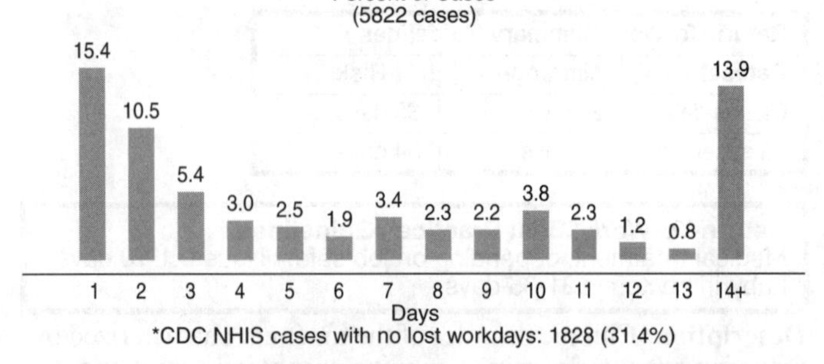

Impact on Total Absence: Prevalence 0.1079% of total lost workdays; Incidence 1.13 days per 100 workers

388 Other disorders of ear

Return-To-Work Summary Guidelines		
Dataset	**Midrange**	**At-Risk**
Claims data	14 days	17 days
All absences	2 days	14 days

388 Other disorders of ear *(cont'd)*

Workers' Comp Costs per Claim (based on 479 claims)					
Quartile	25%	50%	75%	Mean	% no cost
Indemnity	$1,323	$2,205	$4,400	$10,309	91%
Medical	$168	$284	$861	$1,470	4%
Total	$168	$305	$1,197	$2,403	4%

388.3 Tinnitus

Return-To-Work Summary Guidelines		
Dataset	**Midrange**	**At-Risk**
Claims data	14 days	32 days
All absences	3 days	15 days

Return-To-Work "Best Practice" Guidelines
If no safety concerns: 0 days

Description: A noise originating inside the ears often associated with hearing loss. The noise could be in the form of ringing, buzzing, clicking, or other sounds in varying volume.
Other names: Ringing in the ears

Workers' Comp Costs per Claim (based on 184 claims)					
Quartile	25%	50%	75%	Mean	% no cost
Medical	$158	$273	$620	$1,393	2%
Total	$158	$273	$851	$3,419	2%

RTW Claims Data (Calendar-days away from work by decile)										
10%	20%	30%	40%	**50%**	60%	70%	80%	**90%**	100%	Mean
9	10	12	14	**14**	15	17	27	**32**	90	18.83

Integrated Disability Durations, in days*
Median (mid-point) 3.0 Mean (average) 6.07
Mode (most frequent) 1 Calculated rec. 3

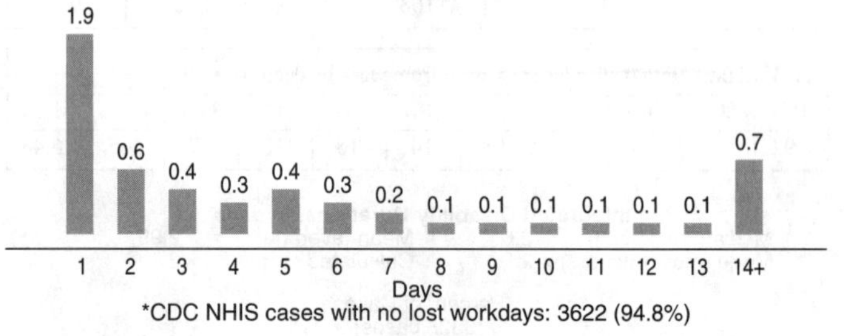

Impact on Total Absence: Prevalence 0.0035% of total lost workdays; Incidence 0.04 days per 100 workers

Occupational Disability Durations, in days
Median (mid-point) 2 - Benchmark Indemnity Costs $1,500

Percent of Cases
(30 cases)

Range of Days	1 day	2 days	3 to 5	6 to 10	11 to 20	21 to 30	31 or more
Percent	18.4	7.5	37.5	2.4	5.9	14.0	14.4

Impact on Occupational Absence: Prevalence 0.0006% of occupational lost workdays

7. DISEASES OF THE CIRCULATORY SYSTEM (390-459)

Impact on Total Absence: Prevalence 9.8921% of total lost workdays; Incidence 103.87 days per 100 workers

RTW Claims Data (Calendar-days away from work by decile)										
10%	20%	30%	40%	**50%**	60%	70%	80%	**90%**	100%	Mean
10	13	14	15	**18**	25	34	46	**69**	365	41.46

HYPERTENSIVE DISEASE (401-405)

Excludes:
that complicating pregnancy, childbirth, or the puerperium (642.0-642.9)
that involving coronary vessels (410.00-414.9)

RTW Claims Data (Calendar-days away from work by decile)										
10%	20%	30%	40%	**50%**	60%	70%	80%	**90%**	100%	Mean
10	11	13	14	**14**	15	17	20	**24**	365	21.25

Impact on Total Absence: Prevalence 1.4172% of total lost workdays; Incidence 14.88 days per 100 workers

Occupational Disability Durations, in days
Median (mid-point) 5 - Benchmark Indemnity Costs $3,750

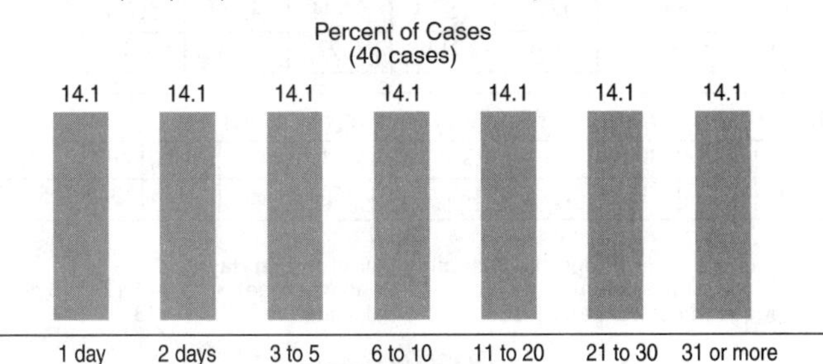

Impact on Occupational Absence: Prevalence 0.0022% of occupational lost workdays

401 Essential hypertension

Return-To-Work Summary Guidelines		
Dataset	**Midrange**	**At-Risk**
Claims data	14 days	25 days
All absences	10 days	21 days

Return-To-Work "Best Practice" Guidelines
Benign, medical treatment: 0 days
Severe (stage 3 - BP>180/110), medical treatment to gain medication control, clerical/modified work: 7-10 days
Severe (stage 3 - BP>180/110), medical treatment, manual work: 10-14 days
Very severe (BP>210/120), with hospitalization, clerical/modified work: 10-14 days
Very severe (BP>210/120), with hospitalization, manual work: 14-21 days
Diabetes comorbidity, multiply by: 1.57
Obesity comorbidity (BMI >= 30), multiply by: 1.22

Description: Abnormally high blood pressure in the arteries which affects the heart, brain, and kidneys, and causes an increase in the risk of stroke, aneurysm, heart failure, heart attack, and kidney damage. High blood pressure is usually without symptoms, although severe cases can experience headaches, blurred vision, and nausea.
Other names: High blood pressure

401 Essential hypertension *(cont'd)*

Includes: high blood pressure
hyperpiesia
hyperpiesis
hypertension (arterial) (essential) (primary) (systemic)
hypertensive vascular:
degeneration
disease

Excludes:
elevated blood pressure without diagnosis of hypertension (796.2)
pulmonary hypertension (416.0-416.9)
that involving vessels of:
brain (430-438)
eye (362.11)

Disability Duration Adjustment Factors by Age						
Age Group	18-24	25-34	35-44	45-54	55-64	65-74
Adjustment Factor	0.52	0.65	0.83	1.20	1.15	1.15

RTW Claims Data (Calendar-days away from work by decile)										
10%	20%	30%	40%	**50%**	60%	70%	80%	**90%**	100%	Mean
10	11	13	14	**14**	15	17	21	**25**	365	21.33

Integrated Disability Durations, in days*
Median (mid-point) 10.0 Mean (average) 13.77
Mode (most frequent) 1 Calculated rec. 9

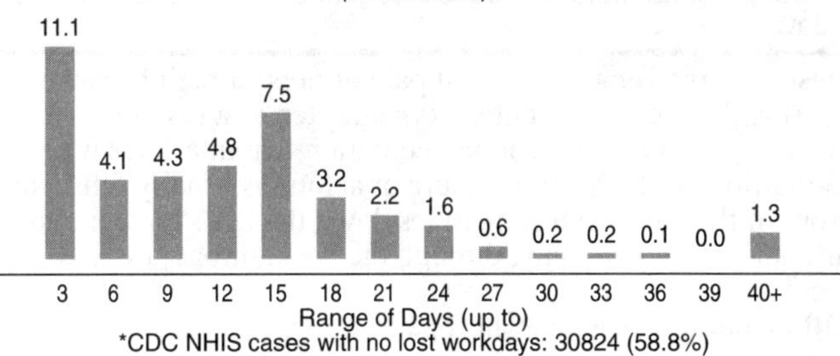

*CDC NHIS cases with no lost workdays: 30824 (58.8%)

Impact on Total Absence: Prevalence 0.8798% of total lost workdays; Incidence 9.24 days per 100 workers

ISCHEMIC HEART DISEASE (410-414)

Includes: that with mention of hypertension
Use additional code to identify presence of hypertension (401.0-405.9)

RTW Claims Data (Calendar-days away from work by decile)										
10%	20%	30%	40%	**50%**	60%	70%	80%	**90%**	100%	Mean
10	12	14	15	**20**	27	31	49	**72**	365	42.81

Impact on Total Absence: Prevalence 2.4118% of total lost workdays; Incidence 25.32 days per 100 workers

ISCHEMIC HEART DISEASE (410-414) *(cont'd)*

Occupational Disability Durations, in days
Median (mid-point) 12 - Benchmark Indemnity Costs $9,000

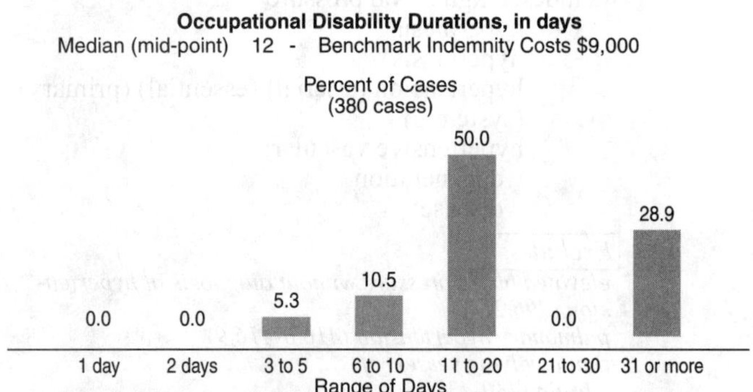

Impact on Occupational Absence: Prevalence 0.0517% of occupational lost workdays; Incidence 0.01 days per 100 workers

413 Angina pectoris

Return-To-Work Summary Guidelines		
Dataset	**Midrange**	**At-Risk**
Claims data	16 days	31 days
All absences	14 days	30 days

Return-To-Work "Best Practice" Guidelines
Asymptomatic: 0 days
Clerical/modified work, without surgery: 7-14 days
Manual work, without surgery, stress test negative: 7-14 days
Heavy manual work, without surgery, stress test negative: 7-28 days

Description: Temporary chest pain or pressure felt because the heart isn't receiving enough oxygen, often as a result of coronary artery disease or any condition that interferes with blood flow to the heart. Pressure or aching is usually felt in the front of the chest, and sometimes down the left shoulder and arm and, less commonly, through the back, throat jaw, and teeth.

Other names: Angina, Chest pain

RTW Claims Data (Calendar-days away from work by decile)

10%	20%	30%	40%	**50%**	60%	70%	80%	**90%**	100%	Mean
11	13	14	15	**16**	17	27	29	**31**	365	25.35

Integrated Disability Durations, in days*

Median (mid-point)	14.0	Mean (average)	19.86
Mode (most frequent)	14	Calculated rec.	15

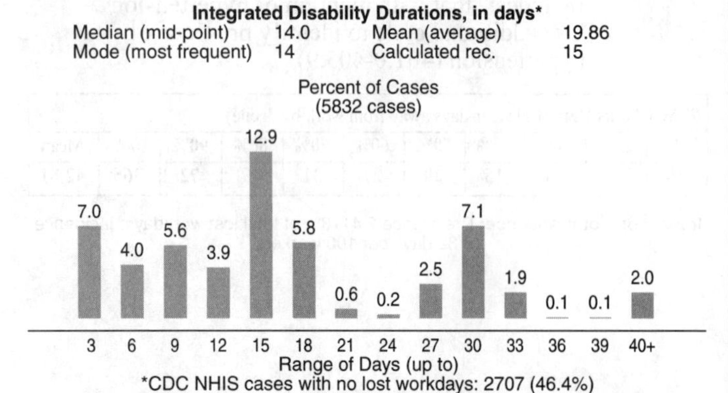

*CDC NHIS cases with no lost workdays: 2707 (46.4%)

Impact on Total Absence: Prevalence 0.1834% of total lost workdays; Incidence 1.93 days per 100 workers

414 Other forms of chronic ischemic heart disease

Return-To-Work Summary Guidelines		
Dataset	**Midrange**	**At-Risk**
Claims data	24 days	84 days
All absences	16 days	74 days

Return-To-Work "Best Practice" Guidelines
See 414.9

Excludes:
arteriosclerotic cardiovascular disease [ASCVD] (429.2)
cardiovascular:
arteriosclerosis or sclerosis (429.2)
degeneration or disease (429.2)

Workers' Comp Costs per Claim (based on 67 claims)

Quartile	25%	50%	75%	Mean	% no cost
Indemnity	$22,796	$50,337	$78,299	$55,407	23%
Medical	$1,124	$5,544	$21,074	$19,789	6%
Total	$17,409	$45,990	$86,982	$61,401	0%

Disability Duration Adjustment Factors by Age

Age Group	18-24	25-34	35-44	45-54	55-64	65-74
Adjustment Factor	NA	NA	0.92	1.11	1.21	0.50

RTW Claims Data (Calendar-days away from work by decile)

10%	20%	30%	40%	**50%**	60%	70%	80%	**90%**	100%	Mean
10	14	15	19	**24**	42	50	69	**84**	365	54.37

Integrated Disability Durations, in days*

Median (mid-point)	16.0	Mean (average)	44.17
Mode (most frequent)	15	Calculated rec.	23

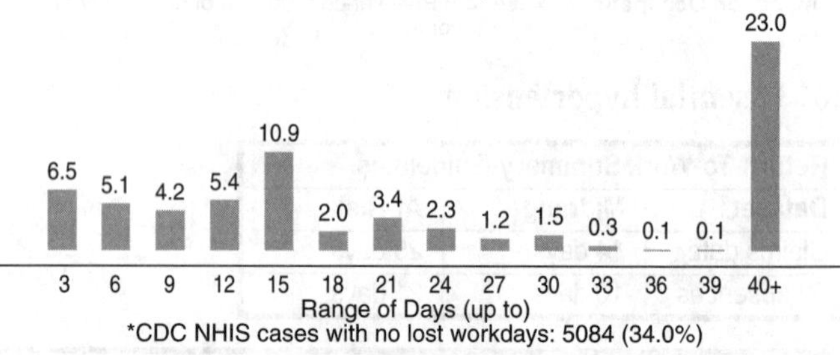

*CDC NHIS cases with no lost workdays: 5084 (34.0%)

Impact on Total Absence: Prevalence 1.2895% of total lost workdays; Incidence 13.54 days per 100 workers

414.0 Coronary atherosclerosis

Return-To-Work Summary Guidelines		
Dataset	**Midrange**	**At-Risk**
Claims data	50 days	364 days
All absences	44 days	128 days

Return-To-Work "Best Practice" Guidelines
Medical treatment: 3 days
Angioplasty/catheter: 7-14 days
Coronary bypass, clerical/modified work: 42-56 days
Coronary bypass, manual work, stress test negative: 56-70 days
Coronary bypass, heavy manual work, stress test negative: 70-112 days
Coronary bypass, heavy manual work, failed stress test: by report
Obesity comorbidity (BMI >= 30), multiply by: 1.22

414.0 Coronary atherosclerosis *(cont'd)*

Description: Accumulation of fatty deposits in the walls of the coronary arteries, which cause blood flow to be obstructed. Eventually the arteries could become so blocked that the heart can't receive enough blood to meet its needs. The main symptom is usually heart pain, although some cases have no symptoms at all.
Other names: Coronary Artery Disease, CAD

Excludes:
embolism of graft (996.72)
occlusion NOS of graft (996.72)
thrombus of graft (996.72)
Arteriosclerotic heart disease [ASHD]
Atherosclerotic heart disease
Coronary (artery):
arteriosclerosis
arteritis or endarteritis
atheroma
sclerosis
stricture

RTW Claims Data (Calendar-days away from work by decile)

10%	20%	30%	40%	**50%**	60%	70%	80%	**90%**	100%	Mean
14	17	41	44	**50**	57	70	84	**364**	365	82.48

Integrated Disability Durations, in days*
Median (mid-point) 44.0 Mean (average) 69.17
Mode (most frequent) 1 Calculated rec. 40

Percent of Cases
(1570 cases)

12.6 9.9 1.0 2.6 7.1 7.3 4.7 6.5 1.1 4.3 0.3 0.1 0.8 6.8
9 18 27 36 45 54 63 72 81 90 99 108 117 118+
Range of Days (up to)
*CDC NHIS cases with no lost workdays: 546 (34.8%)

Impact on Total Absence: Prevalence 0.2093% of total lost workdays; Incidence 2.20 days per 100 workers

OTHER FORMS OF HEART DISEASE (420-429)

RTW Claims Data (Calendar-days away from work by decile)

10%	20%	30%	40%	**50%**	60%	70%	80%	**90%**	100%	Mean
12	14	16	23	**29**	40	45	56	**75**	365	51.26

Impact on Total Absence: Prevalence 1.9548% of total lost workdays; Incidence 20.53 days per 100 workers

424 Other diseases of endocardium

Return-To-Work Summary Guidelines		
Dataset	**Midrange**	**At-Risk**
Claims data	28 days	57 days
All absences	27 days	57 days

Return-To-Work "Best Practice" Guidelines
See 424.9

Excludes:
bacterial endocarditis (421.0-421.9)
rheumatic endocarditis (391.1, 394.0-397.9)
syphilitic endocarditis (093.20-093.24)

424.9 Endocarditis, valve unspecified

Return-To-Work Summary Guidelines		
Dataset	**Midrange**	**At-Risk**
Claims data	28 days	57 days
All absences	27 days	57 days

Return-To-Work "Best Practice" Guidelines
Medical treatment: 0 days
Surgical treatment, clerical/modified work: 14 days
Surgical treatment, manual work: 28 days
Cardiac valve replacement, clerical/modified work: 28 days
Cardiac valve replacement, manual work: 56 days

Description: Inflammation of the interior lining of the heart and heart valves, usually by infection. Sudden high fever, fast heart rate, chills, cough, and fatigue are among the symptoms.
Other names: Infectious endocarditis

RTW Claims Data (Calendar-days away from work by decile)

10%	20%	30%	40%	**50%**	60%	70%	80%	**90%**	100%	Mean
13	15	16	26	**28**	29	32	56	**57**	365	35.17

Integrated Disability Durations, in days*
Median (mid-point) 27.0 Mean (average) 30.78
Mode (most frequent) 28 Calculated rec. 28

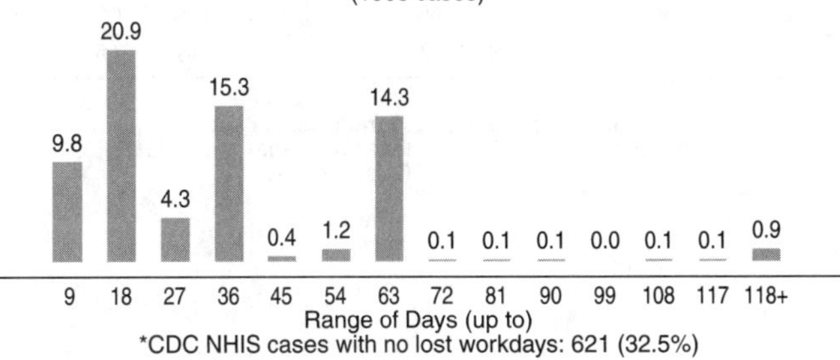

*CDC NHIS cases with no lost workdays: 621 (32.5%)

Impact on Total Absence: Prevalence 0.1171% of total lost workdays; Incidence 1.23 days per 100 workers

428 Heart failure

Return-To-Work Summary Guidelines		
Dataset	**Midrange**	**At-Risk**
Claims data	22 days	44 days
All absences	21 days	44 days

Return-To-Work "Best Practice" Guidelines
See 428.9

Excludes:
rheumatic (398.91)
that complicating:
abortion (634-638 with .7, 639.8)
ectopic or molar pregnancy (639.8)
labor or delivery (668.1, 669.4)
that due to hypertension (402.0-402.9 with fifth-digit 1)

428.0 Congestive heart failure, unspecified

Return-To-Work Summary Guidelines		
Dataset	**Midrange**	**At-Risk**
Claims data	21 days	44 days
All absences	16 days	44 days

428.0 Congestive heart failure, unspecified *(cont'd)*

Return-To-Work "Best Practice" Guidelines
Clerical/modified work: 7-14 days
Manual work, depending on functional capacity, stress test negative: 21 days
Heavy manual work, depending on functional capacity, stress test negative: 42 days
Diabetes comorbidity, multiply by: 1.57
Obesity comorbidity (BMI >= 30), multiply by: 1.22

Description: A condition in which the amount of blood pumped out by the heart isn't enough to meet the normal needs of the body. As a result, blood gathers in the heart causing volume overload, chamber dilation, and increased pressure in the heart. There could also be congestion in the lung. Other symptoms include weakness, shortness of breath, and swelling in the legs and feet, all of which usually develop slowly over time.

Other names: CHF
Congestive heart disease
Right heart failure (secondary to left heart failure)

Disability Duration Adjustment Factors by Age						
Age Group	18-24	25-34	35-44	45-54	55-64	65-74
Adjustment Factor	NA	NA	NA	1.41	1.32	NA

RTW Claims Data (Calendar-days away from work by decile)

10%	20%	30%	40%	**50%**	60%	70%	80%	**90%**	100%	Mean
12	14	15	17	**21**	22	32	42	**44**	365	32.21

Integrated Disability Durations, in days*
Median (mid-point) 16.0 Mean (average) 26.27
Mode (most frequent) 1 Calculated rec. 15

Percent of Cases
(3366 cases)

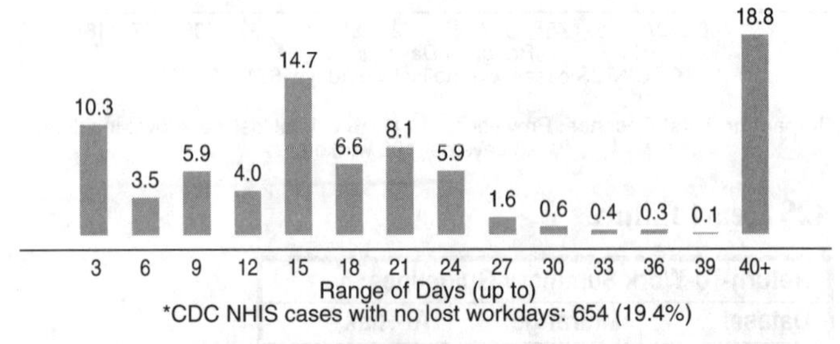

*CDC NHIS cases with no lost workdays: 654 (19.4%)

Impact on Total Absence: Prevalence 0.2106% of total lost workdays; Incidence 2.21 days per 100 workers

CEREBROVASCULAR DISEASE (430-438)

Includes: with mention of hypertension (conditions classifiable to 401-405)
Use additional code to identify presence of hypertension

Excludes:
any condition classifiable to 430-434, 436, 437 occurring during pregnancy, childbirth, or the puerperium, or specified as puerperal (674.0)

RTW Claims Data (Calendar-days away from work by decile)

10%	20%	30%	40%	**50%**	60%	70%	80%	**90%**	100%	Mean
13	14	16	30	**36**	42	46	57	**180**	365	63.20

Impact on Total Absence: Prevalence 2.6073% of total lost workdays; Incidence 27.38 days per 100 workers

Occupational Disability Durations, in days
Median (mid-point) 85 - Benchmark Indemnity Costs $63,750
(80 cases)
Impact on Occupational Absence: Prevalence 0.0771% of occupational lost workdays; Incidence 0.01 days per 100 workers

431 Intracerebral hemorrhage

Return-To-Work Summary Guidelines		
Dataset	**Midrange**	**At-Risk**
Claims data	29 days	45 days
All absences	28 days	45 days

Return-To-Work "Best Practice" Guidelines
Without neurologic deficit, medical treatment: 14 days
Aneurysmectomy, clerical/modified work: 28 days
Aneurysmectomy, manual work: 42 days
Craniectomy, clerical/modified work: 28 days
Craniectomy, manual work: 42 days
Craniotomy, clerical/modified work: 28 days
Craniotomy, manual work: 42 days

Description: Bleeding from a blood vessel in or around the brain causing symptoms of headache, fainting, nausea, confusion, vomiting, or partial paralysis.

Hemorrhage (of):
- basilar
- bulbar
- cerebellar
- cerebral
- cerebromeningeal
- cortical
- internal capsule
- intrapontine
- pontine
- subcortical
- ventricular

Rupture of blood vessel in brain

RTW Claims Data (Calendar-days away from work by decile)

10%	20%	30%	40%	**50%**	60%	70%	80%	**90%**	100%	Mean
14	15	16	28	**29**	31	42	43	**45**	365	39.67

Integrated Disability Durations, in days*
Median (mid-point) 28.0 Mean (average) 37.88
Mode (most frequent) 14 Calculated rec. 27

Percent of Cases
(352 cases)

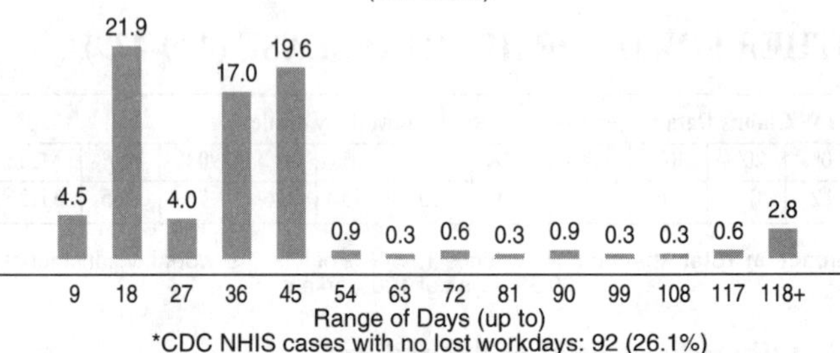

*CDC NHIS cases with no lost workdays: 92 (26.1%)

Impact on Total Absence: Prevalence 0.0291% of total lost workdays; Incidence 0.31 days per 100 workers

434 Occlusion of cerebral arteries

Return-To-Work Summary Guidelines		
Dataset	**Midrange**	**At-Risk**
Claims data	28 days	182 days
All absences	19 days	182 days

Return-To-Work "Best Practice" Guidelines
See 434.9

434 Occlusion of cerebral arteries *(cont'd)*

The following fifth-digit subclassification is for use with category 434:
- 0 without mention of cerebral infarction
- 1 with cerebral infarction

434.0 Cerebral thrombosis

Return-To-Work Summary Guidelines		
Dataset	**Midrange**	**At-Risk**
Claims data	56 days	365 days
All absences	35 days	364 days

Return-To-Work "Best Practice" Guidelines
Completed stroke unimpaired, no brain damage: 14 days
Completed stroke initially unable to walk independently, without neurologic deficit: 55 days
Completed stroke with continuing loss of function, modified work (permanent partial disability): 182 days to indefinite

Description: A blood clot in the cerebral arteries restricting blood flow through the brain. Symptoms may include fainting, headache, confusion, nausea, stroke, and eventual brain damage if not treated.
Other names: CVA
Thrombosis of cerebral arteries

Disability Duration Adjustment Factors by Age						
Age Group	18-24	25-34	35-44	45-54	55-64	65-74
Adjustment Factor	NA	NA	0.87	0.72	1.47	NA

RTW Claims Data (Calendar-days away from work by decile)										
10%	20%	30%	40%	**50%**	60%	70%	80%	**90%**	100%	Mean
14	15	20	54	**56**	75	182	184	**365**	365	115.67

Integrated Disability Durations, in days*
Median (mid-point) 35.0 Mean (average) 91.43
Mode (most frequent) 2 Calculated rec. 41

Percent of Cases
(925 cases)

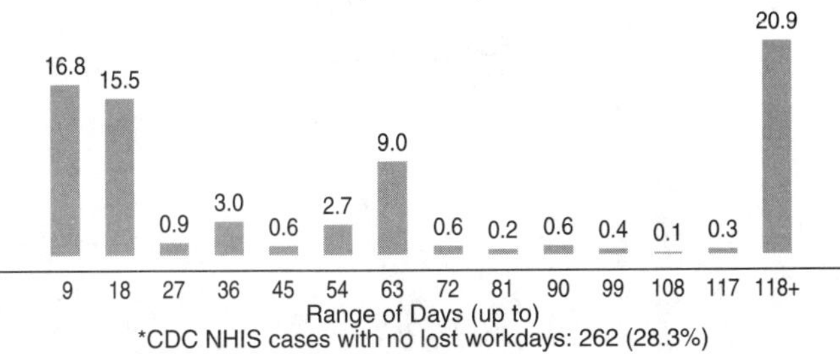

Range of Days (up to)
*CDC NHIS cases with no lost workdays: 262 (28.3%)

Impact on Total Absence: Prevalence 0.1791% of total lost workdays; Incidence 1.88 days per 100 workers

435 Transient cerebral ischemia

Return-To-Work Summary Guidelines		
Dataset	**Midrange**	**At-Risk**
Claims data	17 days	30 days
All absences	15 days	29 days

Return-To-Work "Best Practice" Guidelines
Without hospitalization: 1 day
With hospitalization, medical treatment: 5 days
Carotid endarterectomy, clerical/modified work: 14 days
Carotid endarterectomy, manual work: 28 days

435 Transient cerebral ischemia *(cont'd)*

Description: Temporary loss of blood flow to the brain due to blocked carotid or vertebral arteries typically causing loss of sensation, blurred speech, feelings of spinning, and problems with balance, coordination, speech and thought.

Includes: cerebrovascular insufficiency (acute) with transient focal neurological signs and symptoms
insufficiency of basilar, carotid, and vertebral arteries
spasm of cerebral arteries

Excludes:
acute cerebrovascular insufficiency NOS (437.1)
that due to any condition classifiable to 433 (433.0-433.9)

RTW Claims Data (Calendar-days away from work by decile)										
10%	20%	30%	40%	**50%**	60%	70%	80%	**90%**	100%	Mean
13	14	15	16	**17**	27	28	29	**30**	365	25.42

Integrated Disability Durations, in days*
Median (mid-point) 15.0 Mean (average) 18.72
Mode (most frequent) 1 Calculated rec. 12

Percent of Cases
(246 cases)

11.4 10.2 1.2 1.2 17.5 6.9 1.6 0.8 4.5 14.2 0.8 0.4 0.0 2.0

3 6 9 12 15 18 21 24 27 30 33 36 39 40+
Range of Days (up to)
*CDC NHIS cases with no lost workdays: 67 (27.2%)

Impact on Total Absence: Prevalence 0.0099% of total lost workdays; Incidence 0.10 days per 100 workers

DISEASES OF ARTERIES, ARTERIOLES, AND CAPILLARIES (440-449)

RTW Claims Data (Calendar-days away from work by decile)										
10%	20%	30%	40%	**50%**	60%	70%	80%	**90%**	100%	Mean
10	12	14	16	**28**	35	43	53	**90**	365	52.86

Impact on Total Absence: Prevalence 0.7173% of total lost workdays; Incidence 7.53 days per 100 workers

Occupational Disability Durations, in days
Median (mid-point) 69 - Benchmark Indemnity Costs $51,750

Percent of Cases
(40 cases)

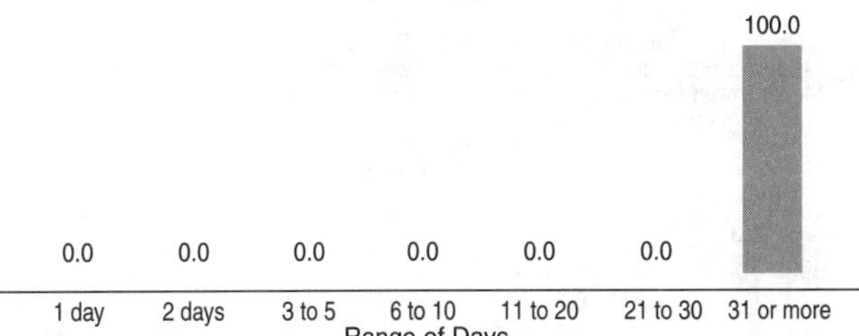

Range of Days

Impact on Occupational Absence: Prevalence 0.0313% of occupational lost workdays; Incidence 0.01 days per 100 workers

440 Atherosclerosis

Return-To-Work Summary Guidelines		
Dataset	**Midrange**	**At-Risk**
Claims data	37 days	300 days
All absences	31 days	110 days

Return-To-Work "Best Practice" Guidelines
Cardiac catheterization: 1 day
Medical treatment: 3 days
Angioplasty: 7-10 days
Angioplasty/stent placement: 10-14 days
Minimally invasive bypass, clerical/modified work: 28 days
Minimally invasive bypass, manual work, stress test negative: 35 days
Minimally invasive bypass, heavy manual work, stress test negative: 42 days
Coronary bypass (open heart surgery/CABG), clerical/modified work: 42-56 days
Coronary bypass, manual work, stress test negative: 56-70 days
Coronary bypass, heavy manual work, stress test negative: 70-112 days
Coronary bypass, heavy manual work, failed stress test: indefinite

Description: Degenerative diseases in which the wall of an artery thickens and becomes less elastic, most often occurring when fatty material accumulates beneath the inner lining of the artery wall. Symptoms depend on where the thickening occurs and usually result in cramps or pain to the part of the body that isn't receiving enough oxygen because of the blocked artery.
Other names: Hardening of the arteries

Includes: arteriolosclerosis
arteriosclerosis (obliterans) (senile)
arteriosclerotic vascular disease
atheroma
degeneration:
arterial
arteriovascular
vascular
endarteritis deformans or obliterans
senile:
arteritis
endarteritis

Excludes:
atherosclerosis of bypass graft of the extremities (440.30-440.32)

RTW Claims Data (Calendar-days away from work by decile)

10%	20%	30%	40%	**50%**	60%	70%	80%	**90%**	100%	Mean
11	14	27	31	**37**	43	49	70	**300**	365	70.95

Integrated Disability Durations, in days*
Median (mid-point) 31.0 Mean (average) 59.14
Mode (most frequent) 1 Calculated rec. 31

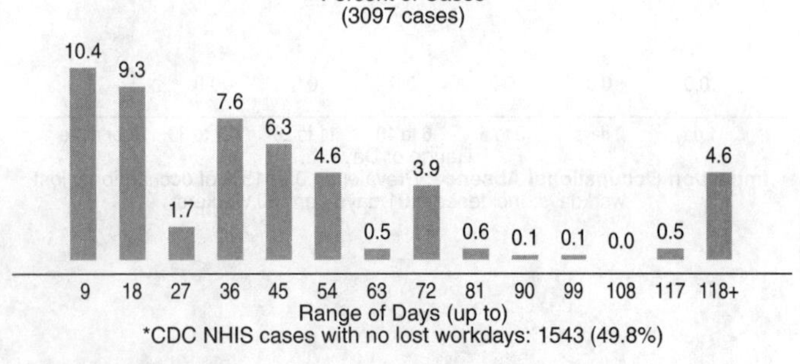

*CDC NHIS cases with no lost workdays: 1543 (49.8%)

Impact on Total Absence: Prevalence 0.2716% of total lost workdays; Incidence 2.85 days per 100 workers

444 Arterial embolism and thrombosis

Return-To-Work Summary Guidelines		
Dataset	**Midrange**	**At-Risk**
Claims data	11 days	25 days
All absences	10 days	16 days

Return-To-Work "Best Practice" Guidelines
Medical treatment: 3 days
Angioplasty: 7-10 days

Description: Blockage of an artery by a piece of a blood clot that has broken off and traveled to another area. Symptoms depend on where the blockage occurs and are reactions to the lessened amount of oxygen, blood, and glucose that are able to travel through the artery to nourish the body and can include pain, numbness, feeling of cold, or a pale pallor.
Other names: Blood clot, Fat emboli, Air emboli

Includes: infarction:
embolic
thrombotic
occlusion

Excludes:
that complicating:
abortion (634-638 with .6, 639.6)
ectopic or molar pregnancy (639.6)
pregnancy, childbirth, or the puerperium (673.0-673.8)

Workers' Comp Costs per Claim (based on 61 claims)

Quartile	25%	50%	75%	Mean	% no cost
Indemnity	$4,337	$11,046	$27,279	$19,157	16%
Medical	$5,565	$10,164	$20,349	$18,582	3%
Total	$10,112	$17,115	$43,607	$35,268	3%

RTW Claims Data (Calendar-days away from work by decile)

10%	20%	30%	40%	**50%**	60%	70%	80%	**90%**	100%	Mean
9	10	10	10	**11**	12	14	15	**25**	325	16.92

Integrated Disability Durations, in days*
Median (mid-point) 10.0 Mean (average) 13.23
Mode (most frequent) 10 Calculated rec. 11

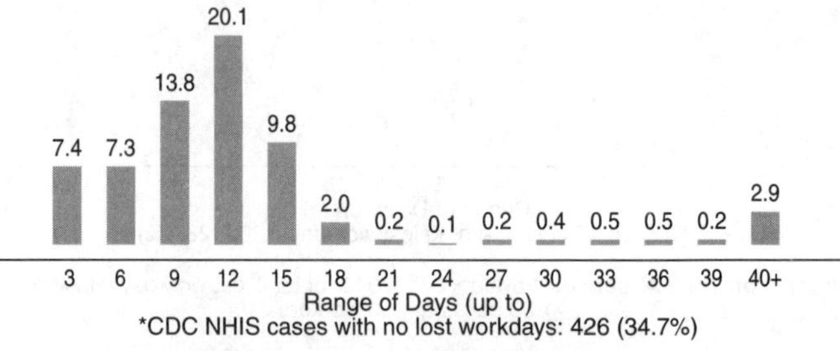

*CDC NHIS cases with no lost workdays: 426 (34.7%)

Impact on Total Absence: Prevalence 0.0314% of total lost workdays; Incidence 0.33 days per 100 workers

DISEASES OF VEINS AND LYMPHATICS, AND OTHER DISEASES OF CIRCULATORY SYSTEM (451-459)

RTW Claims Data (Calendar-days away from work by decile)

10%	20%	30%	40%	**50%**	60%	70%	80%	**90%**	100%	Mean
10	13	14	15	**17**	21	28	30	**56**	365	29.07

Impact on Total Absence: Prevalence 0.5683% of total lost workdays; Incidence 5.97 days per 100 workers

DISEASES OF VEINS AND LYMPHATICS, AND OTHER DISEASES OF CIRCULATORY SYSTEM (451-459) *(cont'd)*

Occupational Disability Durations, in days
Median (mid-point) 13 - Benchmark Indemnity Costs $9,750 (60 cases)
Impact on Occupational Absence: Prevalence 0.0088% of occupational lost workdays

454 Varicose veins of lower extremities

Return-To-Work Summary Guidelines		
Dataset	**Midrange**	**At-Risk**
Claims data	17 days	31 days
All absences	14 days	30 days

Return-To-Work "Best Practice" Guidelines
Medical treatment (support stockings): 0 days
Sclerotherapy, single vein: 0 days
Sclerotherapy, multiple veins, with pressure dressing: 2-5 days
Radio-frequency closure procedure: 1 day
Ligation/stripping, sedentary/modified work: 14 days
Ligation/stripping, standing/manual work: 28 days

Description: Enlarged superficial veins in the legs probably caused by an inherited weakness in the veins resulting in a loss of elasticity over time. The stretched-out veins rapidly fill with blood when the person stands, causing even more enlargement and a visible bulge. Other symptoms may include aching, tired, and/or itchy legs.

Excludes:
that complicating pregnancy, childbirth, or the puerperium (671.0)

RTW Claims Data (Calendar-days away from work by decile)										
10%	20%	30%	40%	**50%**	60%	70%	80%	**90%**	100%	Mean
13	14	14	15	**17**	26	28	29	**31**	365	25.67

Integrated Disability Durations, in days*
Median (mid-point) 14.0 Mean (average) 16.81
Mode (most frequent) 2 Calculated rec. 12

Percent of Cases
(5073 cases)

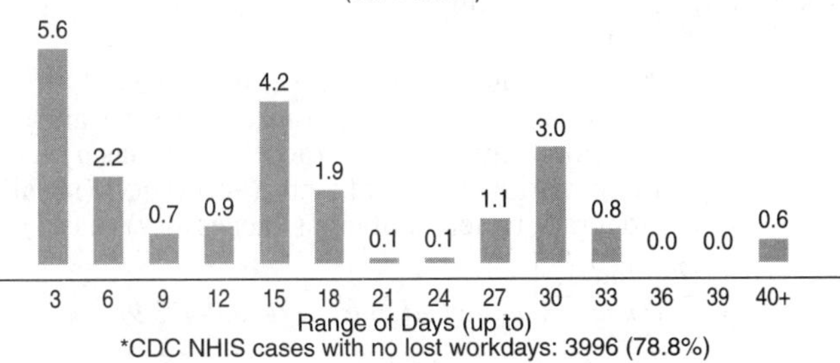

*CDC NHIS cases with no lost workdays: 3996 (78.8%)

Impact on Total Absence: Prevalence 0.0535% of total lost workdays; Incidence 0.56 days per 100 workers

455 Hemorrhoids

Return-To-Work Summary Guidelines		
Dataset	**Midrange**	**At-Risk**
Claims data	17 days	25 days
All absences	10 days	22 days

455 Hemorrhoids *(cont'd)*

Return-To-Work "Best Practice" Guidelines
Medical treatment: 0 days
Sclerotherapy/injection: 1 day
Rubber band ligation: 1 day
Hemorrhoidectomy, simple ligature: 2-14 days
Hemorrhoidectomy, clerical/modified work: 14 days
Hemorrhoidectomy, heavy manual work: 21 days

Description: Swollen veins in the anus and rectum that can be inflamed internally, or can enlarge and protrude. The first symptom is usually a small amount of blood with bowel movements. External hemorrhoids will be visible during a physical exam and may cause pain with bowel movements.

Includes: hemorrhoids (anus) (rectum)
piles
varicose veins, anus or rectum

Excludes:
that complicating pregnancy, childbirth, or the puerperium (671.8)

RTW Claims Data (Calendar-days away from work by decile)										
10%	20%	30%	40%	**50%**	60%	70%	80%	**90%**	100%	Mean
12	14	14	15	**17**	20	21	22	**25**	365	20.84

Integrated Disability Durations, in days*
Median (mid-point) 10.0 Mean (average) 11.89
Mode (most frequent) 2 Calculated rec. 8

Percent of Cases
(6585 cases)

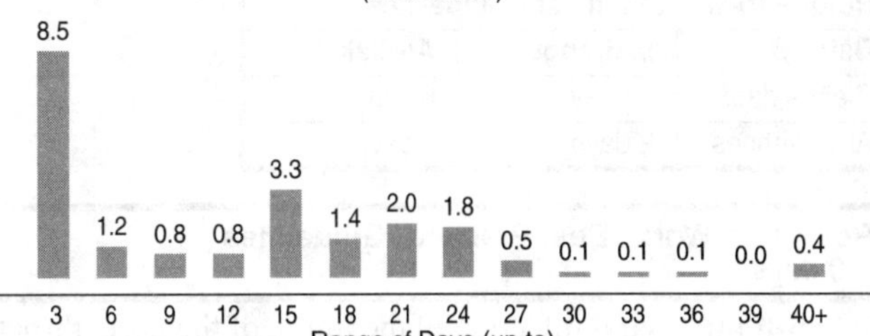

*CDC NHIS cases with no lost workdays: 5205 (79.0%)

Impact on Total Absence: Prevalence 0.0485% of total lost workdays; Incidence 0.51 days per 100 workers

Occupational Disability Durations, in days
Median (mid-point) 20 - Benchmark Indemnity Costs $15,000 (20 cases)
Impact on Occupational Absence: Prevalence 0.0045% of occupational lost workdays

8. DISEASES OF THE RESPIRATORY SYSTEM (460-519)

Impact on Total Absence: Prevalence 6.5371% of total lost workdays; Incidence 68.64 days per 100 workers

RTW Claims Data (Calendar-days away from work by decile)

10%	20%	30%	40%	**50%**	60%	70%	80%	**90%**	100%	Mean
9	10	11	12	**13**	14	15	18	**34**	365	29.95

Use additional code to identify infectious organism

ACUTE RESPIRATORY INFECTIONS (460-466)

Excludes:

pneumonia and influenza (480.0-487.8)

RTW Claims Data (Calendar-days away from work by decile)

10%	20%	30%	40%	**50%**	60%	70%	80%	**90%**	100%	Mean
8	9	10	11	**12**	13	14	15	**21**	365	17.71

Impact on Total Absence: Prevalence 0.7267% of total lost workdays; Incidence 7.63 days per 100 workers

Occupational Disability Durations, in days

Median (mid-point) 6 - Benchmark Indemnity Costs $4,500 (50 cases)

Impact on Occupational Absence: Prevalence 0.0034% of occupational lost workdays

460 Acute nasopharyngitis [common cold]

Return-To-Work Summary Guidelines		
Dataset	**Midrange**	**At-Risk**
Claims data	14 days	62 days
All absences	2 days	6 days

Return-To-Work "Best Practice" Guidelines
0-3 days

Description: A viral infection of the lining of the nose, throat, sinuses, and large airways causing a runny nose, sneezing, sore throat, a stuffed nose, and/or a cough. Symptoms usually appear within 48-72 hours after exposure to the virus, and remain in the upper respiratory tract for about five to seven days.

Other names: Common cold, Head cold, Upper respiratory infection

Coryza (acute)
Nasal catarrh, acute
Nasopharyngitis:
- NOS
- acute
- infective NOS

Rhinitis:
- acute
- infective

Excludes:

nasopharyngitis, chronic (472.2)
pharyngitis:
- *acute or unspecified (462)*
- *chronic (472.1)*

rhinitis:
- *allergic (477.0-477.9)*
- *chronic or unspecified (472.0)*

sore throat:
- *acute or unspecified (462)*
- *chronic (472.1)*

Disability Duration Adjustment Factors by Age

Age Group	18-24	25-34	35-44	45-54	55-64	65-74
Adjustment Factor	0.83	0.77	1.09	1.20	1.12	0.84

460 Acute nasopharyngitis [common cold] *(cont'd)*

RTW Claims Data (Calendar-days away from work by decile)

10%	20%	30%	40%	**50%**	60%	70%	80%	**90%**	100%	Mean
8	10	11	12	**14**	15	20	31	**62**	365	28.50

Integrated Disability Durations, in days*

Median (mid-point)	2.0	Mean (average)	3.94
Mode (most frequent)	1	Calculated rec.	2

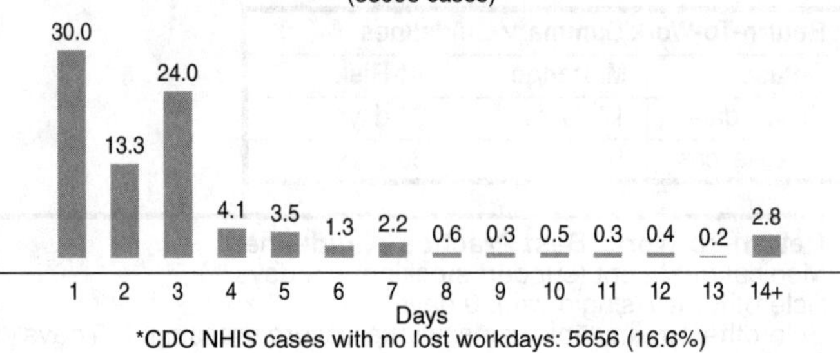

*CDC NHIS cases with no lost workdays: 5656 (16.6%)

Impact on Total Absence: Prevalence 0.3298% of total lost workdays; Incidence 3.46 days per 100 workers

461 Acute sinusitis

Return-To-Work Summary Guidelines		
Dataset	**Midrange**	**At-Risk**
Claims data	14 days	18 days
All absences	4 days	16 days

Return-To-Work "Best Practice" Guidelines
Without hospitalization, mild: 0-1 days
Without hospitalization, severe (fever, headache): 0-3 days
Surgical drainage: 7 days
Caldwell-Luc operation: 14 days

Description: Allergic, viral, bacterial, or fungal infection or inflammation of the sinuses that usually occurs after there has been blockage of the sinuses (such as after a cold or allergy). Common symptoms include a thick discharge from the nose, and headache, facial, or tooth pain.

Other names: Sinus infection

Includes:
- abscess, acute, of sinus (accessory) (nasal)
- empyema, acute, of sinus (accessory) (nasal)
- infection, acute, of sinus (accessory) (nasal)
- inflammation, acute, of sinus (accessory) (nasal)
- suppuration, acute, of sinus (accessory) (nasal)

Excludes:

chronic or unspecified sinusitis (473.0-473.9)

Disability Duration Adjustment Factors by Age

Age Group	18-24	25-34	35-44	45-54	55-64	65-74
Adjustment Factor	1.11	0.81	0.84	1.17	1.16	1.76

RTW Claims Data (Calendar-days away from work by decile)

10%	20%	30%	40%	**50%**	60%	70%	80%	**90%**	100%	Mean
9	11	13	14	**14**	15	16	17	**18**	365	17.57

461 Acute sinusitis *(cont'd)*

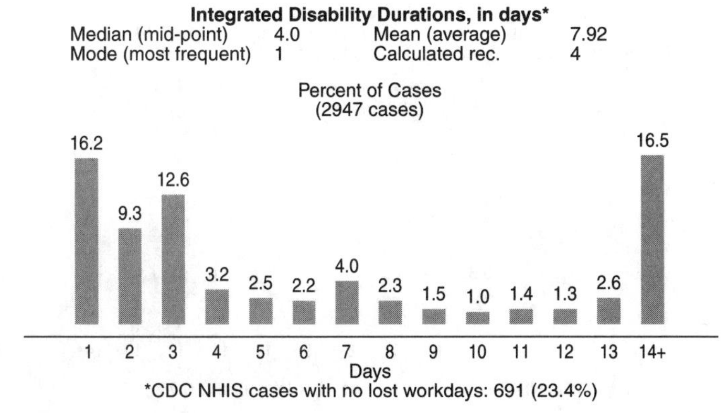

Impact on Total Absence: Prevalence 0.0527% of total lost workdays; Incidence 0.55 days per 100 workers

OTHER DISEASES OF THE UPPER RESPIRATORY TRACT (470-478)

RTW Claims Data (Calendar-days away from work by decile)										
10%	20%	30%	40%	**50%**	60%	70%	80%	**90%**	100%	Mean
9	10	12	13	**14**	15	18	27	**49**	365	26.00

Impact on Total Absence: Prevalence 0.7485% of total lost workdays; Incidence 7.86 days per 100 workers

Occupational Disability Durations, in days
Median (mid-point) 2 - Benchmark Indemnity Costs $1,500 (190 cases)
Impact on Occupational Absence: Prevalence 0.0043% of occupational lost workdays

470 Deviated nasal septum

Return-To-Work Summary Guidelines		
Dataset	**Midrange**	**At-Risk**
Claims data	15 days	26 days
All absences	12 days	21 days

Return-To-Work "Best Practice" Guidelines
Asymptomatic: 0 days
Septoplasty, clerical/modified work: 6 days
Septoplasty, manual work: 14 days

Description: Occurs when the vertical wall (septum) that divides the nasal cavity is deviated either since birth or because of an injury. Usually it causes no symptoms, but in some cases the deviated septum blocks the nose or makes a person prone to a sinus infection or nosebleeds.

Deflected septum (nasal) (acquired)

Excludes:
congenital (754.0)

Workers' Comp Costs per Claim (based on 127 claims)					
Quartile	25%	50%	75%	Mean	% no cost
Indemnity	$1,124	$2,100	$4,232	$3,301	57%
Medical	$2,678	$4,625	$7,004	$5,477	1%
Total	$2,856	$6,001	$8,820	$6,927	1%

RTW Claims Data (Calendar-days away from work by decile)										
10%	20%	30%	40%	**50%**	60%	70%	80%	**90%**	100%	Mean
10	12	14	14	**15**	16	17	19	**26**	309	17.94

470 Deviated nasal septum *(cont'd)*

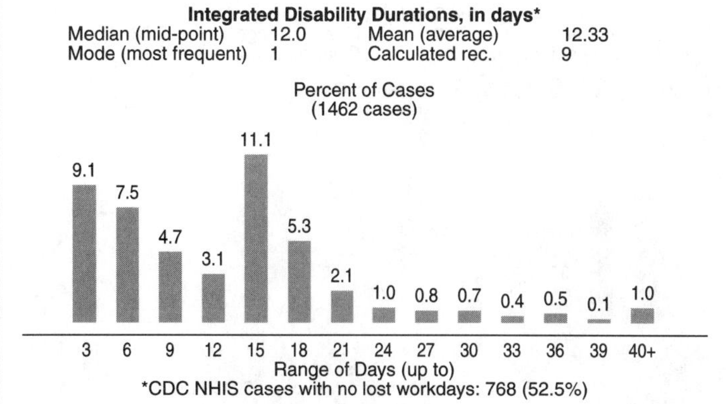

Impact on Total Absence: Prevalence 0.0252% of total lost workdays; Incidence 0.27 days per 100 workers

473 Chronic sinusitis

Return-To-Work Summary Guidelines		
Dataset	**Midrange**	**At-Risk**
Claims data	15 days	77 days
All absences	2 days	9 days

Return-To-Work "Best Practice" Guidelines
0-2 days

Description: A long-lasting infection and inflammation of the sinuses of the face, often occurring after a cold or allergy has blocked the sinuses for long enough for bacteria to gather and multiply. Thick discharge from the nose and a headache and facial pain are among the symptoms.
Other names: Chronic sinus infection

Includes:
abscess (chronic) of sinus (accessory) (nasal)
empyema (chronic) of sinus (accessory) (nasal)
infection (chronic) of sinus (accessory) (nasal)
suppuration (chronic) of sinus (accessory) (nasal)

Excludes:
acute sinusitis (461.0-461.9)

Workers' Comp Costs per Claim (based on 38 claims)					
Quartile	25%	50%	75%	Mean	% no cost
Medical	$284	$1,250	$11,204	$14,767	5%
Total	$420	$2,499	$14,312	$24,566	5%

Disability Duration Adjustment Factors by Age						
Age Group	18-24	25-34	35-44	45-54	55-64	65-74
Adjustment Factor	1.11	0.81	0.84	1.17	1.16	1.76

RTW Claims Data (Calendar-days away from work by decile)										
10%	20%	30%	40%	**50%**	60%	70%	80%	**90%**	100%	Mean
9	10	12	14	**15**	20	26	35	**77**	365	33.12

473 Chronic sinusitis *(cont'd)*

Integrated Disability Durations, in days*

Median (mid-point)	2.0	Mean (average)	5.72
Mode (most frequent)	2	Calculated rec.	3

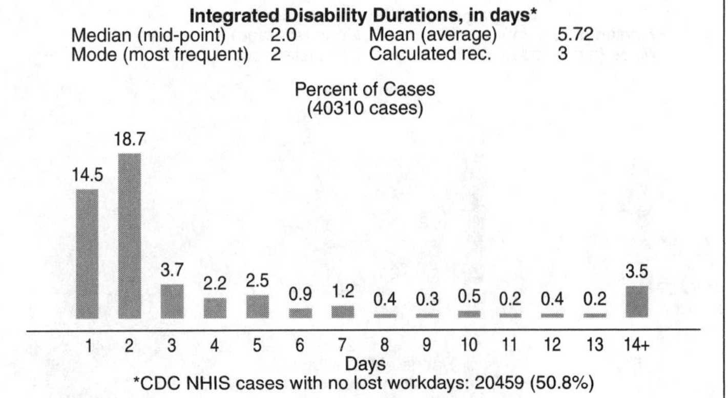

*CDC NHIS cases with no lost workdays: 20459 (50.8%)

Impact on Total Absence: Prevalence 0.3356% of total lost workdays; Incidence 3.52 days per 100 workers

474 Chronic disease of tonsils and adenoids

Return-To-Work Summary Guidelines		
Dataset	**Midrange**	**At-Risk**
Claims data	12 days	15 days
All absences	10 days	15 days

Return-To-Work "Best Practice" Guidelines
See 474.9

474.0 Chronic tonsillitis and adenoiditis

Return-To-Work Summary Guidelines		
Dataset	**Midrange**	**At-Risk**
Claims data	13 days	17 days
All absences	4 days	15 days

Return-To-Work "Best Practice" Guidelines
Medical treatment: 0 days
Radiofrequency shrinkage: 2 days
Tonsillectomy/adenoidectomy, clerical/modified work: 10 days
Tonsillectomy/adenoidectomy, manual work: 14 days

Description: Chronic inflammation of the tonsils due to bacterial or viral infection. Symptoms may include sore throat, earache, pain upon swallowing, headache, fever, malaise, and unpleasant breath.

Excludes:
acute or unspecified tonsillitis (463)

RTW Claims Data (Calendar-days away from work by decile)

10%	20%	30%	40%	**50%**	60%	70%	80%	**90%**	100%	Mean
9	10	11	12	**13**	14	15	15	**17**	123	13.71

474.0 Chronic tonsillitis and adenoiditis *(cont'd)*

Integrated Disability Durations, in days*

Median (mid-point)	4.0	Mean (average)	7.14
Mode (most frequent)	2	Calculated rec.	4

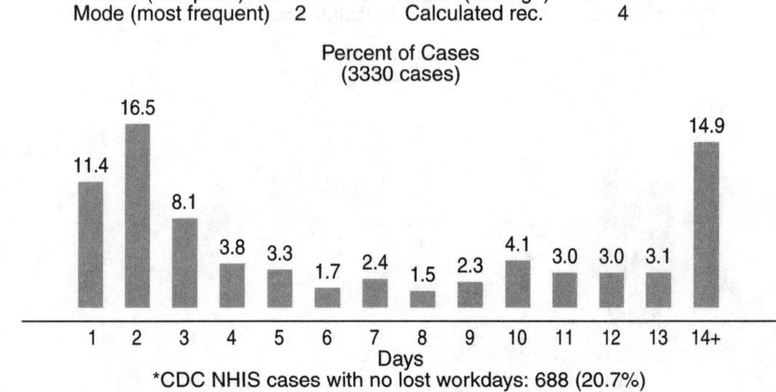

*CDC NHIS cases with no lost workdays: 688 (20.7%)

Impact on Total Absence: Prevalence 0.0557% of total lost workdays; Incidence 0.59 days per 100 workers

476 Chronic laryngitis and laryngotracheitis

Return-To-Work Summary Guidelines		
Dataset	**Midrange**	**At-Risk**
Claims data	14 days	45 days
All absences	2 days	7 days

Return-To-Work "Best Practice" Guidelines
See 476.0

476.0 Chronic laryngitis

Return-To-Work Summary Guidelines		
Dataset	**Midrange**	**At-Risk**
Claims data	14 days	45 days
All absences	2 days	7 days

Return-To-Work "Best Practice" Guidelines
Clerical/modified work (minimize talking): 0 days
Regular work with some talking: 2 days
Regular work with extensive talking/lecturing: 5 days

Description: Chronic inflammation of the voice box, usually because of a viral infection, causing temporary hoarseness or even loss of voice. The throat may also tickle or feel raw and there may be a constant need to clear the throat.

Laryngitis:
- catarrhal
- hypertrophic
- sicca

RTW Claims Data (Calendar-days away from work by decile)

10%	20%	30%	40%	**50%**	60%	70%	80%	**90%**	100%	Mean
8	9	10	12	**14**	16	21	30	**45**	180	24.03

476.0 Chronic laryngitis *(cont'd)*

Integrated Disability Durations, in days*

Median (mid-point)	2.0	Mean (average)	4.56
Mode (most frequent)	2	Calculated rec.	3

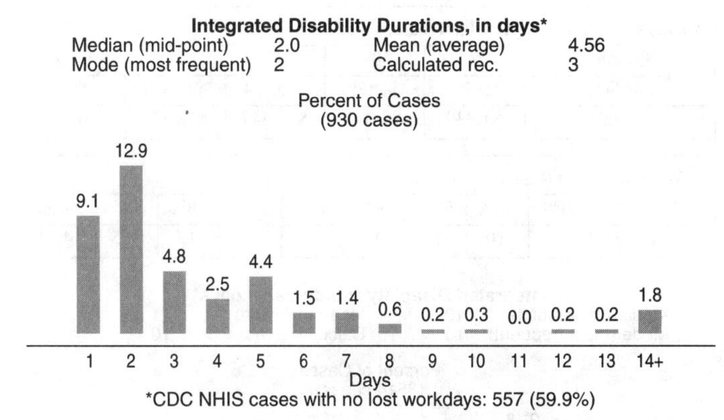

*CDC NHIS cases with no lost workdays: 557 (59.9%)

Impact on Total Absence: Prevalence 0.0050% of total lost workdays; Incidence 0.05 days per 100 workers

477 Allergic rhinitis

Return-To-Work Summary Guidelines		
Dataset	**Midrange**	**At-Risk**
Claims data	15 days	64 days
All absences	2 days	12 days

Return-To-Work "Best Practice" Guidelines
Drug therapy, non-sedating antihistamines, regular work: 0 days
Drug therapy, sedating antihistamines, modified work: 0 days

Description: Inflammation of the nasal mucous membrane usually due to allergies. Symptoms usually include a runny, stuffy nose, itchy eyes, sneezing, and sometimes a mild sore throat.

Other names: Hay fever, Runny nose

Includes: allergic rhinitis (nonseasonal) (seasonal)
hay fever
spasmodic rhinorrhea

Excludes:
allergic rhinitis with asthma (bronchial) (493.0)

Workers' Comp Costs per Claim (based on 122 claims)					
Quartile	25%	50%	75%	Mean	% no cost
Medical	$158	$242	$546	$546	6%
Total	$158	$242	$588	$740	6%

Disability Duration Adjustment Factors by Age						
Age Group	18-24	25-34	35-44	45-54	55-64	65-74
Adjustment Factor	0.88	0.80	0.75	1.12	1.82	1.92

RTW Claims Data (Calendar-days away from work by decile)										
10%	20%	30%	40%	**50%**	60%	70%	80%	**90%**	100%	Mean
9	10	12	14	**15**	20	25	34	**64**	365	30.98

477 Allergic rhinitis *(cont'd)*

Integrated Disability Durations, in days*

Median (mid-point)	2.0	Mean (average)	6.29
Mode (most frequent)	1	Calculated rec.	3

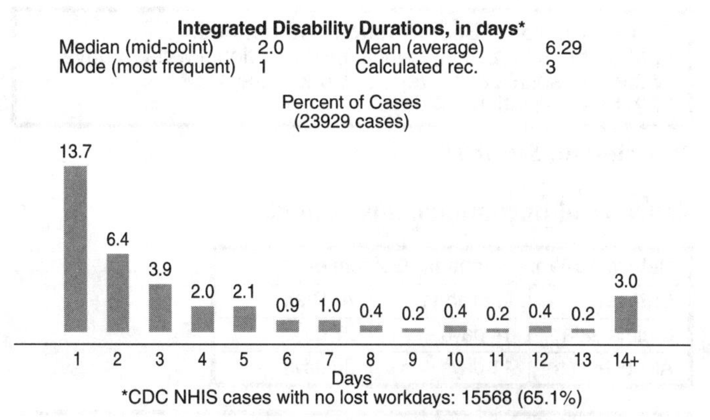

*CDC NHIS cases with no lost workdays: 15568 (65.1%)

Impact on Total Absence: Prevalence 0.1553% of total lost workdays; Incidence 1.63 days per 100 workers

Occupational Disability Durations, in days
Median (mid-point) 4 - Benchmark Indemnity Costs $3,000
(60 cases)
Impact on Occupational Absence: Prevalence 0.0027% of occupational lost workdays

PNEUMONIA AND INFLUENZA (480-488)

Excludes:
pneumonia:
allergic or eosinophilic (518.3)
aspiration:
NOS (507.0)
newborn (770.1)
solids and liquids (507.0-507.8)
congenital (770.0)
lipoid (507.1)
passive (514)
rheumatic (390)

RTW Claims Data (Calendar-days away from work by decile)										
10%	20%	30%	40%	**50%**	60%	70%	80%	**90%**	100%	Mean
9	9	10	10	**11**	11	12	14	**15**	365	12.13

Impact on Total Absence: Prevalence 1.1646% of total lost workdays; Incidence 12.23 days per 100 workers

Occupational Disability Durations, in days
Median (mid-point) 50 - Benchmark Indemnity Costs $37,500

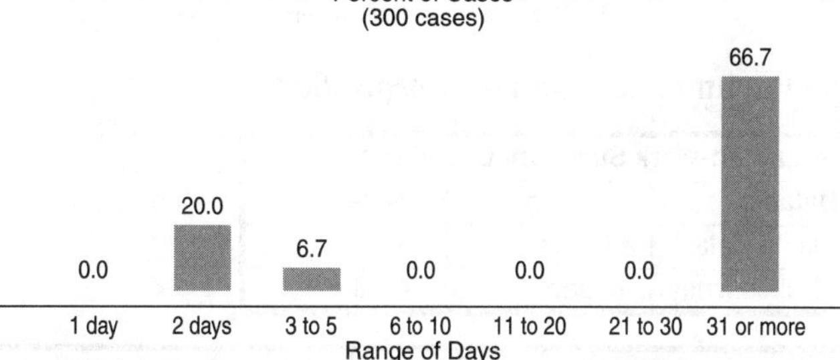

Impact on Occupational Absence: Prevalence 0.1701% of occupational lost workdays; Incidence 0.03 days per 100 workers

480 Viral pneumonia

Return-To-Work Summary Guidelines		
Dataset	**Midrange**	**At-Risk**
Claims data	14 days	27 days
All absences	11 days	20 days

480 Viral pneumonia *(cont'd)*

Return-To-Work "Best Practice" Guidelines
Without hospitalization, clerical/mild exertional work: 4 days
Without hospitalization, regular work: 7 days
With hospitalization: 14 days

Description: See 480.9

480.9 Viral pneumonia, unspecified

Return-To-Work Summary Guidelines		
Dataset	**Midrange**	**At-Risk**
Claims data	14 days	27 days
All absences	11 days	20 days

Return-To-Work "Best Practice" Guidelines
Without hospitalization, clerical/mild exertional work: 4 days
Without hospitalization, regular work: 7 days
With hospitalization: 14 days

Description: Inflammation of the lungs due to a viral infection. Symptoms usually come suddenly and can include fever, chills, shortness of breath, headache, muscle pain, cough, and occasional chest pain.

RTW Claims Data (Calendar-days away from work by decile)										
10%	20%	30%	40%	**50%**	60%	70%	80%	**90%**	100%	Mean
9	11	12	13	**14**	15	16	18	**27**	365	18.93

Integrated Disability Durations, in days*
Median (mid-point) 11.0 Mean (average) 14.09
Mode (most frequent) 14 Calculated rec. 13

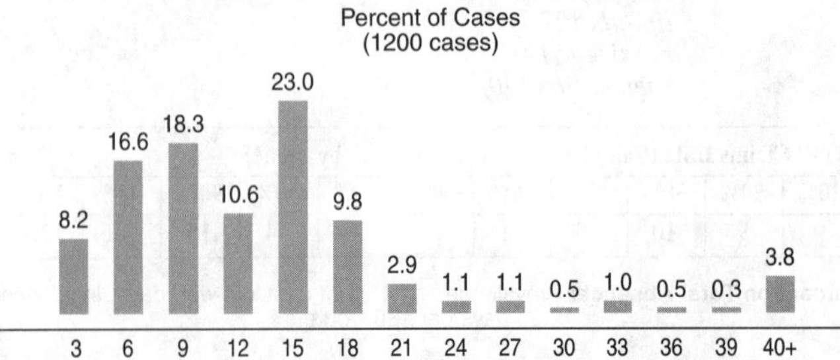

*CDC NHIS cases with no lost workdays: 28 (2.3%)

Impact on Total Absence: Prevalence 0.0488% of total lost workdays; Incidence 0.51 days per 100 workers

486 Pneumonia, organism unspecified

Return-To-Work Summary Guidelines		
Dataset	**Midrange**	**At-Risk**
Claims data	11 days	15 days
All absences	10 days	14 days

Return-To-Work "Best Practice" Guidelines
7-10 days

Description: Inflammation of the lungs due to infection by an unspecified organism. Symptoms usually come suddenly and can include fever, chills, shortness of breath, headache, muscle pain, cough, and occasional chest pain.

Excludes:
hypostatic or passive pneumonia (514)
influenza with pneumonia, any form (487.0)
inhalation or aspiration pneumonia due to foreign materials (507.0-507.8)
pneumonitis due to fumes and vapors (506.0)

486 Pneumonia, organism unspecified *(cont'd)*

Workers' Comp Costs per Claim (based on 55 claims)					
Quartile	25%	50%	75%	Mean	% no cost
Medical	$935	$4,179	$13,524	$12,460	0%
Total	$1,239	$5,082	$25,347	$18,554	0%

RTW Claims Data (Calendar-days away from work by decile)										
10%	20%	30%	40%	**50%**	60%	70%	80%	**90%**	100%	Mean
8	9	10	10	**11**	11	12	14	**15**	365	14.51

Integrated Disability Durations, in days*
Median (mid-point) 10.0 Mean (average) 11.89
Mode (most frequent) 10 Calculated rec. 10

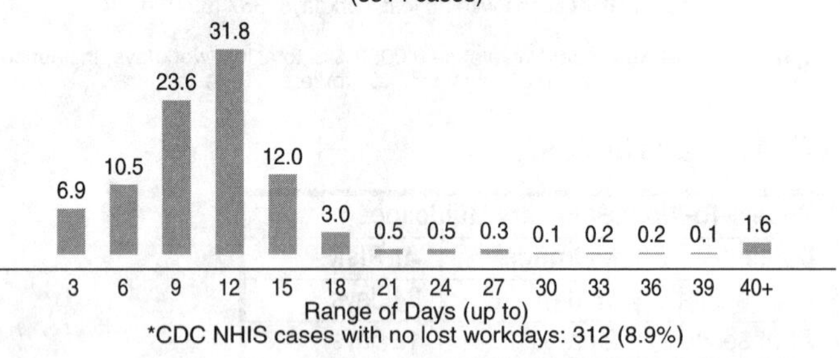

*CDC NHIS cases with no lost workdays: 312 (8.9%)

Impact on Total Absence: Prevalence 0.1125% of total lost workdays; Incidence 1.18 days per 100 workers

Occupational Disability Durations, in days
Median (mid-point) 30 - Benchmark Indemnity Costs $22,500

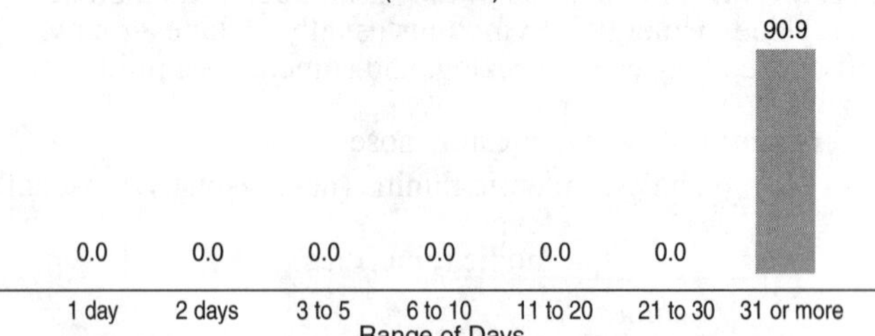

Impact on Occupational Absence: Prevalence 0.0102% of occupational lost workdays

487 Influenza

Return-To-Work Summary Guidelines		
Dataset	**Midrange**	**At-Risk**
Claims data	11 days	14 days
All absences	2 days	12 days

Return-To-Work "Best Practice" Guidelines
2-10 days

Description: A highly contagious viral infection characterized by symptoms of fever, runny nose, cough, headache, malaise, aching, and an inflamed nose and airways. Symptoms are usually sudden and appear 24 to 48 hours after infection, with most lasting two to three days. The fever may last up to five days, and the coughing may last up to 10.
Other names: Flu

Excludes:
Hemophilus influenzae [H. influenzae]:
infection NOS (041.5)
laryngitis (464.0)
meningitis (320.0)
pneumonia (482.2)

487 Influenza *(cont'd)*

Disability Duration Adjustment Factors by Age						
Age Group	18-24	25-34	35-44	45-54	55-64	65-74
Adjustment Factor	0.63	0.79	1.04	1.17	1.89	NA

RTW Claims Data (Calendar-days away from work by decile)										
10%	20%	30%	40%	**50%**	60%	70%	80%	**90%**	100%	Mean
9	9	10	10	**11**	11	12	13	**14**	365	11.13

Integrated Disability Durations, in days*

Median (mid-point)	2.0	Mean (average)	5.19
Mode (most frequent)	2	Calculated rec.	3

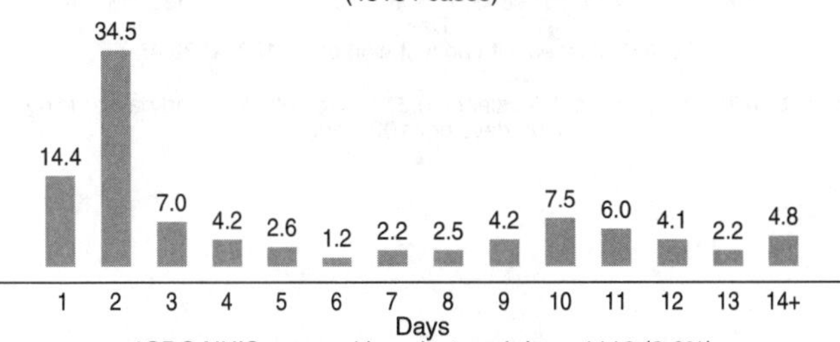

*CDC NHIS cases with no lost workdays: 1116 (2.6%)

Impact on Total Absence: Prevalence 0.6451% of total lost workdays; Incidence 6.77 days per 100 workers

Occupational Disability Durations, in days
Median (mid-point) 2 - Benchmark Indemnity Costs $1,500

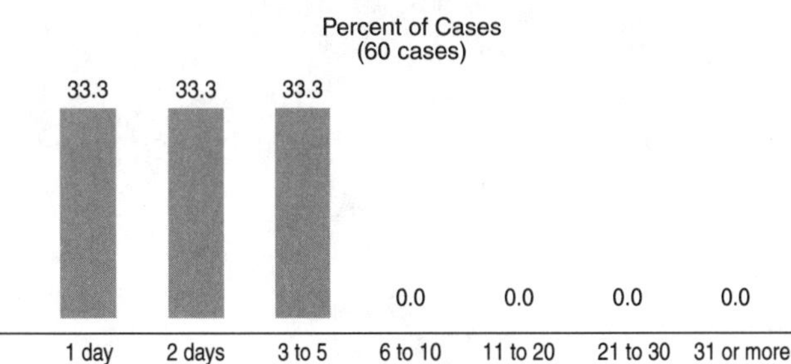

Impact on Occupational Absence: Prevalence 0.0013% of occupational lost workdays

CHRONIC OBSTRUCTIVE PULMONARY DISEASE AND ALLIED CONDITIONS (490-496)

RTW Claims Data (Calendar-days away from work by decile)										
10%	20%	30%	40%	**50%**	60%	70%	80%	**90%**	100%	Mean
9	11	13	14	**15**	16	21	30	**180**	365	52.35

Impact on Total Absence: Prevalence 3.4677% of total lost workdays; Incidence 36.41 days per 100 workers

Occupational Disability Durations, in days
Median (mid-point) 3 - Benchmark Indemnity Costs $2,250

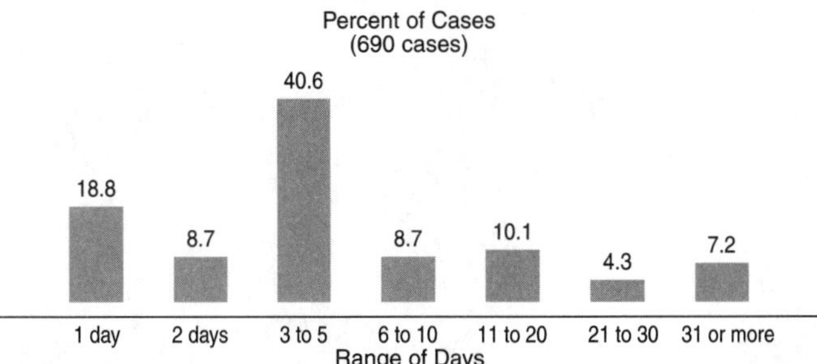

Impact on Occupational Absence: Prevalence 0.0234% of occupational lost workdays

491 Chronic bronchitis

Return-To-Work Summary Guidelines		
Dataset	**Midrange**	**At-Risk**
Claims data	14 days	60 days
All absences	3 days	11 days

Return-To-Work "Best Practice" Guidelines
Pulmonary function testing: 0-1 days
All cases, without work exacerbation (clean environment): 0-3 days

Description: Continuing inflammation of the bronchi (mucous membranes lining the air passages of the lungs) causing secretions to gather in the lungs. This leads to labored breathing, a cough with sputum, or wheezing. The respiratory rate could be elevated and the skin could have a bluish tint.
Other names: Chronic obstructive pulmonary disease (COPD)

Excludes:
chronic obstructive asthma (493.2)

Disability Duration Adjustment Factors by Age						
Age Group	18-24	25-34	35-44	45-54	55-64	65-74
Adjustment Factor	0.49	0.65	1.13	1.28	0.99	0.61

RTW Claims Data (Calendar-days away from work by decile)										
10%	20%	30%	40%	**50%**	60%	70%	80%	**90%**	100%	Mean
9	10	12	14	**14**	15	20	30	**60**	365	29.05

Integrated Disability Durations, in days*

Median (mid-point)	3.0	Mean (average)	6.08
Mode (most frequent)	1	Calculated rec.	3

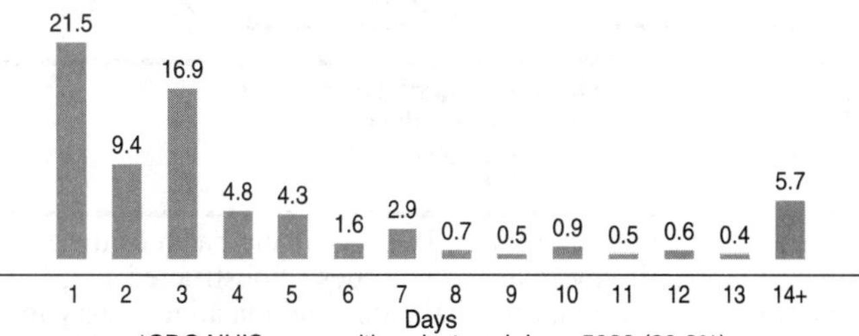

*CDC NHIS cases with no lost workdays: 5088 (29.3%)

Impact on Total Absence: Prevalence 0.2201% of total lost workdays; Incidence 2.31 days per 100 workers

492 Emphysema

Return-To-Work Summary Guidelines		
Dataset	**Midrange**	**At-Risk**
Claims data	16 days	365 days
All absences	15 days	365 days

Return-To-Work "Best Practice" Guidelines
Clerical/modified work: 6 days
Manual work: 14 days
Severe: by report

Description: Enlargement of the tiny air sacs (alveoli) of the lungs, leading to destruction of the alveoli walls and inefficient oxygen absorption and exchange. The main symptom is shortness of breath, which gets worse over time. There could also be a chronic cough, wheezing, and lung infections.

492 Emphysema (cont'd)

Disability Duration Adjustment Factors by Age						
Age Group	18-24	25-34	35-44	45-54	55-64	65-74
Adjustment Factor	NA	NA	NA	1.05	0.51	NA

RTW Claims Data (Calendar-days away from work by decile)										
10%	20%	30%	40%	**50%**	60%	70%	80%	**90%**	100%	Mean
12	14	14	15	**16**	18	364	365	**365**	365	131.47

Integrated Disability Durations, in days*

Median (mid-point)	15.0	Mean (average)	109.79
Mode (most frequent)	14	Calculated rec.	38

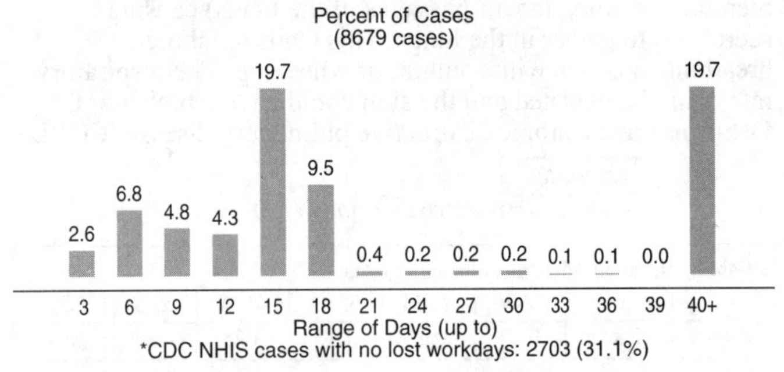

*CDC NHIS cases with no lost workdays: 2703 (31.1%)

Impact on Total Absence: Prevalence 1.9393% of total lost workdays; Incidence 20.36 days per 100 workers

493 Asthma

Return-To-Work Summary Guidelines		
Dataset	**Midrange**	**At-Risk**
Claims data	15 days	32 days
All absences	6 days	28 days

Return-To-Work "Best Practice" Guidelines
Pulmonary function testing: 0-1 days
Without hospitalization: 0-5 days
With hospitalization: 7-28 days

Description: Inflammation of the airways or spasm of the muscles in the airways causing episodes of obstructed breathing, especially upon exhalation. Asthma attacks vary in frequency and severity, and may or may not be triggered by external events.

The following fifth-digit subclassification is for use with category 493:

0 without mention of status asthmaticus
1 with status asthmaticus

Workers' Comp Costs per Claim (based on 302 claims)					
Quartile	25%	50%	75%	Mean	% no cost
Indemnity	$2,940	$7,991	$18,165	$21,835	55%
Medical	$462	$1,040	$4,956	$5,504	8%
Total	$536	$2,846	$11,886	$16,052	7%

Disability Duration Adjustment Factors by Age						
Age Group	18-24	25-34	35-44	45-54	55-64	65-74
Adjustment Factor	0.79	0.65	1.12	1.16	1.67	0.47

RTW Claims Data (Calendar-days away from work by decile)										
10%	20%	30%	40%	**50%**	60%	70%	80%	**90%**	100%	Mean
9	11	13	14	**15**	18	28	29	**32**	365	24.34

493 Asthma (cont'd)

Integrated Disability Durations, in days*

Median (mid-point)	6.0	Mean (average)	11.48
Mode (most frequent)	1	Calculated rec.	6

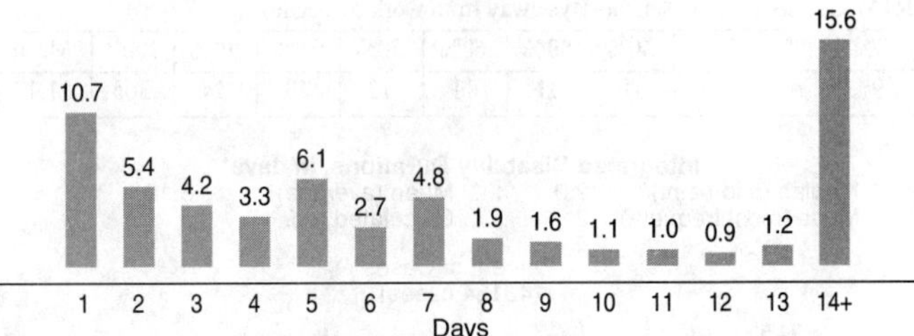

*CDC NHIS cases with no lost workdays: 12884 (39.4%)

Impact on Total Absence: Prevalence 0.6724% of total lost workdays; Incidence 7.06 days per 100 workers

9. DISEASES OF THE DIGESTIVE SYSTEM (520-579)

Impact on Total Absence: Prevalence 3.9374% of total lost workdays; Incidence 41.34 days per 100 workers

RTW Claims Data (Calendar-days away from work by decile)										
10%	20%	30%	40%	**50%**	60%	70%	80%	**90%**	100%	Mean
12	14	18	22	**27**	31	41	43	**55**	365	34.82

DISEASES OF ESOPHAGUS, STOMACH, AND DUODENUM (530-538)

RTW Claims Data (Calendar-days away from work by decile)										
10%	20%	30%	40%	**50%**	60%	70%	80%	**90%**	100%	Mean
11	14	15	20	**21**	24	37	42	**45**	365	31.03

Impact on Total Absence: Prevalence 0.7457% of total lost workdays; Incidence 7.83 days per 100 workers

Occupational Disability Durations, in days
Median (mid-point) 1 - Benchmark Indemnity Costs $750

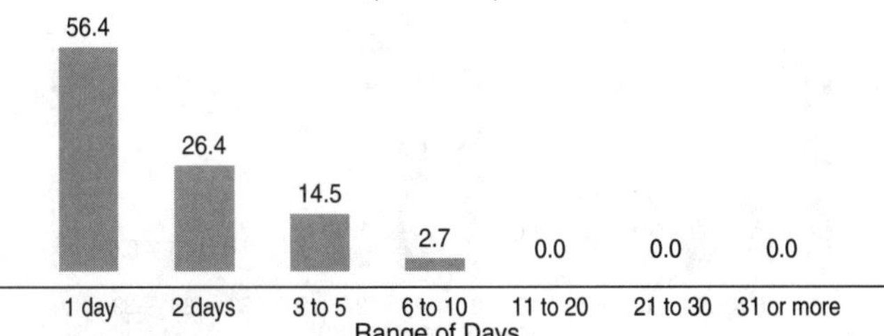

Impact on Occupational Absence: Prevalence 0.0012% of occupational lost workdays

530 Diseases of esophagus

Return-To-Work Summary Guidelines		
Dataset	**Midrange**	**At-Risk**
Claims data	11 days	16 days
All absences	6 days	14 days

Return-To-Work "Best Practice" Guidelines
See 530.0

Excludes:
esophageal varices (456.0-456.2)

Workers' Comp Costs per Claim (based on 30 claims)					
Quartile	25%	50%	75%	Mean	% no cost
Medical	$536	$44,515	$90,069	$141,616	0%
Total	$536	$98,894	$203,207	$205,258	0%

530.1 Esophagitis

Return-To-Work Summary Guidelines		
Dataset	**Midrange**	**At-Risk**
Claims data	13 days	18 days
All absences	9 days	15 days

Return-To-Work "Best Practice" Guidelines
Reflux esophagitis: 0 days
Corrosive esophagitis: 7-14 days

530.1 Esophagitis *(cont'd)*

Description: Inflammation of the esophagus due to infection, ingestion of corrosive chemicals, or acid reflux. Symptoms of infection include painful or difficult swallowing. The ingestion of chemicals causes immediate burning and pain in the mouth and throat. Acid reflux usually causes a burning chest pain that occurs about 30 to 60 minutes after eating.

Abscess of esophagus
Esophagitis:
NOS
chemical
peptic
postoperative
regurgitant
Use additional E code to identify cause, if induced by chemical

Excludes:
tuberculous esophagitis (017.8)

RTW Claims Data (Calendar-days away from work by decile)										
10%	20%	30%	40%	**50%**	60%	70%	80%	**90%**	100%	Mean
8	10	11	12	**13**	14	15	15	**18**	365	16.88

Integrated Disability Durations, in days*
Median (mid-point) 9.0 Mean (average) 11.16
Mode (most frequent) 1 Calculated rec. 8

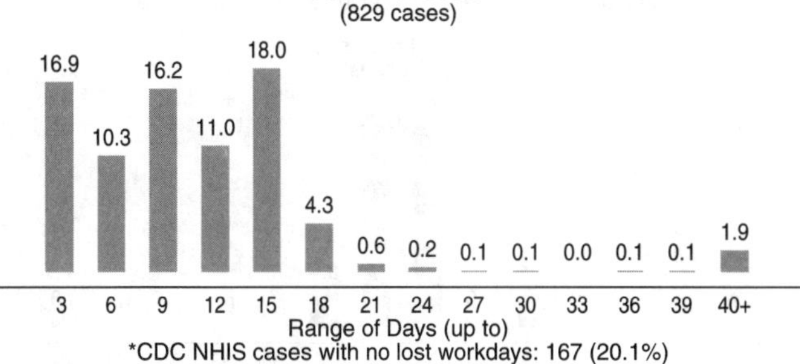

*CDC NHIS cases with no lost workdays: 167 (20.1%)

Impact on Total Absence: Prevalence 0.0218% of total lost workdays; Incidence 0.23 days per 100 workers

531 Gastric ulcer

Return-To-Work Summary Guidelines		
Dataset	**Midrange**	**At-Risk**
Claims data	365 days	365 days
All absences	5 days	365 days

Return-To-Work "Best Practice" Guidelines
See 531.0

Includes: ulcer (peptic):
prepyloric
pylorus
stomach
Use additional E code to identify drug, if drug-induced

Excludes:
peptic ulcer NOS (533.0-533.9)

The following fifth-digit subclassification is for use with category 531:
0 without mention of obstruction
1 with obstruction

531.4 Chronic or unspecified with hemorrhage

Return-To-Work Summary Guidelines		
Dataset	Midrange	At-Risk
Claims data	21 days	24 days
All absences	19 days	23 days

Return-To-Work "Best Practice" Guidelines
Clerical/modified work: 7 days
Manual work: 21 days

Description: Erosion along the upper curve of the stomach caused by stomach acid and digestive juices. Typically an ulcer heals and reoccurs. Some cases are without symptoms. Those that do report symptoms often have an empty, gnawing, hungry feeling, which occurs when the stomach is empty. Some cases also experience belching, bloating, heartburn, nausea, and a sour taste in the mouth. The symptoms may or may not be helped by eating or taking antacids. When hemorrhaging is involved, there could be blood in the stool or vomit.

RTW Claims Data (Calendar-days away from work by decile)										
10%	20%	30%	40%	**50%**	60%	70%	80%	**90%**	100%	Mean
9	11	17	20	**21**	21	22	23	**24**	120	19.36

Integrated Disability Durations, in days*
Median (mid-point) 19.0 Mean (average) 15.87
Mode (most frequent) 21 Calculated rec. 19

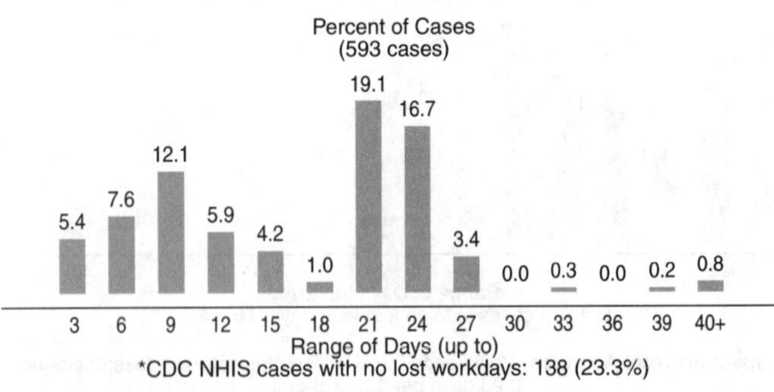

*CDC NHIS cases with no lost workdays: 138 (23.3%)

Impact on Total Absence: Prevalence 0.0213% of total lost workdays; Incidence 0.22 days per 100 workers

532 Duodenal ulcer

Return-To-Work Summary Guidelines		
Dataset	Midrange	At-Risk
Claims data	22 days	44 days
All absences	16 days	43 days

Return-To-Work "Best Practice" Guidelines
Medical treatment: 0 days
Endoscopy: 1 day
Laparoscopic surgery: 7 days
Vagotomy, clerical/modified work: 21 days
Vagotomy, manual work: 42 days

Description: The most common type of ulcer, occurring within the first few inches of the small intestine, just below the stomach. Typically an ulcer heals and reoccurs. Some cases are without symptoms. Those that do report symptoms often have an empty, gnawing, hungry feeling that occurs when the stomach is empty. Some cases also experience belching, bloating, heartburn, nausea, and a sour taste in the mouth. The symptoms may or may not be helped by eating or taking antacids. When hemorrhaging is involved, there could be blood in the stool or vomit.

532 Duodenal ulcer *(cont'd)*

Includes: erosion (acute) of duodenum
ulcer (peptic):
duodenum
postpyloric

Use additional E code to identify drug, if drug-induced

Excludes:
peptic ulcer NOS (533.0-533.9)

The following fifth-digit subclassification is for use with category 532:
0 without mention of obstruction
1 with obstruction

RTW Claims Data (Calendar-days away from work by decile)										
10%	20%	30%	40%	**50%**	60%	70%	80%	**90%**	100%	Mean
10	14	20	21	**22**	24	41	42	**44**	365	27.40

Integrated Disability Durations, in days*
Median (mid-point) 16.0 Mean (average) 19.38
Mode (most frequent) 1 Calculated rec. 13

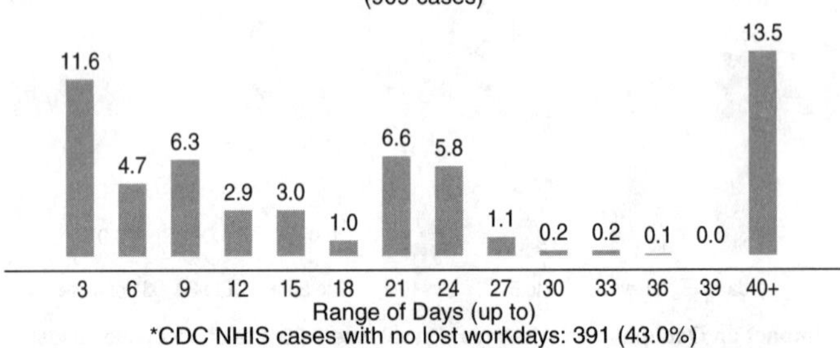

*CDC NHIS cases with no lost workdays: 391 (43.0%)

Impact on Total Absence: Prevalence 0.0296% of total lost workdays; Incidence 0.31 days per 100 workers

533 Peptic ulcer, site unspecified

Return-To-Work Summary Guidelines		
Dataset	Midrange	At-Risk
Claims data	29 days	43 days
All absences	22 days	42 days

Return-To-Work "Best Practice" Guidelines
Medical treatment: 0 days
Endoscopy: 1 day
Vagotomy, clerical/modified work: 21 days
Vagotomy, manual work: 35 days
Gastrectomy, clerical/modified work: 28 days
Gastrectomy, manual work: 42 days

Description: Erosion of the stomach or intestine caused stomach acid and digestive juices. Typically an ulcer heals and reoccurs. Some cases are without symptoms. Those that do report symptoms often have an empty, gnawing, hungry feeling that occurs when the stomach is empty. Some cases also experience belching, bloating, heartburn, nausea, and a sour taste in the mouth. The symptoms may or may not be helped by eating or taking antacids. When hemorrhaging is involved, there could be blood in the stool or vomit.

Includes: gastroduodenal ulcer NOS
peptic ulcer NOS
stress ulcer NOS

Use additional E code to identify drug, if drug-induced

533 Peptic ulcer, site unspecified *(cont'd)*

Excludes:
peptic ulcer:
duodenal (532.0-532.9)
gastric (531.0-531.9)

The following fifth-digit subclassification is for use with category 533:
0 without mention of obstruction
1 with obstruction

RTW Claims Data (Calendar-days away from work by decile)										
10%	20%	30%	40%	**50%**	60%	70%	80%	**90%**	100%	Mean
14	20	22	27	**29**	34	36	41	**43**	351	30.87

Integrated Disability Durations, in days*
Median (mid-point) 22.0 Mean (average) 23.49
Mode (most frequent) 1 Calculated rec. 17

Percent of Cases
(702 cases)

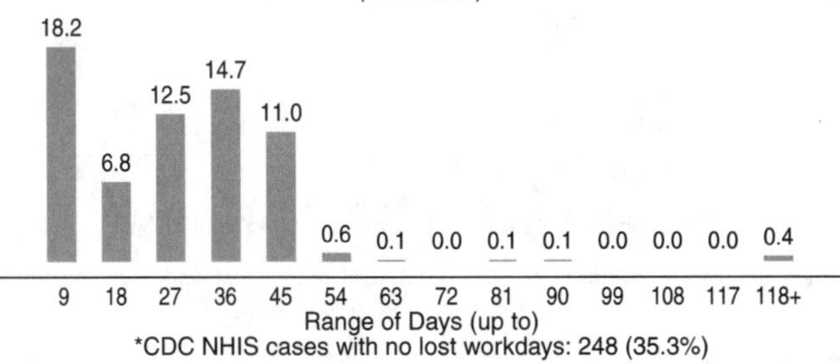

Range of Days (up to)
*CDC NHIS cases with no lost workdays: 248 (35.3%)

Impact on Total Absence: Prevalence 0.0315% of total lost workdays; Incidence 0.33 days per 100 workers

HERNIA OF ABDOMINAL CAVITY (550-553)

Includes: hernia:
acquired
congenital, except diaphragmatic or hiatal

RTW Claims Data (Calendar-days away from work by decile)										
10%	20%	30%	40%	**50%**	60%	70%	80%	**90%**	100%	Mean
14	16	20	23	**28**	36	43	49	**57**	365	33.81

Impact on Total Absence: Prevalence 1.4231% of total lost workdays; Incidence 14.94 days per 100 workers

Occupational Disability Durations, in days
Median (mid-point) 24 - Benchmark Indemnity Costs $18,000

Percent of Cases
(18720 cases)

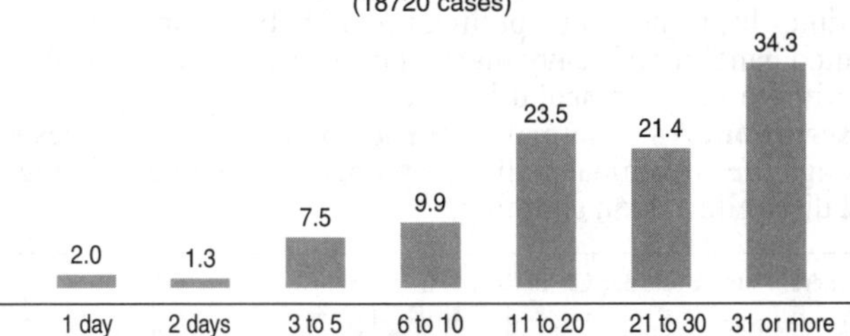

Range of Days

Impact on Occupational Absence: Prevalence 5.0967% of occupational lost workdays; Incidence 0.82 days per 100 workers

550 Inguinal hernia

Return-To-Work Summary Guidelines		
Dataset	**Midrange**	**At-Risk**
Claims data	30 days	58 days
All absences	28 days	57 days

550 Inguinal hernia *(cont'd)*

Return-To-Work "Best Practice" Guidelines
Without surgery (truss), light work: 0 days
With endoscopic surgery, clerical/modified work: 7 days
With endoscopic surgery, manual work: 14 days
With endoscopic surgery, heavy manual work: 28 days
With open surgery, clerical/modified work: 14 days
With open surgery, manual work: 21-28 days
With open surgery, heavy manual work: 42-56 days
With open surgery, bilateral, heavy manual work: 42-56 days
Additional time to re-do hernia repair: 14-28 days

Capabilities & Activity Modifications:
Clerical/modified work: Lifting and carrying not more than 5 lbs up to 3 times/hr; pushing and pulling up to 10 lbs 3 times/hr; no handling of heavy machinery; driving car up to 2 hrs/day.
Manual work: Lifting and carrying not more than 20 lbs up to 10 times/hr; pushing and pulling up to 35 lbs 10 times/hr; limited handling of heavy machinery restricted by physical effort involved; driving car up to 2 hrs/day.
Description: Most likely to happen to men over 40, an inguinal hernia happens when a loop or bulge in the intestine pushes through the abdominal wall near the groin, where the wall is weakest. There could be a swelling in the groin that can cause discomfort when straining or coughing. If a portion of the intestine gets trapped in the scrotum, the blood supply may be cut off and the intestine may become gangrenous.

Includes: bubonocele
inguinal hernia (direct) (double) (indirect) (oblique) (sliding)
scrotal hernia

The following fifth-digit subclassification is for use with category 550:
0 unilateral or unspecified (not specified as recurrent)
Unilateral NOS
1 unilateral or unspecified, recurrent
2 bilateral (not specified as recurrent)
Bilateral NOS
3 bilateral, recurrent

Procedure Summary (from ODG Treatment): Activity restrictions; Antibiotic prophylaxis (for hernia repair); Laparoscopic repair (surgery); Mesh repair (surgery); Physical therapy (PT); Post-herniorrhaphy pain syndrome; Post-op ambulatory infusion pumps (local anesthetic); Return to work; Shouldice repair (surgery); Surgery; Transverse incisions (surgery); Truss (support); Work

Workers' Comp Costs per Claim (based on 7,300 claims)					
Quartile	25%	50%	75%	Mean	% no cost
Indemnity	$1,617	$2,793	$4,788	$3,984	34%
Medical	$2,636	$4,253	$5,733	$4,579	1%
Total	$3,959	$6,038	$8,925	$7,197	1%

RTW Claims Data (Calendar-days away from work by decile)										
10%	20%	30%	40%	**50%**	60%	70%	80%	**90%**	100%	Mean
14	17	21	27	**30**	38	43	49	**58**	365	34.79

RTW Post Surgery (Calendar-days away from work by decile)										
10%	20%	30%	40%	**50%**	60%	70%	80%	**90%**	100%	Mean
Prp i/hern init reduc >5 yr										
13	18	23	27	**32**	38	41	46	**55**	365	36.94
Prp i/hern init block >5 yr										
10	17	25	29	**34**	38	41	45	**55**	125	34.21
Rerepair ing hernia, reduce										
14	21	26	31	**37**	41	46	55	**76**	365	50.17

550 Inguinal hernia *(cont'd)*

Integrated Disability Durations, in days*

Median (mid-point) 28.0 Mean (average) 30.89
Mode (most frequent) 1 Calculated rec. 22

Percent of Cases
(3394 cases)

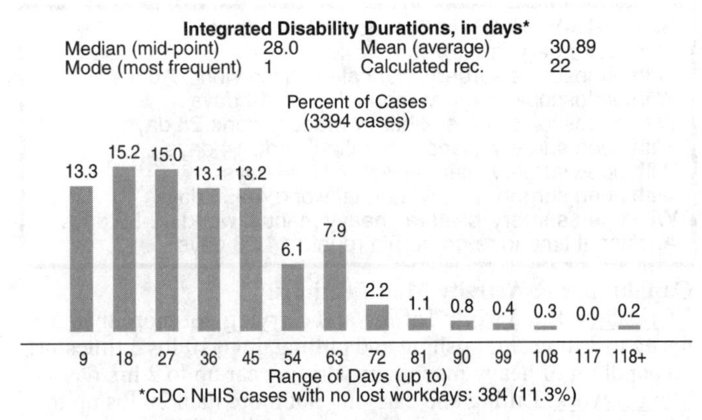

Range of Days (up to)
*CDC NHIS cases with no lost workdays: 384 (11.3%)

Impact on Total Absence: Prevalence 0.2748% of total lost workdays; Incidence 2.89 days per 100 workers

Occupational Disability Durations, in days

Median (mid-point) 24 - Benchmark Indemnity Costs $18,000

Percent of Cases
(7470 cases)

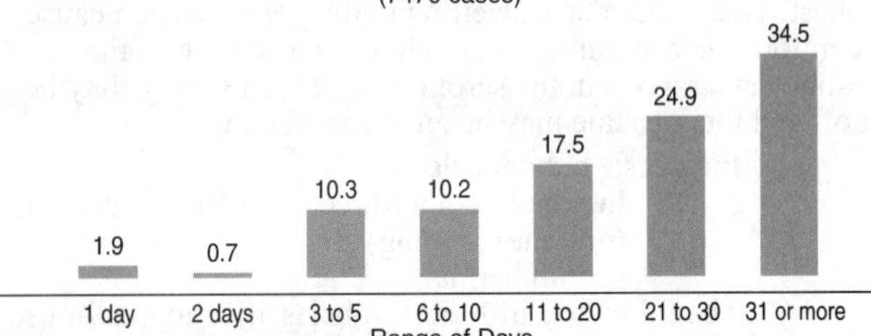

Range of Days

Impact on Occupational Absence: Prevalence 2.0338% of occupational lost workdays; Incidence 0.33 days per 100 workers

553 Other hernia of abdominal cavity without mention of obstruction or gangrene

Return-To-Work Summary Guidelines		
Dataset	**Midrange**	**At-Risk**
Claims data	25 days	56 days
All absences	21 days	56 days

Return-To-Work "Best Practice" Guidelines
See 553.9

Excludes:
the listed conditions with mention of:
gangrene (and obstruction) (551.0-551.9)
obstruction (552.0-552.9)

Workers' Comp Costs per Claim (based on 2,200 claims)					
Quartile	25%	50%	75%	Mean	% no cost
Indemnity	$1,974	$3,145	$5,051	$4,979	35%
Medical	$2,405	$4,200	$6,321	$5,532	2%
Total	$3,749	$6,269	$9,765	$8,763	1%

RTW Claims Data (Calendar-days away from work by decile)										
10%	20%	30%	40%	**50%**	60%	70%	80%	**90%**	100%	Mean
13	15	17	21	**25**	32	42	46	**56**	365	31.78

553 Other hernia of abdominal cavity without mention of obstruction or gangrene *(cont'd)*

RTW Post Surgery (Calendar-days away from work by decile)										
10%	20%	30%	40%	**50%**	60%	70%	80%	**90%**	100%	Mean
Rpr ventral hern init, reduc										
12	20	27	31	**35**	41	45	50	**77**	365	47.18
Rpr umbil hern, block > 5 yr										
12	17	23	27	**32**	37	42	47	**59**	276	40.90

Integrated Disability Durations, in days*

Median (mid-point) 21.0 Mean (average) 26.57
Mode (most frequent) 1 Calculated rec. 17

Percent of Cases
(8058 cases)

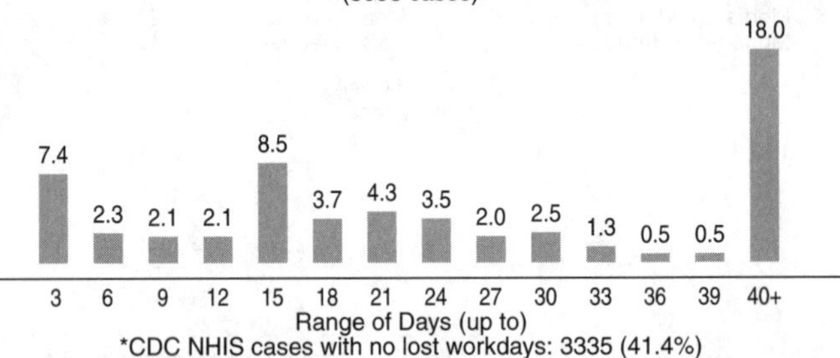

Range of Days (up to)
*CDC NHIS cases with no lost workdays: 3335 (41.4%)

Impact on Total Absence: Prevalence 0.3709% of total lost workdays; Incidence 3.90 days per 100 workers

553.2 Ventral hernia

Return-To-Work Summary Guidelines		
Dataset	**Midrange**	**At-Risk**
Claims data	40 days	61 days
All absences	33 days	60 days

Return-To-Work "Best Practice" Guidelines
Without surgery (truss), light work: 0 days
With surgery, clerical/modified work: 14 days
With surgery, manual work: 21 days
With surgery, heavy manual work: 49-56 days

Capabilities & Activity Modifications:
Clerical/modified work: Lifting and carrying not more than 5 lbs up to 3 times/hr; pushing and pulling up to 10 lbs 3 times/hr; no handling of heavy machinery; personal driving only.
Manual work: Lifting and carrying not more than 20 lbs up to 10 times/hr; pushing and pulling up to 35 lbs 10 times/hr; limited handling of heavy machinery restricted by physical effort involved; personal driving only.
Description: An abnormal protrusion of an organ or tissues through the abdominal wall. Symptoms include unusual bulges and discomfort upon straining.

Workers' Comp Costs per Claim (based on 714 claims)					
Quartile	25%	50%	75%	Mean	% no cost
Indemnity	$2,247	$3,476	$5,964	$6,620	28%
Medical	$3,371	$5,345	$8,873	$7,721	2%
Total	$4,788	$7,980	$13,146	$12,364	0%

RTW Claims Data (Calendar-days away from work by decile)										
10%	20%	30%	40%	**50%**	60%	70%	80%	**90%**	100%	Mean
14	18	22	28	**40**	47	50	56	**61**	365	40.45

553.2 Ventral hernia *(cont'd)*

RTW Post Surgery (Calendar-days away from work by decile)										
10%	20%	30%	40%	**50%**	60%	70%	80%	**90%**	100%	Mean
Rpr ventral hern init, reduc										
12	20	27	30	**34**	41	45	48	**60**	365	44.92

Integrated Disability Durations, in days*

Median (mid-point) 33.0 Mean (average) 36.37
Mode (most frequent) 1 Calculated rec. 26

Percent of Cases
(1014 cases)

10.7 15.2 13.3 6.9 7.3 16.2 10.9 2.1 1.5 1.7 0.5 0.2 0.1 0.8

9 18 27 36 45 54 63 72 81 90 99 108 117 118+
Range of Days (up to)
*CDC NHIS cases with no lost workdays: 129 (12.7%)

Impact on Total Absence: Prevalence 0.0951% of total lost workdays; Incidence 1.00 days per 100 workers

Occupational Disability Durations, in days

Median (mid-point) 18 - Benchmark Indemnity Costs $13,500

Percent of Cases
(1600 cases)

2.5 0.0 8.1 8.1 35.0 15.0 31.3

1 day 2 days 3 to 5 6 to 10 11 to 20 21 to 30 31 or more
Range of Days

Impact on Occupational Absence: Prevalence 0.3267% of occupational lost workdays; Incidence 0.05 days per 100 workers

553.3 Diaphragmatic hernia

Return-To-Work Summary Guidelines		
Dataset	**Midrange**	**At-Risk**
Claims data	28 days	56 days
All absences	22 days	51 days

Return-To-Work "Best Practice" Guidelines
Medical treatment: 0 days
Surgery, endoscopic, clerical/modified work: 14 days
Surgery, endoscopic, manual work: 28 days
Surgery, abdominal, clerical/modified work: 21 days
Surgery, abdominal, manual work: 35 days
Surgery, transthoracic, clerical/modified work: 28 days
Surgery, transthoracic, manual work: 49-56 days

Capabilities & Activity Modifications:
Clerical/modified work: Lifting and carrying not more than 5 lbs up to 3 times/hr; pushing and pulling up to 10 lbs 3 times/hr; no handling of heavy machinery; personal driving only.
Manual work: Lifting and carrying not more than 20 lbs up to 10 times/hr; pushing and pulling up to 35 lbs 10 times/hr; limited handling of heavy machinery restricted by physical effort involved; personal driving only.
Description: Protrusion of the abdominal contents through the chest because of an opening in the respiratory diaphragm through which the esophagus passes, causing stomach acid to

553.3 Diaphragmatic hernia *(cont'd)*

flow backward into the esophagus. Heartburn, chest pain, regurgitation of stomach acid, and/or a feeling that food is stuck in the chest or upper abdomen may be noticed.

Hernia:
- hiatal (esophageal) (sliding)
- paraesophageal

Thoracic stomach

Excludes:
congenital:
- *diaphragmatic hernia (756.6)*
- *hiatal hernia (750.6)*

esophagocele (530.6)

RTW Claims Data (Calendar-days away from work by decile)										
10%	20%	30%	40%	**50%**	60%	70%	80%	**90%**	100%	Mean
13	15	20	22	**28**	31	36	49	**53**	365	31.57

Integrated Disability Durations, in days*

Median (mid-point) 22.0 Mean (average) 25.77
Mode (most frequent) 1 Calculated rec. 18

Percent of Cases
(2933 cases)

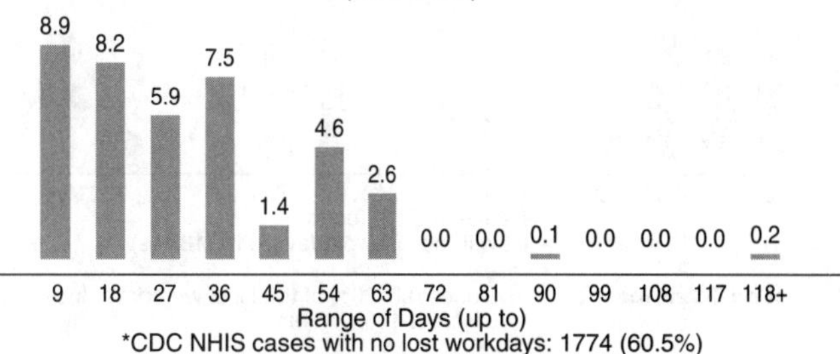

Range of Days (up to)
*CDC NHIS cases with no lost workdays: 1774 (60.5%)

Impact on Total Absence: Prevalence 0.0882% of total lost workdays; Incidence 0.93 days per 100 workers

Occupational Disability Durations, in days

Median (mid-point) 20 - Benchmark Indemnity Costs $15,000

Percent of Cases
(420 cases)

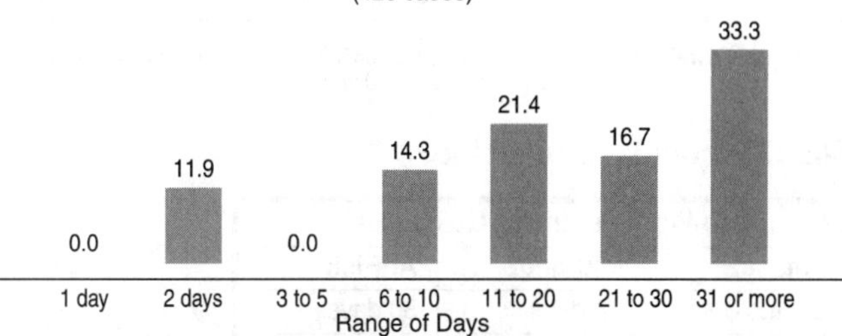

Range of Days

Impact on Occupational Absence: Prevalence 0.0952% of occupational lost workdays; Incidence 0.02 days per 100 workers

NONINFECTIOUS ENTERITIS AND COLITIS (555-558)

RTW Claims Data (Calendar-days away from work by decile)										
10%	20%	30%	40%	**50%**	60%	70%	80%	**90%**	100%	Mean
13	19	27	28	**30**	36	42	43	**49**	365	36.32

Impact on Total Absence: Prevalence 0.3337% of total lost workdays; Incidence 3.50 days per 100 workers

556 Ulcerative colitis

Return-To-Work Summary Guidelines		
Dataset	**Midrange**	**At-Risk**
Claims data	29 days	45 days
All absences	14 days	44 days

556 Ulcerative colitis *(cont'd)*

Return-To-Work "Best Practice" Guidelines
Medical treatment: 0 days
Medical treatment, acute flares: 7 days
Colectomy, clerical/modified work: 28 days
Colectomy, manual work: 42 days

Description: Chronic inflammation of the large colon causing rectal bleeding, violent diarrhea, fever, and abdominal pain. Symptoms could be sudden or gradual.

RTW Claims Data (Calendar-days away from work by decile)										
10%	20%	30%	40%	**50%**	60%	70%	80%	**90%**	100%	Mean
9	12	16	28	**29**	31	42	43	**45**	333	36.89

Integrated Disability Durations, in days*

Median (mid-point)	14.0	Mean (average)	26.66
Mode (most frequent)	1	Calculated rec.	14

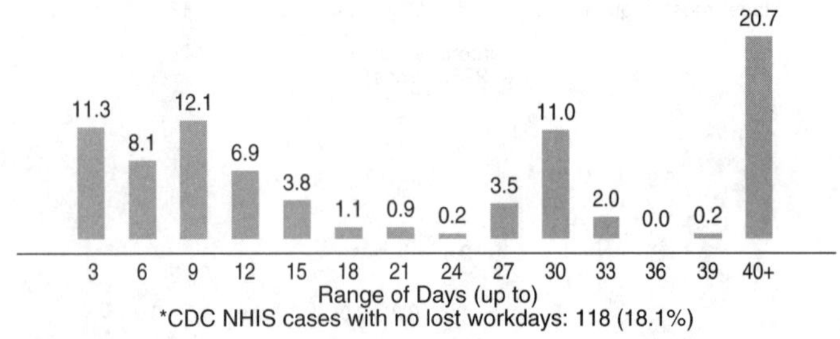

*CDC NHIS cases with no lost workdays: 118 (18.1%)

Impact on Total Absence: Prevalence 0.0420% of total lost workdays; Incidence 0.44 days per 100 workers

OTHER DISEASES OF INTESTINES AND PERITONEUM (560-569)

RTW Claims Data (Calendar-days away from work by decile)										
10%	20%	30%	40%	**50%**	60%	70%	80%	**90%**	100%	Mean
11	14	15	20	**28**	29	40	42	**46**	365	32.78

Impact on Total Absence: Prevalence 0.2984% of total lost workdays; Incidence 3.13 days per 100 workers

562 Diverticula of intestine

Return-To-Work Summary Guidelines

Dataset	Midrange	At-Risk
Claims data	18 days	30 days
All absences	16 days	30 days

Description: Diverticulosis is the presence of pouch-like herniations in the wall of the intestine; Diverticulitis is the inflammation of those herniations.

Use additional code to identify any associated:
peritonitis (567.0-567.9)

Excludes:
congenital diverticulum of colon (751.5)
diverticulum of appendix (543.9)
Meckel's diverticulum (751.0)

562.1 Colon

Return-To-Work Summary Guidelines

Dataset	Midrange	At-Risk
Claims data	30 days	45 days
All absences	28 days	44 days

562.1 Colon *(cont'd)*

Return-To-Work "Best Practice" Guidelines
Medical treatment: 0 days
Sigmoidoscopy: 0-1 days
Colectomy, clerical/modified work: 28 days
Colectomy, manual work: 42 days

Description: Infection and inflammation of the small outpouchings (diverticulum) of the colon. Symptoms may include fever, localized pain, nausea, diarrhea, and/or constipation, although many cases have no symptoms.
Other names: Diverticulitis of the large intestine

RTW Claims Data (Calendar-days away from work by decile)										
10%	20%	30%	40%	**50%**	60%	70%	80%	**90%**	100%	Mean
14	25	28	29	**30**	41	42	43	**45**	365	36.88

Integrated Disability Durations, in days*

Median (mid-point)	28.0	Mean (average)	27.07
Mode (most frequent)	1	Calculated rec.	21

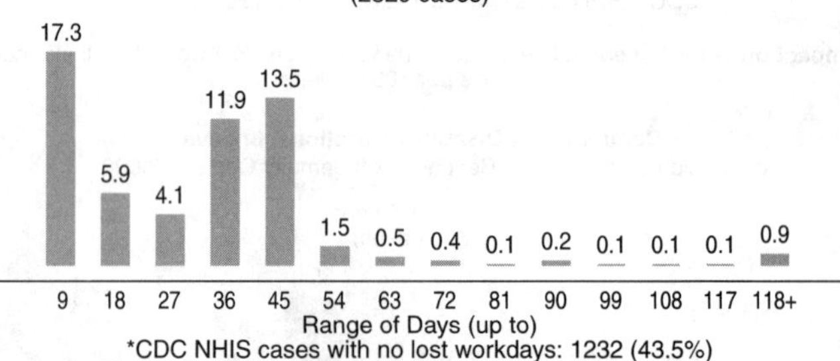

*CDC NHIS cases with no lost workdays: 1232 (43.5%)

Impact on Total Absence: Prevalence 0.1277% of total lost workdays; Incidence 1.34 days per 100 workers

564 Functional digestive disorders, not elsewhere classified

Return-To-Work Summary Guidelines

Dataset	Midrange	At-Risk
Claims data	40 days	119 days
All absences	13 days	119 days

Return-To-Work "Best Practice" Guidelines
See 564.9

Excludes:
functional disorders of stomach (536.0-536.9)
those specified as psychogenic (306.4)

Workers' Comp Costs per Claim (based on 30 claims)					
Quartile	25%	50%	75%	Mean	% no cost
Indemnity	$51,398	$215,891	$315,861	$250,181	6%
Medical	$77,333	$140,616	$246,131	$235,826	0%
Total	$167,024	$341,003	$762,888	$470,371	0%

564.0 Constipation

Return-To-Work Summary Guidelines

Dataset	Midrange	At-Risk
Claims data	15 days	99 days
All absences	2 days	14 days

Return-To-Work "Best Practice" Guidelines
0 days

564.0 Constipation *(cont'd)*

Description: Infrequent or uncomfortable bowel movements, defined by the passage of hard stools or no stools at all. There may also be a feeling the rectum has not been fully emptied.
Other names: Sluggish bowels

RTW Claims Data (Calendar-days away from work by decile)										
10%	20%	30%	40%	**50%**	60%	70%	80%	**90%**	100%	Mean
10	12	13	14	**15**	16	20	25	**99**	365	40.28

Integrated Disability Durations, in days*
Median (mid-point) 2.0 Mean (average) 8.20
Mode (most frequent) 1 Calculated rec. 3

Percent of Cases
(2735 cases)

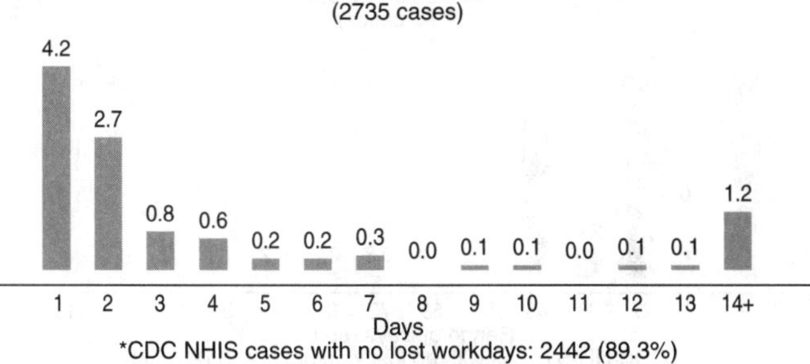

Days
*CDC NHIS cases with no lost workdays: 2442 (89.3%)

Impact on Total Absence: Prevalence 0.0071% of total lost workdays; Incidence 0.07 days per 100 workers

564.1 Irritable bowel syndrome

Return-To-Work Summary Guidelines		
Dataset	**Midrange**	**At-Risk**
Claims data	15 days	27 days
All absences	5 days	17 days

Return-To-Work "Best Practice" Guidelines
Medical treatment: 1-3 days
With hospitalization: 14 days

Description: A disorder of the gastrointestinal tract that causes episodes of bloating, gas, loose stools or constipation, and abdominal pain. The disorder is more frequent in women than men and is often associated with anxiety, stress, or depression, as well as the ingestion of irritants such as coffee or abuse of laxatives.
Other names: Spastic/Irritable colon, IBS, Spastic bowel, Nervous colon, Functional bowel syndrome

Colitis:
- adaptive
- membranous
- mucous

Enterospasm
Irritable bowel syndrome
Spastic colon

RTW Claims Data (Calendar-days away from work by decile)										
10%	20%	30%	40%	**50%**	60%	70%	80%	**90%**	100%	Mean
12	13	14	14	**15**	15	16	18	**27**	365	22.79

564.1 Irritable bowel syndrome *(cont'd)*

Integrated Disability Durations, in days*
Median (mid-point) 5.0 Mean (average) 11.68
Mode (most frequent) 1 Calculated rec. 6

Percent of Cases
(1631 cases)

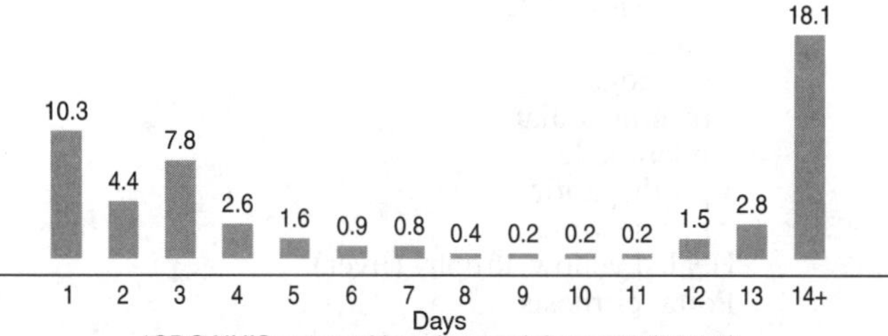

Days
*CDC NHIS cases with no lost workdays: 788 (48.3%)

Impact on Total Absence: Prevalence 0.0291% of total lost workdays; Incidence 0.31 days per 100 workers

OTHER DISEASES OF DIGESTIVE SYSTEM (570-579)

RTW Claims Data (Calendar-days away from work by decile)										
10%	20%	30%	40%	**50%**	60%	70%	80%	**90%**	100%	Mean
12	14	17	21	**27**	29	40	42	**46**	365	41.47

Impact on Total Absence: Prevalence 1.0207% of total lost workdays; Incidence 10.72 days per 100 workers

Occupational Disability Durations, in days
Median (mid-point) 6 - Benchmark Indemnity Costs $4,500

Percent of Cases
(44 cases)

37.9 0.0 0.0 21.9 40.2 0.0 0.0
1 day 2 days 3 to 5 6 to 10 11 to 20 21 to 30 31 or more
Range of Days

Impact on Occupational Absence: Prevalence 0.0029% of occupational lost workdays

571 Chronic liver disease and cirrhosis

Return-To-Work Summary Guidelines		
Dataset	**Midrange**	**At-Risk**
Claims data	16 days	113 days
All absences	14 days	60 days

571.5 Cirrhosis of liver without mention of alcohol

Return-To-Work Summary Guidelines		
Dataset	**Midrange**	**At-Risk**
Claims data	31 days	365 days
All absences	22 days	364 days

Return-To-Work "Best Practice" Guidelines
Asymptomatic, abstinence from alcohol: 0 days
Symptomatic: 5 days
Severe disruption of liver function, clerical/modified work: 21 days
Severe disruption of liver function, manual work: 42 days to indefinite

571.5 Cirrhosis of liver without mention of alcohol *(cont'd)*

Description: Irreversible destruction of liver tissue resulting from a virus or disease. Some people have no symptoms for years, while some cases report a poor appetite, jaundice, malaise, water retention, and weakness.

Cirrhosis of liver:
- NOS
- cryptogenic
- macronodular
- micronodular
- posthepatitic
- postnecrotic

Healed yellow atrophy (liver)
Portal cirrhosis

RTW Claims Data (Calendar-days away from work by decile)

10%	20%	30%	40%	**50%**	60%	70%	80%	**90%**	100%	Mean
15	20	21	22	**31**	42	43	45	**365**	365	75.41

Integrated Disability Durations, in days*

Median (mid-point)	22.0	Mean (average)	61.50
Mode (most frequent)	21	Calculated rec.	32

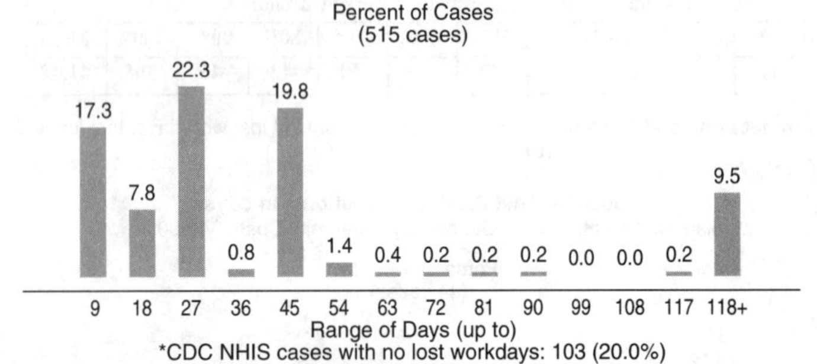

*CDC NHIS cases with no lost workdays: 103 (20.0%)

Impact on Total Absence: Prevalence 0.0748% of total lost workdays; Incidence 0.79 days per 100 workers

573 Other disorders of liver

Return-To-Work Summary Guidelines

Dataset	Midrange	At-Risk
Claims data	41 days	365 days
All absences	23 days	364 days

Return-To-Work "Best Practice" Guidelines
Asymptomatic: 0 days
Severe disruption of liver function, clerical/modified work: 21 days
Severe disruption of liver function, manual work: 42 days to indefinite

Description: Any condition that affects the ability of the liver to function, including metabolic disturbances, tumors, abscesses, cysts, and liver cell disorders or destruction. Symptoms may include jaundice, abdominal pain, weakness, fever, chills, dark urine, loss of appetite, and menstrual problems.

Other names: Liver disease

Excludes:
amyloid or lardaceous degeneration of liver (277.3)
congenital cystic disease of liver (751.62)
glycogen infiltration of liver (271.0)
hepatomegaly NOS (789.1)
portal vein obstruction (452)

573 Other disorders of liver *(cont'd)*

Disability Duration Adjustment Factors by Age

Age Group	18-24	25-34	35-44	45-54	55-64	65-74
Adjustment Factor	NA	0.83	1.27	0.83	0.99	NA

RTW Claims Data (Calendar-days away from work by decile)

10%	20%	30%	40%	**50%**	60%	70%	80%	**90%**	100%	Mean
15	21	22	24	**41**	42	44	90	**365**	365	90.99

Integrated Disability Durations, in days*

Median (mid-point)	23.0	Mean (average)	69.29
Mode (most frequent)	1	Calculated rec.	29

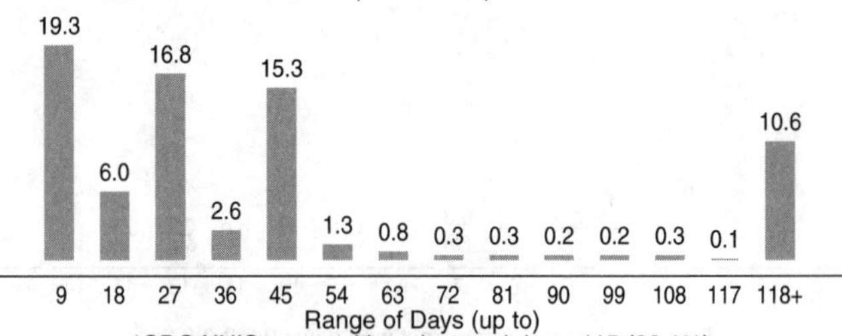

*CDC NHIS cases with no lost workdays: 415 (26.1%)

Impact on Total Absence: Prevalence 0.2406% of total lost workdays; Incidence 2.53 days per 100 workers

574 Cholelithiasis

Return-To-Work Summary Guidelines

Dataset	Midrange	At-Risk
Claims data	25 days	43 days
All absences	20 days	43 days

Return-To-Work "Best Practice" Guidelines
See 574.0

The following fifth-digit subclassification is for use with category 574:
0 without mention of obstruction
1 with obstruction

RTW Claims Data (Calendar-days away from work by decile)

10%	20%	30%	40%	**50%**	60%	70%	80%	**90%**	100%	Mean
13	14	16	21	**25**	28	30	41	**43**	365	26.46

Integrated Disability Durations, in days*

Median (mid-point)	20.0	Mean (average)	22.04
Mode (most frequent)	14	Calculated rec.	19

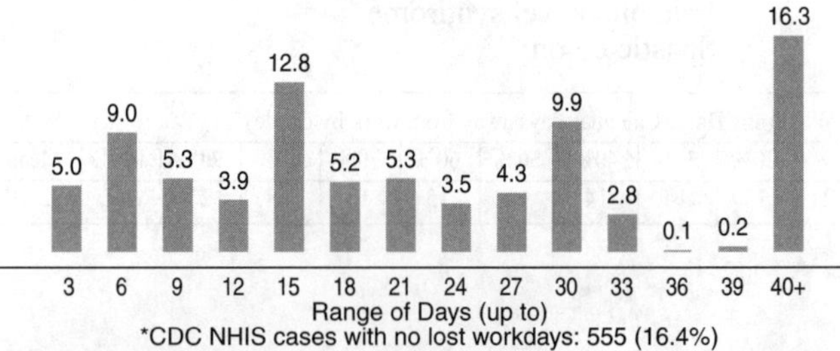

*CDC NHIS cases with no lost workdays: 555 (16.4%)

Impact on Total Absence: Prevalence 0.1841% of total lost workdays; Incidence 1.93 days per 100 workers

574.2 Calculus of gallbladder without mention of cholecystitis

Return-To-Work Summary Guidelines		
Dataset	**Midrange**	**At-Risk**
Claims data	27 days	43 days
All absences	15 days	43 days

Return-To-Work "Best Practice" Guidelines
Medical treatment: 0 days
Lithotripsy: 4 days
Cholecystectomy, laparoscopic: 14 days
Cholecystectomy, open, clerical/modified work: 28 days
Cholecystectomy, open, manual work: 42 days

Description: Collection of crystals formed from cholesterol or calcium salts in the gallbladder. Symptoms may not be present at first, if ever. The gallstones could eventually erode the gallbladder and enter the large or small intestine, causing an intestinal obstruction. If there is pain, it usually follows a large fatty meal.
Other names: Gallstones, Gallbladder calculus
Biliary:
calculus NOS
colic NOS
Calculus of cystic duct
Cholelithiasis NOS
Colic (recurrent) of gallbladder
Gallstone (impacted)

RTW Claims Data (Calendar-days away from work by decile)										
10%	20%	30%	40%	**50%**	60%	70%	80%	**90%**	100%	Mean
12	14	15	18	**27**	29	32	42	**43**	365	26.89

Integrated Disability Durations, in days*

Median (mid-point)	15.0	Mean (average)	20.66
Mode (most frequent)	14	Calculated rec.	16

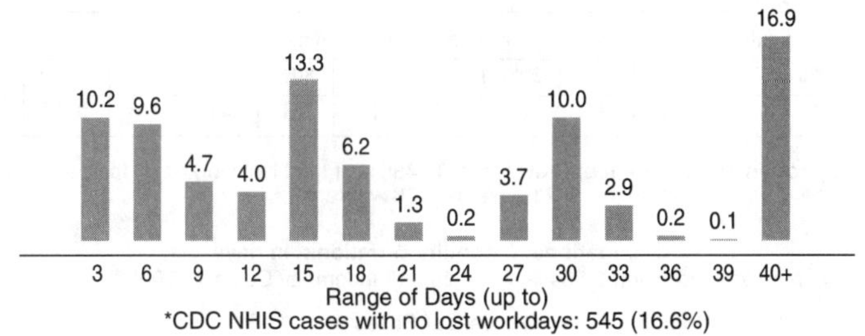

*CDC NHIS cases with no lost workdays: 545 (16.6%)

Impact on Total Absence: Prevalence 0.1666% of total lost workdays; Incidence 1.75 days per 100 workers

10. DISEASES OF THE GENITOURINARY SYSTEM (580-629)

Impact on Total Absence: Prevalence 1.3697% of total lost workdays; Incidence 14.38 days per 100 workers

RTW Claims Data (Calendar-days away from work by decile)										
10%	20%	30%	40%	**50%**	60%	70%	80%	**90%**	100%	Mean
10	11	13	14	**16**	22	28	40	**51**	365	27.45

NEPHRITIS, NEPHROTIC SYNDROME, AND NEPHROSIS (580-589)

Excludes:
hypertensive renal disease (403.00-403.91)

RTW Claims Data (Calendar-days away from work by decile)										
10%	20%	30%	40%	**50%**	60%	70%	80%	**90%**	100%	Mean
10	14	14	16	**26**	28	29	35	**57**	365	33.77

Impact on Total Absence: Prevalence 0.2300% of total lost workdays; Incidence 2.42 days per 100 workers

Occupational Disability Durations, in days
Median (mid-point) 204 - Benchmark Indemnity Costs 153,000

Percent of Cases
(77 cases)

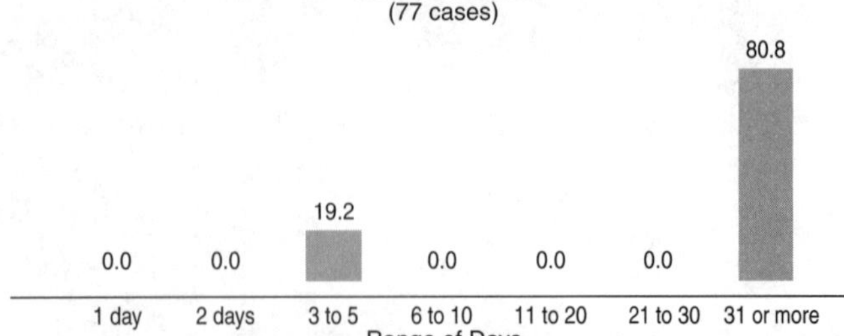

Impact on Occupational Absence: Prevalence 0.1781% of occupational lost workdays; Incidence 0.03 days per 100 workers

585 Chronic kidney disease (CKD)

Return-To-Work Summary Guidelines		
Dataset	**Midrange**	**At-Risk**
Claims data	25 days	58 days
All absences	14 days	57 days

Return-To-Work "Best Practice" Guidelines
Ongoing dialysis: 1 day
Initial dialysis, without hospitalization, based on shunt location, clerical/modified work: 9 days
Initial dialysis, without hospitalization, manual work: 28 days
Initial dialysis, with hospitalization, clerical/modified work: 14 days
Initial dialysis, with hospitalization, manual work: 28 days
Kidney transplant, clerical/modified work: 28 days
Kidney transplant, manual work: 56 days

Description: A slow, progressive decrease in kidney failure causing waste products to build up in the blood. Symptoms are slow to develop and mild at first. They may include a need to urinate many times during the night, weariness, dry, yellow skin, a bad taste in mouth, loss of appetite, brownish discoloration of the tongue, and sometimes seizures.
Other names: Chronic kidney failure
Chronic uremia
Use additional code to identify manifestation as: uremic:
neuropathy (357.4)
pericarditis (420.0)

585 Chronic kidney disease (CKD) *(cont'd)*

Excludes:
that with any condition classifiable to 401 (403.0-403.9 with fifth-digit 1)

Disability Duration Adjustment Factors by Age						
Age Group	18-24	25-34	35-44	45-54	55-64	65-74
Adjustment Factor	0.26	0.73	0.66	1.15	2.62	NA

RTW Claims Data (Calendar-days away from work by decile)										
10%	20%	30%	40%	**50%**	60%	70%	80%	**90%**	100%	Mean
10	13	14	15	**25**	28	30	56	**58**	365	35.49

Integrated Disability Durations, in days*
Median (mid-point) 14.0 Mean (average) 26.92
Mode (most frequent) 1 Calculated rec. 14

Percent of Cases
(1769 cases)

Range of Days (up to)	3	6	9	12	15	18	21	24	27	30	33	36	39	40+
Percent	15.2	4.6	7.5	6.3	13.0	4.1	1.2	0.3	3.0	9.6	2.1	0.3	0.2	15.8

*CDC NHIS cases with no lost workdays: 297 (16.8%)

Impact on Total Absence: Prevalence 0.1171% of total lost workdays; Incidence 1.23 days per 100 workers

OTHER DISEASES OF URINARY SYSTEM (590-599)

Excludes:
conditions classifiable to 590, 595, 597, 599.0 complicating:
abortion (634-638 with .7, 639.8)
ectopic or molar pregnancy (639.8)
pregnancy, childbirth, or the puerperium (646.6)

RTW Claims Data (Calendar-days away from work by decile)										
10%	20%	30%	40%	**50%**	60%	70%	80%	**90%**	100%	Mean
9	10	11	12	**14**	15	17	23	**41**	365	20.80

Impact on Total Absence: Prevalence 0.4486% of total lost workdays; Incidence 4.71 days per 100 workers

Occupational Disability Durations, in days
Median (mid-point) 204 - Benchmark Indemnity Costs 153,000

Percent of Cases
(63 cases)

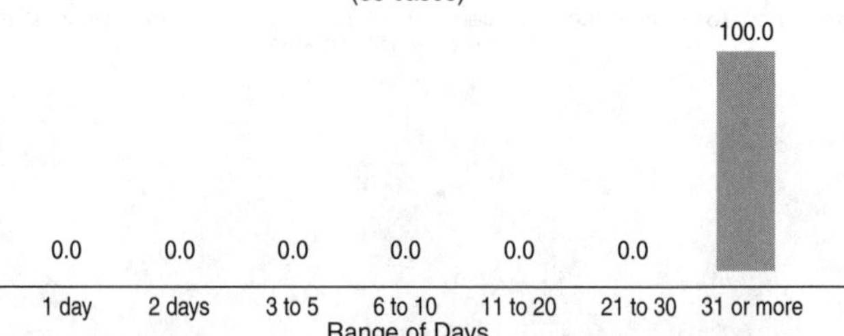

Impact on Occupational Absence: Prevalence 0.1457% of occupational lost workdays; Incidence 0.02 days per 100 workers

590.9 Infection of kidney, unspecified

Return-To-Work Summary Guidelines		
Dataset	**Midrange**	**At-Risk**
Claims data	12 days	16 days
All absences	9 days	15 days

590.9 Infection of kidney, unspecified *(cont'd)*

Return-To-Work "Best Practice" Guidelines
Without hospitalization: 3-7 days
With hospitalization: 10-14 days

Description: Infection of one or both kidneys causing sudden or long-term fever, chills, pain in the lower back, vomiting, nausea, and/or blood in the urine.

Excludes:
urinary tract infection NOS (599.0)

RTW Claims Data (Calendar-days away from work by decile)										
10%	20%	30%	40%	**50%**	60%	70%	80%	**90%**	100%	Mean
9	10	10	11	**12**	13	14	15	**16**	365	14.39

Integrated Disability Durations, in days*

Median (mid-point)	9.0	Mean (average)	9.91
Mode (most frequent)	3	Calculated rec.	8

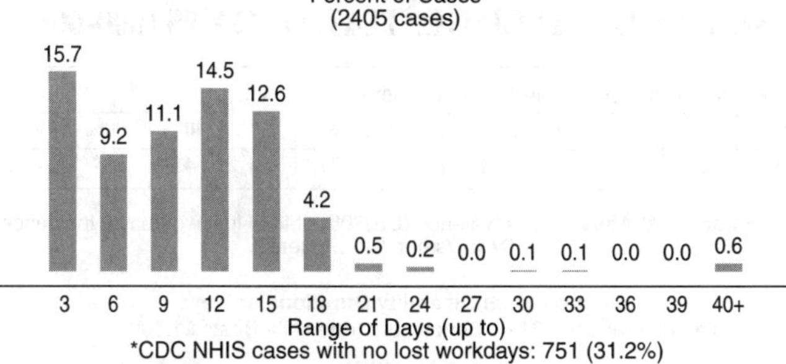

*CDC NHIS cases with no lost workdays: 751 (31.2%)

Impact on Total Absence: Prevalence 0.0484% of total lost workdays; Incidence 0.51 days per 100 workers

592 Calculus of kidney and ureter

Return-To-Work Summary Guidelines

Dataset	Midrange	At-Risk
Claims data	22 days	44 days
All absences	8 days	42 days

Return-To-Work "Best Practice" Guidelines
See 592.0

Excludes:
nephrocalcinosis (275.4)

Disability Duration Adjustment Factors by Age						
Age Group	18-24	25-34	35-44	45-54	55-64	65-74
Adjustment Factor	NA	1.09	0.46	1.14	1.38	NA

RTW Claims Data (Calendar-days away from work by decile)										
10%	20%	30%	40%	**50%**	60%	70%	80%	**90%**	100%	Mean
10	11	14	19	**22**	28	30	42	**44**	365	29.04

592 Calculus of kidney and ureter *(cont'd)*

Integrated Disability Durations, in days*

Median (mid-point)	8.0	Mean (average)	16.70
Mode (most frequent)	2	Calculated rec.	9

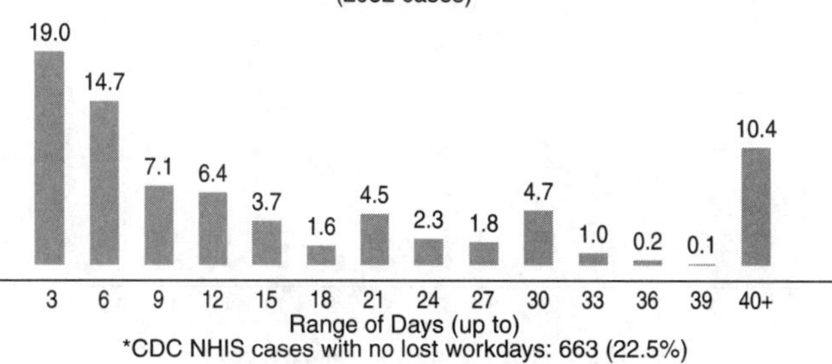

*CDC NHIS cases with no lost workdays: 663 (22.5%)

Impact on Total Absence: Prevalence 0.1130% of total lost workdays; Incidence 1.19 days per 100 workers

592.0 Calculus of kidney

Return-To-Work Summary Guidelines

Dataset	Midrange	At-Risk
Claims data	22 days	43 days
All absences	7 days	41 days

Return-To-Work "Best Practice" Guidelines
Without hospitalization: 0-4 days
With hospitalization, medical treatment: 5 days
Cystoscopy: 2 days
Lithotripsy: 7-10 days
Nephrostomy/lithotomy, percutaneous, clerical/modified work: 20 days
Nephrostomy/lithotomy, percutaneous, manual work: 42 days
Nephrolithotomy/lithotomy, open, clerical/modified work: 28 days
Nephrolithotomy/lithotomy, open, manual work: 42 days

Description: Stones in the kidneys that form due to crystals in the urine sometimes caused by mild, chronic dehydration. Symptoms depend on the size and site of the stones. Small stones may have no symptoms until they start to pass down the ureter, causing a sharp pain that moves from the flank to the groin. The severity of the pain could also cause vomiting.
Other names: Kidney stones
Nephrolithiasis NOS
Renal calculus or stone
Staghorn calculus
Stone in kidney

Excludes:
uric acid nephrolithiasis (274.11)

RTW Claims Data (Calendar-days away from work by decile)										
10%	20%	30%	40%	**50%**	60%	70%	80%	**90%**	100%	Mean
10	11	14	20	**22**	28	30	41	**43**	365	26.54

592.0 Calculus of kidney *(cont'd)*

Integrated Disability Durations, in days*

Median (mid-point)	7.0	Mean (average)	14.75
Mode (most frequent)	2	Calculated rec.	8

Percent of Cases
(2205 cases)

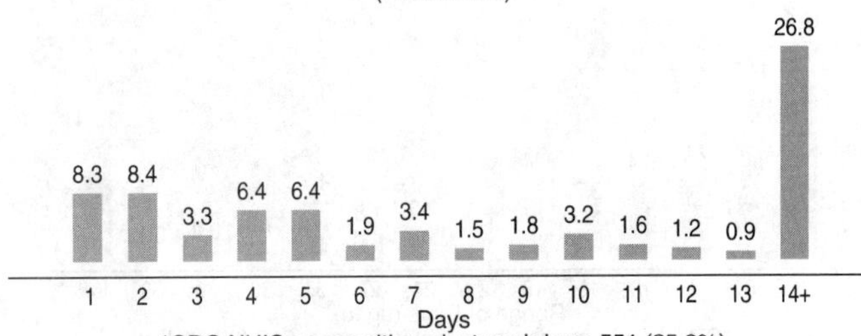

*CDC NHIS cases with no lost workdays: 551 (25.0%)

Impact on Total Absence: Prevalence 0.0721% of total lost workdays; Incidence 0.76 days per 100 workers

595 Cystitis

Return-To-Work Summary Guidelines		
Dataset	**Midrange**	**At-Risk**
Claims data	10 days	14 days
All absences	6 days	12 days

Return-To-Work "Best Practice" Guidelines
See 595.9

Excludes:
prostatocystitis (601.3)
Use additional code to identify organism, such as Escherichia coli [E. coli] (041.4)

595.2 Other chronic cystitis

Return-To-Work Summary Guidelines		
Dataset	**Midrange**	**At-Risk**
Claims data	10 days	14 days
All absences	7 days	12 days

Return-To-Work "Best Practice" Guidelines
Medical treatment: 0 days
Spread of infection beyond bladder: 7-10 days

Description: Long-lasting bladder infection. See 595.0
Other names: Chronic bladder infection
Chronic cystitis NOS
Subacute cystitis

Excludes:
trigonitis (595.3)

RTW Claims Data (Calendar-days away from work by decile)										
10%	20%	30%	40%	**50%**	60%	70%	80%	**90%**	100%	Mean
8	9	10	10	**10**	11	12	13	**14**	90	11.79

595.2 Other chronic cystitis *(cont'd)*

Integrated Disability Durations, in days*

Median (mid-point)	7.0	Mean (average)	7.10
Mode (most frequent)	1	Calculated rec.	6

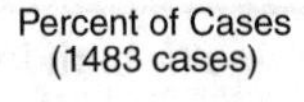
Percent of Cases
(1483 cases)

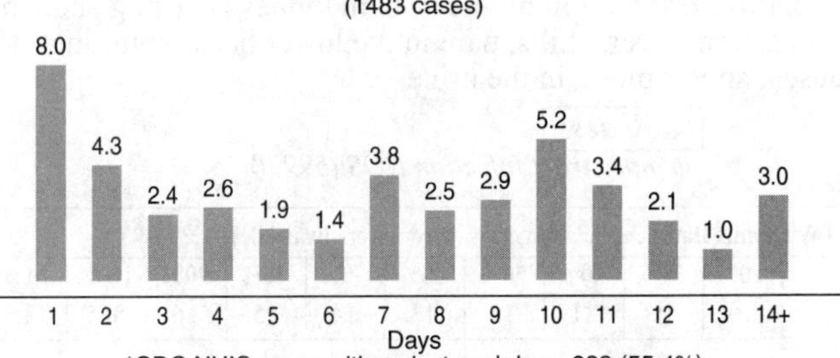

*CDC NHIS cases with no lost workdays: 822 (55.4%)

Impact on Total Absence: Prevalence 0.0138% of total lost workdays; Incidence 0.15 days per 100 workers

DISEASES OF MALE GENITAL ORGANS (600-608)

RTW Claims Data (Calendar-days away from work by decile)										
10%	20%	30%	40%	**50%**	60%	70%	80%	**90%**	100%	Mean
10	11	13	14	**17**	21	27	31	**43**	365	24.84

Impact on Total Absence: Prevalence 0.1020% of total lost workdays; Incidence 1.07 days per 100 workers

Occupational Disability Durations, in days
Median (mid-point) 2 - Benchmark Indemnity Costs $1,500

Percent of Cases
(90 cases)

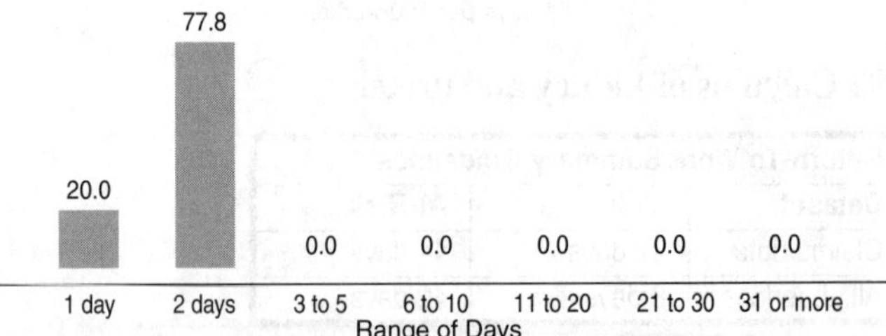

Impact on Occupational Absence: Prevalence 0.0020% of occupational lost workdays

600 Hyperplasia of prostate

Return-To-Work Summary Guidelines		
Dataset	**Midrange**	**At-Risk**
Claims data	27 days	43 days
All absences	20 days	42 days

Return-To-Work "Best Practice" Guidelines
Medical treatment: 0 days
Balloon dilation: 2 days
Transurethral incision of bladder neck: 7 days
Prostatic stent: 5 days
Prostatectomy, transurethral/TURP, clerical/modified work: 21 days
Prostatectomy, transurethral/TURP, manual work: 28-42 days
Prostatectomy, radical, clerical/modified work: 28 days
Prostatectomy, radical, manual work: 42 days

Description: Non-cancerous growth in the prostate gland believed to be a result of hormonal changes associated with aging. Symptoms include difficulty starting urination, decreased force in urine, and a feeling that the urination hasn't been complete.
Other names: Prostate enlargement, Prostate obstruction

600 Hyperplasia of prostate *(cont'd)*

Adenofibromatous hypertrophy of prostate
Adenoma (benign) of prostate
Enlargement (benign) of prostate
Fibroadenoma of prostate
Fibroma of prostate
Hypertrophy (benign) of prostate
Myoma of prostate
Median bar (prostate)
Prostatic obstruction NOS
Use additional code to identify urinary incontinence (788.30-788.39)

Excludes:
benign neoplasms of prostate (222.2)

RTW Claims Data (Calendar-days away from work by decile)										
10%	20%	30%	40%	**50%**	60%	70%	80%	**90%**	100%	Mean
12	16	21	23	**27**	29	31	42	**43**	365	29.62

Integrated Disability Durations, in days*

Median (mid-point)	20.0	Mean (average)	21.65
Mode (most frequent)	2	Calculated rec.	16

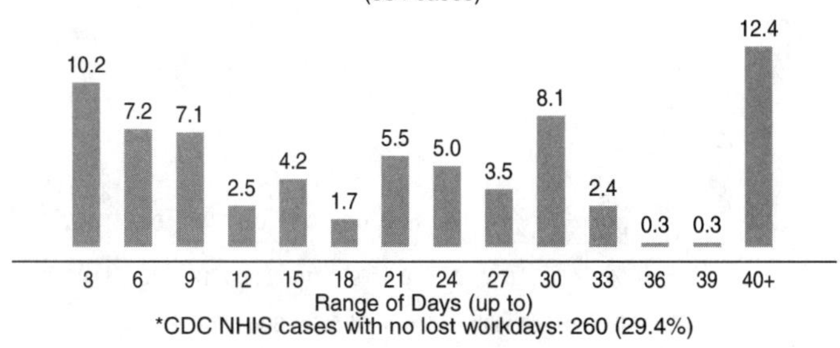

*CDC NHIS cases with no lost workdays: 260 (29.4%)

Impact on Total Absence: Prevalence 0.0399% of total lost workdays; Incidence 0.42 days per 100 workers

INFLAMMATORY DISEASE OF FEMALE PELVIC ORGANS (614-616)

Use additional code to identify organism, such as Staphylococcus (041.1), or Streptococcus (041.0)

Excludes:
that associated with pregnancy, abortion, childbirth, or the puerperium (630-676.9)

RTW Claims Data (Calendar-days away from work by decile)										
10%	20%	30%	40%	**50%**	60%	70%	80%	**90%**	100%	Mean
9	10	13	14	**15**	20	28	41	**55**	365	30.29

Impact on Total Absence: Prevalence 0.0325% of total lost workdays; Incidence 0.34 days per 100 workers

614 Inflammatory disease of ovary, fallopian tube, pelvic cellular tissue, and peritoneum

Return-To-Work Summary Guidelines		
Dataset	**Midrange**	**At-Risk**
Claims data	28 days	57 days
All absences	11 days	55 days

Return-To-Work "Best Practice" Guidelines
See 614.9

614 Inflammatory disease of ovary, fallopian tube, pelvic cellular tissue, and peritoneum *(cont'd)*

Excludes:
endometritis (615.0-615.9)
major infection following delivery (670)
that complicating:
abortion (634-638 with .0, 639.0)
ectopic or molar pregnancy (639.0)
pregnancy or labor (646.6)

614.2 Salpingitis and oophoritis not specified as acute, subacute, or chronic

Return-To-Work Summary Guidelines		
Dataset	**Midrange**	**At-Risk**
Claims data	22 days	56 days
All absences	11 days	43 days

Return-To-Work "Best Practice" Guidelines
Without hospitalization: 1-7 days
Laparoscopy, diagnostic: 1 day
With hospitalization, medical treatment: 10 days
Laparoscopically assisted vaginal hysterectomy/LAVH, clerical/modified work: 21-42 days
Laparoscopically assisted vaginal hysterectomy/LAVH, manual work: 42 days
Abdominal hysterectomy, clerical/modified work: 28-42 days
Abdominal hysterectomy, manual work: 42 days
Salpingo-Oophorectomy, clerical/modified work: 42 days
Salpingo-Oophorectomy, manual work: 56 days

Description: Inflammation of the fallopian tubes usually caused by a bacterial infection that enters through the vagina. The fallopian tubes connect the ovary with the uterus and are also the site of fertilization. Infected tubes can cause scar tissue that might block the passage of an egg to the uterus from the ovary. Symptoms usually begin shortly after menstruation with progressive pain in the lower abdomen and nausea or vomiting. Other symptoms may include fever, headache, malaise, frequent urination, abnormal vaginal discharge, and eventually salpingitis could cause infertility. If the infection is caused by chlamydia, there may be no symptoms at all.

Abscess (of):
  fallopian tube
  ovary
  tubo-ovarian
Oophoritis
Perioophoritis
Perisalpingitis
Pyosalpinx
Salpingitis
Salpingo-oophoritis
Tubo-ovarian inflammatory disease

Excludes:
gonococcal infection (chronic) (098.37)
acute (098.17)
tuberculous (016.6)

RTW Claims Data (Calendar-days away from work by decile)										
10%	20%	30%	40%	**50%**	60%	70%	80%	**90%**	100%	Mean
9	10	13	20	**22**	28	40	42	**44**	57	26.17

614.2 Salpingitis and oophoritis not specified as acute, subacute, or chronic *(cont'd)*

Integrated Disability Durations, in days*

Median (mid-point)	11.0	Mean (average)	18.37
Mode (most frequent)	1	Calculated rec.	10

Percent of Cases
(166 cases)

15.7 8.4 10.8 9.0 3.6 1.8 4.8 3.6 1.8 5.4 0.0 0.0 0.6 16.9

3 6 9 12 15 18 21 24 27 30 33 36 39 40+

Range of Days (up to)

*CDC NHIS cases with no lost workdays: 29 (17.5%)

Impact on Total Absence: Prevalence 0.0074% of total lost workdays; Incidence 0.08 days per 100 workers

OTHER DISORDERS OF FEMALE GENITAL TRACT (617-629)

RTW Claims Data (Calendar-days away from work by decile)										
10%	20%	30%	40%	**50%**	60%	70%	80%	**90%**	100%	Mean
11	14	16	21	**28**	34	42	45	**57**	365	33.67

Impact on Total Absence: Prevalence 0.5236% of total lost workdays; Incidence 5.50 days per 100 workers

Occupational Disability Durations, in days

Median (mid-point) 22 - Benchmark Indemnity Costs $16,500

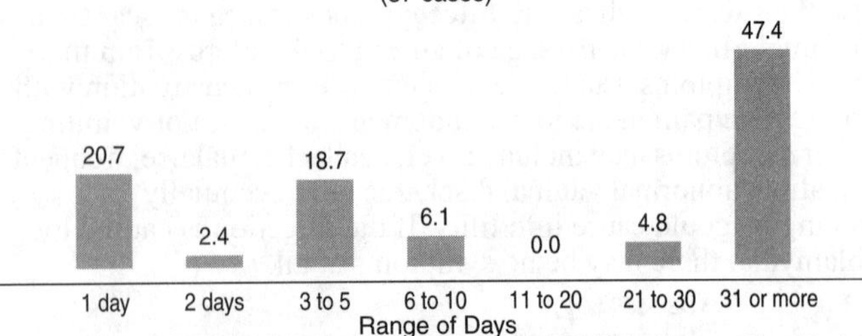

Impact on Occupational Absence: Prevalence 0.0217% of occupational lost workdays

625 Pain and other symptoms associated with female genital organs

Return-To-Work Summary Guidelines		
Dataset	**Midrange**	**At-Risk**
Claims data	18 days	111 days
All absences	12 days	90 days

625.3 Dysmenorrhea

Return-To-Work Summary Guidelines		
Dataset	**Midrange**	**At-Risk**
Claims data	15 days	60 days
All absences	2 days	7 days

Return-To-Work "Best Practice" Guidelines
Medical treatment: 0 days
Dilation & curettage/D&C: 3 days
Other causes: see primary diagnosis

625.3 Dysmenorrhea *(cont'd)*

Description: Abdominal pain stemming from uterine cramps just before or during menstruation. Over 50 percent of women are affected and five to 15 percent are affected severely enough to interfere with everyday activities. The pain in the lower abdomen may extend to the lower back or legs and could come and go as cramps, or be experienced as a constant, dull ache. Pain usually peaks after 24 hours and subsides within two days. Other symptoms include headache, nausea, constipation or diarrhea, irritability, depression, bloating, and/or frequent urination.

Painful menstruation

Excludes:

psychogenic dysmenorrhea (306.52)

RTW Claims Data (Calendar-days away from work by decile)										
10%	20%	30%	40%	**50%**	60%	70%	80%	**90%**	100%	Mean
10	12	12	14	**15**	24	34	42	**60**	365	31.02

Integrated Disability Durations, in days*

Median (mid-point)	2.0	Mean (average)	4.78
Mode (most frequent)	1	Calculated rec.	2

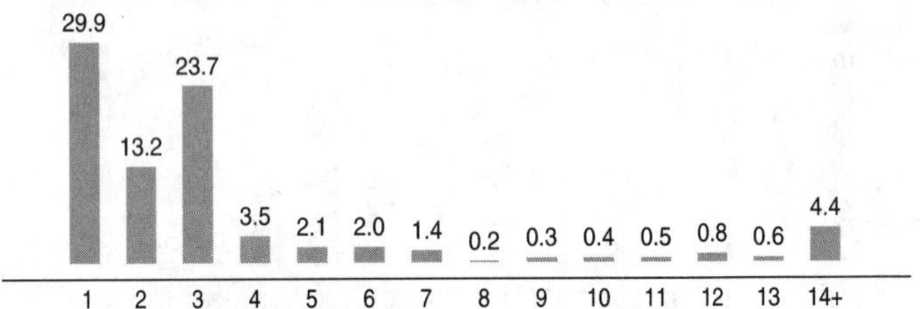

*CDC NHIS cases with no lost workdays: 304 (17.0%)

Impact on Total Absence: Prevalence 0.0208% of total lost workdays; Incidence 0.22 days per 100 workers

11. COMPLICATIONS OF PREGNANCY, CHILDBIRTH, AND THE PUERPERIUM (630-679)

Impact on Total Absence: Prevalence 18.5101% of total lost workdays; Incidence 194.36 days per 100 workers

RTW Claims Data (Calendar-days away from work by decile)										
10%	20%	30%	40%	**50%**	60%	70%	80%	**90%**	100%	Mean
22	34	41	43	**46**	49	53	61	**67**	365	48.95

NORMAL DELIVERY, AND OTHER INDICATIONS FOR CARE IN PREGNANCY, LABOR, AND DELIVERY (650-659)

The following fifth-digit subclassification is for use with categories 651-659 to denote the current episode of care:

0 unspecified as to episode of care or not applicable
1 delivered, with or without mention of antepartum condition
2 delivered, with mention of postpartum complication
3 antepartum condition or complication
4 postpartum condition or complication

RTW Claims Data (Calendar-days away from work by decile)										
10%	20%	30%	40%	**50%**	60%	70%	80%	**90%**	100%	Mean
22	37	42	43	**45**	48	50	57	**64**	365	46.57

Impact on Total Absence: Prevalence 13.8921% of total lost workdays; Incidence 145.87 days per 100 workers

650 Normal delivery

Return-To-Work Summary Guidelines		
Dataset	**Midrange**	**At-Risk**
Claims data	45 days	64 days
All absences	45 days	64 days

Return-To-Work "Best Practice" Guidelines
Modified work, days after delivery: 21 days
Regular work, days after delivery (also allowing newborn care): 42 days
Postpartum depression comorbidity: 49-63 days

Delivery without abnormality or complication classifiable elsewhere in categories 630-676, and with spontaneous cephalic delivery, without mention of fetal manipulation [e.g., rotation, version] or instrumentation [forceps]

Excludes:
breech delivery (assisted) (spontaneous) NOS (652.2)
delivery by vacuum extractor, forceps, cesarean section, or breech extraction, without specified complication (669.5-669.7)

RTW Claims Data (Calendar-days away from work by decile)										
10%	20%	30%	40%	**50%**	60%	70%	80%	**90%**	100%	Mean
22	37	42	43	**45**	48	50	56	**64**	365	46.55

650 Normal delivery *(cont'd)*

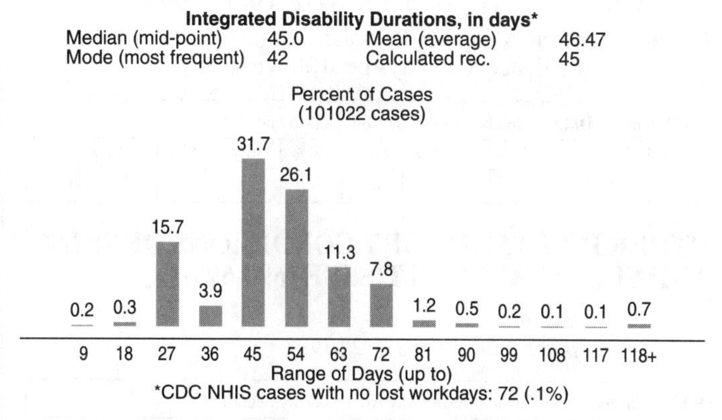

Impact on Total Absence: Prevalence 13.8660% of total lost workdays; Incidence 145.59 days per 100 workers

12. DISEASES OF THE SKIN AND SUBCUTANEOUS TISSUE (680-709)

Impact on Total Absence: Prevalence 0.8245% of total lost workdays; Incidence 8.66 days per 100 workers

RTW Claims Data (Calendar-days away from work by decile)										
10%	20%	30%	40%	**50%**	60%	70%	80%	**90%**	100%	Mean
9	11	13	14	**16**	20	23	33	**72**	365	40.64

OTHER INFLAMMATORY CONDITIONS OF SKIN AND SUBCUTANEOUS TISSUE (690-698)

Excludes:
panniculitis (729.30-729.39)

RTW Claims Data (Calendar-days away from work by decile)										
10%	20%	30%	40%	**50%**	60%	70%	80%	**90%**	100%	Mean
10	13	14	16	**19**	21	22	29	**365**	365	65.01

Impact on Total Absence: Prevalence 0.4173% of total lost workdays; Incidence 4.38 days per 100 workers

Occupational Disability Durations, in days
Median (mid-point) 3 - Benchmark Indemnity Costs $2,250

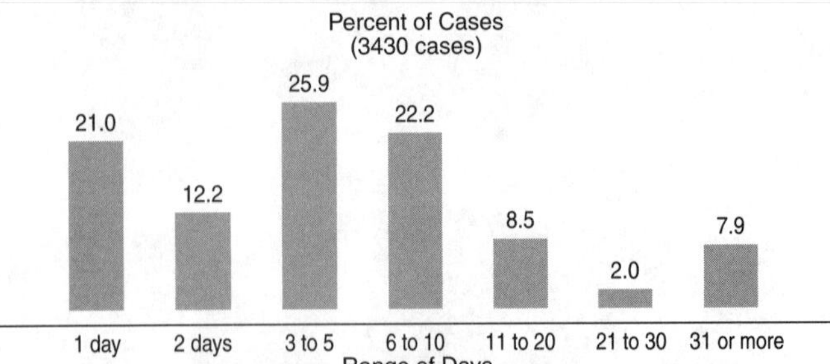

Impact on Occupational Absence: Prevalence 0.1167% of occupational lost workdays; Incidence 0.02 days per 100 workers

692 Contact dermatitis and other eczema

Return-To-Work Summary Guidelines		
Dataset	**Midrange**	**At-Risk**
Claims data	20 days	365 days
All absences	4 days	23 days

Return-To-Work "Best Practice" Guidelines
Limited surface area: 0 days
Extensive surface area, clerical/modified work: 5 days
Extensive surface area, regular work (if not cause): 15 days
Regular work (if work related): 21 days to indefinite

Description: Inflammation of the skin resulting from direct contact with an irritant such as soap, chemicals, detergents, or abrasives. Symptoms may include itchy, swollen, red patches on the skin and/or blisters.

Other names: Allergic contact dermatitis, Irritant contact dermatitis

Includes: dermatitis:
- NOS
- contact
- occupational
- venenata

eczema (acute) (chronic):
- NOS
- allergic
- erythematous
- occupational

692 Contact dermatitis and other eczema *(cont'd)*

Excludes:
allergy NOS (995.3)
contact dermatitis of eyelids (373.32)
dermatitis due to substances taken internally (693.0-693.9)
eczema of external ear (380.22)
perioral dermatitis (695.3)
urticarial reactions (708.0-708.9, 995.1)

Workers' Comp Costs per Claim (based on 13,186 claims)					
Quartile	25%	50%	75%	Mean	% no cost
Indemnity	$788	$1,974	$4,358	$4,515	96%
Medical	$105	$158	$252	$274	8%
Total	$105	$158	$263	$458	7%

RTW Claims Data (Calendar-days away from work by decile)										
10%	20%	30%	40%	**50%**	60%	70%	80%	**90%**	100%	Mean
11	14	15	17	**20**	22	24	363	**365**	365	89.16

Integrated Disability Durations, in days*
Median (mid-point) 4.0 Mean (average) 30.63
Mode (most frequent) 1 Calculated rec. 10

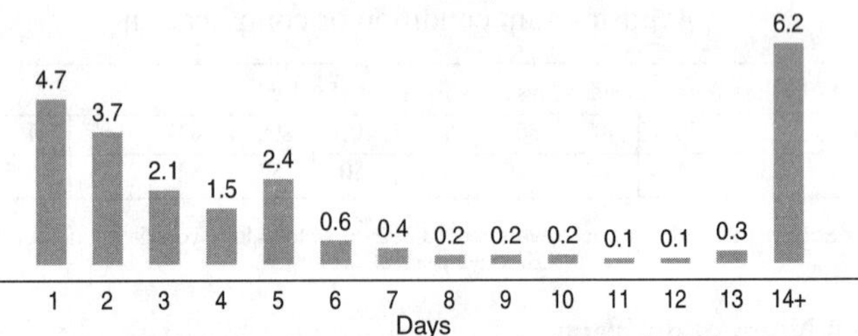

*CDC NHIS cases with no lost workdays: 9948 (77.1%)

Impact on Total Absence: Prevalence 0.2670% of total lost workdays; Incidence 2.80 days per 100 workers

Occupational Disability Durations, in days
Median (mid-point) 5 - Benchmark Indemnity Costs $3,750

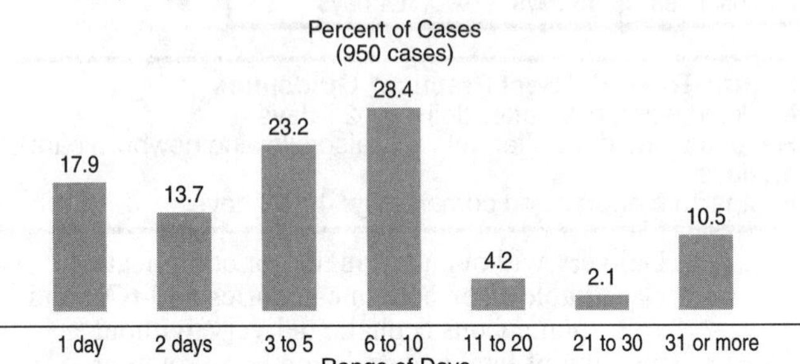

Impact on Occupational Absence: Prevalence 0.0538% of occupational lost workdays; Incidence 0.01 days per 100 workers

692.9 Unspecified cause

Return-To-Work Summary Guidelines		
Dataset	**Midrange**	**At-Risk**
Claims data	21 days	27 days
All absences	3 days	21 days

Return-To-Work "Best Practice" Guidelines
Limited surface area: 0 days
Extensive surface area: 3-5 days
If problem agent in workplace, modified work: 5 days
If problem agent in workplace, regular work: 21 days

Description: See 692

692.9 Unspecified cause *(cont'd)*

Dermatitis:
NOS
contact NOS
venenata NOS
Eczema NOS

Workers' Comp Costs per Claim (based on 5,269 claims)					
Quartile	25%	50%	75%	Mean	% no cost
Indemnity	$651	$1,979	$4,274	$3,548	95%
Medical	$105	$168	$273	$296	8%
Total	$105	$168	$284	$484	8%

RTW Claims Data (Calendar-days away from work by decile)

10%	20%	30%	40%	**50%**	60%	70%	80%	**90%**	100%	Mean
10	13	17	20	**21**	21	22	23	**27**	261	21.94

Integrated Disability Durations, in days*
Median (mid-point) 3.0 Mean (average) 7.84
Mode (most frequent) 1 Calculated rec. 4

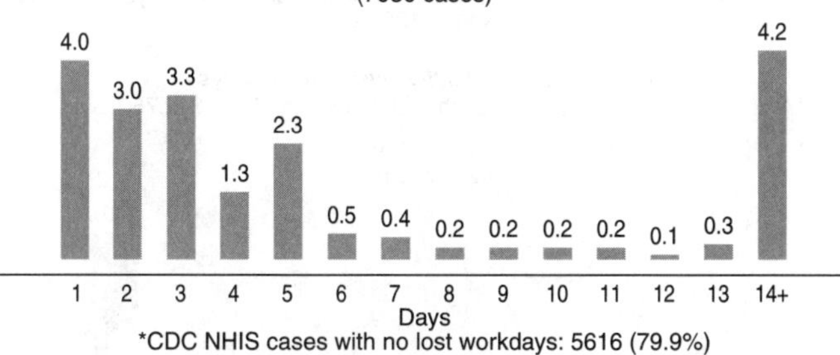

*CDC NHIS cases with no lost workdays: 5616 (79.9%)

Impact on Total Absence: Prevalence 0.0327% of total lost workdays; Incidence 0.34 days per 100 workers

696 Psoriasis and similar disorders

Return-To-Work Summary Guidelines		
Dataset	Midrange	At-Risk
Claims data	12 days	18 days
All absences	7 days	14 days

RTW Claims Data (Calendar-days away from work by decile)

10%	20%	30%	40%	**50%**	60%	70%	80%	**90%**	100%	Mean
8	9	10	11	**12**	13	14	15	**18**	365	21.79

Integrated Disability Durations, in days*
Median (mid-point) 7.0 Mean (average) 12.32
Mode (most frequent) 1 Calculated rec. 7

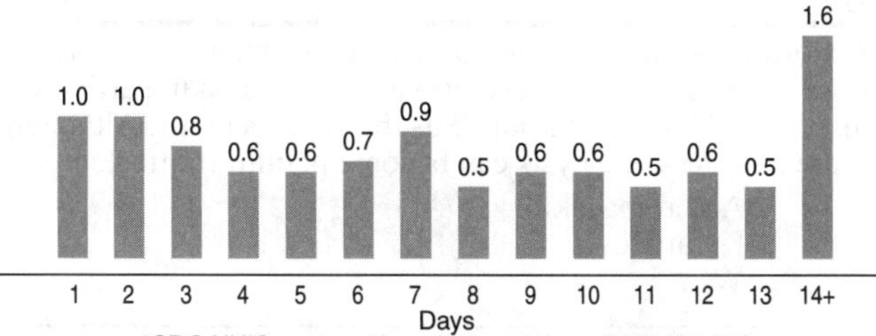

*CDC NHIS cases with no lost workdays: 1360 (89.6%)

Impact on Total Absence: Prevalence 0.0057% of total lost workdays; Incidence 0.06 days per 100 workers

696.1 Other psoriasis

Return-To-Work Summary Guidelines		
Dataset	Midrange	At-Risk
Claims data	15 days	32 days
All absences	6 days	22 days

Return-To-Work "Best Practice" Guidelines
Without hospitalization: 0 days

Description: A chronic, recurring disease characterized by inflamed, red skin with silvery, scaly bumps and raised patches. It is usually seen on the scalp, elbows, knees, back, and buttocks, and comes and goes with varying severity. The bumps and patches rarely itch, and flaking is the most obvious sign.

Acrodermatitis continua
Dermatitis repens
Psoriasis:
NOS
any type, except arthropathic

Excludes:
psoriatic arthropathy (696.0)

RTW Claims Data (Calendar-days away from work by decile)

10%	20%	30%	40%	**50%**	60%	70%	80%	**90%**	100%	Mean
11	12	13	14	**15**	16	20	25	**32**	223	29.18

Integrated Disability Durations, in days*
Median (mid-point) 6.5 Mean (average) 14.41
Mode (most frequent) 1 Calculated rec. 7

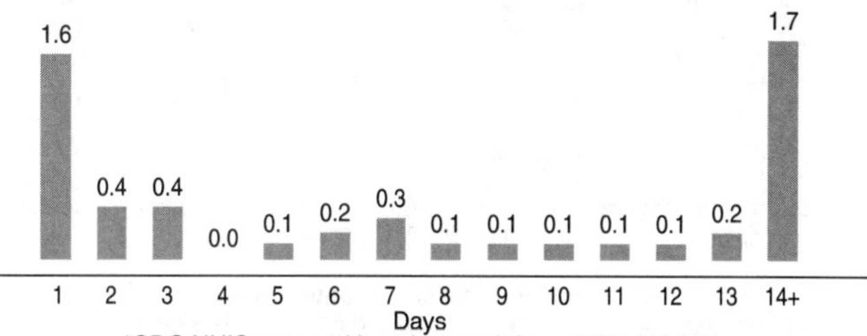

*CDC NHIS cases with no lost workdays: 1272 (94.5%)

Impact on Total Absence: Prevalence 0.0031% of total lost workdays; Incidence 0.03 days per 100 workers

OTHER DISEASES OF SKIN AND SUBCUTANEOUS TISSUE (700-709)

Excludes:
conditions confined to eyelids (373.0-374.9)
congenital conditions of skin, hair, and nails (757.0-757.9)

RTW Claims Data (Calendar-days away from work by decile)

10%	20%	30%	40%	**50%**	60%	70%	80%	**90%**	100%	Mean
9	10	11	12	**14**	15	16	26	**65**	365	28.20

Impact on Total Absence: Prevalence 0.1674% of total lost workdays; Incidence 1.76 days per 100 workers

Occupational Disability Durations, in days
Median (mid-point) 5 - Benchmark Indemnity Costs $3,750
(60 cases)
Impact on Occupational Absence: Prevalence 0.0034% of occupational lost workdays

700 Corns and callosities

Return-To-Work Summary Guidelines		
Dataset	Midrange	At-Risk
Claims data	14 days	36 days
All absences	3 days	14 days

Return-To-Work "Best Practice" Guidelines
Sedentary/modified work: 0-2 days
Standing/manual work: 0-5 days

Description: An area on the top layer of skin that becomes thick and toughened as a result of repeated rubbing or pressure on the foot. Everyday pressure on the foot may aggravate the condition, causing modest to extensive pain.

Callus
Clavus

RTW Claims Data (Calendar-days away from work by decile)										
10%	20%	30%	40%	**50%**	60%	70%	80%	**90%**	100%	Mean
8	11	12	13	**14**	15	16	18	**36**	145	21.72

Integrated Disability Durations, in days*
Median (mid-point) 3.0 Mean (average) 6.43
Mode (most frequent) 2 Calculated rec. 4

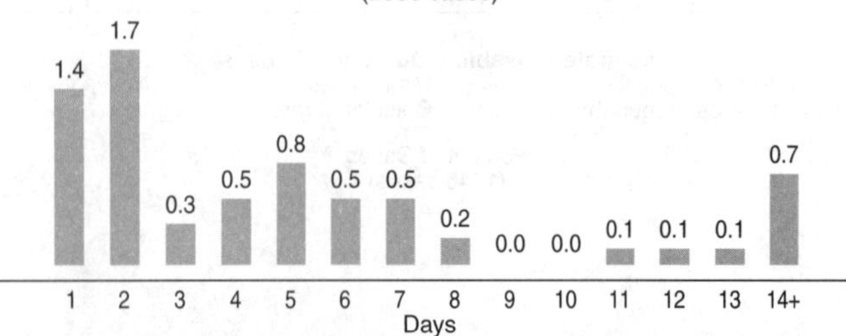

*CDC NHIS cases with no lost workdays: 2485 (93.2%)

Impact on Total Absence: Prevalence 0.0034% of total lost workdays; Incidence 0.04 days per 100 workers

Occupational Disability Durations, in days
Median (mid-point) 3 - Benchmark Indemnity Costs $2,250

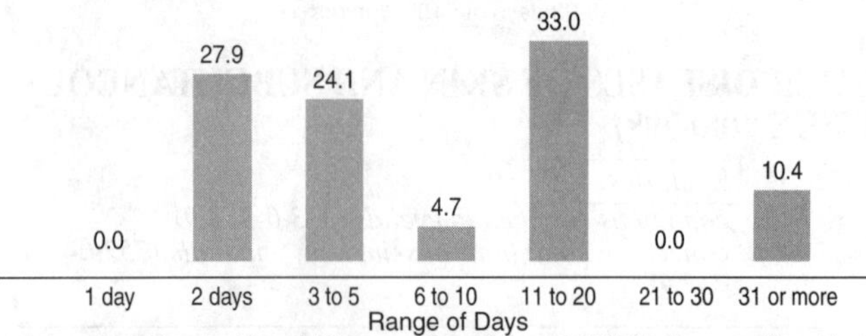

Impact on Occupational Absence: Prevalence 0.0020% of occupational lost workdays

706 Diseases of sebaceous glands

Return-To-Work Summary Guidelines		
Dataset	Midrange	At-Risk
Claims data	14 days	21 days
All absences	3 days	14 days

Workers' Comp Costs per Claim (based on 99 claims)					
Quartile	25%	50%	75%	Mean	% no cost
Medical	$378	$840	$3,108	$1,922	0%
Total	$410	$982	$3,822	$3,241	0%

706 Diseases of sebaceous glands *(cont'd)*

RTW Claims Data (Calendar-days away from work by decile)										
10%	20%	30%	40%	**50%**	60%	70%	80%	**90%**	100%	Mean
8	10	12	13	**14**	15	15	16	**21**	90	15.76

Integrated Disability Durations, in days*
Median (mid-point) 3.0 Mean (average) 5.84
Mode (most frequent) 1 Calculated rec. 3

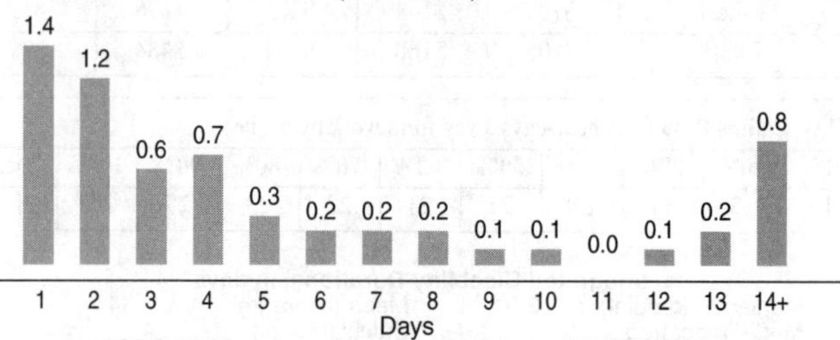

*CDC NHIS cases with no lost workdays: 3761 (93.9%)

Impact on Total Absence: Prevalence 0.0042% of total lost workdays; Incidence 0.04 days per 100 workers

Occupational Disability Durations, in days
Median (mid-point) 57 - Benchmark Indemnity Costs $42,750

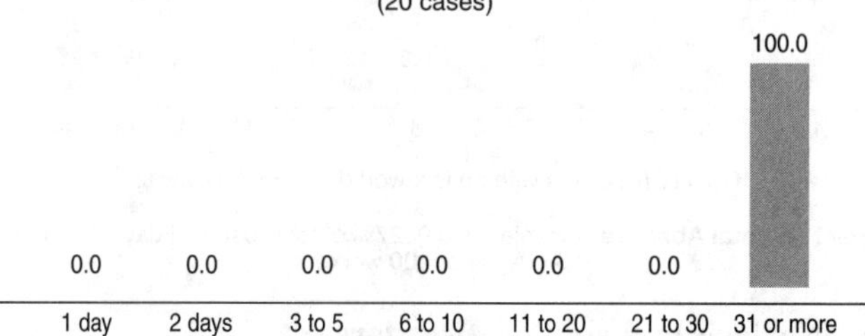

Impact on Occupational Absence: Prevalence 0.0129% of occupational lost workdays

706.2 Sebaceous cyst

Return-To-Work Summary Guidelines		
Dataset	Midrange	At-Risk
Claims data	14 days	19 days
All absences	8 days	17 days

Return-To-Work "Best Practice" Guidelines
Without treatment: 0 days
Surgical removal, depending on surgery site: 1-7 day
Infected cyst, sedentary/modified work: 7 days
Infected cyst, standing/regular work (if located on foot): 14 days

Description: Slow-growing, non-cancerous bump on the skin filled with dead skin, skin excretions, and other skin particles occurring usually on the scalp, ears, back, or genitals. Although they are harmless, the cysts can become painful if infected.

Atheroma, skin
Keratin cyst
Wen

Workers' Comp Costs per Claim (based on 95 claims)					
Quartile	25%	50%	75%	Mean	% no cost
Medical	$410	$914	$3,455	$1,987	0%
Total	$483	$982	$3,822	$2,829	0%

706.2 Sebaceous cyst *(cont'd)*

RTW Claims Data (Calendar-days away from work by decile)										
10%	20%	30%	40%	**50%**	60%	70%	80%	**90%**	100%	Mean
9	11	13	14	**14**	15	15	17	**19**	365	17.81

Integrated Disability Durations, in days*

Median (mid-point)	8.0	Mean (average)	10.49
Mode (most frequent)	1	Calculated rec.	7

Percent of Cases
(1548 cases)

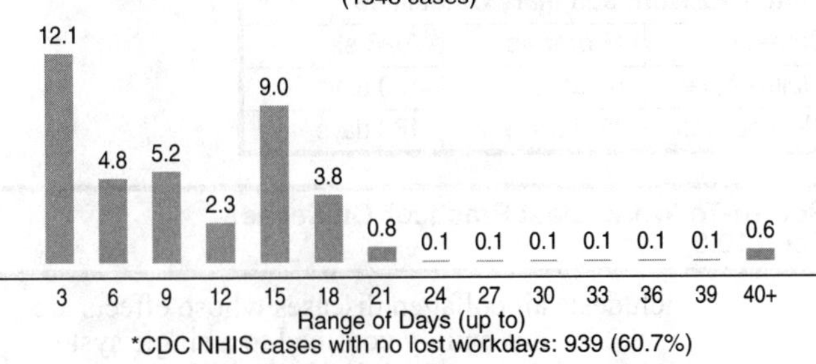

Range of Days (up to)

*CDC NHIS cases with no lost workdays: 939 (60.7%)

Impact on Total Absence: Prevalence 0.0188% of total lost workdays; Incidence 0.20 days per 100 workers

Occupational Disability Durations, in days

Median (mid-point) 57 - Benchmark Indemnity Costs $42,750

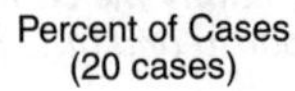

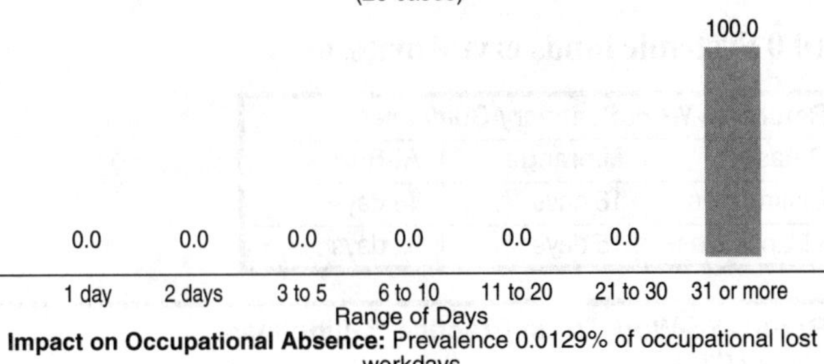

Range of Days

Impact on Occupational Absence: Prevalence 0.0129% of occupational lost workdays

13. DISEASES OF THE MUSCULOSKELETAL SYSTEM AND CONNECTIVE TISSUE (710-739)

Impact on Total Absence: Prevalence 24.4208% of total lost workdays; Incidence 256.42 days per 100 workers

RTW Claims Data (Calendar-days away from work by decile)										
10%	20%	30%	40%	**50%**	60%	70%	80%	**90%**	100%	Mean
12	15	21	25	**35**	43	58	83	**93**	365	52.94

The following fifth-digit subclassification is for use with categories 711-712, 715-716, 718-719, and 730:

0 site unspecified
1 shoulder region
  Acromioclavicular joint(s)
  Glenohumeral joint(s)
  Sternoclavicular joint(s)
  Clavicle
  Scapula
2 upper arm
  Elbow joint
  Humerus
3 forearm
  Radius
  Ulna
  Wrist joint
4 hand
  Carpus
  Metacarpus
  Phalanges [fingers]
5 pelvic region and thigh
  Buttock
  Femur
  Hip (joint)
6 lower leg
  Fibula
  Knee joint
  Patella
  Tibia
7 ankle and foot
  Ankle joint
  Digits [toes]
  Metatarsus
  Phalanges, foot
  Tarsus
  Other joints in foot
8 other specified sites
  Head
  Neck
  Ribs
  Skull
  Trunk
  Vertebral column
9 multiple sites

ARTHROPATHIES AND RELATED DISORDERS (710-719)

Excludes:
disorders of spine (720.0-724.9)

RTW Claims Data (Calendar-days away from work by decile)										
10%	20%	30%	40%	**50%**	60%	70%	80%	**90%**	100%	Mean
14	20	22	40	**43**	50	77	85	**90**	365	55.23

Impact on Total Absence: Prevalence 9.9855% of total lost workdays; Incidence 104.85 days per 100 workers

ARTHROPATHIES AND RELATED DISORDERS (710-719) *(cont'd)*

Occupational Disability Durations, in days
Median (mid-point) 31 - Benchmark Indemnity Costs $23,250
(140 cases)
Impact on Occupational Absence: Prevalence 0.0492% of occupational lost workdays; Incidence 0.01 days per 100 workers

710 Diffuse diseases of connective tissue

Return-To-Work Summary Guidelines		
Dataset	**Midrange**	**At-Risk**
Claims data	51 days	180 days
All absences	17 days	180 days

Return-To-Work "Best Practice" Guidelines
See 710.0

Includes: all collagen diseases whose effects are not mainly confined to a single system
Use additional code to identify manifestation, as:
lung involvement (517.8)
myopathy (359.6)

Excludes:
those affecting mainly the cardiovascular system, i.e., polyarteritis nodosa and allied conditions (446.0-446.7)

710.0 Systemic lupus erythematosus

Return-To-Work Summary Guidelines		
Dataset	**Midrange**	**At-Risk**
Claims data	18 days	48 days
All absences	15 days	32 days

Return-To-Work "Best Practice" Guidelines
Mild: 0 days
Severe, clerical/modified work: 14 days
Severe, manual work: 28 days

Description: Auto-immune disease that affects the connective tissue of the joints, skin, kidneys, nervous system, and mucous membranes causing mild to debilitating inflammation which usually flares up intermittently. Joint and muscle pain, fever, skin rash (especially in a butterfly shape across the nose and cheeks), temporary hair loss, and skin sensitivity to sunlight are common symptoms.
Other names: Lupus

Disseminated lupus erythematosus
Libman-Sacks disease
Use additional code to identify manifestation, as:
endocarditis (424.91)
nephritis (583.81)
  chronic (582.81)
nephrotic syndrome (581.81)

Excludes:
lupus erythematosus (discoid) NOS (695.4)

RTW Claims Data (Calendar-days away from work by decile)										
10%	20%	30%	40%	**50%**	60%	70%	80%	**90%**	100%	Mean
12	14	14	15	**18**	28	29	30	**48**	365	36.45

710.0 Systemic lupus erythematosus *(cont'd)*

Integrated Disability Durations, in days*

Median (mid-point)	15.0	Mean (average)	29.68
Mode (most frequent)	14	Calculated rec.	18

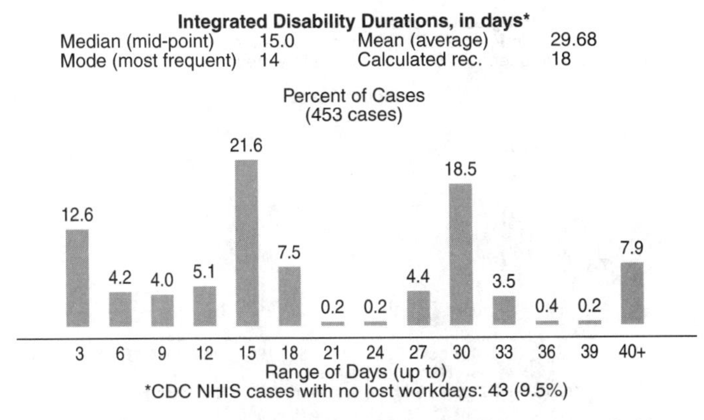

*CDC NHIS cases with no lost workdays: 43 (9.5%)

Impact on Total Absence: Prevalence 0.0359% of total lost workdays; Incidence 0.38 days per 100 workers

710.1 Systemic sclerosis

Return-To-Work Summary Guidelines		
Dataset	**Midrange**	**At-Risk**
Claims data	28 days	41 days
All absences	28 days	41 days

Return-To-Work "Best Practice" Guidelines
28 days

Description: A chronic disease characterized by progressive hardening and thickening of the skin as well as degeneration of the internal organs and blood vessels. The first symptom is usually thickening and swelling at the ends of the fingers. Other symptoms usually appear later and can include joint aches, heartburn, difficulty swallowing, shortness of breath and eventually more serious damage to the internal organs.

Acrosclerosis
CRST syndrome
Progressive systemic sclerosis
Scleroderma

Excludes:
circumscribed scleroderma (701.0)

RTW Claims Data (Calendar-days away from work by decile)

10%	20%	30%	40%	**50%**	60%	70%	80%	**90%**	100%	Mean
26	27	28	28	**28**	29	30	30	**41**	200	33.81

Integrated Disability Durations, in days*

Median (mid-point)	28.0	Mean (average)	32.33
Mode (most frequent)	28	Calculated rec.	29

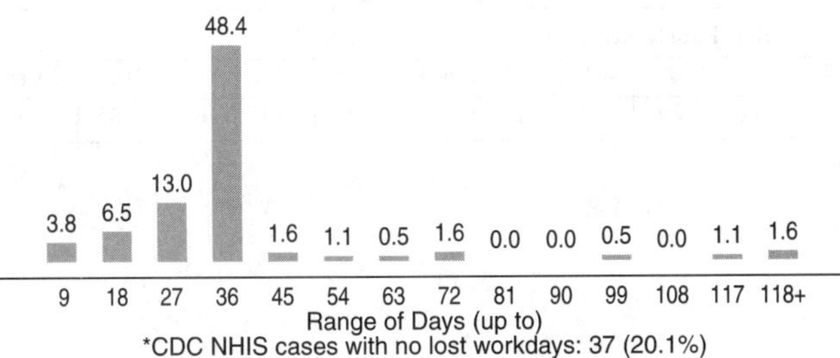

*CDC NHIS cases with no lost workdays: 37 (20.1%)

Impact on Total Absence: Prevalence 0.0140% of total lost workdays; Incidence 0.15 days per 100 workers

710.2 Sicca syndrome

Return-To-Work Summary Guidelines		
Dataset	**Midrange**	**At-Risk**
Claims data	49 days	53 days
All absences	49 days	53 days

Return-To-Work "Best Practice" Guidelines
49 days

Description: An autoimmune disorder characterized by excessive dryness of the eyes, mouth, and mucous membranes. The eyes may be especially sensitive to light and there may be painful swallowing, dulled taste and smell, and joint inflammation.

Other names: Sjogren's disease

Keratoconjunctivitis sicca
Sjogren's disease

RTW Claims Data (Calendar-days away from work by decile)

10%	20%	30%	40%	**50%**	60%	70%	80%	**90%**	100%	Mean
17	48	49	49	**49**	50	50	51	**53**	326	51.35

Integrated Disability Durations, in days*

Median (mid-point)	49.0	Mean (average)	47.91
Mode (most frequent)	49	Calculated rec.	49

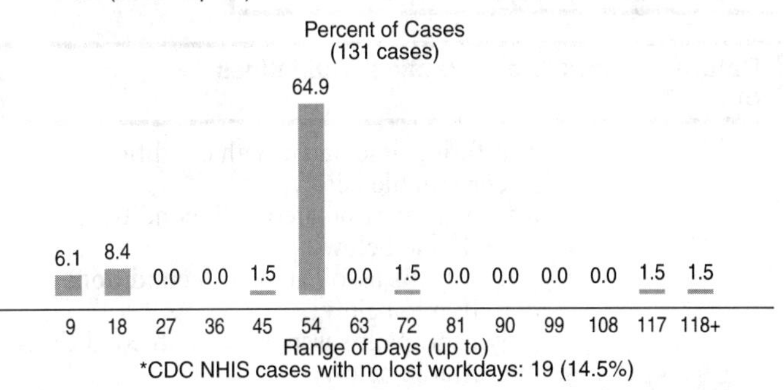

*CDC NHIS cases with no lost workdays: 19 (14.5%)

Impact on Total Absence: Prevalence 0.0158% of total lost workdays; Incidence 0.17 days per 100 workers

710.3 Dermatomyositis

Return-To-Work Summary Guidelines		
Dataset	**Midrange**	**At-Risk**
Claims data	41 days	70 days
All absences	17 days	70 days

Return-To-Work "Best Practice" Guidelines
Clerical/modified work: 14 days
Manual work: 42 days

Description: Chronic inflammation of the connective tissue causing painful inflammation and degeneration of the muscles accompanied by skin inflammation. Muscle weakness, especially in the legs, difficulty breathing or swallowing, red scaly rash, and swelling around the eye are among the symptoms.

Poikilodermatomyositis
Polymyositis with skin involvement

RTW Claims Data (Calendar-days away from work by decile)

10%	20%	30%	40%	**50%**	60%	70%	80%	**90%**	100%	Mean
13	14	15	15	**41**	42	42	43	**70**	180	37.76

710.3 Dermatomyositis *(cont'd)*

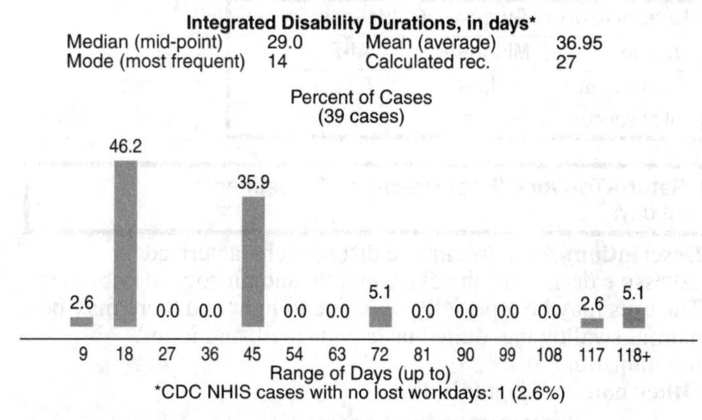

Impact on Total Absence: Prevalence 0.0041% of total lost workdays; Incidence 0.04 days per 100 workers

711 Arthropathy associated with infections

Return-To-Work Summary Guidelines		
Dataset	**Midrange**	**At-Risk**
Claims data	28 days	73 days
All absences	27 days	67 days

Return-To-Work "Best Practice" Guidelines
See 711.0

Includes: arthritis associated with conditions classifiable below
arthropathy associated with conditions classifiable below
polyarthritis associated with conditions classifiable below
polyarthropathy associated with conditions classifiable below

Excludes:
rheumatic fever (390)

The following fifth-digit subclassification is for use with category 711; valid digits are in [brackets] under each code. See list at beginning of chapter for definitions:

0 site unspecified
1 shoulder region
2 upper arm
3 forearm
4 hand
5 pelvic region and thigh
6 lower leg
7 ankle and foot
8 other specified sites
9 multiple sites

Workers' Comp Costs per Claim (based on 57 claims)

Quartile	25%	50%	75%	Mean	% no cost
Indemnity	$1,218	$1,491	$4,074	$8,586	30%
Medical	$2,342	$7,497	$17,882	$17,469	0%
Total	$3,192	$8,951	$17,882	$23,480	0%

RTW Claims Data (Calendar-days away from work by decile)

10%	20%	30%	40%	**50%**	60%	70%	80%	**90%**	100%	Mean
13	20	22	26	**28**	28	29	33	**73**	195	37.37

711 Arthropathy associated with infections *(cont'd)*

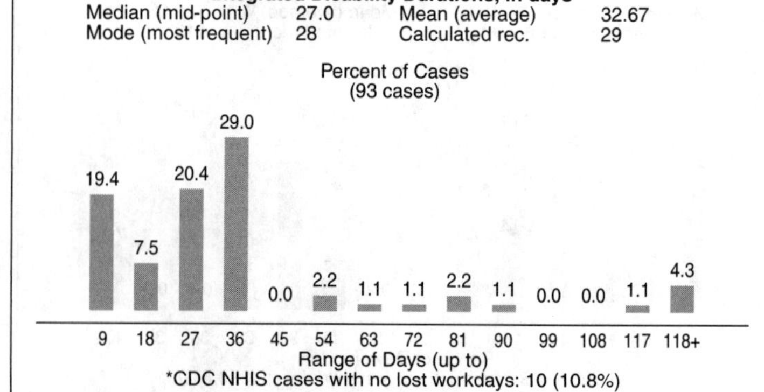

Impact on Total Absence: Prevalence 0.0080% of total lost workdays; Incidence 0.08 days per 100 workers

711.0 Pyogenic arthritis

Return-To-Work Summary Guidelines		
Dataset	**Midrange**	**At-Risk**
Claims data	25 days	60 days
All absences	20 days	35 days

Return-To-Work "Best Practice" Guidelines
Medical treatment: 7 days
Medical treatment, extensive IV antibiotics: 21 days
With surgery: 28 days

Description: Inflammation of one or more joints that is caused by infection. Swelling and pain in the joint(s), along with chills, fever, and rash are among the symptoms.
Other names: Infectious arthritis

[0-9] Arthritis or polyarthritis (due to):
coliform [Escherichia coli]
Hemophilus influenzae [H. influenzae]
pneumococcal
Pseudomonas
staphylococcal
streptococcal
Pyarthrosis
Use additional code to identify infectious organism (041.0-041.8)

Workers' Comp Costs per Claim (based on 49 claims)

Quartile	25%	50%	75%	Mean	% no cost
Indemnity	$1,218	$1,460	$4,074	$9,386	31%
Medical	$3,192	$8,101	$17,882	$18,677	0%
Total	$4,673	$9,209	$17,882	$25,176	0%

RTW Claims Data (Calendar-days away from work by decile)

10%	20%	30%	40%	**50%**	60%	70%	80%	**90%**	100%	Mean
10	14	20	22	**25**	28	29	33	**60**	365	37.88

711.0 Pyogenic arthritis *(cont'd)*

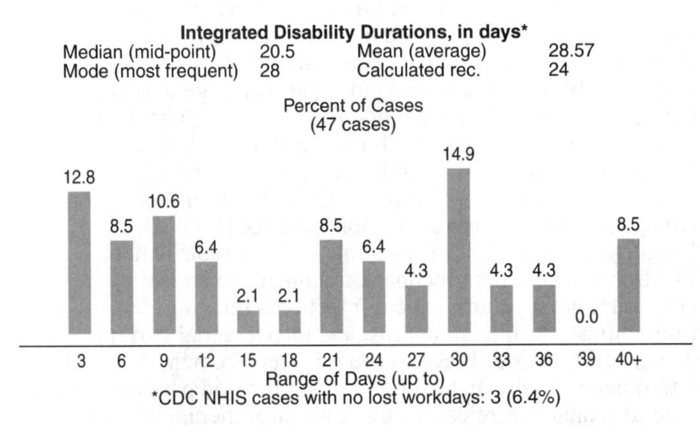

Impact on Total Absence: Prevalence 0.0037% of total lost workdays; Incidence 0.04 days per 100 workers

714 Rheumatoid arthritis and other inflammatory polyarthropathies

Return-To-Work Summary Guidelines		
Dataset	**Midrange**	**At-Risk**
Claims data	43 days	93 days
All absences	30 days	90 days

Return-To-Work "Best Practice" Guidelines
See 714.0

Excludes:
rheumatic fever (390)
rheumatoid arthritis of spine NOS (720.0)

Disability Duration Adjustment Factors by Age						
Age Group	18-24	25-34	35-44	45-54	55-64	65-74
Adjustment Factor	NA	0.77	0.77	1.43	0.96	0.46

RTW Claims Data (Calendar-days away from work by decile)

10%	20%	30%	40%	**50%**	60%	70%	80%	**90%**	100%	Mean
15	21	23	32	**43**	49	79	85	**93**	365	70.91

Integrated Disability Durations, in days*
Median (mid-point) 30.0 Mean (average) 57.77
Mode (most frequent) 21 Calculated rec. 35

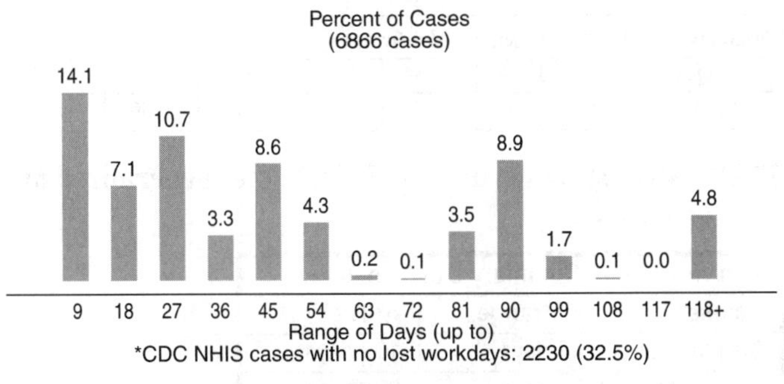

Impact on Total Absence: Prevalence 0.7916% of total lost workdays; Incidence 8.31 days per 100 workers

714.0 Rheumatoid arthritis

Return-To-Work Summary Guidelines		
Dataset	**Midrange**	**At-Risk**
Claims data	43 days	92 days
All absences	31 days	90 days

714.0 Rheumatoid arthritis *(cont'd)*

Return-To-Work "Best Practice" Guidelines
Medical treatment: 0 days
Active, inflammatory, clerical/modified work: 6 days
Active, inflammatory, manual work: 21 days
Arthroplasty, elbow, clerical/modified work: 42 days
Arthroplasty, knee, clerical/modified work: 42 days
Arthroplasty, hip, clerical/modified work: 42-90 days
Arthroplasty, shoulder, arthroscopic, clerical/modified work: 28 days
Arthroplasty, shoulder, open, clerical/modified work: 49 days
Arthroplasty, shoulder, arthroscopic, manual work: 77 days
Arthroplasty, shoulder, open, manual work: indefinite
Arthroplasty, manual work: 84-90 days
Wrist fusion, clerical/modified work: 21 days
Wrist fusion, manual work: 84 days

Description: Autoimmune disease in which the joints are inflamed, causing swelling, pain, and eventual destruction of the joint. Usually the small joints in the hands, feet, wrists, elbows and ankles become inflamed first. Morning stiffness and stiffness after prolonged inactivity, fatigue, and symmetric inflammation (when one finger on one hand is affected, the corresponding finger on the other hand is as well) are among the symptoms.

Arthritis or polyarthritis:
atrophic
rheumatic (chronic)
Use additional code to identify manifestation, as:
myopathy (359.6)
polyneuropathy (357.1)

Excludes:
juvenile rheumatoid arthritis NOS (714.30)

Physical Therapy Guidelines:
Allow for fading of treatment frequency (from up to 3 visits per week to 1 or less), plus active self-directed home PT
Medical treatment: 9 visits over 8 weeks
Post-surgical treatment: 18 visits over 12 weeks

RTW Claims Data (Calendar-days away from work by decile)

10%	20%	30%	40%	**50%**	60%	70%	80%	**90%**	100%	Mean
15	21	23	32	**43**	48	79	85	**92**	365	69.21

Integrated Disability Durations, in days*
Median (mid-point) 31.0 Mean (average) 57.62
Mode (most frequent) 21 Calculated rec. 35

Percent of Cases
(5954 cases)

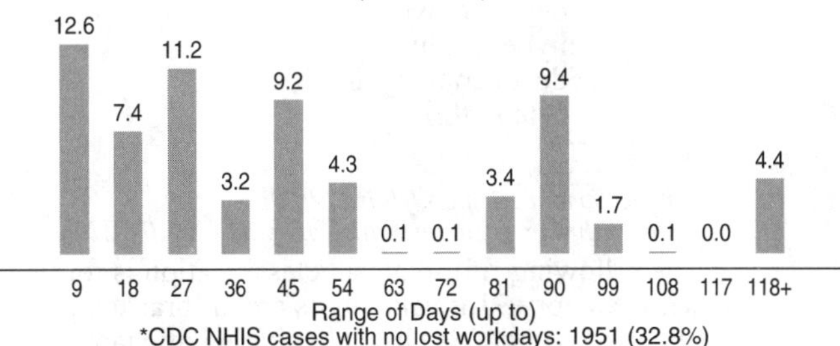

Impact on Total Absence: Prevalence 0.6817% of total lost workdays; Incidence 7.16 days per 100 workers

715 Osteoarthrosis and allied disorders

Return-To-Work Summary Guidelines		
Dataset	**Midrange**	**At-Risk**
Claims data	43 days	103 days
All absences	30 days	92 days

715 Osteoarthrosis and allied disorders *(cont'd)*

Return-To-Work "Best Practice" Guidelines
Medical treatment: 0 days
Visco injection, knee: 7 days
Partial arthroplasty, knee: 28 days
Arthroplasty, wrist, clerical/modified work: 21 days
Arthroplasty, elbow, clerical/modified work: 21 days
Arthroplasty, knee, clerical/modified work: 42 days
Arthroplasty, hip, arthroscopic, clerical/modified work: 21 days
Arthroplasty, hip, clerical/modified work: 42 days
Arthroplasty, shoulder, arthroscopic, clerical/modified work: 28 days
Arthroplasty, shoulder, open, clerical/modified work: 49 days
Arthroplasty, shoulder, arthroscopic, manual work: 77 days
Arthroplasty, shoulder, open, manual work: indefinite
Arthroplasty, other, manual work: 84 days
Wrist fusion, clerical/modified work: 21 days
Wrist fusion, manual work: 84 days
Obesity comorbidity (BMI >= 30), multiply by: 1.31

Capabilities & Activity Modifications:
Sedentary/modified work: Standing limited to 5-10 min/hr; walking only on a smooth surface using crutches with limited pressure on the foot; no walking on an irregular surface; no climbing stairs; no climbing ladders or hill climbing requiring frequent knee flexion; no activities requiring balance; no applying strength against bent knee (squatting, kneeling, crouching, stooping, pedaling, etc.); elevate leg half of time; may need immobilization; limited weight bearing.
Manual/standing work: Standing not more than 50 min/hr; walking on a smooth surface up to 1,200 ft/hr carrying up to 25 lbs; walking on an irregular surface up to 900 ft/hr carrying up to 25 lbs; climbing stairs up to 8 flights/hr carrying up to 40 lbs; climbing ladders up to 50 rungs/hr carrying up to 25 lbs; activities requiring balance up to 45 min/hr (if able to work with two hands without assistance for balance); applying strength against bent knee (pedaling, squatting, kneeling, etc.) up to 60 times/hr; may need brace for uneven ground or ladders.
Description: The most common joint disorder, osteoarthritis is a chronic joint disorder characterized by degeneration of joint cartilage and bone causing pain and stiffness. Morning stiffness, swollen joints that are aggravated by activity, and frozen joints are among the symptoms.
Other names: Degenerative arthritis

Note: Localized, in the subcategories below, includes bilateral involvement of the same site.

Includes: arthritis or polyarthritis:
degenerative
hypertrophic
degenerative joint disease
osteoarthritis

Excludes:
Marie-Strumpell spondylitis (720.0)
osteoarthrosis [osteoarthritis] of spine (721.0-721.9)

The following fifth-digit subclassification is for use with category 715; valid digits are in [brackets] under each code. See list at beginning of chapter for definitions:
0 site unspecified
1 shoulder region
2 upper arm
3 forearm
4 hand
5 pelvic region and thigh
6 lower leg
7 ankle and foot
8 other specified sites
9 multiple sites

715 Osteoarthrosis and allied disorders *(cont'd)*

Procedure Summary (from ODG Treatment): ACI; Activity restrictions; Anterior cruciate ligament (ACL) repair; ACL diagnostic tests; ACL injury rehabilitation; Acupuncture; Arthroplasty; Arthroscopy; Autologous cartilage implantation (ACI); Bone-growth stimulators; Braces; Canes; Cetylated fatty acids (CFA) topical cream; Chiropractic; Chondroplasty; Cold/heat packs; Cold lasers; Continuous-flow cryotherapy; Continuous passive motion (CPM); Corticosteroid injections; Crutches; Deep transverse friction massage (DTFM); Diagnostic arthroscopy; Education for knee replacement; Electromyographic biofeedback treatment; Exercise; Glucosamine; Hyaluronic acid injections; Imaging; Immobilization; Injections; Insoles; Interferential current therapy (IFC); Knee brace; Knee joint replacement; KT 1000 arthrometer; Lachman test; Lateral pull test and patellar tilt test; Lateral retinacular release; Low level laser therapy (LLLT); Magnet therapy; Manipulation; Meniscal allograft transplantation; Meniscectomy; Microprocessor-controlled knee prostheses; Modified duty; Mosaicplasty; MRI's (magnetic resonance imaging); Non-surgical intervention for PFPS (patellofemoral pain syndrome); Occupational therapy; Orthoses; Osteochondral autograft transplant system (OATS); Osteotomy; Pharmacotherapy; Physical therapy; Pivot shift test (MacIntosh test) ; Posterior cruciate ligament (PCL) repair; Post-op ambulatory infusion pumps (local anesthetic); Prolotherapy; Prostheses (artificial limb); Pulsed magnetic field therapy (PMFT); Radiography; Return to work; SAMe (S-adenosylmethionine); Single photon emission computed tomography (SPECT); Static progressive stretch (SPS) therapy; Stretching and flexibility; Surgery; SynviscÒ; Therapeutic knee splint; Therapeutic ultrasound; Transcutaneous electrical neurostimulation (TENS); Ultrasound, diagnostic; Ultrasound, therapeutic; Ultrasound fracture healing (bone-growth stimulators); Viscosupplementation; Walkers; Walking aids (canes, crutches, braces, orthoses, & walkers); Work
Physical Therapy Guidelines:
Medical treatment: 9 visits over 8 weeks
Post-injection treatment: 1-2 visits over 1 week
Post-surgical treatment: 18 visits over 12 weeks

Workers' Comp Costs per Claim (based on 3,939 claims)

Quartile	25%	50%	75%	Mean	% no cost
Indemnity	$6,311	$14,117	$31,721	$23,554	13%
Medical	$8,505	$16,485	$32,939	$23,936	0%
Total	$14,574	$29,836	$62,118	$44,382	0%

Disability Duration Adjustment Factors by Age

Age Group	18-24	25-34	35-44	45-54	55-64	65-74
Adjustment Factor	NA	0.50	1.10	1.10	0.86	1.47

715.9 Osteoarthrosis, unspecified whether generalized or localized

Return-To-Work Summary Guidelines

Dataset	Midrange	At-Risk
Claims data	43 days	103 days
All absences	30 days	92 days

715.9 Osteoarthrosis, unspecified whether generalized or localized *(cont'd)*

Return-To-Work "Best Practice" Guidelines
Medical treatment: 0 days
Visco injection, knee: 7 days
Partial arthroplasty, knee: 28 days
Arthroplasty, wrist, clerical/modified work: 21 days
Arthroplasty, elbow, clerical/modified work: 21 days
Arthroplasty, knee, clerical/modified work: 42 days
Arthroplasty, hip, arthroscopic, clerical/modified work: 21 days
Arthroplasty, hip replacement, clerical/modified work: 42-90 days
Arthroplasty, shoulder, arthroscopic, clerical/modified work: 28 days
Arthroplasty, shoulder, open, clerical/modified work: 49 days
Arthroplasty, shoulder, arthroscopic, manual work: 77 days
Arthroplasty, shoulder, open, manual work: indefinite
Arthroplasty, manual work: 84-90 days
Wrist fusion, clerical/modified work: 21 days
Wrist fusion, manual work: 84 days

Description: See 715
[0-8]

Physical Therapy Guidelines:
Allow for fading of treatment frequency (from up to 3 visits per week to 1 or less), plus active self-directed home PT
Medical treatment: 9 visits over 8 weeks
Post-surgical treatment: 18 visits over 12 weeks

Chiropractic Guidelines:
Allow for fading of treatment frequency (from up to 3 visits per week to 1 or less), plus active self-directed home therapy
Medical treatment: 9 visits over 6 weeks
Post-surgical treatment: 18 visits over 12 weeks

Workers' Comp Costs per Claim (based on 2,312 claims)

Quartile	25%	50%	75%	Mean	% no cost
Indemnity	$5,838	$13,025	$30,755	$22,779	12%
Medical	$7,739	$15,535	$33,968	$23,723	0%
Total	$13,430	$29,106	$62,622	$43,768	0%

Disability Duration Adjustment Factors by Age

Age Group	18-24	25-34	35-44	45-54	55-64	65-74
Adjustment Factor	NA	0.50	1.10	1.10	0.86	1.47

RTW Claims Data (Calendar-days away from work by decile)

10%	20%	30%	40%	**50%**	60%	70%	80%	**90%**	100%	Mean
14	21	24	32	**43**	50	79	86	**103**	365	71.10

RTW Post Surgery (Calendar-days away from work by decile)

10%	20%	30%	40%	**50%**	60%	70%	80%	**90%**	100%	Mean
Total knee arthroplasty										
72	96	109	117	**131**	144	194	293	**365**	365	171.49

715.9 Osteoarthrosis, unspecified whether generalized or localized *(cont'd)*

Integrated Disability Durations, in days*

Median (mid-point)	30.0	Mean (average)	58.75
Mode (most frequent)	1	Calculated rec.	30

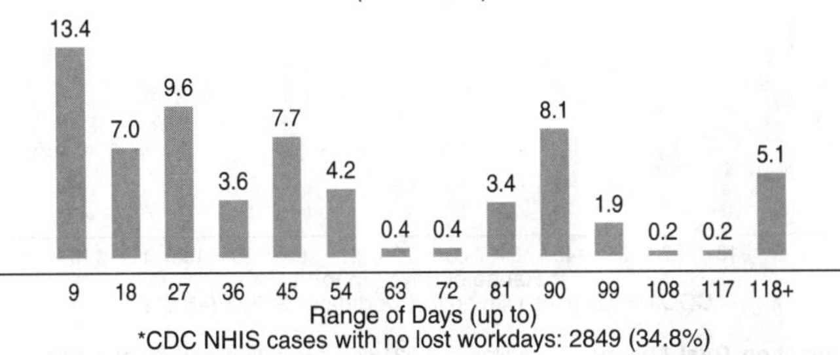

*CDC NHIS cases with no lost workdays: 2849 (34.8%)

Impact on Total Absence: Prevalence 0.9261% of total lost workdays; Incidence 9.72 days per 100 workers

716 Other and unspecified arthropathies

Return-To-Work Summary Guidelines

Dataset	Midrange	At-Risk
Claims data	43 days	90 days
All absences	23 days	88 days

Return-To-Work "Best Practice" Guidelines
See 716.9

Excludes:
cricoarytenoid arthropathy (478.79)

The following fifth-digit subclassification is for use with category 716; valid digits are in [brackets] under each code. See list at beginning of chapter for definitions:
0 site unspecified
1 shoulder region
2 upper arm
3 forearm
4 hand
5 pelvic region and thigh
6 lower leg
7 ankle and foot
8 other specified sites
9 multiple sites

Workers' Comp Costs per Claim (based on 2,168 claims)

Quartile	25%	50%	75%	Mean	% no cost
Indemnity	$7,214	$16,464	$36,824	$27,344	13%
Medical	$7,728	$17,399	$35,417	$27,248	0%
Total	$14,606	$32,918	$70,791	$51,101	0%

Disability Duration Adjustment Factors by Age

Age Group	18-24	25-34	35-44	45-54	55-64	65-74
Adjustment Factor	0.80	0.84	0.93	1.08	1.28	1.36

RTW Claims Data (Calendar-days away from work by decile)

10%	20%	30%	40%	**50%**	60%	70%	80%	**90%**	100%	Mean
14	21	24	42	**43**	60	83	85	**90**	365	53.25

716 Other and unspecified arthropathies *(cont'd)*

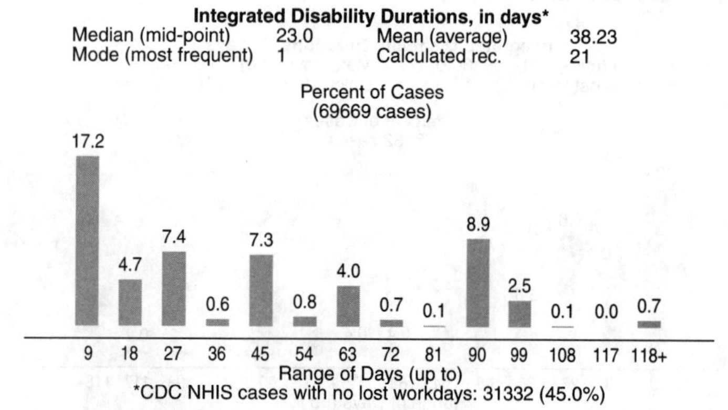

Impact on Total Absence: Prevalence 4.3316% of total lost workdays; Incidence 45.48 days per 100 workers

716.9 Arthropathy, unspecified

Return-To-Work Summary Guidelines		
Dataset	**Midrange**	**At-Risk**
Claims data	43 days	90 days
All absences	41 days	88 days

Return-To-Work "Best Practice" Guidelines
Medical treatment: 0 days
Arthroplasty, elbow, clerical/modified work: 21 days
Arthroplasty, knee, clerical/modified work: 42 days
Arthroplasty, hip, clerical/modified work: 42-90 days
Arthroplasty, manual work: 84-90 days
Wrist fusion, clerical/modified work: 21 days
Wrist fusion, manual work: 84 days
Ankle arthrodesis: 60-90 days

Description: Any disease or abnormal condition that affects a joint.

[0-9] Arthritis, (acute) (chronic) (subacute)
Arthropathy, (acute) (chronic) (subacute)
Articular rheumatism, (chronic)
Inflammation of joint, NOS

Physical Therapy Guidelines:
Post-injection treatment: 1-2 visits over 1 week
Post-surgical treatment: 24 visits over 10 weeks
Post-surgical treatment, arthroplasty, knee: 24 visits over 10 weeks
Post-surgical treatment, arthroplasty, shoulder: 24 visits over 10 weeks
Post-surgical treatment, arthroplasty, elbow: 24 visits over 10 weeks
Post-surgical treatment, arthroplasty/fusion, hip: 24 visits over 10 weeks
Post-surgical treatment, arthroplasty/fusion, wrist/finger: 24 visits over 10 weeks
Chiropractic Guidelines:
Post-surgical treatment: 24 visits over 8 weeks

Workers' Comp Costs per Claim (based on 1,032 claims)

Quartile	25%	50%	75%	Mean	% no cost
Indemnity	$6,059	$13,624	$31,952	$24,239	16%
Medical	$5,912	$13,587	$30,219	$22,106	1%
Total	$11,435	$24,633	$60,774	$42,701	1%

RTW Claims Data (Calendar-days away from work by decile)

10%	20%	30%	40%	**50%**	60%	70%	80%	**90%**	100%	Mean
15	21	23	41	**43**	58	82	85	**89**	365	51.90

716.9 Arthropathy, unspecified *(cont'd)*

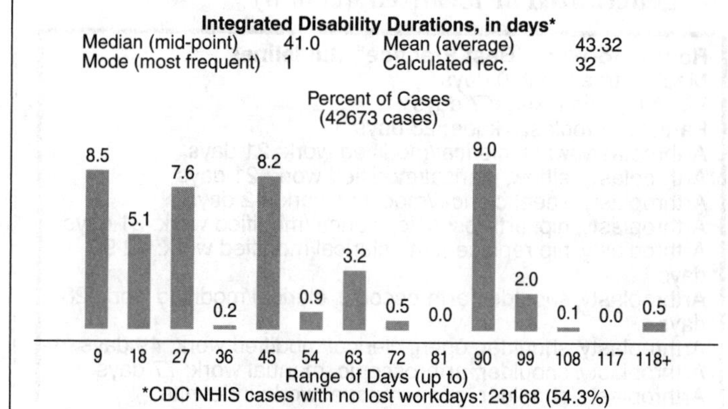

Impact on Total Absence: Prevalence 2.4976% of total lost workdays; Incidence 26.23 days per 100 workers

717 Internal derangement of knee

Return-To-Work Summary Guidelines		
Dataset	**Midrange**	**At-Risk**
Claims data	53 days	194 days
All absences	45 days	126 days

Return-To-Work "Best Practice" Guidelines
See 717.0

Includes: degeneration of articular cartilage or meniscus of knee
rupture, old of articular cartilage or meniscus of knee
tear, old of articular cartilage or meniscus of knee

Excludes:
acute derangement of knee (836.0-836.6)
ankylosis (718.5)
contracture (718.4)
current injury (836.0-836.6)
deformity (736.4-736.6)
recurrent dislocation (718.3)

Workers' Comp Costs per Claim (based on 2,386 claims)

Quartile	25%	50%	75%	Mean	% no cost
Indemnity	$3,182	$6,521	$15,971	$13,587	30%
Medical	$3,350	$7,203	$13,083	$11,619	1%
Total	$5,156	$11,739	$23,993	$21,134	1%

717.0 Old bucket handle tear of medial meniscus

Return-To-Work Summary Guidelines		
Dataset	**Midrange**	**At-Risk**
Claims data	46 days	140 days
All absences	36 days	105 days

717.0 Old bucket handle tear of medial meniscus *(cont'd)*

Return-To-Work "Best Practice" Guidelines
Without surgery, if condition resolves, clerical/modified work: 0-1 days
Without surgery, if condition resolves, manual work: 7 days
Meniscectomy, arthroscopy, clerical/modified work: 10 days
Meniscectomy, arthroscopy, manual work: 35 days
Meniscectomy, arthrotomy (open), clerical/modified work: 21 days
Meniscectomy, arthrotomy (open), manual work: 56 days
Meniscectomy, heavy manual work: 84 days
Meniscus repair (transplant), clerical/modified work: 28 days
Meniscus repair (transplant), manual work: 63 days
Meniscus repair (transplant), heavy manual work: 140 days

Capabilities & Activity Modifications:
Sedentary/modified work: Standing limited to 5-10 min/hr; walking only on a smooth surface using crutches with limited pressure on the foot; no walking on an irregular surface; no climbing stairs; no climbing ladders or hill climbing requiring frequent knee flexion; no activities requiring balance; no applying strength against bent knee (squatting, kneeling, crouching, stooping, pedaling, etc.); elevate leg half of time; may need immobilization; limited weight bearing.
Manual/standing work: Standing not more than 50 min/hr; walking on a smooth surface up to 1,200 ft/hr carrying up to 25 lbs; walking on an irregular surface up to 900 ft/hr carrying up to 25 lbs; climbing stairs up to 8 flights/hr carrying up to 40 lbs; climbing ladders up to 50 rungs/hr carrying up to 25 lbs; activities requiring balance up to 45 min/hr (if able to work with two hands without assistance for balance); applying strength against bent knee (pedaling, squatting, kneeling, etc.) up to 60 times/hr; may need brace for uneven ground or ladders.
Description: Tear of the medial meniscus (one of the two pads of cartilage in the knee between the place where the tibia and femur meet) causing pain, swelling, limitation of movement, and/or buckling of the knee.

Old bucket handle tear of unspecified cartilage

Procedure Summary (from ODG Treatment): ACI; Activity restrictions; Anterior cruciate ligament (ACL) repair; ACL diagnostic tests; ACL injury rehabilitation; Acupuncture; Arthroplasty; Arthroscopy; Autologous cartilage implantation (ACI); Bone-growth stimulators; Braces; Canes; Cetylated fatty acids (CFA) topical cream; Chiropractic; Chondroplasty; Cold/heat packs; Cold lasers; Continuous-flow cryotherapy; Continuous passive motion (CPM); Corticosteroid injections; Crutches; Deep transverse friction massage (DTFM); Diagnostic arthroscopy; Education for knee replacement; Electromyographic biofeedback treatment; Exercise; Glucosamine; Hyaluronic acid injections; Imaging; Immobilization; Injections; Insoles; Interferential current therapy (IFC); Knee brace; Knee joint replacement; KT 1000 arthrometer; Lachman test; Lateral pull test and patellar tilt test; Lateral retinacular release; Low level laser therapy (LLLT); Magnet therapy; Manipulation; Meniscal allograft transplantation; Meniscectomy; Microprocessor-controlled knee prostheses; Modified duty; Mosaicplasty; MRI's (magnetic resonance imaging); Non-surgical intervention for PFPS (patellofemoral pain syndrome); Occupational therapy; Orthoses; Osteochondral autograft transplant system (OATS); Osteotomy; Pharmacotherapy; Physical therapy; Pivot shift test (MacIntosh test) ; Posterior cruciate ligament (PCL) repair; Post-op ambulatory infusion pumps (local anesthetic); Prolotherapy; Prostheses (artificial limb); Pulsed magnetic field therapy (PMFT); Radiography; Return to work; SAMe (S-adenosylmethionine); Single photon emission computed tomography (SPECT); Static progressive stretch (SPS) therapy; Stretching and flexibility; Surgery; SynviscÒ; Therapeutic knee

717.0 Old bucket handle tear of medial meniscus *(cont'd)*

splint; Therapeutic ultrasound; Transcutaneous electrical neurostimulation (TENS); Ultrasound, diagnostic; Ultrasound, therapeutic; Ultrasound fracture healing (bone-growth stimulators); Viscosupplementation; Walkers; Walking aids (canes, crutches, braces, orthoses, & walkers); Work
Physical Therapy Guidelines:
Allow for fading of treatment frequency (from up to 3 visits per week to 1 or less), plus active self-directed home PT
Medical treatment: 9 visits over 8 weeks
Post-surgical treatment: 12 visits over 12 weeks

RTW Claims Data (Calendar-days away from work by decile)

10%	20%	30%	40%	**50%**	60%	70%	80%	**90%**	100%	Mean
13	22	31	35	**46**	56	64	83	**139**	365	66.27

Integrated Disability Durations, in days*
Median (mid-point) 36.0 Mean (average) 58.77
Mode (most frequent) 1 Calculated rec. 33

Percent of Cases (179 cases)

Range of Days (up to)	9	18	27	36	45	54	63	72	81	90	99	108	117	118+
Percent of Cases	15.1	8.4	9.5	16.8	4.5	7.3	10.1	4.5	3.4	6.1	1.1	1.7	0.0	9.5

*CDC NHIS cases with no lost workdays: 4 (2.2%)

Impact on Total Absence: Prevalence 0.0303% of total lost workdays; Incidence 0.32 days per 100 workers

717.5 Derangement of meniscus, not elsewhere classified

Return-To-Work Summary Guidelines

Dataset	Midrange	At-Risk
Claims data	33 days	208 days
All absences	28 days	180 days

Return-To-Work "Best Practice" Guidelines
Without surgery, if condition resolves, clerical/modified work: 0-1 days
Without surgery, if condition resolves, manual work: 7 days
Meniscectomy, arthroscopy, clerical/modified work: 10 days
Meniscectomy, arthroscopy, manual work: 35 days
Meniscectomy, arthrotomy (open), clerical/modified work: 21 days
Meniscectomy, arthrotomy (open), manual work: 56 days
Meniscectomy, heavy manual work: 84 days
Meniscus repair (transplant), clerical/modified work: 28 days
Meniscus repair (transplant), manual work: 63 days
Meniscus repair (transplant), heavy manual work: 140 days

Capabilities & Activity Modifications:
Sedentary/modified work: Standing limited to 5-10 min/hr; walking only on a smooth surface using crutches with limited pressure on the foot; no walking on an irregular surface; no climbing stairs; no climbing ladders or hill climbing requiring frequent knee flexion; no activities requiring balance; no applying strength against bent knee (squatting, kneeling, crouching, stooping, pedaling, etc.); elevate leg half of time; may need immobilization; limited weight bearing.
Manual/standing work: Standing not more than 50 min/hr; walking on a smooth surface up to 1,200 ft/hr carrying up to 25 lbs; walking on an irregular surface up to 900 ft/hr carrying up to 25 lbs; climbing stairs up to 8 flights/hr carrying up to 40 lbs;

717.5 Derangement of meniscus, not elsewhere classified *(cont'd)*

climbing ladders up to 50 rungs/hr carrying up to 25 lbs; activities requiring balance up to 45 min/hr (if able to work with two hands without assistance for balance); applying strength against bent knee (pedaling, squatting, kneeling, etc.) up to 60 times/hr; may need brace for uneven ground or ladders.

Description: Tear or other form of derangement of one of the meniscus (pads of cartilage in the knee between the place where the tibia and femur meet) causing pain, swelling, limitation of movement, and/or buckling of the knee.

Other names: Injured knee cartilage, Torn knee cartilage
Congenital discoid meniscus
Cyst of semilunar cartilage
Derangement of semilunar cartilage NOS

Procedure Summary (from ODG Treatment): ACI; Activity restrictions; Anterior cruciate ligament (ACL) repair; ACL diagnostic tests; ACL injury rehabilitation; Acupuncture; Arthroplasty; Arthroscopy; Autologous cartilage implantation (ACI); Bone-growth stimulators; Braces; Canes; Cetylated fatty acids (CFA) topical cream; Chiropractic; Chondroplasty; Cold/heat packs; Cold lasers; Continuous-flow cryotherapy; Continuous passive motion (CPM); Corticosteroid injections; Crutches; Deep transverse friction massage (DTFM); Diagnostic arthroscopy; Education for knee replacement; Electromyographic biofeedback treatment; Exercise; Glucosamine; Hyaluronic acid injections; Imaging; Immobilization; Injections; Insoles; Interferential current therapy (IFC); Knee brace; Knee joint replacement; KT 1000 arthrometer; Lachman test; Lateral pull test and patellar tilt test; Lateral retinacular release; Low level laser therapy (LLLT); Magnet therapy; Manipulation; Meniscal allograft transplantation; Meniscectomy; Microprocessor-controlled knee prostheses; Modified duty; Mosaicplasty; MRI's (magnetic resonance imaging); Non-surgical intervention for PFPS (patellofemoral pain syndrome); Occupational therapy; Orthoses; Osteochondral autograft transplant system (OATS); Osteotomy; Pharmacotherapy; Physical therapy; Pivot shift test (MacIntosh test) ; Posterior cruciate ligament (PCL) repair; Post-op ambulatory infusion pumps (local anesthetic); Prolotherapy; Prostheses (artificial limb); Pulsed magnetic field therapy (PMFT); Radiography; Return to work; SAMe (S-adenosylmethionine); Single photon emission computed tomography (SPECT); Static progressive stretch (SPS) therapy; Stretching and flexibility; Surgery; SynviscÒ; Therapeutic knee splint; Therapeutic ultrasound; Transcutaneous electrical neurostimulation (TENS); Ultrasound, diagnostic; Ultrasound, therapeutic; Ultrasound fracture healing (bone-growth stimulators); Viscosupplementation; Walkers; Walking aids (canes, crutches, braces, orthoses, & walkers); Work

Physical Therapy Guidelines:
Allow for fading of treatment frequency (from up to 3 visits per week to 1 or less), plus active self-directed home PT
9 visits over 8 weeks

Workers' Comp Costs per Claim (based on 99 claims)

Quartile	25%	50%	75%	Mean	% no cost
Indemnity	$3,518	$7,938	$24,476	$16,965	25%
Medical	$4,998	$8,411	$23,531	$17,153	2%
Total	$6,836	$15,467	$39,984	$30,126	2%

RTW Claims Data (Calendar-days away from work by decile)

10%	20%	30%	40%	**50%**	60%	70%	80%	**90%**	100%	Mean
13	20	24	27	**33**	56	64	85	**208**	365	70.90

717.5 Derangement of meniscus, not elsewhere classified *(cont'd)*

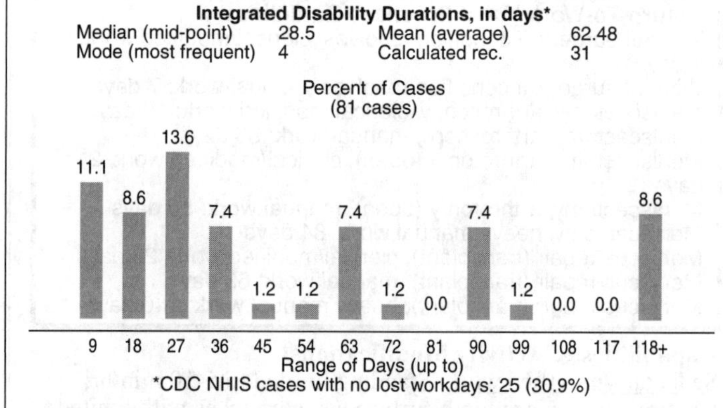

Impact on Total Absence: Prevalence 0.0103% of total lost workdays; Incidence 0.11 days per 100 workers

717.6 Loose body in knee

Return-To-Work Summary Guidelines

Dataset	Midrange	At-Risk
Claims data	35 days	87 days
All absences	32 days	68 days

Return-To-Work "Best Practice" Guidelines
Arthroscopic surgery, clerical/modified work: 21 days
Arthroscopic surgery, manual work: 35 days
Open surgery, clerical/modified work: 35 days
Open surgery, manual work: 56 days

Capabilities & Activity Modifications:
Sedentary/modified work: Standing limited to 5-10 min/hr; walking only on a smooth surface using crutches with limited pressure on the foot; no walking on an irregular surface; no climbing stairs; no climbing ladders or hill climbing requiring frequent knee flexion; no activities requiring balance; no applying strength against bent knee (squatting, kneeling, crouching, stooping, pedaling, etc.); elevate leg half of time; may need immobilization; limited weight bearing.
Manual/standing work: Standing not more than 50 min/hr; walking on a smooth surface up to 1,200 ft/hr carrying up to 25 lbs; walking on an irregular surface up to 900 ft/hr carrying up to 25 lbs; climbing stairs up to 8 flights/hr carrying up to 40 lbs; climbing ladders up to 50 rungs/hr carrying up to 25 lbs; activities requiring balance up to 45 min/hr (if able to work with two hands without assistance for balance); applying strength against bent knee (pedaling, squatting, kneeling, etc.) up to 60 times/hr; may need brace for uneven ground or ladders.

Description: Detached pieces of bone or cartilage in the joint space of the knee causing pain or swelling of the joint with occasional locking or catching. There could be a grating sound and/or a history of osteoarthritis.
Joint mice, knee
Rice bodies, knee (joint)

Procedure Summary (from ODG Treatment): ACI; Activity restrictions; Anterior cruciate ligament (ACL) repair; ACL diagnostic tests; ACL injury rehabilitation; Acupuncture; Arthroplasty; Arthroscopy; Autologous cartilage implantation (ACI); Bone-growth stimulators; Braces; Canes; Cetylated fatty acids (CFA) topical cream; Chiropractic; Chondroplasty; Cold/heat packs; Cold lasers; Continuous-flow cryotherapy; Continuous passive motion (CPM); Corticosteroid injections; Crutches; Deep transverse friction massage (DTFM); Diagnostic arthroscopy; Education for knee replacement;

717.6 Loose body in knee *(cont'd)*

Electromyographic biofeedback treatment; Exercise; Glucosamine; Hyaluronic acid injections; Imaging; Immobilization; Injections; Insoles; Interferential current therapy (IFC); Knee brace; Knee joint replacement; KT 1000 arthrometer; Lachman test; Lateral pull test and patellar tilt test; Lateral retinacular release; Low level laser therapy (LLLT); Magnet therapy; Manipulation; Meniscal allograft transplantation; Meniscectomy; Microprocessor-controlled knee prostheses; Modified duty; Mosaicplasty; MRI's (magnetic resonance imaging); Non-surgical intervention for PFPS (patellofemoral pain syndrome); Occupational therapy; Orthoses; Osteochondral autograft transplant system (OATS); Osteotomy; Pharmacotherapy; Physical therapy; Pivot shift test (MacIntosh test) ; Posterior cruciate ligament (PCL) repair; Post-op ambulatory infusion pumps (local anesthetic); Prolotherapy; Prostheses (artificial limb); Pulsed magnetic field therapy (PMFT); Radiography; Return to work; SAMe (S-adenosylmethionine); Single photon emission computed tomography (SPECT); Static progressive stretch (SPS) therapy; Stretching and flexibility; Surgery; SynviscÒ; Therapeutic knee splint; Therapeutic ultrasound; Transcutaneous electrical neurostimulation (TENS); Ultrasound, diagnostic; Ultrasound, therapeutic; Ultrasound fracture healing (bone-growth stimulators); Viscosupplementation; Walkers; Walking aids (canes, crutches, braces, orthoses, & walkers); Work

Physical Therapy Guidelines:
9 visits over 8 weeks

Workers' Comp Costs per Claim (based on 219 claims)					
Quartile	25%	50%	75%	Mean	% no cost
Indemnity	$3,161	$4,935	$9,849	$10,675	30%
Medical	$4,935	$6,920	$12,117	$10,851	0%
Total	$6,531	$11,088	$18,228	$18,370	0%

RTW Claims Data (Calendar-days away from work by decile)										
10%	20%	30%	40%	**50%**	60%	70%	80%	**90%**	100%	Mean
11	16	21	32	**35**	36	46	57	**87**	336	44.46

Integrated Disability Durations, in days*

Median (mid-point)	32.0	Mean (average)	38.40
Mode (most frequent)	35	Calculated rec.	34

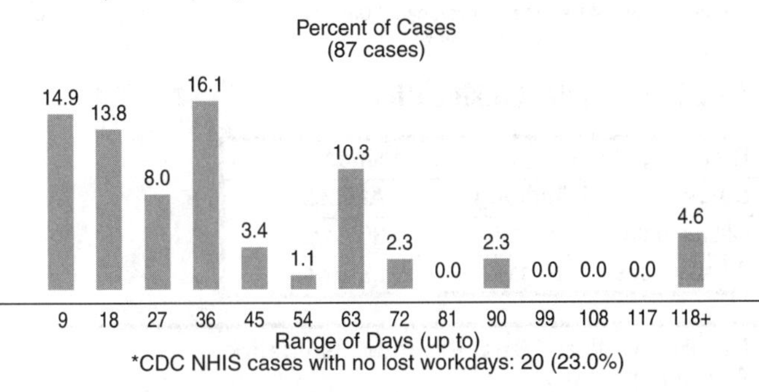

*CDC NHIS cases with no lost workdays: 20 (23.0%)

Impact on Total Absence: Prevalence 0.0076% of total lost workdays; Incidence 0.08 days per 100 workers

717.7 Chondromalacia of patella

Return-To-Work Summary Guidelines		
Dataset	**Midrange**	**At-Risk**
Claims data	35 days	139 days
All absences	27 days	112 days

717.7 Chondromalacia of patella *(cont'd)*

Return-To-Work "Best Practice" Guidelines
Initial conservative medical treatment, clerical/modified work: 0 days
Initial conservative medical treatment, manual work: 10 days
Arthroscopy, clerical/modified work: 7-10 days
Arthroscopy, manual work: 28 days
Arthroscopy, debridement of cartilage, clerical/modified work: 7-14 days
Arthroscopy, debridement of cartilage, manual work: 30 days
Arthrotomy, clerical/modified work: 21 days
Arthrotomy, manual work: 49 days

Capabilities & Activity Modifications:
Sedentary/modified work: Standing limited to 5-10 min/hr; walking only on a smooth surface using crutches with limited pressure on the foot; no walking on an irregular surface; no climbing stairs; no climbing ladders or hill climbing requiring frequent knee flexion; no activities requiring balance; no applying strength against bent knee (squatting, kneeling, crouching, stooping, pedaling, etc.); elevate leg half of time; may need immobilization; limited weight bearing.
Manual/standing work: Standing not more than 50 min/hr; walking on a smooth surface up to 1,200 ft/hr carrying up to 25 lbs; walking on an irregular surface up to 900 ft/hr carrying up to 25 lbs; climbing stairs up to 8 flights/hr carrying up to 40 lbs; climbing ladders up to 50 rungs/hr carrying up to 25 lbs; activities requiring balance up to 45 min/hr (if able to work with two hands without assistance for balance); applying strength against bent knee (pedaling, squatting, kneeling, etc.) up to 60 times/hr; may need brace for uneven ground or ladders.
Description: Occurs when the cartilage in the knee (patella) becomes worn from age or injury causing knee pain and stiffening with movement because of the roughened surface rubbing against the femur as the knee bends and straightens. There is also pain from sitting with the knee bent for long periods and climbing stairs.
Other names: Chondromalacia knee, Post patellofemoral syndrome

Chondromalacia patellae
Degeneration [softening] of articular cartilage of patella

Procedure Summary (from ODG Treatment): ACI; Activity restrictions; Anterior cruciate ligament (ACL) repair; ACL diagnostic tests; ACL injury rehabilitation; Acupuncture; Arthroplasty; Arthroscopy; Autologous cartilage implantation (ACI); Bone-growth stimulators; Braces; Canes; Cetylated fatty acids (CFA) topical cream; Chiropractic; Chondroplasty; Cold/heat packs; Cold lasers; Continuous-flow cryotherapy; Continuous passive motion (CPM); Corticosteroid injections; Crutches; Deep transverse friction massage (DTFM); Diagnostic arthroscopy; Education for knee replacement; Electromyographic biofeedback treatment; Exercise; Glucosamine; Hyaluronic acid injections; Imaging; Immobilization; Injections; Insoles; Interferential current therapy (IFC); Knee brace; Knee joint replacement; KT 1000 arthrometer; Lachman test; Lateral pull test and patellar tilt test; Lateral retinacular release; Low level laser therapy (LLLT); Magnet therapy; Manipulation; Meniscal allograft transplantation; Meniscectomy; Microprocessor-controlled knee prostheses; Modified duty; Mosaicplasty; MRI's (magnetic resonance imaging); Non-surgical intervention for PFPS (patellofemoral pain syndrome); Occupational therapy; Orthoses; Osteochondral autograft transplant system (OATS); Osteotomy; Pharmacotherapy; Physical therapy; Pivot shift test (MacIntosh test) ; Posterior cruciate ligament (PCL) repair; Post-op ambulatory infusion pumps (local anesthetic); Prolotherapy; Prostheses (artificial limb); Pulsed magnetic field therapy (PMFT); Radiography; Return to work; SAMe

717.7 Chondromalacia of patella *(cont'd)*

(S-adenosylmethionine); Single photon emission computed tomography (SPECT); Static progressive stretch (SPS) therapy; Stretching and flexibility; Surgery; SynviscÒ; Therapeutic knee splint; Therapeutic ultrasound; Transcutaneous electrical neurostimulation (TENS); Ultrasound, diagnostic; Ultrasound, therapeutic; Ultrasound fracture healing (bone-growth stimulators); Viscosupplementation; Walkers; Walking aids (canes, crutches, braces, orthoses, & walkers); Work

Physical Therapy Guidelines:
Allow for fading of treatment frequency (from up to 3 visits per week to 1 or less), plus active self-directed home PT
9 visits over 8 weeks

Workers' Comp Costs per Claim (based on 1,455 claims)					
Quartile	25%	50%	75%	Mean	% no cost
Indemnity	$3,161	$6,500	$14,879	$11,890	29%
Medical	$3,339	$7,156	$12,264	$10,390	0%
Total	$5,145	$11,739	$22,953	$18,841	0%

RTW Claims Data (Calendar-days away from work by decile)										
10%	20%	30%	40%	**50%**	60%	70%	80%	**90%**	100%	Mean
13	19	25	30	**35**	49	61	88	**139**	365	58.71

RTW Post Surgery (Calendar-days away from work by decile)										
10%	20%	30%	40%	**50%**	60%	70%	80%	**90%**	100%	Mean
Knee arthroscopy/surgery										
18	27	34	42	**53**	61	88	128	**226**	365	89.41

Integrated Disability Durations, in days*
Median (mid-point) 27.0 Mean (average) 44.15
Mode (most frequent) 1 Calculated rec. 25

Percent of Cases
(503 cases)

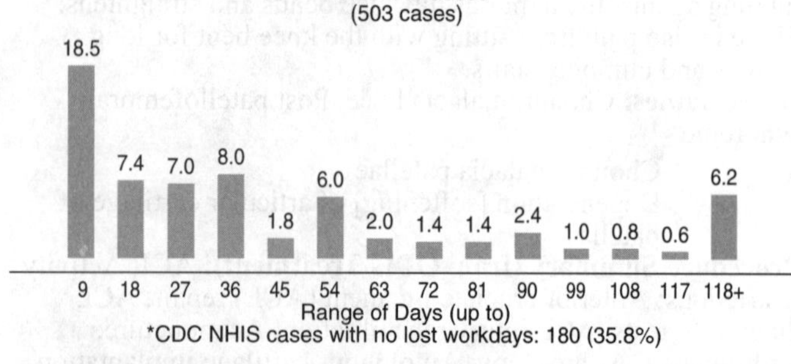

Range of Days (up to)
*CDC NHIS cases with no lost workdays: 180 (35.8%)

Impact on Total Absence: Prevalence 0.0421% of total lost workdays; Incidence 0.44 days per 100 workers

718 Other derangement of joint

Return-To-Work Summary Guidelines		
Dataset	**Midrange**	**At-Risk**
Claims data	19 days	76 days
All absences	8 days	48 days

Excludes:
current injury (830.0-848.9)
jaw (524.6)

718 Other derangement of joint *(cont'd)*

The following fifth-digit subclassification is for use with category 718; valid digits are in [brackets] under each code. See list at beginning of chapter for definitions:
0 site unspecified
1 shoulder region
2 upper arm
3 forearm
4 hand
5 pelvic region and thigh
6 lower leg
7 ankle and foot
8 other specified sites
9 multiple sites

Workers' Comp Costs per Claim (based on 2,415 claims)					
Quartile	25%	50%	75%	Mean	% no cost
Indemnity	$6,962	$16,580	$34,934	$31,618	23%
Medical	$5,649	$14,553	$29,001	$26,531	1%
Total	$11,435	$26,313	$56,543	$51,069	1%

RTW Claims Data (Calendar-days away from work by decile)										
10%	20%	30%	40%	**50%**	60%	70%	80%	**90%**	100%	Mean
10	13	14	16	**19**	28	38	47	**76**	365	35.11

Integrated Disability Durations, in days*
Median (mid-point) 8.0 Mean (average) 19.82
Mode (most frequent) 2 Calculated rec. 9

Percent of Cases
(938 cases)

14.9 8.8 5.0 2.5 5.7 3.4 1.5 0.9 0.5 1.2 1.3 0.6 0.3 8.2
3 6 9 12 15 18 21 24 27 30 33 36 39 40+
Range of Days (up to)
*CDC NHIS cases with no lost workdays: 424 (45.2%)

Impact on Total Absence: Prevalence 0.0301% of total lost workdays; Incidence 0.32 days per 100 workers

718.2 Pathological dislocation

Return-To-Work Summary Guidelines		
Dataset	**Midrange**	**At-Risk**
Claims data	16 days	30 days
All absences	14 days	29 days

Return-To-Work "Best Practice" Guidelines
Arthrography: 0-1 days
Clerical/modified work: 14 days
Manual work: 28 days

Description: Dislocation caused by or involving a disease process.

[0-9] Dislocation or displacement of joint, not recurrent and not current

RTW Claims Data (Calendar-days away from work by decile)										
10%	20%	30%	40%	**50%**	60%	70%	80%	**90%**	100%	Mean
13	14	14	15	**16**	26	28	29	**30**	46	20.20

718.2 Pathological dislocation *(cont'd)*

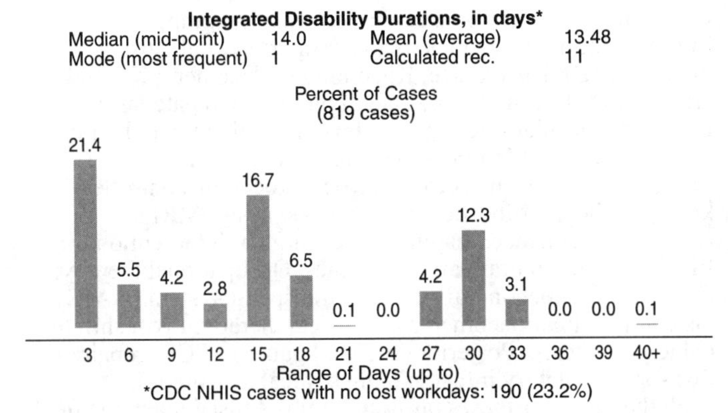

Impact on Total Absence: Prevalence 0.0250% of total lost workdays; Incidence 0.26 days per 100 workers

719 Other and unspecified disorders of joint

Return-To-Work Summary Guidelines		
Dataset	**Midrange**	**At-Risk**
Claims data	15 days	96 days
All absences	11 days	50 days

Return-To-Work "Best Practice" Guidelines
See 719.0

Excludes:
jaw (524.6)

The following fifth-digit subclassification is for use with category 719; valid digits are in [brackets] under each code. See list at beginning of chapter for definitions:

0 site unspecified
1 shoulder region
2 upper arm
3 forearm
4 hand
5 pelvic region and thigh
6 lower leg
7 ankle and foot
8 other specified sites
9 multiple sites

Workers' Comp Costs per Claim (based on 1,438 claims)					
Quartile	25%	50%	75%	Mean	% no cost
Indemnity	$2,016	$5,418	$13,997	$12,960	55%
Medical	$462	$1,491	$7,329	$6,398	2%
Total	$525	$2,336	$12,999	$12,338	2%

719.0 Effusion of joint

Return-To-Work Summary Guidelines		
Dataset	**Midrange**	**At-Risk**
Claims data	13 days	47 days
All absences	10 days	26 days

Return-To-Work "Best Practice" Guidelines
Without surgery, clerical/modified work: 0 days
Without surgery, manual work: 12 days

Capabilities & Activity Modifications:

719.0 Effusion of joint *(cont'd)*

Sedentary/modified work: Standing limited to 5-10 min/hr; walking only on a smooth surface using crutches with limited pressure on the foot; no walking on an irregular surface; no climbing stairs; no climbing ladders or hill climbing requiring frequent knee flexion; no activities requiring balance; no applying strength against bent knee (squatting, kneeling, crouching, stooping, pedaling, etc.); elevate leg half of time; may need immobilization; limited weight bearing.
Manual/standing work: Standing not more than 50 min/hr; walking on a smooth surface up to 1,200 ft/hr carrying up to 25 lbs; walking on an irregular surface up to 900 ft/hr carrying up to 25 lbs; climbing stairs up to 8 flights/hr carrying up to 40 lbs; climbing ladders up to 50 rungs/hr carrying up to 25 lbs; activities requiring balance up to 45 min/hr (if able to work with two hands without assistance for balance); applying strength against bent knee (pedaling, squatting, kneeling, etc.) up to 60 times/hr; may need brace for uneven ground or ladders.
Description: Leakage or swelling of a joint causing joint pain, stiffness, cracking, popping, and/or grinding.

[0-9] Hydrarthrosis
Swelling of joint, with or without pain

Excludes:
intermittent hydrarthrosis (719.3)

Procedure Summary (from ODG Treatment): ACI; Activity restrictions; Anterior cruciate ligament (ACL) repair; ACL diagnostic tests; ACL injury rehabilitation; Acupuncture; Arthroplasty; Arthroscopy; Autologous cartilage implantation (ACI); Bone-growth stimulators; Braces; Canes; Cetylated fatty acids (CFA) topical cream; Chiropractic; Chondroplasty; Cold/heat packs; Cold lasers; Continuous-flow cryotherapy; Continuous passive motion (CPM); Corticosteroid injections; Crutches; Deep transverse friction massage (DTFM); Diagnostic arthroscopy; Education for knee replacement; Electromyographic biofeedback treatment; Exercise; Glucosamine; Hyaluronic acid injections; Imaging; Immobilization; Injections; Insoles; Interferential current therapy (IFC); Knee brace; Knee joint replacement; KT 1000 arthrometer; Lachman test; Lateral pull test and patellar tilt test; Lateral retinacular release; Low level laser therapy (LLLT); Magnet therapy; Manipulation; Meniscal allograft transplantation; Meniscectomy; Microprocessor-controlled knee prostheses; Modified duty; Mosaicplasty; MRI's (magnetic resonance imaging); Non-surgical intervention for PFPS (patellofemoral pain syndrome); Occupational therapy; Orthoses; Osteochondral autograft transplant system (OATS); Osteotomy; Pharmacotherapy; Physical therapy; Pivot shift test (MacIntosh test) ; Posterior cruciate ligament (PCL) repair; Post-op ambulatory infusion pumps (local anesthetic); Prolotherapy; Prostheses (artificial limb); Pulsed magnetic field therapy (PMFT); Radiography; Return to work; SAMe (S-adenosylmethionine); Single photon emission computed tomography (SPECT); Static progressive stretch (SPS) therapy; Stretching and flexibility; Surgery; SynviscÒ; Therapeutic knee splint; Therapeutic ultrasound; Transcutaneous electrical neurostimulation (TENS); Ultrasound, diagnostic; Ultrasound, therapeutic; Ultrasound fracture healing (bone-growth stimulators); Viscosupplementation; Walkers; Walking aids (canes, crutches, braces, orthoses, & walkers); Work
Physical Therapy Guidelines:
9 visits over 8 weeks

Workers' Comp Costs per Claim (based on 825 claims)					
Quartile	25%	50%	75%	Mean	% no cost
Indemnity	$1,302	$3,245	$8,957	$7,115	69%
Medical	$378	$840	$2,405	$2,571	3%
Total	$399	$1,050	$3,686	$4,831	2%

719.0 Effusion of joint *(cont'd)*

RTW Claims Data (Calendar-days away from work by decile)										
10%	20%	30%	40%	**50%**	60%	70%	80%	**90%**	100%	Mean
10	11	12	12	**13**	14	15	23	**47**	302	22.68

Integrated Disability Durations, in days*

Median (mid-point) 10.0 Mean (average) 14.09
Mode (most frequent) 1 Calculated rec. 9

Percent of Cases (1074 cases)

23.3 7.6 6.0 15.2 12.6 2.6 1.0 0.9 0.7 0.5 0.6 0.6 0.6 5.4

3 6 9 12 15 18 21 24 27 30 33 36 39 40+

Range of Days (up to)

*CDC NHIS cases with no lost workdays: 242 (22.5%)

Impact on Total Absence: Prevalence 0.0346% of total lost workdays; Incidence 0.36 days per 100 workers

719.4 Pain in joint

Return-To-Work Summary Guidelines		
Dataset	**Midrange**	**At-Risk**
Claims data	14 days	60 days
All absences	12 days	28 days

Return-To-Work "Best Practice" Guidelines
Medical treatment, modified work: 0 days
Medical treatment, regular work: 0-12 days
With surgery, depending on underlying condition, modified work: 14 days
With surgery, depending on underlying condition, regular work: 21 days

Capabilities & Activity Modifications:
Modified work: Repetitive motion activities (w or w/o splint) not more than 4 times/hr; repetitive keying up to 15 keystrokes/min not more than 2 hrs/day; gripping and using light tools (pens, scissors, etc.) with 5-minute break at least every 20 min; no pinching; driving car up to 2 hrs/day; light work up to 5 lbs 3 times/hr; avoidance of prolonged periods in wrist flexion or extension.
Regular work (if not cause or aggravating to disability): Repetitive motion activities not more than 25 times/hr; repetitive keying up to 45 keystrokes/min 8 hrs/day; gripping and using moderate tools (pliers, screwdrivers, etc.) fulltime; pinching up to 5 times/min; driving car or light truck up to 6 hrs/day or heavy truck up to 3 hrs/day; moderate to heavy work up to 35 lbs not more than 7 times/hr.
Description: Pain in the joints as a symptom of something else. There could be pain in one joint or multiple joints, and other symptoms depend on what is causing the pain.
[0-9] Arthralgia
Procedure Summary (from ODG Treatment): ACI; Activity restrictions; Anterior cruciate ligament (ACL) repair; ACL diagnostic tests; ACL injury rehabilitation; Acupuncture; Arthroplasty; Arthroscopy; Autologous cartilage implantation (ACI); Bone-growth stimulators; Braces; Canes; Cetylated fatty acids (CFA) topical cream; Chiropractic; Chondroplasty; Cold/heat packs; Cold lasers; Continuous-flow cryotherapy; Continuous passive motion (CPM); Corticosteroid injections; Crutches; Deep transverse friction massage (DTFM); Diagnostic arthroscopy; Education for knee replacement;

719.4 Pain in joint *(cont'd)*

Electromyographic biofeedback treatment; Exercise; Glucosamine; Hyaluronic acid injections; Imaging; Immobilization; Injections; Insoles; Interferential current therapy (IFC); Knee brace; Knee joint replacement; KT 1000 arthrometer; Lachman test; Lateral pull test and patellar tilt test; Lateral retinacular release; Low level laser therapy (LLLT); Magnet therapy; Manipulation; Meniscal allograft transplantation; Meniscectomy; Microprocessor-controlled knee prostheses; Modified duty; Mosaicplasty; MRI's (magnetic resonance imaging); Non-surgical intervention for PFPS (patellofemoral pain syndrome); Occupational therapy; Orthoses; Osteochondral autograft transplant system (OATS); Osteotomy; Pharmacotherapy; Physical therapy; Pivot shift test (MacIntosh test) ; Posterior cruciate ligament (PCL) repair; Post-op ambulatory infusion pumps (local anesthetic); Prolotherapy; Prostheses (artificial limb); Pulsed magnetic field therapy (PMFT); Radiography; Return to work; SAMe (S-adenosylmethionine); Single photon emission computed tomography (SPECT); Static progressive stretch (SPS) therapy; Stretching and flexibility; Surgery; SynviscÒ; Therapeutic knee splint; Therapeutic ultrasound; Transcutaneous electrical neurostimulation (TENS); Ultrasound, diagnostic; Ultrasound, therapeutic; Ultrasound fracture healing (bone-growth stimulators); Viscosupplementation; Walkers; Walking aids (canes, crutches, braces, orthoses, & walkers); Work
Physical Therapy Guidelines:
9 visits over 8 weeks

Workers' Comp Costs per Claim (based on 203 claims)					
Quartile	25%	50%	75%	Mean	% no cost
Indemnity	$1,733	$5,996	$12,674	$9,108	47%
Medical	$515	$1,517	$7,833	$6,838	3%
Total	$557	$2,510	$14,249	$11,607	1%

RTW Claims Data (Calendar-days away from work by decile)										
10%	20%	30%	40%	**50%**	60%	70%	80%	**90%**	100%	Mean
10	12	12	13	**14**	16	21	23	**60**	365	29.88

Integrated Disability Durations, in days*

Median (mid-point) 12.0 Mean (average) 20.62
Mode (most frequent) 1 Calculated rec. 11

Percent of Cases (2271 cases)

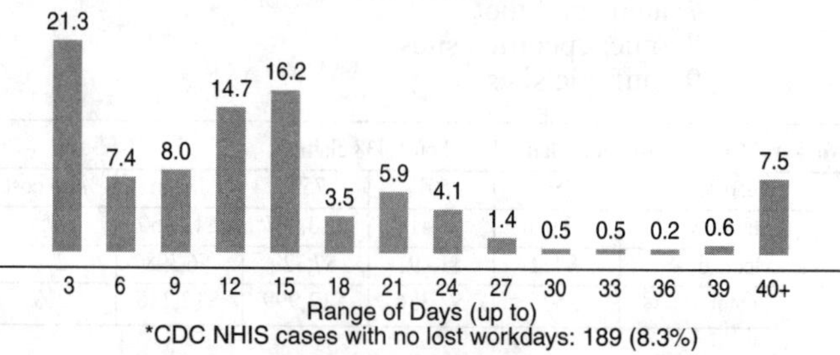

Impact on Total Absence: Prevalence 0.1269% of total lost workdays; Incidence 1.33 days per 100 workers

719.5 Stiffness of joint, not elsewhere classified

Return-To-Work Summary Guidelines		
Dataset	**Midrange**	**At-Risk**
Claims data	14 days	45 days
All absences	4 days	15 days

719.5 Stiffness of joint, not elsewhere classified

Return-To-Work "Best Practice" Guidelines
Medical treatment, depending on cause, modified work: 0 days
Medical treatment, depending on cause, regular work: 0-7 days

Capabilities & Activity Modifications:
Modified work: No overhead work (reaching above shoulder) plus no reaching to shoulder level (90 degree position); no holding arm in abduction or flexion; pulling and pushing not more than 8 lbs up to 4 times/hr; lifting and carrying up to 5 lbs 3 times/hr; single arm upper extremity work using injured arm for light work only; possible immobilization by abduction brace, sling, or clavicle brace; no climbing ladders.
Manual work: Reaching above shoulder not more than 12 times/hr with up to 15 lbs of weight; reaching to shoulder up to 15 times/hr with up to 25 lbs of weight; holding arm in abduction or flexion up to 12 times/hr with up to 15 lbs of weight; pulling and pushing up to 60 lbs 20 times/hr; lifting and carrying up to 40 lbs 15 times/hr; single upper extremity work using injured arm for moderate work only (full use of non-injured arm); possible immobilization by abduction brace, sling, or clavicle brace; climbing ladders up to 50 rungs/hr.
Description: Stiffness in the joint(s), usually as a symptom of something else.
[0-9]
Procedure Summary (from ODG Treatment): ACI; Activity restrictions; Anterior cruciate ligament (ACL) repair; ACL diagnostic tests; ACL injury rehabilitation; Acupuncture; Arthroplasty; Arthroscopy; Autologous cartilage implantation (ACI); Bone-growth stimulators; Braces; Canes; Cetylated fatty acids (CFA) topical cream; Chiropractic; Chondroplasty; Cold/heat packs; Cold lasers; Continuous-flow cryotherapy; Continuous passive motion (CPM); Corticosteroid injections; Crutches; Deep transverse friction massage (DTFM); Diagnostic arthroscopy; Education for knee replacement; Electromyographic biofeedback treatment; Exercise; Glucosamine; Hyaluronic acid injections; Imaging; Immobilization; Injections; Insoles; Interferential current therapy (IFC); Knee brace; Knee joint replacement; KT 1000 arthrometer; Lachman test; Lateral pull test and patellar tilt test; Lateral retinacular release; Low level laser therapy (LLLT); Magnet therapy; Manipulation; Meniscal allograft transplantation; Meniscectomy; Microprocessor-controlled knee prostheses; Modified duty; Mosaicplasty; MRI's (magnetic resonance imaging); Non-surgical intervention for PFPS (patellofemoral pain syndrome); Occupational therapy; Orthoses; Osteochondral autograft transplant system (OATS); Osteotomy; Pharmacotherapy; Physical therapy; Pivot shift test (MacIntosh test) ; Posterior cruciate ligament (PCL) repair; Post-op ambulatory infusion pumps (local anesthetic); Prolotherapy; Prostheses (artificial limb); Pulsed magnetic field therapy (PMFT); Radiography; Return to work; SAMe (S-adenosylmethionine); Single photon emission computed tomography (SPECT); Static progressive stretch (SPS) therapy; Stretching and flexibility; Surgery; SynviscÒ; Therapeutic knee splint; Therapeutic ultrasound; Transcutaneous electrical neurostimulation (TENS); Ultrasound, diagnostic; Ultrasound, therapeutic; Ultrasound fracture healing (bone-growth stimulators); Viscosupplementation; Walkers; Walking aids (canes, crutches, braces, orthoses, & walkers); Work

RTW Claims Data (Calendar-days away from work by decile)

10%	20%	30%	40%	**50%**	60%	70%	80%	**90%**	100%	Mean
8	8	9	11	**14**	15	16	18	**45**	90	20.53

719.5 Stiffness of joint, not elsewhere classified

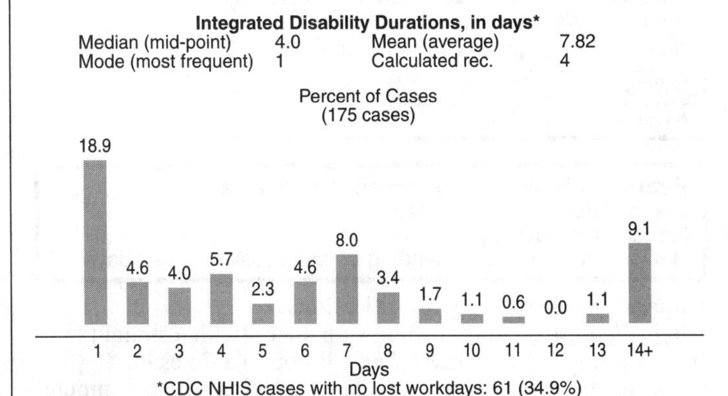

Impact on Total Absence: Prevalence 0.0026% of total lost workdays; Incidence 0.03 days per 100 workers

DORSOPATHIES (720-724)

Excludes:
curvature of spine (737.0-737.9)
osteochondrosis of spine (juvenile) (732.0) adult (732.8)

RTW Claims Data (Calendar-days away from work by decile)

10%	20%	30%	40%	**50%**	60%	70%	80%	**90%**	100%	Mean
12	15	20	26	**31**	40	54	74	**122**	365	54.44

Impact on Total Absence: Prevalence 10.3841% of total lost workdays; Incidence 109.03 days per 100 workers

Occupational Disability Durations, in days
Median (mid-point) 6 - Benchmark Indemnity Costs $4,500

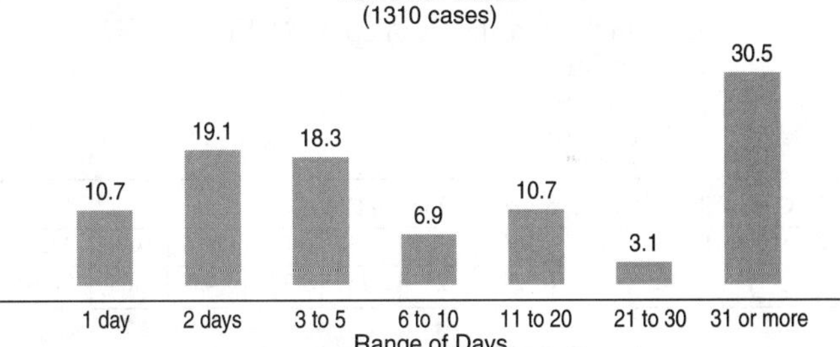

Impact on Occupational Absence: Prevalence 0.0891% of occupational lost workdays; Incidence 0.01 days per 100 workers

720 Ankylosing spondylitis and other inflammatory spondylopathies

Return-To-Work Summary Guidelines

Dataset	Midrange	At-Risk
Claims data	15 days	57 days
All absences	14 days	48 days

Return-To-Work "Best Practice" Guidelines
See 720.9

Workers' Comp Costs per Claim (based on 274 claims)

Quartile	25%	50%	75%	Mean	% no cost
Indemnity	$2,205	$4,337	$12,348	$11,937	55%
Medical	$294	$2,048	$10,259	$7,560	3%
Total	$399	$3,297	$13,776	$13,143	3%

720.0 Ankylosing spondylitis

Return-To-Work Summary Guidelines		
Dataset	**Midrange**	**At-Risk**
Claims data	21 days	43 days
All absences	14 days	42 days

Return-To-Work "Best Practice" Guidelines
Clerical/modified work: 1 day
Manual work: 10 days
Heavy manual work, depending on progression: 21-42 days

Capabilities & Activity Modifications:
Clerical/modified work: Lifting with knees (with a straight back, no stooping) not more than 5 lbs up to 3 times/hr; squatting up to 4 times/hr; standing or walking with a 5-minute break at least every 20 minutes; sitting with a 5-minute break every 30 minutes; no extremes of extension or flexion; no extremes of twisting; no climbing ladders; driving car only up to 2 hrs/day.
Manual work: Lifting with knees (with a straight back) not more than 25 lbs up to 15 times/hr; squatting up to 16 times/hr; standing or walking with a 10-minute break at least every 1-2 hours; sitting with a 10-minute break every 1-2 hours; extremes of flexion or extension allowed up to 12 times/hr; extremes of twisting allowed up to 16 times/hr; climbing ladders allowed up to 25 rungs 6 times/hr; driving car or light truck up to a full work day; driving heavy truck up to 4 hrs/day.
Description: Chronic connective tissue disease causing inflammation of the spine and joints. Back pain (often worse at night), stiffness which is often relieved by activity, pain in the hips, knees, and shoulders, and/or weight loss, fatigue, and a stopped or stiff posture are among the symptoms.
Other names: Marie-Strumpell arthritis
Rheumatoid arthritis of spine NOS
Spondylitis:
Marie-Str
rheumatoid

RTW Claims Data (Calendar-days away from work by decile)										
10%	20%	30%	40%	**50%**	60%	70%	80%	**90%**	100%	Mean
10	11	12	15	**21**	23	25	32	**43**	365	28.63

Integrated Disability Durations, in days*
Median (mid-point) 14.0 Mean (average) 23.17
Mode (most frequent) 1 Calculated rec. 13

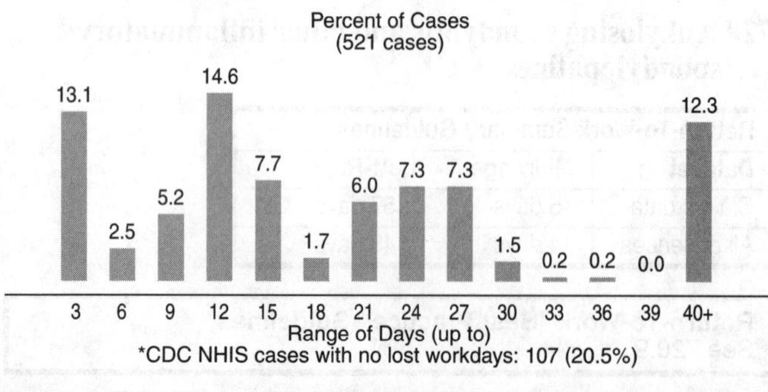

Impact on Total Absence: Prevalence 0.0283% of total lost workdays; Incidence 0.30 days per 100 workers

720.9 Unspecified inflammatory spondylopathy

Return-To-Work Summary Guidelines		
Dataset	**Midrange**	**At-Risk**
Claims data	15 days	57 days
All absences	14 days	48 days

720.9 Unspecified inflammatory spondylopathy

Return-To-Work "Best Practice" Guidelines
Asymptomatic: 0 days
Clerical/modified work: 5 days
Manual work: 14 days

Description: Inflammation of the joints between the vertebrae, which may or may not be infectious. Symptoms include back pain, fatigue, morning stiffness that is relieved by activity, and low fever.
Other names: Infectious spondylitis, Noninfectious spondylitis
Spondylitis NOS

RTW Claims Data (Calendar-days away from work by decile)										
10%	20%	30%	40%	**50%**	60%	70%	80%	**90%**	100%	Mean
13	14	14	14	**15**	16	17	27	**57**	180	25.90

Integrated Disability Durations, in days*
Median (mid-point) 14.0 Mean (average) 19.91
Mode (most frequent) 14 Calculated rec. 15

Percent of Cases
(85 cases)
7.1 14.1 0.0 1.2 31.8 10.6 2.4 0.0 1.2 1.2 0.0 1.2 0.0 8.2
3 6 9 12 15 18 21 24 27 30 33 36 39 40+
Range of Days (up to)
*CDC NHIS cases with no lost workdays: 18 (21.2%)

Impact on Total Absence: Prevalence 0.0039% of total lost workdays; Incidence 0.04 days per 100 workers

721 Spondylosis and allied disorders

Return-To-Work Summary Guidelines		
Dataset	**Midrange**	**At-Risk**
Claims data	14 days	27 days
All absences	12 days	27 days

Return-To-Work "Best Practice" Guidelines
See 721.9

Workers' Comp Costs per Claim (based on 1,881 claims)					
Quartile	25%	50%	75%	Mean	% no cost
Indemnity	$7,329	$19,399	$41,003	$30,660	9%
Medical	$9,797	$20,370	$39,617	$29,339	0%
Total	$18,197	$39,680	$81,060	$57,330	0%

721.0 Cervical spondylosis without myelopathy

Return-To-Work Summary Guidelines		
Dataset	**Midrange**	**At-Risk**
Claims data	15 days	29 days
All absences	11 days	28 days

Return-To-Work "Best Practice" Guidelines
Clerical/modified work: 1 day
Manual work: 10 days
Heavy manual work: 25 days

Capabilities & Activity Modifications:

721.0 Cervical spondylosis without myelopathy

Clerical/modified work: No lifting over shoulder; lifting to level of shoulder not more than 5 lbs up to 2 times/hr; standing or walking with a 5-minute break at least every 20 minutes; sitting with a 5-minute break every 30 minutes (using an operator head set if extended phone operations); no extremes of motion including extension or flexion; no extremes of twisting or lateral rotation; no climbing ladders; driving car only up to 2 hrs/day; possible use of cervical collar with change of position and stretching every 30 min; modify workstation or position to eliminate lifting away from body or using twisting motion.
Manual work: Lifting over shoulder not more than 25 lbs up to 15 times/hr; lifting to level of shoulder up to 30 lbs of weight not more than 15 times/hr; standing or walking with a 10-minute break at least every 1-2 hours; sitting with a 10-minute break every 1-2 hours; extremes of flexion or extension allowed up to 20 times/hr; extremes of twisting allowed up to 16 times/hr; climbing ladders allowed up to 40 rungs 8 times/hr; driving car or light truck up to a full work day; driving heavy truck up to 4 hrs/day.
Description: Inflammation joints between the vertebrae of the neck resulting in neck and back stiffness, pain, fatigue, and/or low fever.

Cervical or cervicodorsal:
arthritis
osteoarthritis
spondylarthritis

Procedure Summary (from ODG Treatment): Activity restrictions; Acupuncture; Arthrodesis (fusion); Arthroplasty; Back schools; Bed rest; Biofeedback; Bone scan; Botulinum toxin (injection); Cervical orthosis; Chiropractic care; Chymopapain (injection); Cognitive behavioral rehabilitation; Cold packs; Collars (cervical); Computed tomography (CT); Computerized range of motion (ROM); Corticosteroid injection; Decompression; Diathermy; Discography; Disc prosthesis; Discectomy/laminectomy; Education (patient); Electromyography (EMG); Electrotherapies; Electromagnetic therapy (PEMT); Epidural steroid injection (ESI); Ergonomics; Exercise; Facet-joint injections; Facet rhizotomy; Flexibility; Fluoroscopy (for ESI's); Fusion (spinal); H-Reflex tests; Heat/cold applications; High-dose methylprednisolone; Imaging; Immobilization (collars); Injections; Laminectomy; Laminoplasty; Laser therapy; Magnetic resonance imaging (MRI); Manipulation; Manipulation under anesthesia (MUA) ; Massage; Methylprednisolone; Multidisciplinary biopsychosocial (rehabilitation); Myelography; Nonprescription medications; Occupational therapy (OT); Opioids; Oral corticosteroids; Patient education; Percutaneous electrical nerve stimulation (PENS); Percutaneous neuromodulation therapy (PNT); Percutaneous radio-frequency neurotomy; Physical therapy (PT); Prolotherapy (also known as sclerotherapy); Pulsed electromagnetic therapy (PEMT); Radiofrequency neurotomy; Radiography (x-rays); Range of motion (ROM); Rest; Return to work; Sensory evoked potentials (SEPs); Soft collars; Steroids; Stretching; Surface EMG (electromyography); Surgery; Therapeutic exercises; Thermography (diagnostic); Traction; Transcutaneous electrical neurostimulation (TENS); Trigger point injections; Ultrasound, diagnostic (imaging); Ultrasound, therapeutic; Videofluoroscopy (for range of motion); Work
Physical Therapy Guidelines:
9 visits over 8 weeks
Chiropractic Guidelines:
(If not contraindicated by risk of stroke)
12-15 visits over 8 weeks

721.0 Cervical spondylosis without myelopathy

Workers' Comp Costs per Claim (based on 794 claims)

Quartile	25%	50%	75%	Mean	% no cost
Indemnity	$8,253	$20,538	$42,525	$31,827	9%
Medical	$10,458	$24,287	$43,239	$30,617	0%
Total	$20,223	$42,635	$84,683	$59,766	0%

RTW Claims Data (Calendar-days away from work by decile)

10%	20%	30%	40%	**50%**	60%	70%	80%	**90%**	100%	Mean
10	10	11	13	**15**	24	25	26	**29**	365	26.33

Integrated Disability Durations, in days*

Median (mid-point)	11.0	Mean (average)	19.47
Mode (most frequent)	1	Calculated rec.	11

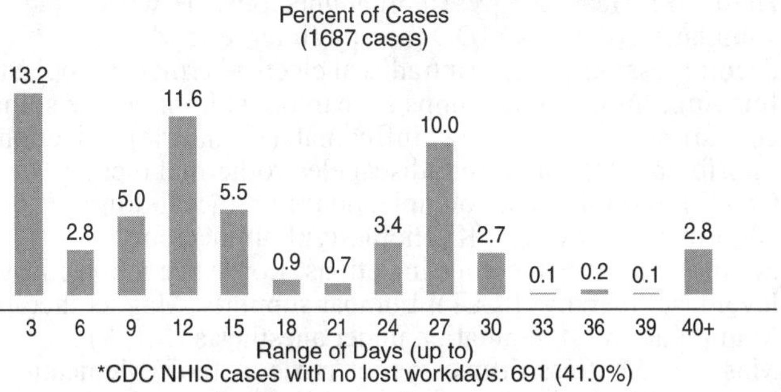

Percent of Cases
(1687 cases)

Range of Days (up to)	3	6	9	12	15	18	21	24	27	30	33	36	39	40+
Percent of Cases	13.2	2.8	5.0	11.6	5.5	0.9	0.7	3.4	10.0	2.7	0.1	0.2	0.1	2.8

*CDC NHIS cases with no lost workdays: 691 (41.0%)

Impact on Total Absence: Prevalence 0.0573% of total lost workdays; Incidence 0.60 days per 100 workers

721.9 Spondylosis of unspecified site

Return-To-Work Summary Guidelines

Dataset	Midrange	At-Risk
Claims data	14 days	27 days
All absences	12 days	27 days

Return-To-Work "Best Practice" Guidelines
Clerical/modified work: 1 day
Manual work: 5-10 days
Heavy manual work: 14-25 days

Capabilities & Activity Modifications:
Clerical/modified work: Lifting with knees (with a straight back, no stooping) not more than 5 lbs up to 3 times/hr; squatting up to 4 times/hr; standing or walking with a 5-minute break at least every 20 minutes; sitting with a 5-minute break every 30 minutes; no extremes of extension or flexion; no extremes of twisting; no climbing ladders; driving car only up to 2 hrs/day.
Manual work: Lifting with knees (with a straight back) not more than 25 lbs up to 15 times/hr; squatting up to 16 times/hr; standing or walking with a 10-minute break at least every 1-2 hours; sitting with a 10-minute break every 1-2 hours; extremes of flexion or extension allowed up to 12 times/hr; extremes of twisting allowed up to 16 times/hr; climbing ladders allowed up to 25 rungs 6 times/hr; driving car or light truck up to a full work day; driving heavy truck up to 4 hrs/day.
Description: Inflammation of one or more vertebrae causing stiffness that is relieved by activity, back pain, fatigue, and low fever.
Procedure Summary (from ODG Treatment): Activity restrictions; Acupuncture; Adhesiolysis; Aerobic exercise; Age adjustment factors; Annuloplasty (IDET); Antidepressants; Anti-inflammatory medications; Aquatic therapy; Arthrodesis; Arthroplasty; Artificial disk; Back brace; Back schools; Bed rest; Behavioral treatment; Biofeedback; Bone-growth stimulators (BGS); Bone scan; Botulinum toxin (Botox);

721.9 Spondylosis of unspecified site *(cont'd)*

Chemonucleolysis (chymopapain); Chiropractic; Coblation nucleoplasty; Cognitive intervention; Colchicine; Cold/heat packs; Computerized range of motion (ROM); Corsets; CT & CT Myelography (computed tomography); Cutaneous laser treatment; Decompression; Diagnostic imaging; Diathermy; Differential Diagnosis; Disc prosthesis; Discectomy/laminectomy; Discography; DRX (traction); Dynamic neutralization system (Dynesys); Education; Electrical stimulators (E-stim); Electromagnetic pulsed therapy; EMG's (electromyography); Epidural steroid injections (ESI's); Ergonomics interventions; Etanercept (Enbrel); Exercise; Facet-joint injections; Facet rhizotomy (radio frequency medial branch neurotomy); Feldenkrais; Flexibility; Fluoroscopy (for ESI's); Foraminotomy; Fusion (spinal); Fusion, endoscopic; Hardware; Heat therapy; Hemilaminectomy; H-wave stimulation (devices); IDD therapy (intervertebral disc decompression); IDET (intradiscal electrothermal anuloplasty); Imaging; Implantable pumps for narcotics; Implantable spinal cord stimulators; Implants; Infliximab (Remicade); Injections; Interferential therapy; Intradiscal electrothermal therapy (IDET); Intradiscal steroid injection; Intrathecal drug administration system; Kyphoplasty; Laminectomy/laminotomy; Ligamentous injections; Lordex (traction); Low level laser therapy (LLLT); Lumbar supports; Magnet therapy; Manipulation; Manipulation under anesthesia (MUA) ; Massage; Mattress firmness; McKenzie method; Medications; MedX lumbar extension machine; Microcurrent electrical stimulation (MENS devices); Microdiscectomy; Modified duty; MR neurography; MRI's (magnetic resonance imaging); Muscle relaxants ; Myelography; Neuromodulation devices; Neuromuscular electrical stimulators (NMES); Neuroplasty; Neuroreflexotherapy; Nonprescription medications; Narcotics; Nucleoplasty; Occupational therapy (OT); Opioids; Oral corticosteroids; Percutaneous diskectomy (PCD); Percutaneous electrical nerve stimulation (PENS) ; Percutaneous endoscopic laser discectomy (PELD); Percutaneous epidural neuroplasty; Percutaneous intradiscal radiofrequency (thermocoagulation); Percutaneous neuromodulation therapy (PNT); Percutaneous vertebroplasty (PV); Physical therapy (PT); Pilates; Powered traction devices; Prolotherapy, also known as sclerotherapy; Psychological screening; Racz neurolysis; Radiofrequency neurotomy; Radiography (x-rays); Range of motion (ROM); Return to work; Sclerotherapy; Shoe insoles/shoe lifts; SPECT (single photon emission computed tomography); Spinal cord stimulation (SCS); Standing MRI; Stimulators, electrical; Stretching; Supports & braces; Surface electromyography (SEMG); Surgery; Sympathetic therapy; Thermography (infrared stress thermography); Traction; Transcutaneous electrical neurostimulation (TENS) ; Trigger point injections; Tumor necrosis factor (TNF) modifiers; Ultrasound, diagnostic (imaging); Ultrasound, therapeutic; Vertebral axial decompression (VAX-D); Vertebroplasty; Videofluoroscopy (for range of motion); Work conditioning, work hardening; Work; X-rays; Yoga

RTW Claims Data (Calendar-days away from work by decile)										
10%	20%	30%	40%	**50%**	60%	70%	80%	**90%**	100%	Mean
10	10	12	13	**14**	17	24	26	**27**	365	23.91

721.9 Spondylosis of unspecified site *(cont'd)*

Integrated Disability Durations, in days*

Median (mid-point)	12.0	Mean (average)	17.89
Mode (most frequent)	1	Calculated rec.	11

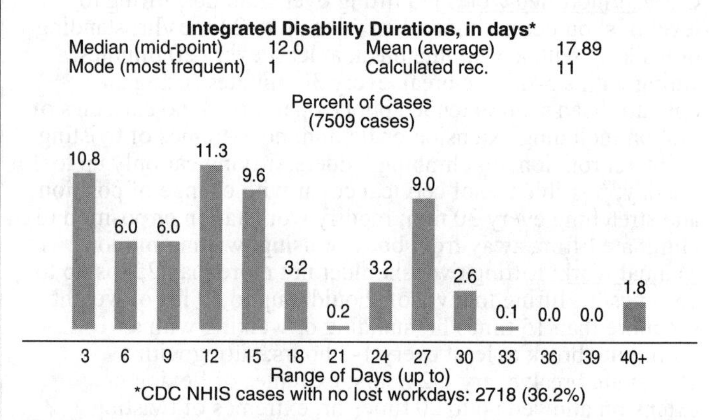

*CDC NHIS cases with no lost workdays: 2718 (36.2%)

Impact on Total Absence: Prevalence 0.2533% of total lost workdays; Incidence 2.66 days per 100 workers

722 Intervertebral disc disorders

Return-To-Work Summary Guidelines		
Dataset	**Midrange**	**At-Risk**
Claims data	38 days	119 days
All absences	28 days	91 days

Return-To-Work "Best Practice" Guidelines
See 722.9

Other names: Herniated disc, Herniated nucleus pulposus (HNP), Disc bulge, Disc rupture, Disc protrusion, Degenerative disc disease (DDD), Spondylosis

Workers' Comp Costs per Claim (based on 22,946 claims)					
Quartile	25%	50%	75%	Mean	% no cost
Indemnity	$6,594	$16,212	$36,330	$26,246	15%
Medical	$8,705	$18,018	$34,314	$26,532	0%
Total	$14,690	$32,293	$68,145	$48,859	0%

Disability Duration Adjustment Factors by Age						
Age Group	18-24	25-34	35-44	45-54	55-64	65-74
Adjustment Factor	0.66	0.74	1.07	1.10	1.35	1.64

RTW Claims Data (Calendar-days away from work by decile)										
10%	20%	30%	40%	**50%**	60%	70%	80%	**90%**	100%	Mean
15	20	23	29	**38**	41	55	67	**119**	365	53.57

722 Intervertebral disc disorders *(cont'd)*

RTW Post Surgery (Calendar-days away from work by decile)										
10%	20%	30%	40%	**50%**	60%	70%	80%	**90%**	100%	Mean
Neck spine fusion										
40	56	68	87	**103**	131	181	251	**365**	365	147.41
Lumbar spine fusion										
88	144	184	222	**278**	326	365	365	**365**	365	254.78
Lumbar spine fusion										
83	124	152	184	**229**	277	353	365	**365**	365	233.50
Insert spine fixation device										
105	143	177	207	**244**	292	365	365	**365**	365	245.53
Insert spine fixation device										
74	130	164	209	**271**	324	365	365	**365**	365	245.27
Insert spine fixation device										
39	55	71	89	**102**	129	174	242	**365**	365	144.87
Apply spine prosth device										
62	97	138	181	**223**	287	365	365	**365**	365	227.06
Epidural lysis mult sessions										
21	56	90	189	**259**	365	365	365	**365**	365	229.00
Percutaneous diskectomy										
32	61	103	124	**183**	251	331	365	**365**	365	201.37
Low back disk surgery										
36	48	62	79	**97**	122	166	240	**365**	365	139.59
Laminotomy, single lumbar										
34	55	92	104	**138**	178	250	365	**365**	365	175.73
Removal of spinal lamina										
43	61	80	97	**116**	163	214	298	**365**	365	164.15
Neck spine disk surgery										
44	56	72	90	**104**	131	179	254	**365**	365	149.37
Removal of vertebral body										
31	50	74	96	**109**	151	198	236	**311**	365	146.43
Removal of vertebral body										
82	116	189	223	**309**	328	363	365	**365**	365	257.89

Integrated Disability Durations, in days*

Median (mid-point)	28.0	Mean (average)	42.55
Mode (most frequent)	1	Calculated rec.	25

Percent of Cases
(29892 cases)

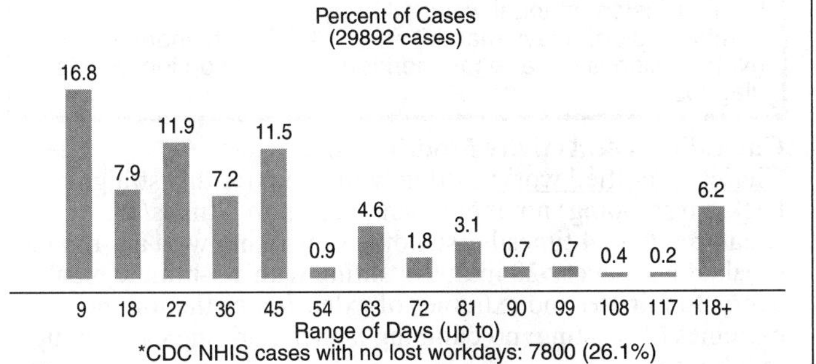

*CDC NHIS cases with no lost workdays: 7800 (26.1%)

Impact on Total Absence: Prevalence 2.7784% of total lost workdays; Incidence 29.17 days per 100 workers

Occupational Disability Durations, in days
Median (mid-point) 55 - Benchmark Indemnity Costs $41,250
(130 cases)
Impact on Occupational Absence: Prevalence 0.0811% of occupational lost workdays; Incidence 0.01 days per 100 workers

722.0 Displacement of cervical intervertebral disc without myelopathy

Return-To-Work Summary Guidelines		
Dataset	**Midrange**	**At-Risk**
Claims data	62 days	128 days
All absences	49 days	125 days

Return-To-Work "Best Practice" Guidelines
Mild cases with back pain, avoid strenuous activity: 0 days
Initial conservative medical treatment, clerical/modified work: 0-3 days
Initial conservative medical treatment, manual/heavy manual work: 35 days
Cervical discectomy, clerical/modified work: 28-56 days
Cervical discectomy, manual work: 56 days
Cervical discectomy, heavy manual work: 126 days to indefinite
Cervical laminectomy/decompression, clerical/modified work: 28 days
Cervical laminectomy/decompression, manual work: 63 days
Cervical laminectomy/decompression, heavy manual work: 105 days to indefinite
Cervical fusion, anterior, clerical/modified work: 28-56 days
Cervical fusion, anterior, manual work: 77 days
Cervical fusion, anterior, heavy manual work: indefinite
Cervical fusion, posterior, clerical/modified work: 35-56 days
Cervical fusion, posterior, manual work: 90-120 days
Cervical fusion, posterior, heavy manual work: indefinite

Capabilities & Activity Modifications:
Clerical/modified work: No lifting over shoulder; lifting to level of shoulder not more than 5 lbs up to 2 times/hr; standing or walking with a 5-minute break at least every 20 minutes; sitting with a 5-minute break every 30 minutes (using an operator head set if extended phone operations); no extremes of motion including extension or flexion; no extremes of twisting or lateral rotation; no climbing ladders; driving car only up to 2 hrs/day; possible use of cervical collar with change of position and stretching every 30 min; modify workstation or position to eliminate lifting away from body or using twisting motion.
Manual work: Lifting over shoulder not more than 25 lbs up to 15 times/hr; lifting to level of shoulder up to 30 lbs of weight not more than 15 times/hr; standing or walking with a 10-minute break at least every 1-2 hours; sitting with a 10-minute break every 1-2 hours; extremes of flexion or extension allowed up to 20 times/hr; extremes of twisting allowed up to 16 times/hr; climbing ladders allowed up to 40 rungs 8 times/hr; driving car or light truck up to a full work day; driving heavy truck up to 4 hrs/day.
Description: Displacement of a disc in the neck that may cause it to press against a nerve of the upper extremities. The pressure on the nerve could cause pain in the shoulder, arm, or hand, which is aggravated by movement, coughing, or sneezing.
Other names: Cervical disc protrusion, Herniated disc, Disc bulge, Disc rupture

Neuritis (brachial) or radiculitis due to displacement or rupture of cervical intervertebral disc
Any condition classifiable to 722.2 of the cervical or cervicothoracic intervertebral disc

Procedure Summary (from ODG Treatment): Activity restrictions; Acupuncture; Arthrodesis (fusion); Arthroplasty; Back schools; Bed rest; Biofeedback; Bone scan; Botulinum toxin (injection); Cervical orthosis; Chiropractic care; Chymopapain (injection); Cognitive behavioral rehabilitation; Cold packs; Collars (cervical); Computed tomography (CT); Computerized range of motion (ROM); Corticosteroid injection; Decompression; Diathermy; Discography; Disc prosthesis; Discectomy/laminectomy; Education (patient); Electromyography (EMG); Electrotherapies; Electromagnetic

722.0 Displacement of cervical intervertebral disc without myelopathy *(cont'd)*

therapy (PEMT); Epidural steroid injection (ESI); Ergonomics; Exercise; Facet-joint injections; Facet rhizotomy; Flexibility; Fluoroscopy (for ESI's); Fusion (spinal); H-Reflex tests; Heat/cold applications; High-dose methylprednisolone; Imaging; Immobilization (collars); Injections; Laminectomy; Laminoplasty; Laser therapy; Magnetic resonance imaging (MRI); Manipulation; Manipulation under anesthesia (MUA) ; Massage; Methylprednisolone; Multidisciplinary biopsychosocial (rehabilitation); Myelography; Nonprescription medications; Occupational therapy (OT); Opioids; Oral corticosteroids; Patient education; Percutaneous electrical nerve stimulation (PENS); Percutaneous neuromodulation therapy (PNT); Percutaneous radio-frequency neurotomy; Physical therapy (PT); Prolotherapy (also known as sclerotherapy); Pulsed electromagnetic therapy (PEMT); Radiofrequency neurotomy; Radiography (x-rays); Range of motion (ROM); Rest; Return to work; Sensory evoked potentials (SEPs); Soft collars; Steroids; Stretching; Surface EMG (electromyography); Surgery; Therapeutic exercises; Thermography (diagnostic); Traction; Transcutaneous electrical neurostimulation (TENS); Trigger point injections; Ultrasound, diagnostic (imaging); Ultrasound, therapeutic; Videofluoroscopy (for range of motion); Work

Physical Therapy Guidelines:
Allow for fading of treatment frequency (from up to 3 visits per week to 1 or less), plus active self-directed home PT
Medical treatment: 10 visits over 8 weeks
Post-injection treatment: 1-2 visits over 1 week
Post-surgical treatment (discectomy/laminectomy): 16 visits over 8 weeks
Post-surgical treatment (fusion): 24 visits over 16 weeks

Chiropractic Guidelines:
(If not contraindicated by risk of stroke)
10 visits over 8 weeks

Workers' Comp Costs per Claim (based on 3,450 claims)

Quartile	25%	50%	75%	Mean	% no cost
Indemnity	$7,791	$17,126	$37,191	$27,114	14%
Medical	$10,406	$23,326	$40,383	$28,111	0%
Total	$17,808	$38,619	$71,484	$51,432	0%

RTW Claims Data (Calendar-days away from work by decile)

10%	20%	30%	40%	**50%**	60%	70%	80%	**90%**	100%	Mean
16	28	34	54	**62**	76	90	119	**128**	365	80.19

RTW Post Surgery (Calendar-days away from work by decile)

10%	20%	30%	40%	**50%**	60%	70%	80%	**90%**	100%	Mean
Neck spine fusion										
40	55	67	83	**101**	125	174	247	**365**	365	145.11
Insert spine fixation device										
39	54	70	86	**100**	122	164	237	**365**	365	141.78
Neck spine disk surgery										
43	55	71	89	**102**	127	166	243	**365**	365	145.97
Removal of vertebral body										
30	45	73	94	**108**	133	174	235	**277**	365	139.37

722.0 Displacement of cervical intervertebral disc without myelopathy *(cont'd)*

Integrated Disability Durations, in days*

Median (mid-point)	49.0	Mean (average)	66.44
Mode (most frequent)	3	Calculated rec.	42

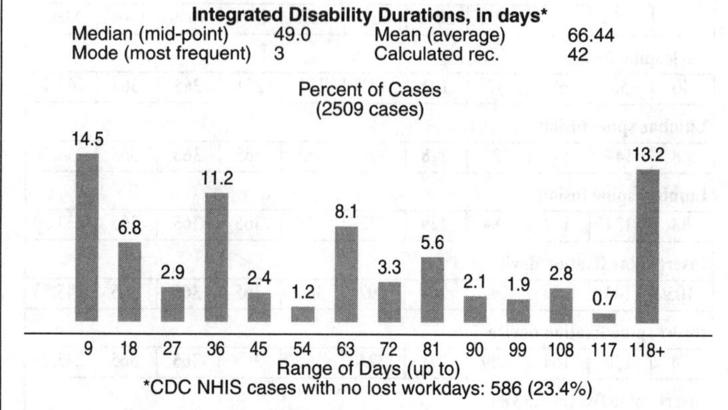

*CDC NHIS cases with no lost workdays: 586 (23.4%)

Impact on Total Absence: Prevalence 0.3776% of total lost workdays; Incidence 3.97 days per 100 workers

722.1 Displacement of thoracic or lumbar intervertebral disc without myelopathy

Return-To-Work Summary Guidelines

Dataset	Midrange	At-Risk
Claims data	66 days	144 days
All absences	55 days	142 days

Return-To-Work "Best Practice" Guidelines
Disc bulge —
Mild cases with back pain, avoid strenuous activity: 0 days
Herniated disc —
Initial conservative medical treatment, clerical/modified work: 0-3 days
Initial conservative medical treatment, manual/heavy manual work: 28 days
Initial conservative medical treatment, regular work if cause of disability: 84 days
Discectomy, clerical/modified work: 28-42 days
Discectomy, manual work: 56 days
Discectomy, heavy manual work: 126 days to indefinite
Laminectomy, clerical/modified work: 28 days
Laminectomy, manual work: 70 days
Laminectomy, heavy manual work: 105 days to indefinite
Lumbar fusion, clerical/modified work: 56 days
Lumbar fusion, manual work: 140 days
Lumbar fusion, heavy manual work: 140 days to indefinite
(Note: fusion is not a recommended treatment option for this diagnosis)

Capabilities & Activity Modifications:
Clerical/modified work: Lifting with knees (with a straight back, no stooping) not more than 5 lbs up to 3 times/hr; squatting up to 4 times/hr; standing or walking with a 5-minute break at least every 20 minutes; sitting with a 5-minute break every 30 minutes; no extremes of extension or flexion; no extremes of twisting; no climbing ladders; driving car only up to 2 hrs/day.
Manual work: Lifting with knees (with a straight back) not more than 25 lbs up to 15 times/hr; squatting up to 16 times/hr; standing or walking with a 10-minute break at least every 1-2 hours; sitting with a 10-minute break every 1-2 hours; extremes of flexion or extension allowed up to 12 times/hr; extremes of

722.1 Displacement of thoracic or lumbar intervertebral disc without myelopathy *(cont'd)*

twisting allowed up to 16 times/hr; climbing ladders allowed up to 25 rungs 6 times/hr; driving car or light truck up to a full work day; driving heavy truck up to 4 hrs/day.

Description: Displacement of a disc in the upper or lower back which may put pressure on the adjacent spinal nerve causing pain and sometimes sensory loss.

Other names: Herniated disc, Herniated nucleus pulposus (HNP), Disc bulge, Disc rupture, Disc protrusion, Degenerative disc disease (DDD), Spondylosis

Procedure Summary (from ODG Treatment): Activity restrictions; Acupuncture; Adhesiolysis; Aerobic exercise; Age adjustment factors; Annuloplasty (IDET); Antidepressants; Anti-inflammatory medications; Aquatic therapy; Arthrodesis; Arthroplasty; Artificial disk; Back brace; Back schools; Bed rest; Behavioral treatment; Biofeedback; Bone-growth stimulators (BGS); Bone scan; Botulinum toxin (Botox); Chemonucleolysis (chymopapain); Chiropractic; Coblation nucleoplasty; Cognitive intervention; Colchicine; Cold/heat packs; Computerized range of motion (ROM); Corsets; CT & CT Myelography (computed tomography); Cutaneous laser treatment; Decompression; Diagnostic imaging; Diathermy; Differential Diagnosis; Disc prosthesis; Discectomy/ laminectomy; Discography; DRX (traction); Dynamic neutralization system (Dynesys); Education; Electrical stimulators (E-stim); Electromagnetic pulsed therapy; EMG's (electromyography); Epidural steroid injections (ESI's); Ergonomics interventions; Etanercept (Enbrel); Exercise; Facet-joint injections; Facet rhizotomy (radio frequency medial branch neurotomy); Feldenkrais; Flexibility; Fluoroscopy (for ESI's); Foraminotomy; Fusion (spinal); Fusion, endoscopic; Hardware; Heat therapy; Hemilaminectomy; H-wave stimulation (devices); IDD therapy (intervertebral disc decompression); IDET (intradiscal electrothermal anuloplasty); Imaging; Implantable pumps for narcotics; Implantable spinal cord stimulators; Implants; Infliximab (Remicade); Injections; Interferential therapy; Intradiscal electrothermal therapy (IDET); Intradiscal steroid injection; Intrathecal drug administration system; Kyphoplasty; Laminectomy/ laminotomy; Ligamentous injections; Lordex (traction); Low level laser therapy (LLLT); Lumbar supports; Magnet therapy; Manipulation; Manipulation under anesthesia (MUA) ; Massage; Mattress firmness; McKenzie method; Medications; MedX lumbar extension machine; Microcurrent electrical stimulation (MENS devices); Microdiscectomy; Modified duty; MR neurography; MRI's (magnetic resonance imaging); Muscle relaxants ; Myelography; Neuromodulation devices; Neuromuscular electrical stimulators (NMES); Neuroplasty; Neuroreflexotherapy; Nonprescription medications; Narcotics; Nucleoplasty; Occupational therapy (OT); Opioids; Oral corticosteroids; Percutaneous diskectomy (PCD); Percutaneous electrical nerve stimulation (PENS) ; Percutaneous endoscopic laser discectomy (PELD); Percutaneous epidural neuroplasty; Percutaneous intradiscal radiofrequency (thermocoagulation); Percutaneous neuromodulation therapy (PNT); Percutaneous vertebroplasty (PV); Physical therapy (PT); Pilates; Powered traction devices; Prolotherapy, also known as sclerotherapy; Psychological screening; Racz neurolysis; Radiofrequency neurotomy; Radiography (x-rays); Range of motion (ROM); Return to work; Sclerotherapy; Shoe insoles/shoe lifts; SPECT (single photon emission computed tomography); Spinal cord stimulation (SCS); Standing MRI; Stimulators, electrical; Stretching; Supports & braces; Surface electromyography (SEMG); Surgery; Sympathetic therapy; Thermography (infrared stress thermography); Traction; Transcutaneous electrical neurostimulation (TENS) ; Trigger point injections; Tumor necrosis factor (TNF) modifiers; Ultrasound, diagnostic

722.1 Displacement of thoracic or lumbar intervertebral disc without myelopathy *(cont'd)*

(imaging); Ultrasound, therapeutic; Vertebral axial decompression (VAX-D); Vertebroplasty; Videofluoroscopy (for range of motion); Work conditioning, work hardening; Work; X-rays; Yoga

Physical Therapy Guidelines:

Allow for fading of treatment frequency (from up to 3 visits per week to 1 or less), plus active self-directed home PT

Medical treatment: 10 visits over 8 weeks

Post-injection treatment: 1-2 visits over 1 week

Post-surgical treatment (discectomy/laminectomy): 16 visits over 8 weeks

Post-surgical treatment (arthroplasty): 26 visits over 16 weeks

Post-surgical treatment (fusion): 34 visits over 16 weeks

Chiropractic Guidelines:

Patient selection based on previous chiropractic success -- Trial of 6 visits over 2-3 weeks

With evidence of objective functional improvement, total of up to 18 visits over 6-8 weeks, avoid chronicity and gradually fade the patient into active self-directed care

Workers' Comp Costs per Claim (based on 11,174 claims)

Quartile	25%	50%	75%	Mean	% no cost
Indemnity	$6,185	$14,522	$32,970	$23,991	18%
Medical	$7,581	$15,960	$30,282	$23,927	0%
Total	$12,905	$27,484	$59,514	$43,539	0%

Disability Duration Adjustment Factors by Age

Age Group	18-24	25-34	35-44	45-54	55-64	65-74
Adjustment Factor	0.66	0.74	1.07	1.10	1.35	1.64

RTW Claims Data (Calendar-days away from work by decile)

10%	20%	30%	40%	**50%**	60%	70%	80%	**90%**	100%	Mean
15	28	34	55	**66**	75	88	128	**144**	365	87.54

RTW Post Surgery (Calendar-days away from work by decile)

10%	20%	30%	40%	**50%**	60%	70%	80%	**90%**	100%	Mean
Lumbar spine fusion										
88	142	184	213	**277**	326	365	365	**365**	365	252.04
Lumbar spine fusion										
83	115	143	181	**221**	277	352	365	**365**	365	229.23
Insert spine fixation device										
88	138	174	200	**233**	282	365	365	**365**	365	242.21
Insert spine fixation device										
89	131	159	209	**278**	352	365	365	**365**	365	249.60
Apply spine prosth device										
83	116	156	189	**244**	322	365	365	**365**	365	241.37
Epidural lysis mult sessions										
56	72	131	205	**259**	365	365	365	**365**	365	241.41
Percutaneous diskectomy										
46	62	103	124	**183**	251	331	365	**365**	365	203.53
Low back disk surgery										
34	48	61	79	**96**	120	164	242	**365**	365	138.81
Laminotomy, single lumbar										
34	54	75	102	**124**	168	215	347	**365**	365	167.49
Removal of spinal lamina										
42	58	75	96	**114**	153	202	292	**365**	365	159.24

722.1 Displacement of thoracic or lumbar intervertebral disc without myelopathy *(cont'd)*

Integrated Disability Durations, in days*

Median (mid-point)	55.0	Mean (average)	71.71
Mode (most frequent)	3	Calculated rec.	46

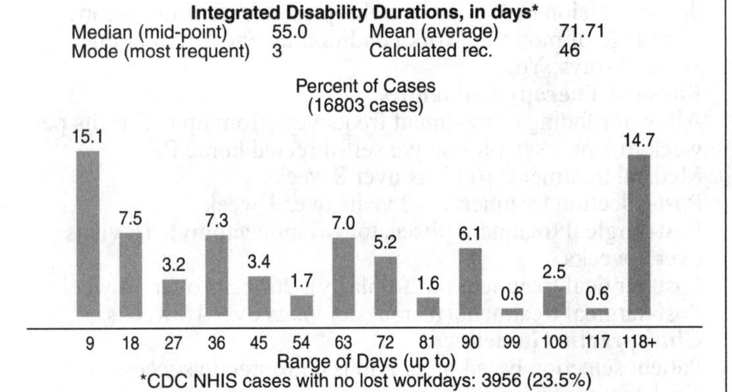

*CDC NHIS cases with no lost workdays: 3956 (23.5%)

Impact on Total Absence: Prevalence 2.7229% of total lost workdays; Incidence 28.59 days per 100 workers

723 Other disorders of cervical region

Return-To-Work Summary Guidelines

Dataset	Midrange	At-Risk
Claims data	57 days	143 days
All absences	17 days	133 days

Excludes:
conditions due to:
intervertebral disc disorders (722.0-722.9)
spondylosis (721.0-721.9)

Workers' Comp Costs per Claim (based on 1,473 claims)

Quartile	25%	50%	75%	Mean	% no cost
Indemnity	$3,896	$7,502	$17,283	$15,099	54%
Medical	$903	$3,386	$10,353	$8,946	2%
Total	$1,071	$5,696	$18,186	$16,080	2%

723.1 Cervicalgia

Return-To-Work Summary Guidelines

Dataset	Midrange	At-Risk
Claims data	17 days	34 days
All absences	12 days	31 days

Return-To-Work "Best Practice" Guidelines
Vague diagnosis —
Clerical/modified work: 1 day
Manual work: 10 days
Heavy manual work: 20-30 days

Capabilities & Activity Modifications:
Clerical/modified work: No lifting over shoulder; lifting to level of shoulder not more than 5 lbs up to 2 times/hr; standing or walking with a 5-minute break at least every 20 minutes; sitting with a 5-minute break every 30 minutes (using an operator head set if extended phone operations); no extremes of motion including extension or flexion; no extremes of twisting or lateral rotation; no climbing ladders; driving car only up to 2 hrs/day; possible use of cervical collar with change of position and stretching every 30 min; modify workstation or position to eliminate lifting away from body or using twisting motion.
Manual work: Lifting over shoulder not more than 25 lbs up to 15 times/hr; lifting to level of shoulder up to 30 lbs of weight not more than 15 times/hr; standing or walking with a 10-minute break at least every 1-2 hours; sitting with a

723.1 Cervicalgia *(cont'd)*

10-minute break every 1-2 hours; extremes of flexion or extension allowed up to 20 times/hr; extremes of twisting allowed up to 16 times/hr; climbing ladders allowed up to 40 rungs 8 times/hr; driving car or light truck up to a full work day; driving heavy truck up to 4 hrs/day.

Description: Pain in the neck caused by degenerative changes in the spine, muscle strain, or tension.

Pain in neck

Procedure Summary (from ODG Treatment): Activity restrictions; Acupuncture; Arthrodesis (fusion); Arthroplasty; Back schools; Bed rest; Biofeedback; Bone scan; Botulinum toxin (injection); Cervical orthosis; Chiropractic care; Chymopapain (injection); Cognitive behavioral rehabilitation; Cold packs; Collars (cervical); Computed tomography (CT); Computerized range of motion (ROM); Corticosteroid injection; Decompression; Diathermy; Discography; Disc prosthesis; Discectomy/laminectomy; Education (patient); Electromyography (EMG); Electrotherapies; Electromagnetic therapy (PEMT); Epidural steroid injection (ESI); Ergonomics; Exercise; Facet-joint injections; Facet rhizotomy; Flexibility; Fluoroscopy (for ESI's); Fusion (spinal); H-Reflex tests; Heat/cold applications; High-dose methylprednisolone; Imaging; Immobilization (collars); Injections; Laminectomy; Laminoplasty; Laser therapy; Magnetic resonance imaging (MRI); Manipulation; Manipulation under anesthesia (MUA) ; Massage; Methylprednisolone; Multidisciplinary biopsychosocial (rehabilitation); Myelography; Nonprescription medications; Occupational therapy (OT); Opioids; Oral corticosteroids; Patient education; Percutaneous electrical nerve stimulation (PENS); Percutaneous neuromodulation therapy (PNT); Percutaneous radio-frequency neurotomy; Physical therapy (PT); Prolotherapy (also known as sclerotherapy); Pulsed electromagnetic therapy (PEMT); Radiofrequency neurotomy; Radiography (x-rays); Range of motion (ROM); Rest; Return to work; Sensory evoked potentials (SEPs); Soft collars; Steroids; Stretching; Surface EMG (electromyography); Surgery; Therapeutic exercises; Thermography (diagnostic); Traction; Transcutaneous electrical neurostimulation (TENS); Trigger point injections; Ultrasound, diagnostic (imaging); Ultrasound, therapeutic; Videofluoroscopy (for range of motion); Work

Physical Therapy Guidelines:
Allow for fading of treatment frequency (from up to 3 visits per week to 1 or less), plus active self-directed home PT
9 visits over 8 weeks

Chiropractic Guidelines:
(If not contraindicated by risk of stroke)
9 visits over 8 weeks

Workers' Comp Costs per Claim (based on 150 claims)

Quartile	25%	50%	75%	Mean	% no cost
Indemnity	$3,087	$4,400	$8,369	$7,256	73%
Medical	$389	$1,239	$4,190	$3,085	5%
Total	$452	$1,281	$6,689	$5,117	5%

RTW Claims Data (Calendar-days away from work by decile)

10%	20%	30%	40%	**50%**	60%	70%	80%	**90%**	100%	Mean
10	11	12	14	**17**	21	28	30	**34**	365	28.24

723.1 Cervicalgia *(cont'd)*

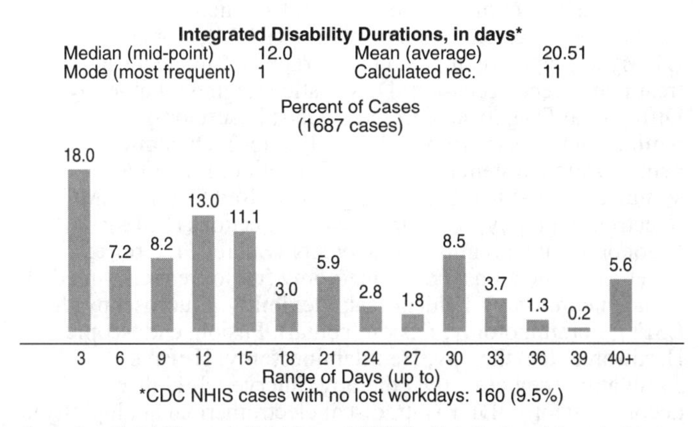

Impact on Total Absence: Prevalence 0.0925% of total lost workdays; Incidence 0.97 days per 100 workers

723.4 Brachia neuritis or radiculitis NOS

Return-To-Work Summary Guidelines		
Dataset	**Midrange**	**At-Risk**
Claims data	28 days	83 days
All absences	26 days	72 days

Return-To-Work "Best Practice" Guidelines
Diagnostic testing: 0 days
Treatment, clerical/modified work: 14 days
Treatment, manual work: 21-28 days
Treatment, manual work, delayed recovery: 35-42 days

Capabilities & Activity Modifications:
Clerical/modified work: Lifting with knees (with a straight back, no stooping) not more than 5 lbs up to 3 times/hr; squatting up to 4 times/hr; standing or walking with a 5-minute break at least every 20 minutes; sitting with a 5-minute break every 30 minutes; no extremes of extension or flexion; no extremes of twisting; no climbing ladders; driving car only up to 2 hrs/day.
Manual work: Lifting with knees (with a straight back) not more than 25 lbs up to 15 times/hr; squatting up to 16 times/hr; standing or walking with a 10-minute break at least every 1-2 hours; sitting with a 10-minute break every 1-2 hours; extremes of flexion or extension allowed up to 12 times/hr; extremes of twisting allowed up to 16 times/hr; climbing ladders allowed up to 25 rungs 6 times/hr; driving car or light truck up to a full work day; driving heavy truck up to 4 hrs/day.
Description: Inflammation in the brachial nerves in the shoulder area causing pain and changes in sensation along the pathway. Symptoms include a severe shoulder ache that sometimes extends to the arm and neck. The pain is constant for about a day and then disappears, and is followed by weakness in the upper arm and shoulder three to ten days later.
Other names: Brachial neuropathy
Cervical radiculitis
Radicular syndrome of upper limbs
Procedure Summary (from ODG Treatment): Activity restrictions; Acupuncture; Arthrodesis (fusion); Arthroplasty; Back schools; Bed rest; Biofeedback; Bone scan; Botulinum toxin (injection); Cervical orthosis; Chiropractic care; Chymopapain (injection); Cognitive behavioral rehabilitation; Cold packs; Collars (cervical); Computed tomography (CT); Computerized range of motion (ROM); Corticosteroid injection; Decompression; Diathermy; Discography; Disc prosthesis; Discectomy/laminectomy; Education (patient); Electromyography (EMG); Electrotherapies; Electromagnetic

723.4 Brachia neuritis or radiculitis NOS *(cont'd)*

therapy (PEMT); Epidural steroid injection (ESI); Ergonomics; Exercise; Facet-joint injections; Facet rhizotomy; Flexibility; Fluoroscopy (for ESI's); Fusion (spinal); H-Reflex tests; Heat/cold applications; High-dose methylprednisolone; Imaging; Immobilization (collars); Injections; Laminectomy; Laminoplasty; Laser therapy; Magnetic resonance imaging (MRI); Manipulation; Manipulation under anesthesia (MUA) ; Massage; Methylprednisolone; Multidisciplinary biopsychosocial (rehabilitation); Myelography; Nonprescription medications; Occupational therapy (OT); Opioids; Oral corticosteroids; Patient education; Percutaneous electrical nerve stimulation (PENS); Percutaneous neuromodulation therapy (PNT); Percutaneous radio-frequency neurotomy; Physical therapy (PT); Prolotherapy (also known as sclerotherapy); Pulsed electromagnetic therapy (PEMT); Radiofrequency neurotomy; Radiography (x-rays); Range of motion (ROM); Rest; Return to work; Sensory evoked potentials (SEPs); Soft collars; Steroids; Stretching; Surface EMG (electromyography); Surgery; Therapeutic exercises; Thermography (diagnostic); Traction; Transcutaneous electrical neurostimulation (TENS); Trigger point injections; Ultrasound, diagnostic (imaging); Ultrasound, therapeutic; Videofluoroscopy (for range of motion); Work
Physical Therapy Guidelines:
12 visits over 10 weeks
See 722.0 for post-surgical visits
Chiropractic Guidelines:
Patient selection based on previous chiropractic success --
Trial of 6 visits over 2-3 weeks
With evidence of objective functional improvement, total of up to 18 visits over 6-8 weeks, avoid chronicity and gradually fade the patient into active self-directed care

Workers' Comp Costs per Claim (based on 941 claims)					
Quartile	25%	50%	75%	Mean	% no cost
Indemnity	$3,822	$7,649	$17,063	$13,691	57%
Medical	$777	$2,951	$9,587	$7,122	2%
Total	$966	$4,599	$15,110	$13,082	2%

RTW Claims Data (Calendar-days away from work by decile)										
10%	20%	30%	40%	**50%**	60%	70%	80%	**90%**	100%	Mean
13	15	18	26	**28**	32	38	46	**83**	365	42.83

Integrated Disability Durations, in days*
Median (mid-point) 26.0 Mean (average) 36.04
Mode (most frequent) 1 Calculated rec. 22

Percent of Cases
(1290 cases)

13.1 17.2 8.2 14.1 7.1 1.7 1.5 1.6 1.0 1.0 0.9 0.7 0.4 3.2

9 18 27 36 45 54 63 72 81 90 99 108 117 118+
Range of Days (up to)
*CDC NHIS cases with no lost workdays: 366 (28.4%)

Impact on Total Absence: Prevalence 0.0984% of total lost workdays; Incidence 1.03 days per 100 workers

724 Other and unspecified disorders of back

Return-To-Work Summary Guidelines		
Dataset	**Midrange**	**At-Risk**
Claims data	16 days	30 days
All absences	14 days	29 days

Return-To-Work "Best Practice" Guidelines
See 724.9

Excludes:
collapsed vertebra (code to cause, e.g., osteoporosis, 733.00-733.09)
conditions due to:
intervertebral disc disorders (722.0-722.9)
spondylosis (721.0-721.9)

Workers' Comp Costs per Claim (based on 3,751 claims)					
Quartile	25%	50%	75%	Mean	% no cost
Indemnity	$3,665	$10,595	$29,862	$21,970	40%
Medical	$1,208	$5,156	$18,165	$14,199	2%
Total	$1,596	$8,988	$36,099	$27,510	1%

724.0 Spinal stenosis, other than cervical

Return-To-Work Summary Guidelines		
Dataset	**Midrange**	**At-Risk**
Claims data	31 days	300 days
All absences	28 days	192 days

Return-To-Work "Best Practice" Guidelines
Medical treatment, clerical/modified work: 1 day
Medical treatment, manual work: 14 days
Medical treatment, heavy manual work: 14-28 days
Surgical decompression, clerical/modified work: 35 days
Surgical decompression, manual work: 70 days
Surgical decompression, heavy manual work: indefinite

Capabilities & Activity Modifications:
Clerical/modified work: Lifting with knees (with a straight back, no stooping) not more than 5 lbs up to 3 times/hr; squatting up to 4 times/hr; standing or walking with a 5-minute break at least every 20 minutes; sitting with a 5-minute break every 30 minutes; no extremes of extension or flexion; no extremes of twisting; no climbing ladders; driving car only up to 2 hrs/day.
Manual work: Lifting with knees (with a straight back) not more than 25 lbs up to 15 times/hr; squatting up to 16 times/hr; standing or walking with a 10-minute break at least every 1-2 hours; sitting with a 10-minute break every 1-2 hours; extremes of flexion or extension allowed up to 12 times/hr; extremes of twisting allowed up to 16 times/hr; climbing ladders allowed up to 25 rungs 6 times/hr; driving car or light truck up to a full work day; driving heavy truck up to 4 hrs/day.
Description: Narrowing of the space around the spinal cord caused by a congenital or developmental abnormality or because of degenerative changes that occur naturally with aging. The main symptom is an intense pain in one or both legs that is brought on by walking or standing.
Procedure Summary (from ODG Treatment): Activity restrictions; Acupuncture; Adhesiolysis; Aerobic exercise; Age adjustment factors; Annuloplasty (IDET); Antidepressants; Anti-inflammatory medications; Aquatic therapy; Arthrodesis; Arthroplasty; Artificial disk; Back brace; Back schools; Bed rest; Behavioral treatment; Biofeedback; Bone-growth stimulators (BGS); Bone scan; Botulinum toxin (Botox); Chemonucleolysis (chymopapain); Chiropractic; Coblation

724.0 Spinal stenosis, other than cervical *(cont'd)*

nucleoplasty; Cognitive intervention; Colchicine; Cold/heat packs; Computerized range of motion (ROM); Corsets; CT & CT Myelography (computed tomography); Cutaneous laser treatment; Decompression; Diagnostic imaging; Diathermy; Differential Diagnosis; Disc prosthesis; Discectomy/laminectomy; Discography; DRX (traction); Dynamic neutralization system (Dynesys); Education; Electrical stimulators (E-stim); Electromagnetic pulsed therapy; EMG's (electromyography); Epidural steroid injections (ESI's); Ergonomics interventions; Etanercept (Enbrel); Exercise; Facet-joint injections; Facet rhizotomy (radio frequency medial branch neurotomy); Feldenkrais; Flexibility; Fluoroscopy (for ESI's); Foraminotomy; Fusion (spinal); Fusion, endoscopic; Hardware; Heat therapy; Hemilaminectomy; H-wave stimulation (devices); IDD therapy (intervertebral disc decompression); IDET (intradiscal electrothermal anuloplasty); Imaging; Implantable pumps for narcotics; Implantable spinal cord stimulators; Implants; Infliximab (Remicade); Injections; Interferential therapy; Intradiscal electrothermal therapy (IDET); Intradiscal steroid injection; Intrathecal drug administration system; Kyphoplasty; Laminectomy/laminotomy; Ligamentous injections; Lordex (traction); Low level laser therapy (LLLT); Lumbar supports; Magnet therapy; Manipulation; Manipulation under anesthesia (MUA) ; Massage; Mattress firmness; McKenzie method; Medications; MedX lumbar extension machine; Microcurrent electrical stimulation (MENS devices); Microdiscectomy; Modified duty; MR neurography; MRI's (magnetic resonance imaging); Muscle relaxants ; Myelography; Neuromodulation devices; Neuromuscular electrical stimulators (NMES); Neuroplasty; Neuroreflexotherapy; Nonprescription medications; Narcotics; Nucleoplasty; Occupational therapy (OT); Opioids; Oral corticosteroids; Percutaneous diskectomy (PCD); Percutaneous electrical nerve stimulation (PENS) ; Percutaneous endoscopic laser discectomy (PELD); Percutaneous epidural neuroplasty; Percutaneous intradiscal radiofrequency (thermocoagulation); Percutaneous neuromodulation therapy (PNT); Percutaneous vertebroplasty (PV); Physical therapy (PT); Pilates; Powered traction devices; Prolotherapy, also known as sclerotherapy; Psychological screening; Racz neurolysis; Radiofrequency neurotomy; Radiography (x-rays); Range of motion (ROM); Return to work; Sclerotherapy; Shoe insoles/shoe lifts; SPECT (single photon emission computed tomography); Spinal cord stimulation (SCS); Standing MRI; Stimulators, electrical; Stretching; Supports & braces; Surface electromyography (SEMG); Surgery; Sympathetic therapy; Thermography (infrared stress thermography); Traction; Transcutaneous electrical neurostimulation (TENS) ; Trigger point injections; Tumor necrosis factor (TNF) modifiers; Ultrasound, diagnostic (imaging); Ultrasound, therapeutic; Vertebral axial decompression (VAX-D); Vertebroplasty; Videofluoroscopy (for range of motion); Work conditioning, work hardening; Work; X-rays; Yoga
Physical Therapy Guidelines:
10-12 visits over 8 weeks
See 722.1 for post-surgical visits

Workers' Comp Costs per Claim (based on 996 claims)					
Quartile	25%	50%	75%	Mean	% no cost
Indemnity	$7,854	$25,421	$48,773	$34,328	6%
Medical	$10,458	$22,654	$41,444	$33,173	0%
Total	$21,693	$49,009	$94,794	$65,272	0%

RTW Claims Data (Calendar-days away from work by decile)										
10%	20%	30%	40%	**50%**	60%	70%	80%	**90%**	100%	Mean
13	14	17	28	**31**	37	70	92	**300**	365	76.65

724.0 Spinal stenosis, other than cervical *(cont'd)*

RTW Post Surgery (Calendar-days away from work by decile)										
10%	20%	30%	40%	**50%**	60%	70%	80%	**90%**	100%	Mean
Removal of spinal lamina										
49	80	90	124	**130**	151	188	227	**365**	365	158.69

Integrated Disability Durations, in days*

Median (mid-point) 28.0 Mean (average) 64.64
Mode (most frequent) 1 Calculated rec. 30

Percent of Cases (1153 cases)

Range of Days (up to)	9	18	27	36	45	54	63	72	81	90	99	108	117	118+
Percent	17.2	22.1	4.5	16.1	2.7	1.7	1.5	6.4	1.8	1.2	1.4	0.4	1.0	12.7

*CDC NHIS cases with no lost workdays: 105 (9.1%)

Impact on Total Absence: Prevalence 0.2002% of total lost workdays; Incidence 2.10 days per 100 workers

724.2 Lumbago

Return-To-Work Summary Guidelines		
Dataset	**Midrange**	**At-Risk**
Claims data	18 days	52 days
All absences	7 days	47 days

Return-To-Work "Best Practice" Guidelines
Vague, descriptive diagnosis with multiple causes —
Mild, clerical/modified work: 0 days
Mild, manual work: 7-10 days
Severe, clerical/modified work: 0-3 days
Severe, manual work: 14-17 days
Severe, heavy manual work: 35 days
Severe, heavy manual work, chemical dependence comorbidity: 49 days
With radicular signs, see 722.1 (disc disorders)
With radiating pain, no radicular signs, see 847.2 (sprains & strains)
Obesity comorbidity (BMI >= 30), multiply by: 1.31

Capabilities & Activity Modifications:
Clerical/modified work: Lifting with knees (with a straight back, no stooping) not more than 5 lbs up to 3 times/hr; squatting up to 4 times/hr; standing or walking with a 5-minute break at least every 20 minutes; sitting with a 5-minute break every 30 minutes; no extremes of extension or flexion; no extremes of twisting; no climbing ladders; driving car only up to 2 hrs/day.
Manual work: Lifting with knees (with a straight back) not more than 25 lbs up to 15 times/hr; squatting up to 16 times/hr; standing or walking with a 10-minute break at least every 1-2 hours; sitting with a 10-minute break every 1-2 hours; extremes of flexion or extension allowed up to 12 times/hr; extremes of twisting allowed up to 16 times/hr; climbing ladders allowed up to 25 rungs 6 times/hr; driving car or light truck up to a full work day; driving heavy truck up to 4 hrs/day.
Description: Pain, discomfort, stiffness, and weakness of the lower back which may or may not extend to the legs, hips, and buttocks. This is a symptom of many diagnoses but it is not a disease in itself. Lumbago and other back problems are second only to upper respiratory infections as a reason for lost work.

724.2 Lumbago *(cont'd)*

Low back pain
Low back syndrome
Lumbalgia

Procedure Summary (from ODG Treatment): Activity restrictions; Acupuncture; Adhesiolysis; Aerobic exercise; Age adjustment factors; Annuloplasty (IDET); Antidepressants; Anti-inflammatory medications; Aquatic therapy; Arthrodesis; Arthroplasty; Artificial disk; Back brace; Back schools; Bed rest; Behavioral treatment; Biofeedback; Bone-growth stimulators (BGS); Bone scan; Botulinum toxin (Botox); Chemonucleolysis (chymopapain); Chiropractic; Coblation nucleoplasty; Cognitive intervention; Colchicine; Cold/heat packs; Computerized range of motion (ROM); Corsets; CT & CT Myelography (computed tomography); Cutaneous laser treatment; Decompression; Diagnostic imaging; Diathermy; Differential Diagnosis; Disc prosthesis; Discectomy/ laminectomy; Discography; DRX (traction); Dynamic neutralization system (Dynesys); Education; Electrical stimulators (E-stim); Electromagnetic pulsed therapy; EMG's (electromyography); Epidural steroid injections (ESI's); Ergonomics interventions; Etanercept (Enbrel); Exercise; Facet-joint injections; Facet rhizotomy (radio frequency medial branch neurotomy); Feldenkrais; Flexibility; Fluoroscopy (for ESI's); Foraminotomy; Fusion (spinal); Fusion, endoscopic; Hardware; Heat therapy; Hemilaminectomy; H-wave stimulation (devices); IDD therapy (intervertebral disc decompression); IDET (intradiscal electrothermal anuloplasty); Imaging; Implantable pumps for narcotics; Implantable spinal cord stimulators; Implants; Infliximab (Remicade); Injections; Interferential therapy; Intradiscal electrothermal therapy (IDET); Intradiscal steroid injection; Intrathecal drug administration system; Kyphoplasty; Laminectomy/ laminotomy; Ligamentous injections; Lordex (traction); Low level laser therapy (LLLT); Lumbar supports; Magnet therapy; Manipulation; Manipulation under anesthesia (MUA) ; Massage; Mattress firmness; McKenzie method; Medications; MedX lumbar extension machine; Microcurrent electrical stimulation (MENS devices); Microdiscectomy; Modified duty; MR neurography; MRI's (magnetic resonance imaging); Muscle relaxants ; Myelography; Neuromodulation devices; Neuromuscular electrical stimulators (NMES); Neuroplasty; Neuroreflexotherapy; Nonprescription medications; Narcotics; Nucleoplasty; Occupational therapy (OT); Opioids; Oral corticosteroids; Percutaneous diskectomy (PCD); Percutaneous electrical nerve stimulation (PENS) ; Percutaneous endoscopic laser discectomy (PELD); Percutaneous epidural neuroplasty; Percutaneous intradiscal radiofrequency (thermocoagulation); Percutaneous neuromodulation therapy (PNT); Percutaneous vertebroplasty (PV); Physical therapy (PT); Pilates; Powered traction devices; Prolotherapy, also known as sclerotherapy; Psychological screening; Racz neurolysis; Radiofrequency neurotomy; Radiography (x-rays); Range of motion (ROM); Return to work; Sclerotherapy; Shoe insoles/shoe lifts; SPECT (single photon emission computed tomography); Spinal cord stimulation (SCS); Standing MRI; Stimulators, electrical; Stretching; Supports & braces; Surface electromyography (SEMG); Surgery; Sympathetic therapy; Thermography (infrared stress thermography); Traction; Transcutaneous electrical neurostimulation (TENS) ; Trigger point injections; Tumor necrosis factor (TNF) modifiers; Ultrasound, diagnostic (imaging); Ultrasound, therapeutic; Vertebral axial

724.2 Lumbago *(cont'd)*

decompression (VAX-D); Vertebroplasty; Videofluoroscopy (for range of motion); Work conditioning, work hardening; Work; X-rays; Yoga

Physical Therapy Guidelines:
Allow for fading of treatment frequency (from up to 3 visits per week to 1 or less), plus active self-directed home PT
9 visits over 8 weeks

Chiropractic Guidelines:
Therapeutic care --
Mild: 6 visits over 2 weeks
Severe: Trial of 6 visits over 2 weeks
Severe: With evidence of objective functional improvement, total of up to 18 visits (12 additional) over 6-8 weeks, avoid chronicity of care
Elective care -- As needed

Workers' Comp Costs per Claim (based on 175 claims)					
Quartile	25%	50%	75%	Mean	% no cost
Indemnity	$1,082	$2,793	$7,361	$7,821	60%
Medical	$315	$830	$4,106	$3,603	8%
Total	$378	$1,334	$6,164	$6,693	3%

Disability Duration Adjustment Factors by Age						
Age Group	18-24	25-34	35-44	45-54	55-64	65-74
Adjustment Factor	0.66	0.74	1.07	1.10	1.35	1.64

RTW Claims Data (Calendar-days away from work by decile)										
10%	20%	30%	40%	**50%**	60%	70%	80%	**90%**	100%	Mean
10	11	14	15	**18**	28	35	47	**52**	365	32.71

Integrated Disability Durations, in days*
Median (mid-point) 7.0 Mean (average) 17.87
Mode (most frequent) 1 Calculated rec. 8

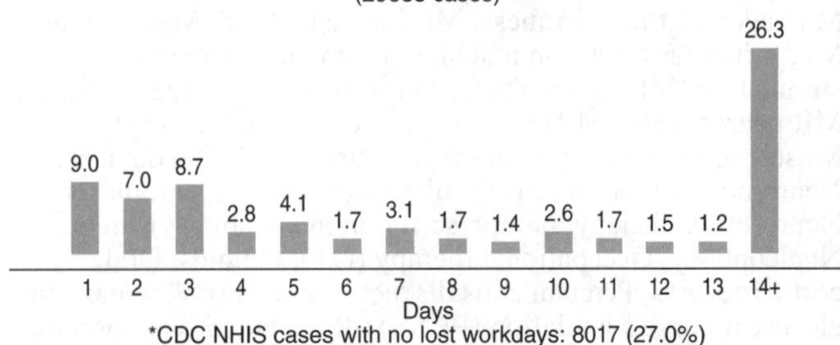

*CDC NHIS cases with no lost workdays: 8017 (27.0%)

Impact on Total Absence: Prevalence 1.1445% of total lost workdays; Incidence 12.02 days per 100 workers

Occupational Disability Durations, in days
Median (mid-point) 19 - Benchmark Indemnity Costs $14,250

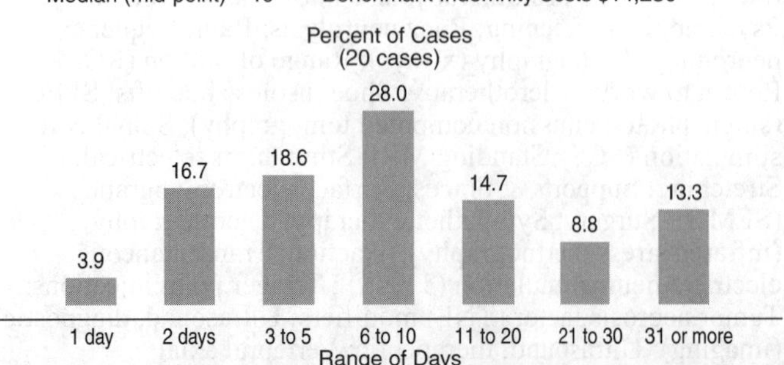

Impact on Occupational Absence: Prevalence 0.0043% of occupational lost workdays

724.3 Sciatica

Return-To-Work Summary Guidelines		
Dataset	**Midrange**	**At-Risk**
Claims data	24 days	77 days
All absences	8 days	38 days

Return-To-Work "Best Practice" Guidelines
Clerical/modified work: 2-5 days
Manual work: 21 days
Heavy manual work: 35 days
As a symptom of herniated disc, see 722 (disc disorders)

Capabilities & Activity Modifications:
Clerical/modified work: Lifting with knees (with a straight back, no stooping) not more than 5 lbs up to 3 times/hr; squatting up to 4 times/hr; standing or walking with a 5-minute break at least every 20 minutes; sitting with a 5-minute break every 30 minutes; no extremes of extension or flexion; no extremes of twisting; no climbing ladders; driving car only up to 2 hrs/day.
Manual work: Lifting with knees (with a straight back) not more than 25 lbs up to 15 times/hr; squatting up to 16 times/hr; standing or walking with a 10-minute break at least every 1-2 hours; sitting with a 10-minute break every 1-2 hours; extremes of flexion or extension allowed up to 12 times/hr; extremes of twisting allowed up to 16 times/hr; climbing ladders allowed up to 25 rungs 6 times/hr; driving car or light truck up to a full work day; driving heavy truck up to 4 hrs/day.

Description: The sciatic nerve runs from the lower back through to the foot. Pain, tingling, and muscle weakness are all symptoms of sciatica, although sciatica is actually a symptom itself and is usually caused by pressure on the nerve by a displaced lumbar disc or inflamed tissue near the nerve.

Other names: Radiculopathy
Neuralgia or neuritis of sciatic nerve
Excludes:
specified lesion of sciatic nerve (355.0)

Procedure Summary (from ODG Treatment): Activity restrictions; Acupuncture; Adhesiolysis; Aerobic exercise; Age adjustment factors; Annuloplasty (IDET); Antidepressants; Anti-inflammatory medications; Aquatic therapy; Arthrodesis; Arthroplasty; Artificial disk; Back brace; Back schools; Bed rest; Behavioral treatment; Biofeedback; Bone-growth stimulators (BGS); Bone scan; Botulinum toxin (Botox); Chemonucleolysis (chymopapain); Chiropractic; Coblation nucleoplasty; Cognitive intervention; Colchicine; Cold/heat packs; Computerized range of motion (ROM); Corsets; CT & CT Myelography (computed tomography); Cutaneous laser treatment; Decompression; Diagnostic imaging; Diathermy; Differential Diagnosis; Disc prosthesis; Discectomy/ laminectomy; Discography; DRX (traction); Dynamic neutralization system (Dynesys); Education; Electrical stimulators (E-stim); Electromagnetic pulsed therapy; EMG's (electromyography); Epidural steroid injections (ESI's); Ergonomics interventions; Etanercept (Enbrel); Exercise; Facet-joint injections; Facet rhizotomy (radio frequency medial branch neurotomy); Feldenkrais; Flexibility; Fluoroscopy (for ESI's); Foraminotomy; Fusion (spinal); Fusion, endoscopic; Hardware; Heat therapy; Hemilaminectomy; H-wave stimulation (devices); IDD therapy (intervertebral disc decompression); IDET (intradiscal electrothermal anuloplasty); Imaging; Implantable pumps for narcotics; Implantable spinal cord stimulators; Implants; Infliximab (Remicade); Injections; Interferential therapy; Intradiscal electrothermal therapy (IDET); Intradiscal steroid injection; Intrathecal drug administration system; Kyphoplasty; Laminectomy/ laminotomy; Ligamentous injections; Lordex (traction); Low

724.3 Sciatica *(cont'd)*

level laser therapy (LLLT); Lumbar supports; Magnet therapy; Manipulation; Manipulation under anesthesia (MUA) ; Massage; Mattress firmness; McKenzie method; Medications; MedX lumbar extension machine; Microcurrent electrical stimulation (MENS devices); Microdiscectomy; Modified duty; MR neurography; MRI's (magnetic resonance imaging); Muscle relaxants ; Myelography; Neuromodulation devices; Neuromuscular electrical stimulators (NMES); Neuroplasty; Neuroreflexotherapy; Nonprescription medications; Narcotics; Nucleoplasty; Occupational therapy (OT); Opioids; Oral corticosteroids; Percutaneous diskectomy (PCD); Percutaneous electrical nerve stimulation (PENS) ; Percutaneous endoscopic laser discectomy (PELD); Percutaneous epidural neuroplasty; Percutaneous intradiscal radiofrequency (thermocoagulation); Percutaneous neuromodulation therapy (PNT); Percutaneous vertebroplasty (PV); Physical therapy (PT); Pilates; Powered traction devices; Prolotherapy, also known as sclerotherapy; Psychological screening; Racz neurolysis; Radiofrequency neurotomy; Radiography (x-rays); Range of motion (ROM); Return to work; Sclerotherapy; Shoe insoles/shoe lifts; SPECT (single photon emission computed tomography); Spinal cord stimulation (SCS); Standing MRI; Stimulators, electrical; Stretching; Supports & braces; Surface electromyography (SEMG); Surgery; Sympathetic therapy; Thermography (infrared stress thermography); Traction; Transcutaneous electrical neurostimulation (TENS) ; Trigger point injections; Tumor necrosis factor (TNF) modifiers; Ultrasound, diagnostic (imaging); Ultrasound, therapeutic; Vertebral axial decompression (VAX-D); Vertebroplasty; Videofluoroscopy (for range of motion); Work conditioning, work hardening; Work; X-rays; Yoga

Physical Therapy Guidelines:
10-12 visits over 8 weeks
See 722.1 for post-surgical visits

Chiropractic Guidelines:
Trial of 6 visits over 2 weeks
With evidence of objective functional improvement, total of up to 18 visits (12 additional) over 6-8 weeks, avoid chronicity of care

Workers' Comp Costs per Claim (based on 876 claims)					
Quartile	25%	50%	75%	Mean	% no cost
Indemnity	$2,006	$3,990	$11,739	$8,694	54%
Medical	$557	$2,006	$5,030	$4,875	3%
Total	$735	$2,982	$9,629	$8,902	2%

Disability Duration Adjustment Factors by Age						
Age Group	18-24	25-34	35-44	45-54	55-64	65-74
Adjustment Factor	0.49	0.80	1.10	1.00	1.34	0.89

RTW Claims Data (Calendar-days away from work by decile)										
10%	20%	30%	40%	**50%**	60%	70%	80%	**90%**	100%	Mean
10	14	20	21	**24**	33	35	38	**77**	365	40.44

724.3 Sciatica *(cont'd)*

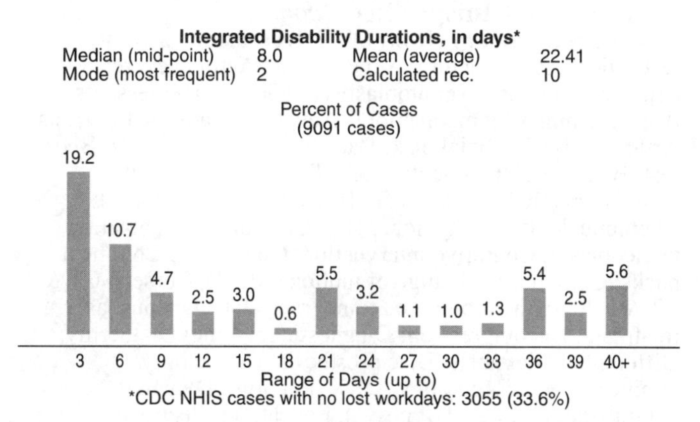

Impact on Total Absence: Prevalence 0.3997% of total lost workdays; Incidence 4.20 days per 100 workers

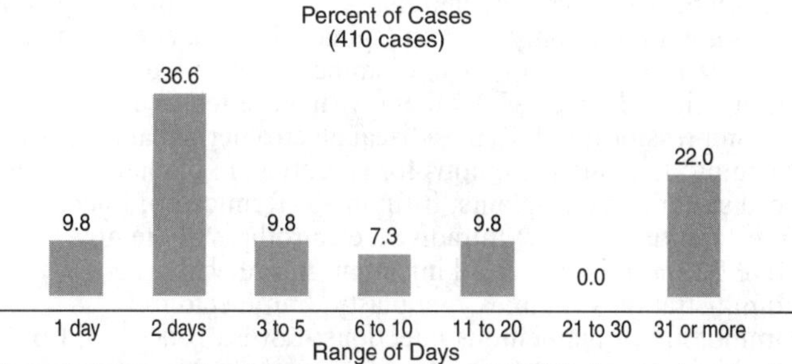

Impact on Occupational Absence: Prevalence 0.0139% of occupational lost workdays

724.4 Thoracic or lumbosacral neuritis or radiculitis, unspecified

Return-To-Work Summary Guidelines		
Dataset	**Midrange**	**At-Risk**
Claims data	27 days	131 days
All absences	21 days	95 days

Return-To-Work "Best Practice" Guidelines
Clerical/modified work: 7 days
Manual work: 21 days
Heavy manual work: 42 days

Capabilities & Activity Modifications:
Clerical/modified work: Lifting with knees (with a straight back, no stooping) not more than 5 lbs up to 3 times/hr; squatting up to 4 times/hr; standing or walking with a 5-minute break at least every 20 minutes; sitting with a 5-minute break every 30 minutes; no extremes of extension or flexion; no extremes of twisting; no climbing ladders; driving car only up to 2 hrs/day.
Manual work: Lifting with knees (with a straight back) not more than 25 lbs up to 15 times/hr; squatting up to 16 times/hr; standing or walking with a 10-minute break at least every 1-2 hours; sitting with a 10-minute break every 1-2 hours; extremes of flexion or extension allowed up to 12 times/hr; extremes of twisting allowed up to 16 times/hr; climbing ladders allowed up to 25 rungs 6 times/hr; driving car or light truck up to a full work day; driving heavy truck up to 4 hrs/day.
Description: Disorder or inflammation of the spinal nerve roots causing burning or dull pain in the abdomen, buttocks, legs, and groin, which may be increased by movements or coughing.

Radicular syndrome of lower limbs

724.4 Thoracic or lumbosacral neuritis or radiculitis, unspecified *(cont'd)*

Procedure Summary (from ODG Treatment): Activity restrictions; Acupuncture; Adhesiolysis; Aerobic exercise; Age adjustment factors; Annuloplasty (IDET); Antidepressants; Anti-inflammatory medications; Aquatic therapy; Arthrodesis; Arthroplasty; Artificial disk; Back brace; Back schools; Bed rest; Behavioral treatment; Biofeedback; Bone-growth stimulators (BGS); Bone scan; Botulinum toxin (Botox); Chemonucleolysis (chymopapain); Chiropractic; Coblation nucleoplasty; Cognitive intervention; Colchicine; Cold/heat packs; Computerized range of motion (ROM); Corsets; CT & CT Myelography (computed tomography); Cutaneous laser treatment; Decompression; Diagnostic imaging; Diathermy; Differential Diagnosis; Disc prosthesis; Discectomy/ laminectomy; Discography; DRX (traction); Dynamic neutralization system (Dynesys); Education; Electrical stimulators (E-stim); Electromagnetic pulsed therapy; EMG's (electromyography); Epidural steroid injections (ESI's); Ergonomics interventions; Etanercept (Enbrel); Exercise; Facet-joint injections; Facet rhizotomy (radio frequency medial branch neurotomy); Feldenkrais; Flexibility; Fluoroscopy (for ESI's); Foraminotomy; Fusion (spinal); Fusion, endoscopic; Hardware; Heat therapy; Hemilaminectomy; H-wave stimulation (devices); IDD therapy (intervertebral disc decompression); IDET (intradiscal electrothermal anuloplasty); Imaging; Implantable pumps for narcotics; Implantable spinal cord stimulators; Implants; Infliximab (Remicade); Injections; Interferential therapy; Intradiscal electrothermal therapy (IDET); Intradiscal steroid injection; Intrathecal drug administration system; Kyphoplasty; Laminectomy/ laminotomy; Ligamentous injections; Lordex (traction); Low level laser therapy (LLLT); Lumbar supports; Magnet therapy; Manipulation; Manipulation under anesthesia (MUA) ; Massage; Mattress firmness; McKenzie method; Medications; MedX lumbar extension machine; Microcurrent electrical stimulation (MENS devices); Microdiscectomy; Modified duty; MR neurography; MRI's (magnetic resonance imaging); Muscle relaxants ; Myelography; Neuromodulation devices; Neuromuscular electrical stimulators (NMES); Neuroplasty; Neuroreflexotherapy; Nonprescription medications; Narcotics; Nucleoplasty; Occupational therapy (OT); Opioids; Oral corticosteroids; Percutaneous diskectomy (PCD); Percutaneous electrical nerve stimulation (PENS) ; Percutaneous endoscopic laser discectomy (PELD); Percutaneous epidural neuroplasty; Percutaneous intradiscal radiofrequency (thermocoagulation); Percutaneous neuromodulation therapy (PNT); Percutaneous vertebroplasty (PV); Physical therapy (PT); Pilates; Powered traction devices; Prolotherapy, also known as sclerotherapy; Psychological screening; Racz neurolysis; Radiofrequency neurotomy; Radiography (x-rays); Range of motion (ROM); Return to work; Sclerotherapy; Shoe insoles/shoe lifts; SPECT (single photon emission computed tomography); Spinal cord stimulation (SCS); Standing MRI; Stimulators, electrical; Stretching; Supports & braces; Surface electromyography (SEMG); Surgery; Sympathetic therapy; Thermography (infrared stress thermography); Traction; Transcutaneous electrical neurostimulation (TENS) ; Trigger point injections; Tumor necrosis factor (TNF) modifiers; Ultrasound, diagnostic (imaging); Ultrasound, therapeutic; Vertebral axial

724.4 Thoracic or lumbosacral neuritis or radiculitis, unspecified *(cont'd)*

decompression (VAX-D); Vertebroplasty; Videofluoroscopy (for range of motion); Work conditioning, work hardening; Work; X-rays; Yoga

Physical Therapy Guidelines:
10-12 visits over 8 weeks
See 722.1 for post-surgical visits

Chiropractic Guidelines:
Trial of 6 visits over 2 weeks
With evidence of objective functional improvement, total of up to 16 visits (10 additional) over 6-8 weeks, avoid chronicity of care

Workers' Comp Costs per Claim (based on 1,336 claims)

Quartile	25%	50%	75%	Mean	% no cost
Indemnity	$3,014	$6,836	$21,011	$15,241	51%
Medical	$1,050	$3,528	$11,235	$8,216	2%
Total	$1,218	$4,998	$19,908	$15,793	2%

RTW Claims Data (Calendar-days away from work by decile)

10%	20%	30%	40%	**50%**	60%	70%	80%	**90%**	100%	Mean
11	14	19	22	**27**	38	43	59	**131**	365	50.71

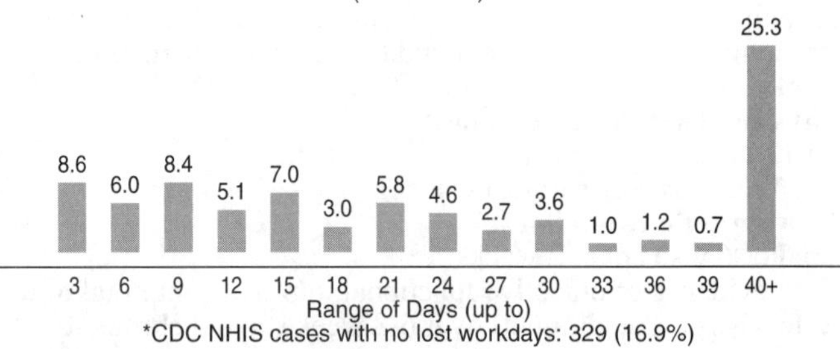

Impact on Total Absence: Prevalence 0.1910% of total lost workdays; Incidence 2.01 days per 100 workers

724.5 Backache, unspecified

Return-To-Work Summary Guidelines

Dataset	Midrange	At-Risk
Claims data	14 days	62 days
All absences	9 days	31 days

Return-To-Work "Best Practice" Guidelines
Vague symptom, see more specific diagnosis
Clerical/modified work: 0-3 days
Manual work: 7-14 days
Heavy manual work: 14-28 days
With radicular signs, see 722
With radiating pain, no radicular signs, see 847 (sprains & strains)

Capabilities & Activity Modifications:
Clerical/modified work: Lifting with knees (with a straight back, no stooping) not more than 5 lbs up to 3 times/hr; squatting up to 4 times/hr; standing or walking with a 5-minute break at least every 20 minutes; sitting with a 5-minute break every 30 minutes; no extremes of extension or flexion; no extremes of twisting; no climbing ladders; driving car only up to 2 hrs/day.

724.5 Backache, unspecified *(cont'd)*

Manual work: Lifting with knees (with a straight back) not more than 25 lbs up to 15 times/hr; squatting up to 16 times/hr; standing or walking with a 10-minute break at least every 1-2 hours; sitting with a 10-minute break every 1-2 hours; extremes of flexion or extension allowed up to 12 times/hr; extremes of twisting allowed up to 16 times/hr; climbing ladders allowed up to 25 rungs 6 times/hr; driving car or light truck up to a full work day; driving heavy truck up to 4 hrs/day.

Description: Backache is a symptom and not a disease. See 724.2 (lumbago) for more information.

Vertebrogenic (pain) syndrome NOS

Procedure Summary (from ODG Treatment): Activity restrictions; Acupuncture; Adhesiolysis; Aerobic exercise; Age adjustment factors; Annuloplasty (IDET); Antidepressants; Anti-inflammatory medications; Aquatic therapy; Arthrodesis; Arthroplasty; Artificial disk; Back brace; Back schools; Bed rest; Behavioral treatment; Biofeedback; Bone-growth stimulators (BGS); Bone scan; Botulinum toxin (Botox); Chemonucleolysis (chymopapain); Chiropractic; Coblation nucleoplasty; Cognitive intervention; Colchicine; Cold/heat packs; Computerized range of motion (ROM); Corsets; CT & CT Myelography (computed tomography); Cutaneous laser treatment; Decompression; Diagnostic imaging; Diathermy; Differential Diagnosis; Disc prosthesis; Discectomy/ laminectomy; Discography; DRX (traction); Dynamic neutralization system (Dynesys); Education; Electrical stimulators (E-stim); Electromagnetic pulsed therapy; EMG's (electromyography); Epidural steroid injections (ESI's); Ergonomics interventions; Etanercept (Enbrel); Exercise; Facet-joint injections; Facet rhizotomy (radio frequency medial branch neurotomy); Feldenkrais; Flexibility; Fluoroscopy (for ESI's); Foraminotomy; Fusion (spinal); Fusion, endoscopic; Hardware; Heat therapy; Hemilaminectomy; H-wave stimulation (devices); IDD therapy (intervertebral disc decompression); IDET (intradiscal electrothermal anuloplasty); Imaging; Implantable pumps for narcotics; Implantable spinal cord stimulators; Implants; Infliximab (Remicade); Injections; Interferential therapy; Intradiscal electrothermal therapy (IDET); Intradiscal steroid injection; Intrathecal drug administration system; Kyphoplasty; Laminectomy/ laminotomy; Ligamentous injections; Lordex (traction); Low level laser therapy (LLLT); Lumbar supports; Magnet therapy; Manipulation; Manipulation under anesthesia (MUA) ; Massage; Mattress firmness; McKenzie method; Medications; MedX lumbar extension machine; Microcurrent electrical stimulation (MENS devices); Microdiscectomy; Modified duty; MR neurography; MRI's (magnetic resonance imaging); Muscle relaxants ; Myelography; Neuromodulation devices; Neuromuscular electrical stimulators (NMES); Neuroplasty; Neuroreflexotherapy; Nonprescription medications; Narcotics; Nucleoplasty; Occupational therapy (OT); Opioids; Oral corticosteroids; Percutaneous diskectomy (PCD); Percutaneous electrical nerve stimulation (PENS) ; Percutaneous endoscopic laser discectomy (PELD); Percutaneous epidural neuroplasty; Percutaneous intradiscal radiofrequency (thermocoagulation); Percutaneous neuromodulation therapy (PNT); Percutaneous vertebroplasty (PV); Physical therapy (PT); Pilates; Powered traction devices; Prolotherapy, also known as sclerotherapy; Psychological screening; Racz neurolysis; Radiofrequency neurotomy; Radiography (x-rays); Range of motion (ROM); Return to work; Sclerotherapy; Shoe insoles/shoe lifts; SPECT (single photon emission computed tomography); Spinal cord stimulation (SCS); Standing MRI; Stimulators, electrical; Stretching; Supports & braces; Surface electromyography (SEMG); Surgery; Sympathetic therapy; Thermography (infrared stress thermography); Traction; Transcutaneous electrical neurostimulation (TENS) ; Trigger point injections;

724.5 Backache, unspecified *(cont'd)*

Tumor necrosis factor (TNF) modifiers; Ultrasound, diagnostic (imaging); Ultrasound, therapeutic; Vertebral axial decompression (VAX-D); Vertebroplasty; Videofluoroscopy (for range of motion); Work conditioning, work hardening; Work; X-rays; Yoga

Physical Therapy Guidelines:
Allow for fading of treatment frequency (from up to 3 visits per week to 1 or less), plus active self-directed home PT
9 visits over 8 weeks

Chiropractic Guidelines:
Trial of 6 visits over 2 weeks
With evidence of objective functional improvement, total of up to 16 visits (10 additional) over 6-8 weeks, avoid chronicity

Disability Duration Adjustment Factors by Age						
Age Group	18-24	25-34	35-44	45-54	55-64	65-74
Adjustment Factor	0.66	0.74	1.07	1.10	1.35	1.64

RTW Claims Data (Calendar-days away from work by decile)										
10%	20%	30%	40%	**50%**	60%	70%	80%	**90%**	100%	Mean
9	11	13	14	**14**	17	27	30	**62**	365	31.60

Integrated Disability Durations, in days*

Median (mid-point)	9.0	Mean (average)	19.41
Mode (most frequent)	1	Calculated rec.	10

Percent of Cases
(1958 cases)

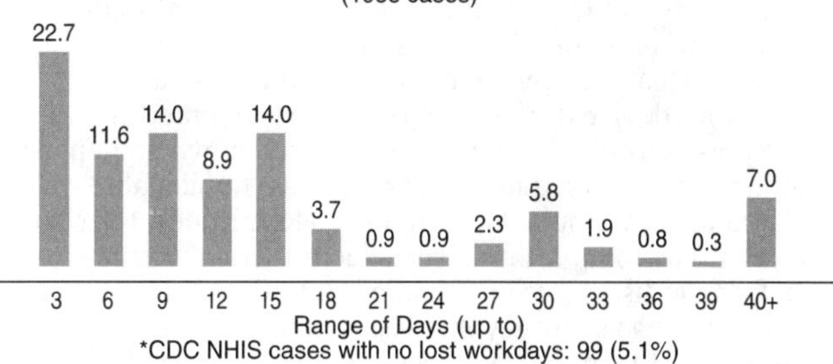

Range of Days (up to)
*CDC NHIS cases with no lost workdays: 99 (5.1%)

Impact on Total Absence: Prevalence 0.1066% of total lost workdays; Incidence 1.12 days per 100 workers

724.9 Other unspecified back disorders

Return-To-Work Summary Guidelines		
Dataset	**Midrange**	**At-Risk**
Claims data	16 days	30 days
All absences	14 days	29 days

Return-To-Work "Best Practice" Guidelines
Clerical/modified work: 1 day
Manual work: 14 days
Heavy manual work: 28 days

Capabilities & Activity Modifications:
Clerical/modified work: Lifting with knees (with a straight back, no stooping) not more than 5 lbs up to 3 times/hr; squatting up to 4 times/hr; standing or walking with a 5-minute break at least every 20 minutes; sitting with a 5-minute break every 30 minutes; no extremes of extension or flexion; no extremes of twisting; no climbing ladders; driving car only up to 2 hrs/day.
Manual work: Lifting with knees (with a straight back) not more than 25 lbs up to 15 times/hr; squatting up to 16 times/hr; standing or walking with a 10-minute break at least every 1-2 hours; sitting with a 10-minute break every 1-2 hours; extremes of flexion or extension allowed up to 12 times/hr; extremes of

724.9 Other unspecified back disorders *(cont'd)*

twisting allowed up to 16 times/hr; climbing ladders allowed up to 25 rungs 6 times/hr; driving car or light truck up to a full work day; driving heavy truck up to 4 hrs/day.

Ankylosis of spine NOS
Compression of spinal nerve root NEC
Spinal disorder NOS
Excludes: sacroiliitis (720.2)

Procedure Summary (from ODG Treatment): Activity restrictions; Acupuncture; Adhesiolysis; Aerobic exercise; Age adjustment factors; Annuloplasty (IDET); Antidepressants; Anti-inflammatory medications; Aquatic therapy; Arthrodesis; Arthroplasty; Artificial disk; Back brace; Back schools; Bed rest; Behavioral treatment; Biofeedback; Bone-growth stimulators (BGS); Bone scan; Botulinum toxin (Botox); Chemonucleolysis (chymopapain); Chiropractic; Coblation nucleoplasty; Cognitive intervention; Colchicine; Cold/heat packs; Computerized range of motion (ROM); Corsets; CT & CT Myelography (computed tomography); Cutaneous laser treatment; Decompression; Diagnostic imaging; Diathermy; Differential Diagnosis; Disc prosthesis; Discectomy/ laminectomy; Discography; DRX (traction); Dynamic neutralization system (Dynesys); Education; Electrical stimulators (E-stim); Electromagnetic pulsed therapy; EMG's (electromyography); Epidural steroid injections (ESI's); Ergonomics interventions; Etanercept (Enbrel); Exercise; Facet-joint injections; Facet rhizotomy (radio frequency medial branch neurotomy); Feldenkrais; Flexibility; Fluoroscopy (for ESI's); Foraminotomy; Fusion (spinal); Fusion, endoscopic; Hardware; Heat therapy; Hemilaminectomy; H-wave stimulation (devices); IDD therapy (intervertebral disc decompression); IDET (intradiscal electrothermal anuloplasty); Imaging; Implantable pumps for narcotics; Implantable spinal cord stimulators; Implants; Infliximab (Remicade); Injections; Interferential therapy; Intradiscal electrothermal therapy (IDET); Intradiscal steroid injection; Intrathecal drug administration system; Kyphoplasty; Laminectomy/ laminotomy; Ligamentous injections; Lordex (traction); Low level laser therapy (LLLT); Lumbar supports; Magnet therapy; Manipulation; Manipulation under anesthesia (MUA) ; Massage; Mattress firmness; McKenzie method; Medications; MedX lumbar extension machine; Microcurrent electrical stimulation (MENS devices); Microdiscectomy; Modified duty; MR neurography; MRI's (magnetic resonance imaging); Muscle relaxants ; Myelography; Neuromodulation devices; Neuromuscular electrical stimulators (NMES); Neuroplasty; Neuroreflexotherapy; Nonprescription medications; Narcotics; Nucleoplasty; Occupational therapy (OT); Opioids; Oral corticosteroids; Percutaneous diskectomy (PCD); Percutaneous electrical nerve stimulation (PENS) ; Percutaneous endoscopic laser discectomy (PELD); Percutaneous epidural neuroplasty; Percutaneous intradiscal radiofrequency (thermocoagulation); Percutaneous neuromodulation therapy (PNT); Percutaneous vertebroplasty (PV); Physical therapy (PT); Pilates; Powered traction devices; Prolotherapy, also known as sclerotherapy; Psychological screening; Racz neurolysis; Radiofrequency neurotomy; Radiography (x-rays); Range of motion (ROM); Return to work; Sclerotherapy; Shoe insoles/shoe lifts; SPECT (single photon emission computed tomography); Spinal cord stimulation (SCS); Standing MRI; Stimulators, electrical; Stretching; Supports & braces; Surface electromyography (SEMG); Surgery; Sympathetic therapy; Thermography (infrared stress thermography); Traction; Transcutaneous electrical neurostimulation (TENS) ; Trigger point injections; Tumor necrosis factor (TNF) modifiers; Ultrasound, diagnostic (imaging); Ultrasound, therapeutic; Vertebral axial decompression (VAX-D); Vertebroplasty; Videofluoroscopy (for range of motion); Work conditioning, work hardening; Work; X-rays; Yoga

RTW Claims Data (Calendar-days away from work by decile)

10%	20%	30%	40%	**50%**	60%	70%	80%	**90%**	100%	Mean
12	14	14	15	**16**	27	28	29	**30**	365	23.48

Integrated Disability Durations, in days*

Median (mid-point) 14.0 Mean (average) 17.32
Mode (most frequent) 1 Calculated rec. 12

Percent of Cases
(562 cases)

Range of Days (up to)	3	6	9	12	15	18	21	24	27	30	33	36	39	40+
Percent	18.5	3.2	2.5	4.6	18.7	7.8	0.2	0.2	4.8	14.9	3.0	0.0	0.0	0.9

*CDC NHIS cases with no lost workdays: 116 (20.6%)

Impact on Total Absence: Prevalence 0.0228% of total lost workdays; Incidence 0.24 days per 100 workers

Occupational Disability Durations, in days

Median (mid-point) 5 - Benchmark Indemnity Costs $3,750

Percent of Cases
(720 cases)

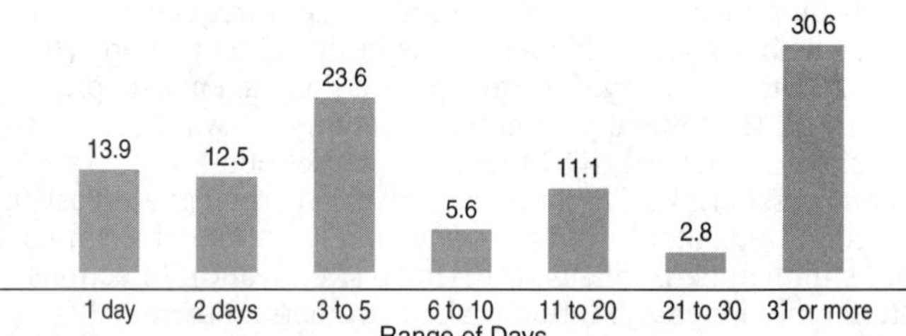

Impact on Occupational Absence: Prevalence 0.0408% of occupational lost workdays; Incidence 0.01 days per 100 workers

RHEUMATISM, EXCLUDING THE BACK (725-729)

Includes: disorders of muscles and tendons and their attachments, and of other soft tissues

RTW Claims Data (Calendar-days away from work by decile)

10%	20%	30%	40%	**50%**	60%	70%	80%	**90%**	100%	Mean
10	13	15	20	**23**	30	41	52	**88**	365	42.76

Impact on Total Absence: Prevalence 3.0090% of total lost workdays; Incidence 31.60 days per 100 workers

Occupational Disability Durations, in days

Median (mid-point) 14 - Benchmark Indemnity Costs $10,500

Percent of Cases
(9800 cases)

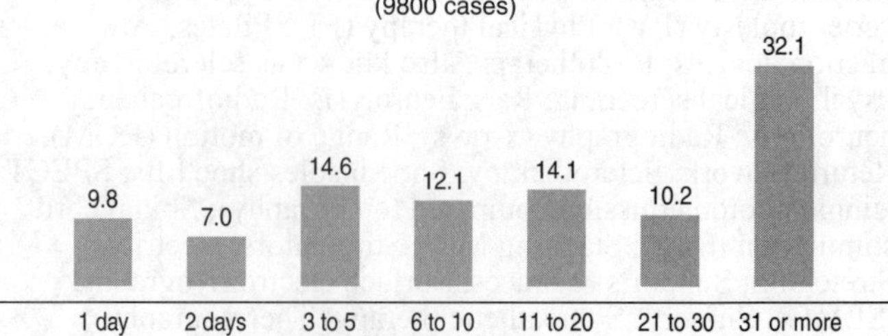

Impact on Occupational Absence: Prevalence 1.5564% of occupational lost workdays; Incidence 0.25 days per 100 workers

726 Peripheral enthesopathies and allied syndromes

Return-To-Work Summary Guidelines		
Dataset	**Midrange**	**At-Risk**
Claims data	21 days	69 days
All absences	12 days	49 days

Return-To-Work "Best Practice" Guidelines
See 726.9

Description: Inflammatory process involving the area where a ligament or tendon is inserted into bone. Pain and other symptoms depend on where the inflammation occurs.
Other names: Tendonitis, Bursitis

Note: Enthesopathies are disorders of peripheral ligamentous or muscular attachments.

Excludes:
spinal enthesopathy (720.1)

Workers' Comp Costs per Claim (based on 28,035 claims)

Quartile	25%	50%	75%	Mean	% no cost
Indemnity	$2,667	$6,342	$16,538	$13,443	59%
Medical	$452	$1,880	$8,862	$6,902	2%
Total	$494	$2,625	$14,112	$12,573	2%

Disability Duration Adjustment Factors by Age

Age Group	18-24	25-34	35-44	45-54	55-64	65-74
Adjustment Factor	0.80	0.84	0.93	1.08	1.28	1.36

RTW Claims Data (Calendar-days away from work by decile)

10%	20%	30%	40%	**50%**	60%	70%	80%	**90%**	100%	Mean
10	12	14	17	**21**	25	36	43	**69**	365	35.90

RTW Post Surgery (Calendar-days away from work by decile)

10%	20%	30%	40%	**50%**	60%	70%	80%	**90%**	100%	Mean
Partial removal, collar bone										
28	46	61	79	**93**	117	158	216	**333**	365	131.76
Remove shoulder bone, part										
31	43	62	79	**95**	128	160	214	**353**	365	137.42
Repair rotator cuff, chronic										
40	51	77	108	**123**	158	201	267	**363**	365	159.17
Release of shoulder ligament										
32	61	73	86	**113**	128	157	234	**333**	365	140.61
Repair of shoulder										
32	68	97	103	**121**	153	200	318	**365**	365	166.04
Repair of tennis elbow										
25	37	52	60	**74**	94	130	188	**300**	365	116.06
Repair of tennis elbow										
14	32	45	58	**71**	84	106	284	**365**	365	124.47
Revision of tennis elbow										
16	34	46	61	**75**	101	131	201	**296**	365	118.38
Shoulder arthroscopy/surgery										
34	50	73	88	**117**	144	198	257	**360**	365	149.72
Shoulder arthroscopy/surgery										
23	45	55	70	**94**	123	160	209	**293**	365	127.90
Shoulder arthroscopy/surgery										
27	48	60	76	**89**	121	166	201	**326**	365	129.09
Shoulder arthroscopy/surgery										
20	40	53	66	**84**	102	138	189	**285**	365	117.92

726 Peripheral enthesopathies and allied syndromes *(cont'd)*

Integrated Disability Durations, in days*

Median (mid-point)	12.0	Mean (average)	23.80
Mode (most frequent)	1	Calculated rec.	12

Percent of Cases
(13211 cases)

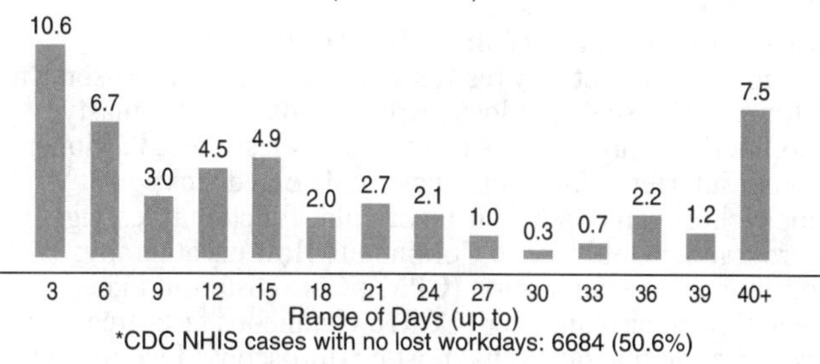

*CDC NHIS cases with no lost workdays: 6684 (50.6%)

Impact on Total Absence: Prevalence 0.4592% of total lost workdays; Incidence 4.82 days per 100 workers

Occupational Disability Durations, in days
Median (mid-point) 14 - Benchmark Indemnity Costs $10,500

Percent of Cases
(4750 cases)

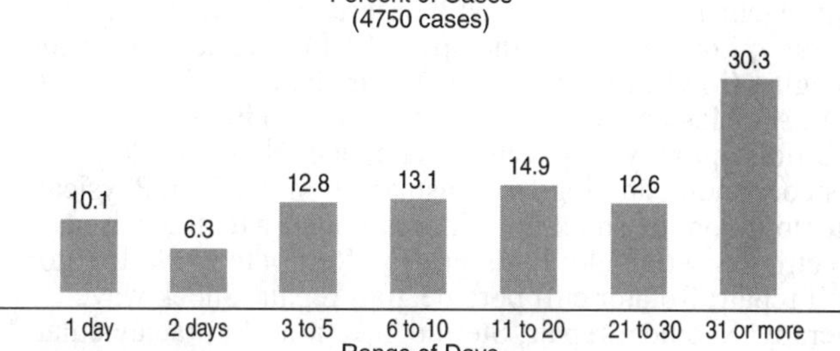

Impact on Occupational Absence: Prevalence 0.7543% of occupational lost workdays; Incidence 0.12 days per 100 workers

726.0 Adhesive capsulitis of shoulder

Return-To-Work Summary Guidelines		
Dataset	**Midrange**	**At-Risk**
Claims data	35 days	69 days
All absences	17 days	66 days

Return-To-Work "Best Practice" Guidelines
Clerical/modified work (concurrent physical therapy - no overhead work): 5 days
Manual work, non-dominant arm: 14 days
Manual work, dominant arm: 35-42 days
Manual work, dominant arm, significant loss of range of motion: 49 days to indefinite

Capabilities & Activity Modifications:
Modified work: No overhead work (reaching above shoulder) plus no reaching to shoulder level (90 degree position); no holding arm in abduction or flexion; pulling and pushing not more than 8 lbs up to 4 times/hr; lifting and carrying up to 5 lbs 3 times/hr; single arm upper extremity work using injured arm for light work only; possible immobilization by abduction brace, sling, or clavicle brace; no climbing ladders.
Manual work: Reaching above shoulder not more than 12 times/hr with up to 15 lbs of weight; reaching to shoulder up to 15 times/hr with up to 25 lbs of weight; holding arm in abduction or flexion up to 12 times/hr with up to 15 lbs of weight; pulling and pushing up to 60 lbs 20 times/hr; lifting and carrying up to 40 lbs 15 times/hr; single upper extremity work

726.0 Adhesive capsulitis of shoulder *(cont'd)*

using injured arm for moderate work only (full use of non-injured arm); possible immobilization by abduction brace, sling, or clavicle brace; climbing ladders up to 50 rungs/hr.
Description: Chronic inflammation of the shoulder joint tissue. The "freezing" of the shoulder starts gradually and causes loss of motion and constant pain.
Other names: Frozen shoulder
Procedure Summary (from ODG Treatment):
Acromioplasty; Activity restrictions; Acupuncture; Adson's test (AT); Anterior scalene block; Arthrography; Arthroplasty (shoulder); Arthroscopy; Arthroscopic release of adhesions; Bipolar interferential electrotherapy; Biofeedback; Biopsychosocial rehab; Cardiovascular functional testing; Chiropractic; Cold lasers; Continuous-flow cryotherapy; Continuous passive motion (CPM); Corticosteroid injections; Costoclavicular maneuver (CCM); Cutaneous laser treatment; Deep friction massage; Diagnostic arthroscopy; Diathermy; Distension arthrography; Electrical stimulation; Electrodiagnostic testing for TOS (thoracic outlet syndrome); Elevated arm stress test (EAST); Ergonomic interventions; Exercises; Extracorporeal shock wave therapy (ESWT); Hydroplasty/ hydrodilation; Imaging; Immobilization; Impingement test; Injections; Interferential therapy; Laser therapy; Low level laser therapy (LLLT); Magnetic resonance imaging (MRI); Manipulation; Manipulation under anesthesia (MUA); Massage; Mechanical traction; Modified duty; Multidisciplinary biopsychosocial rehab; Nerve blocks; Osteochondral autologous transplantation (OATS); Physical therapy; Porcine small intestinal submucosa (SIS); Pulsed electromagnetic field; Radiography; Return to work; Rotator cuff repair; Rotator cuff porcine graft repair; Shock wave therapy; Shoulder repair; Steroid injections; Supraclavicular pressure (SCP); Surgery for AC joint separation; Surgery for adhesive capsulitis; Surgery for impingement syndrome; Surgery for rotator cuff repair; Surgery for ruptured biceps tendon; Surgery for shoulder dislocation; Surgery for Thoracic Outlet Syndrome; Thermal capsulorrhaphy; Thermotherapy; Transcutaneous electrical neurostimulation (TENS); Transdermal nitroglycerin; Ultrasound, diagnostic; Ultrasound, therapeutic; Work
Physical Therapy Guidelines:
Allow for fading of treatment frequency (from up to 3 visits per week to 1 or less), plus active self-directed home PT
Medical treatment: 16 visits over 8 weeks
Post-surgical treatment: 24 visits over 14 weeks

Workers' Comp Costs per Claim (based on 1,189 claims)					
Quartile	25%	50%	75%	Mean	% no cost
Indemnity	$6,321	$13,650	$30,240	$22,588	31%
Medical	$4,127	$13,939	$26,156	$17,761	1%
Total	$5,408	$23,074	$45,612	$33,521	1%

RTW Claims Data (Calendar-days away from work by decile)										
10%	20%	30%	40%	**50%**	60%	70%	80%	**90%**	100%	Mean
13	14	16	27	**35**	41	44	51	**69**	365	52.32

726.0 Adhesive capsulitis of shoulder *(cont'd)*

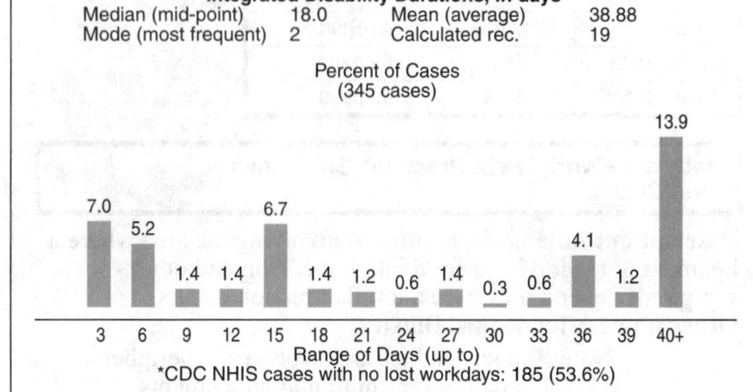

Impact on Total Absence: Prevalence 0.0183% of total lost workdays; Incidence 0.19 days per 100 workers

726.1 Rotator cuff syndrome of shoulder and allied disorders

Return-To-Work Summary Guidelines		
Dataset	**Midrange**	**At-Risk**
Claims data	52 days	180 days
All absences	28 days	115 days

Return-To-Work "Best Practice" Guidelines
Medical treatment (Grade I or II, impingement, no tear), modified work: 0 days
Medical treatment (impingement, no tear), manual work: 7-14 days
Medical treatment (impingement, no tear), manual overhead work: 28 days
Medical treatment, regular work if cause of disability: 42 days
Medical treatment, heavy manual work: 42 days
Arthroscopic surgical repair/acromioplasty (Grade III), clerical/ modified work: 28-56 days
Arthroscopic surgical repair/acromioplasty, manual work, non-dominant arm: 56-90 days
Arthroscopic surgical repair/acromioplasty, manual work, dominant arm: 70-90 days
Open surgery (Grade III), clerical/modified work: 42-56 days
Open surgery, manual work, non-dominant arm: 70-90 days
Open surgery, manual work, dominant arm: 106-180 days
Open surgery, heavy manual work if cause of disability: indefinite

Capabilities & Activity Modifications:
Modified work: No overhead work (reaching above shoulder) plus no reaching to shoulder level (90 degree position); no holding arm in abduction or flexion; pulling and pushing not more than 8 lbs up to 4 times/hr; lifting and carrying up to 5 lbs 3 times/hr; single arm upper extremity work using injured arm for light work only; possible immobilization by abduction brace, sling, or clavicle brace; no climbing ladders.
Manual work: Reaching above shoulder not more than 12 times/hr with up to 15 lbs of weight; reaching to shoulder up to 15 times/hr with up to 25 lbs of weight; holding arm in abduction or flexion up to 12 times/hr with up to 15 lbs of weight; pulling and pushing up to 60 lbs 20 times/hr; lifting and carrying up to 40 lbs 15 times/hr; single upper extremity work using injured arm for moderate work only (full use of non-injured arm); possible immobilization by abduction brace, sling, or clavicle brace; climbing ladders up to 50 rungs/hr.
Description: Tearing and swelling of the muscles and joints that hold the upper arm in the shoulder joint caused by repeatedly moving the arm over the head such as in sports. The movement causes the top of the arm bone to rub against part of

726.1 Rotator cuff syndrome of shoulder and allied disorders *(cont'd)*

the shoulder joint and its tendons, which tears individual fibers. Shoulder pain (especially with movement) and sometimes a squeaking sound when moving the arm are among the symptoms.

Other names: Swimmer's shoulder, Tennis shoulder, Pitcher's shoulder, Shoulder impingement syndrome

Procedure Summary (from ODG Treatment):
Acromioplasty; Activity restrictions; Acupuncture; Adson's test (AT); Anterior scalene block; Arthrography; Arthroplasty (shoulder); Arthroscopy; Arthroscopic release of adhesions; Bipolar interferential electrotherapy; Biofeedback; Biopsychosocial rehab; Cardiovascular functional testing; Chiropractic; Cold lasers; Continuous-flow cryotherapy; Continuous passive motion (CPM); Corticosteroid injections; Costoclavicular maneuver (CCM); Cutaneous laser treatment; Deep friction massage; Diagnostic arthroscopy; Diathermy; Distension arthrography; Electrical stimulation; Electrodiagnostic testing for TOS (thoracic outlet syndrome); Elevated arm stress test (EAST); Ergonomic interventions; Exercises; Extracorporeal shock wave therapy (ESWT); Hydroplasty/ hydrodilation; Imaging; Immobilization; Impingement test; Injections; Interferential therapy; Laser therapy; Low level laser therapy (LLLT); Magnetic resonance imaging (MRI); Manipulation; Manipulation under anesthesia (MUA); Massage; Mechanical traction; Modified duty; Multidisciplinary biopsychosocial rehab; Nerve blocks; Osteochondral autologous transplantation (OATS); Physical therapy; Porcine small intestinal submucosa (SIS); Pulsed electromagnetic field; Radiography; Return to work; Rotator cuff repair; Rotator cuff porcine graft repair; Shock wave therapy; Shoulder repair; Steroid injections; Supraclavicular pressure (SCP); Surgery for AC joint separation; Surgery for adhesive capsulitis; Surgery for impingement syndrome; Surgery for rotator cuff repair; Surgery for ruptured biceps tendon; Surgery for shoulder dislocation; Surgery for Thoracic Outlet Syndrome; Thermal capsulorrhaphy; Thermotherapy; Transcutaneous electrical neurostimulation (TENS); Transdermal nitroglycerin; Ultrasound, diagnostic; Ultrasound, therapeutic; Work

Physical Therapy Guidelines:
Allow for fading of treatment frequency (from up to 3 visits per week to 1 or less), plus active self-directed home PT
Medical treatment: 10 visits over 8 weeks
Post-injection treatment: 1-2 visits over 1 week
Post-surgical treatment, arthroscopic: 24 visits over 14 weeks
Post-surgical treatment, open: 30 visits over 18 weeks

Workers' Comp Costs per Claim (based on 6,732 claims)					
Quartile	25%	50%	75%	Mean	% no cost
Indemnity	$2,678	$5,849	$14,144	$11,788	61%
Medical	$515	$2,111	$8,222	$6,245	2%
Total	$588	$2,846	$12,401	$10,953	2%

RTW Claims Data (Calendar-days away from work by decile)										
10%	20%	30%	40%	**50%**	60%	70%	80%	**90%**	100%	Mean
14	20	29	41	**52**	67	84	105	**152**	365	74.19

726.1 Rotator cuff syndrome of shoulder and allied disorders *(cont'd)*

RTW Post Surgery (Calendar-days away from work by decile)										
10%	20%	30%	40%	**50%**	60%	70%	80%	**90%**	100%	Mean
Partial removal, collar bone										
39	53	67	88	**104**	138	168	234	**365**	365	145.78
Remove shoulder bone, part										
39	53	73	93	**115**	144	199	234	**365**	365	144.41
Repair rotator cuff, chronic										
31	63	84	108	**131**	158	193	264	**363**	365	158.52
Shoulder arthroscopy/surgery										
33	50	66	79	**102**	147	230	264	**365**	365	153.78
Shoulder arthroscopy/surgery										
30	46	59	82	**97**	122	175	209	**249**	365	127.11
Shoulder arthroscopy/surgery										
33	50	61	86	**116**	151	180	258	**365**	365	148.36
Shoulder arthroscopy/surgery										
19	37	50	65	**82**	108	151	200	**291**	365	120.10

Integrated Disability Durations, in days*
Median (mid-point) 28.0 Mean (average) 52.21
Mode (most frequent) 1 Calculated rec. 27

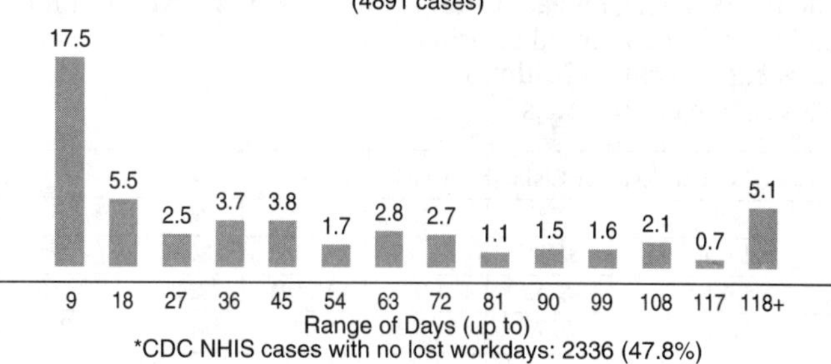

*CDC NHIS cases with no lost workdays: 2336 (47.8%)

Impact on Total Absence: Prevalence 0.3943% of total lost workdays; Incidence 4.14 days per 100 workers

Occupational Disability Durations, in days
Median (mid-point) 11 - Benchmark Indemnity Costs $8,250

Percent of Cases
(2904 cases)

Range of Days	1 day	2 days	3 to 5	6 to 10	11 to 20	21 to 30	31 or more
Percent of Cases	5.8	8.6	25.3	9.3	12.5	7.3	31.2

Impact on Occupational Absence: Prevalence 0.3623% of occupational lost workdays; Incidence 0.06 days per 100 workers

726.12 Bicipital tenosynovitis

Return-To-Work Summary Guidelines		
Dataset	**Midrange**	**At-Risk**
Claims data	35 days	109 days
All absences	14 days	78 days

726.12 Bicipital tenosynovitis *(cont'd)*

Return-To-Work "Best Practice" Guidelines
Medical treatment, clerical/modified work: 0 days
Medical treatment, manual work: 7 days
Medical treatment, heavy manual work: 35 days
Surgical repair, clerical/modified work: 28 days
Surgical repair, manual work, non-dominant arm: 42 days
Surgical repair, manual work, dominant arm: 56 days

Capabilities & Activity Modifications:
Modified work: No overhead work (reaching above shoulder) plus no reaching to shoulder level (90 degree position); no holding arm in abduction or flexion; pulling and pushing not more than 8 lbs up to 4 times/hr; lifting and carrying up to 5 lbs 3 times/hr; single arm upper extremity work using injured arm for light work only; possible immobilization by abduction brace, sling, or clavicle brace; no climbing ladders.
Manual work: Reaching above shoulder not more than 12 times/hr with up to 15 lbs of weight; reaching to shoulder up to 15 times/hr with up to 25 lbs of weight; holding arm in abduction or flexion up to 12 times/hr with up to 15 lbs of weight; pulling and pushing up to 60 lbs 20 times/hr; lifting and carrying up to 40 lbs 15 times/hr; single upper extremity work using injured arm for moderate work only (full use of non-injured arm); possible immobilization by abduction brace, sling, or clavicle brace; climbing ladders up to 50 rungs/hr.
Description: Inflammation of a tendon sheath caused by calcium deposits, repeated strain or trauma, high levels of blood cholesterol, rheumatoid arthritis, gout, or gonorrhea.
Physical Therapy Guidelines:
6-8 visits over 10 weeks

Workers' Comp Costs per Claim (based on 927 claims)

Quartile	25%	50%	75%	Mean	% no cost
Indemnity	$1,407	$3,087	$8,148	$6,579	78%
Medical	$252	$851	$2,594	$2,823	2%
Total	$273	$1,029	$3,497	$4,324	2%

RTW Claims Data (Calendar-days away from work by decile)

10%	20%	30%	40%	**50%**	60%	70%	80%	**90%**	100%	Mean
12	17	25	29	**35**	42	55	75	**109**	211	49.27

Integrated Disability Durations, in days*

Median (mid-point)	14.0	Mean (average)	29.53
Mode (most frequent)	1	Calculated rec.	15

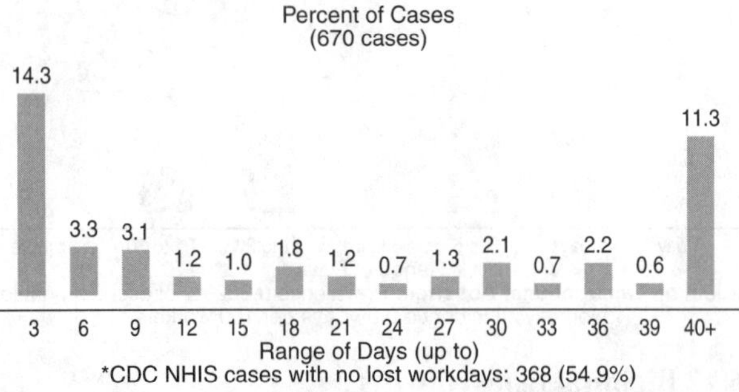

Percent of Cases
(670 cases)

Range of Days (up to)	3	6	9	12	15	18	21	24	27	30	33	36	39	40+
Percent	14.3	3.3	3.1	1.2	1.0	1.8	1.2	0.7	1.3	2.1	0.7	2.2	0.6	11.3

*CDC NHIS cases with no lost workdays: 368 (54.9%)

Impact on Total Absence: Prevalence 0.0263% of total lost workdays; Incidence 0.28 days per 100 workers

726.2 Other affections of shoulder region, not elsewhere classified

Return-To-Work Summary Guidelines

Dataset	Midrange	At-Risk
Claims data	61 days	212 days
All absences	46 days	177 days

726.2 Other affections of shoulder region, not elsewhere classified *(cont'd)*

Return-To-Work "Best Practice" Guidelines
Impingement, medical treatment, modified work: 0 days
Impingement, medical treatment, manual work: 7 days
Impingement, medical treatment, manual overhead work: 28 days
Impingement, medical treatment, heavy manual work: 42 days
Impingement, arthroscopic surgical repair/acromioplasty, clerical/modified work: 28 days
Impingement, arthroscopic surgical repair/acromioplasty, manual work, non-dominant arm: 56 days
Impingement, arthroscopic surgical repair/acromioplasty, manual work, dominant arm: 70 days
Impingement, open surgery, clerical/modified work: 42 days
Impingement, open surgery, manual work, non-dominant arm: 70 days
Impingement, open surgery, manual work, dominant arm: 106 days
Impingement, open surgery, heavy manual work if cause of disability: indefinite

Capabilities & Activity Modifications:
Modified work: No overhead work (reaching above shoulder) plus no reaching to shoulder level (90 degree position); no holding arm in abduction or flexion; pulling and pushing not more than 8 lbs up to 4 times/hr; lifting and carrying up to 5 lbs 3 times/hr; single arm upper extremity work using injured arm for light work only; possible immobilization by abduction brace, sling, or clavicle brace; no climbing ladders.
Manual work: Reaching above shoulder not more than 12 times/hr with up to 15 lbs of weight; reaching to shoulder up to 15 times/hr with up to 25 lbs of weight; holding arm in abduction or flexion up to 12 times/hr with up to 15 lbs of weight; pulling and pushing up to 60 lbs 20 times/hr; lifting and carrying up to 40 lbs 15 times/hr; single upper extremity work using injured arm for moderate work only (full use of non-injured arm); possible immobilization by abduction brace, sling, or clavicle brace; climbing ladders up to 50 rungs/hr.

Periarthritis of shoulder
Scapulohumeral fibrositis

Procedure Summary (from ODG Treatment):
Acromioplasty; Activity restrictions; Acupuncture; Adson's test (AT); Anterior scalene block; Arthrography; Arthroplasty (shoulder); Arthroscopy; Arthroscopic release of adhesions; Bipolar interferential electrotherapy; Biofeedback; Biopsychosocial rehab; Cardiovascular functional testing; Chiropractic; Cold lasers; Continuous-flow cryotherapy; Continuous passive motion (CPM); Corticosteroid injections; Costoclavicular maneuver (CCM); Cutaneous laser treatment; Deep friction massage; Diagnostic arthroscopy; Diathermy; Distension arthrography; Electrical stimulation; Electrodiagnostic testing for TOS (thoracic outlet syndrome); Elevated arm stress test (EAST); Ergonomic interventions; Exercises; Extracorporeal shock wave therapy (ESWT); Hydroplasty/ hydrodilation; Imaging; Immobilization; Impingement test; Injections; Interferential therapy; Laser therapy; Low level laser therapy (LLLT); Magnetic resonance imaging (MRI); Manipulation; Manipulation under anesthesia (MUA); Massage; Mechanical traction; Modified duty; Multidisciplinary biopsychosocial rehab; Nerve blocks; Osteochondral autologous transplantation (OATS); Physical therapy; Porcine small intestinal submucosa (SIS); Pulsed electromagnetic field; Radiography; Return to work; Rotator cuff repair; Rotator cuff porcine graft repair; Shock wave therapy; Shoulder repair; Steroid injections; Supraclavicular pressure (SCP); Surgery for AC joint separation; Surgery for adhesive capsulitis; Surgery for impingement syndrome; Surgery for rotator cuff repair; Surgery for ruptured biceps tendon; Surgery for shoulder dislocation; Surgery for Thoracic

726.2 Other affections of shoulder region, not elsewhere classified *(cont'd)*

Outlet Syndrome; Thermal capsulorrhaphy; Thermotherapy; Transcutaneous electrical neurostimulation (TENS); Transdermal nitroglycerin; Ultrasound, diagnostic; Ultrasound, therapeutic; Work

Workers' Comp Costs per Claim (based on 4,786 claims)					
Quartile	25%	50%	75%	Mean	% no cost
Indemnity	$5,019	$10,962	$24,035	$18,160	24%
Medical	$5,901	$13,346	$22,617	$16,623	0%
Total	$9,366	$21,221	$41,349	$30,505	0%

RTW Claims Data (Calendar-days away from work by decile)										
10%	20%	30%	40%	**50%**	60%	70%	80%	**90%**	100%	Mean
15	28	41	48	**61**	76	101	122	**212**	365	90.56

RTW Post Surgery (Calendar-days away from work by decile)										
10%	20%	30%	40%	**50%**	60%	70%	80%	**90%**	100%	Mean
Partial removal, collar bone										
27	46	58	74	**87**	110	150	207	**311**	365	125.10
Remove shoulder bone, part										
26	40	55	74	**86**	121	159	214	**348**	365	131.83
Shoulder arthroscopy/surgery										
30	47	74	88	**117**	139	159	216	**325**	365	139.45
Shoulder arthroscopy/surgery										
19	41	51	59	**72**	103	150	204	**365**	365	122.03
Shoulder arthroscopy/surgery										
24	40	54	68	**79**	96	131	179	**236**	365	112.05
Shoulder arthroscopy/surgery										
24	40	54	67	**85**	100	133	182	**276**	365	115.95

Integrated Disability Durations, in days*

Median (mid-point)	46.0	Mean (average)	72.38
Mode (most frequent)	1	Calculated rec.	41

Percent of Cases
(1257 cases)

Range of Days (up to)	9	18	27	36	45	54	63	72	81	90	99	108	117	118+
Percent	14.9	5.5	3.1	4.4	5.0	3.0	4.5	3.7	1.8	2.1	2.0	3.9	1.0	11.0

*CDC NHIS cases with no lost workdays: 429 (34.1%)

Impact on Total Absence: Prevalence 0.1771% of total lost workdays; Incidence 1.86 days per 100 workers

726.3 Enthesopathy of elbow region

Return-To-Work Summary Guidelines		
Dataset	**Midrange**	**At-Risk**
Claims data	28 days	75 days
All absences	16 days	54 days

726.3 Enthesopathy of elbow region *(cont'd)*

Return-To-Work "Best Practice" Guidelines
Without surgery, modified work: 0 day
Without surgery, regular manual work: 4 days
Without surgery, regular work if cause of disability: 28 days
Without surgery, heavy manual work: 42 days
With surgery, modified work, non-dominant arm: 6 days
With surgery, modified work, dominant arm: 21 days
With surgery, regular work, non-dominant arm: 28 days
With surgery, regular work, dominant arm: 42 days

Capabilities & Activity Modifications:
Modified work: Repetitive motion activities not more than 4 times/hr; single upper extremity work if injured arm is non-dominant arm; lifting and carrying up to 3 lbs not more than 4 times/hr; pulling and pushing up to 5 lbs 3 times/hr; gripping using light tools (pens, scissors, etc) with 5-minute break at least every 20 min; avoid direct pressure on the elbow area; limit repetitive keying up to 15 keystrokes/min not more than 2 hrs/day; driving car up to 2 hrs/day; no full extension activities; possible immobilization by long arm splint or cast, tennis elbow splint, or wrist splint; no climbing ladders.
Regular manual work: Repetitive motion activities not more than 8 times/hr; use of injured dominant arm for moderate work; lifting and carrying up to 20 lbs not more than 15 times/hr; pulling and pushing up to 40 lbs 15 times/hr; gripping using moderate tools (pliers, screwdrivers, etc) full time; driving car or light truck up to 6 hrs/day or heavy truck up to 4 hrs/day; full extension activities up to 12 times/hr with up to 10 lbs of weight; possible immobilization by sling, wrist splint, or tennis elbow splint; climbing ladders up to 50 rungs/hr.
Description: Occurs when tendons in the elbow develop microscopic tears and inflammation. Pain, swelling, and inability to use the wrist may be sudden or gradual symptoms.
Procedure Summary (from ODG Treatment): Activity restrictions; Acupuncture; Arthroplasty (elbow); Augmented soft tissue mobilization (ASTM); Autologous blood injection; Band; Biofeedback; Botulinum toxin injection; Brace; Chiropractic; Cold packs; Corticosteroid injections; Deep transverse friction massage; Diathermy; Education; Electrical stimulation (E-STIM); Exercise; Extracorporeal shockwave therapy (ESWT); Fatty acid supplements; Friction massage; Imaging; Injections; Iontophoresis; Laser doppler imaging (LDI); Light therapy; Laser treatment (LLLT); Manipulation; Massage; MRI's; Neural tension; Night splints; Nonprescription medications; Orthotic devices; Patient education; Phonophoresis; Physical therapy; Pulsed electromagnetic field therapy; Radial shockwave therapy (RSWT); Radiography; Return to work; Shockwave therapy; Soft tissue mobilization; Splinting; Stretching; Surgery for cubital tunnel syndrome; Surgery for epicondylitis; Surgery for pronator syndrome ; Tennis elbow band; Tests for cubital tunnel syndrome; Tests for epicondylitis; Tests for pronator syndrome ; Total elbow replacement (TER); Transcutaneous electrical neurostimulation (TENS); Ulnar motor nerve conduction velocity at the elbow; Ultrasound, diagnostic; Ultrasound, therapeutic; Work
Physical Therapy Guidelines:
Allow for fading of treatment frequency (from up to 3 visits per week to 1 or less), plus active self-directed home PT
Medical treatment: 10 visits over 8 weeks
Post-surgical treatment: 12 visits over 12 weeks

Workers' Comp Costs per Claim (based on 10,878 claims)					
Quartile	25%	50%	75%	Mean	% no cost
Indemnity	$1,659	$3,308	$8,033	$8,103	71%
Medical	$326	$914	$2,898	$2,970	3%
Total	$336	$1,197	$4,347	$5,387	3%

726.3 Enthesopathy of elbow region *(cont'd)*

RTW Claims Data (Calendar-days away from work by decile)										
10%	20%	30%	40%	**50%**	60%	70%	80%	**90%**	100%	Mean
14	18	21	25	**28**	33	42	47	**75**	365	38.36

RTW Post Surgery (Calendar-days away from work by decile)										
10%	20%	30%	40%	**50%**	60%	70%	80%	**90%**	100%	Mean
Repair of tennis elbow										
25	37	52	60	**74**	94	130	188	**300**	365	116.06
Repair of tennis elbow										
14	32	45	58	**71**	84	106	284	**365**	365	124.47
Revision of tennis elbow										
16	34	46	61	**75**	101	130	200	**296**	365	117.26

Integrated Disability Durations, in days*

Median (mid-point) 16.0 Mean (average) 24.27
Mode (most frequent) 1 Calculated rec. 14

Percent of Cases
(941 cases)

9.2 7.0 1.4 1.0 2.2 1.5 2.7 1.8 1.5 3.2 0.9 0.6 0.4 9.0

3 6 9 12 15 18 21 24 27 30 33 36 39 40+
Range of Days (up to)

*CDC NHIS cases with no lost workdays: 542 (57.6%)

Impact on Total Absence: Prevalence 0.0286% of total lost workdays; Incidence 0.30 days per 100 workers

726.31 Medial epicondylitis

Return-To-Work Summary Guidelines		
Dataset	**Midrange**	**At-Risk**
Claims data	28 days	54 days
All absences	8 days	44 days

Return-To-Work "Best Practice" Guidelines
Without surgery, modified work: 0 day
Without surgery, regular manual work: 7 days
Without surgery, heavy manual work: 42 days

Capabilities & Activity Modifications:
Modified work: Repetitive motion activities not more than 4 times/hr; single upper extremity work if injured arm is non-dominant arm; lifting and carrying up to 3 lbs not more than 4 times/hr; pulling and pushing up to 5 lbs 3 times/hr; gripping using light tools (pens, scissors, etc) with 5-minute break at least every 20 min; avoid direct pressure on the elbow area; limit repetitive keying up to 15 keystrokes/min not more than 2 hrs/day; driving car up to 2 hrs/day; no full extension activities; possible immobilization by long arm splint or cast, tennis elbow splint, or wrist splint; no climbing ladders.
Regular manual work: Repetitive motion activities not more than 8 times/hr; use of injured dominant arm for moderate work; lifting and carrying up to 20 lbs not more than 15 times/hr; pulling and pushing up to 40 lbs 15 times/hr; gripping using moderate tools (pliers, screwdrivers, etc) full time; driving car or light truck up to 6 hrs/day or heavy truck up to 4 hrs/day; full extension activities up to 12 times/hr with up to 10 lbs of weight; possible immobilization by sling, wrist splint, or tennis elbow splint; climbing ladders up to 50 rungs/hr.

Description: Painful inflammation of the muscle and tissues of the elbow caused by repeated strain or violent extension of the wrist against a resisting force.

Golfers' elbow

Procedure Summary (from ODG Treatment): Activity restrictions; Acupuncture; Arthroplasty (elbow); Augmented soft tissue mobilization (ASTM); Autologous blood injection; Band; Biofeedback; Botulinum toxin injection; Brace; Chiropractic; Cold packs; Corticosteroid injections; Deep transverse friction massage; Diathermy; Education; Electrical stimulation (E-STIM); Exercise; Extracorporeal shockwave therapy (ESWT); Fatty acid supplements; Friction massage; Imaging; Injections; Iontophoresis; Laser doppler imaging (LDI); Light therapy; Laser treatment (LLLT); Manipulation; Massage; MRI's; Neural tension; Night splints; Nonprescription medications; Orthotic devices; Patient education; Phonophoresis; Physical therapy; Pulsed electromagnetic field therapy; Radial shockwave therapy (RSWT); Radiography; Return to work; Shockwave therapy; Soft tissue mobilization; Splinting; Stretching; Surgery for cubital tunnel syndrome; Surgery for epicondylitis; Surgery for pronator syndrome ; Tennis elbow band; Tests for cubital tunnel syndrome; Tests for epicondylitis; Tests for pronator syndrome ; Total elbow replacement (TER); Transcutaneous electrical neurostimulation (TENS); Ulnar motor nerve conduction velocity at the elbow; Ultrasound, diagnostic; Ultrasound, therapeutic; Work

Physical Therapy Guidelines:
Medical treatment: 10 visits over 8 weeks
Post-surgical treatment: 12 visits over 12 weeks

Workers' Comp Costs per Claim (based on 1,495 claims)					
Quartile	25%	50%	75%	Mean	% no cost
Indemnity	$1,659	$3,617	$9,398	$9,371	67%
Medical	$378	$1,134	$3,423	$3,564	3%
Total	$399	$1,428	$5,565	$6,674	2%

RTW Claims Data (Calendar-days away from work by decile)										
10%	20%	30%	40%	**50%**	60%	70%	80%	**90%**	100%	Mean
10	13	17	22	**28**	35	42	44	**54**	68	30.06

Integrated Disability Durations, in days*

Median (mid-point) 8.0 Mean (average) 16.65
Mode (most frequent) 1 Calculated rec. 8

Percent of Cases
(763 cases)

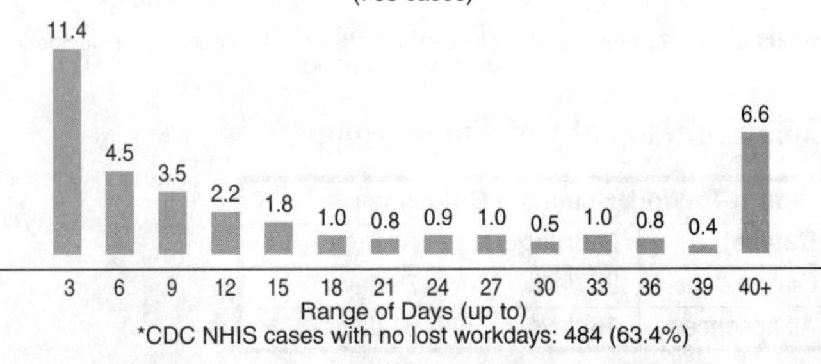

*CDC NHIS cases with no lost workdays: 484 (63.4%)

Impact on Total Absence: Prevalence 0.0137% of total lost workdays; Incidence 0.14 days per 100 workers

726.32 Lateral epicondylitis

Return-To-Work Summary Guidelines		
Dataset	**Midrange**	**At-Risk**
Claims data	31 days	125 days
All absences	14 days	96 days

Return-To-Work "Best Practice" Guidelines
Without surgery, modified work: 0 day
Without surgery, regular manual work: 7 days
Without surgery, heavy manual work: 42 days
Without surgery, heavy manual vibrating work, if cause of disability: indefinite
With surgery (rare), modified work, non-dominant arm: 6 days
With surgery (rare), modified work, dominant arm: 21 days
With surgery (rare), heavy manual work, non-dominant arm: 28 days
With surgery (rare), heavy manual work, dominant arm: 42 days
Acupuncture (3-6 treatments): 7-21 days

Capabilities & Activity Modifications:
Modified work: Repetitive motion activities not more than 4 times/hr; single upper extremity work if injured arm is non-dominant arm; lifting and carrying up to 3 lbs not more than 4 times/hr; pulling and pushing up to 5 lbs 3 times/hr; gripping using light tools (pens, scissors, etc) with 5-minute break at least every 20 min; avoid direct pressure on the elbow area; limit repetitive keying up to 15 keystrokes/min not more than 2 hrs/day; driving car up to 2 hrs/day; no full extension activities; possible immobilization by long arm splint or cast, tennis elbow splint, or wrist splint; no climbing ladders.
Regular manual work: Repetitive motion activities not more than 8 times/hr; use of injured dominant arm for moderate work; lifting and carrying up to 20 lbs not more than 15 times/hr; pulling and pushing up to 40 lbs 15 times/hr; gripping using moderate tools (pliers, screwdrivers, etc) full time; driving car or light truck up to 6 hrs/day or heavy truck up to 4 hrs/day; full extension activities up to 12 times/hr with up to 10 lbs of weight; possible immobilization by sling, wrist splint, or tennis elbow splint; climbing ladders up to 50 rungs/hr.
Description: Painful inflammation of the muscle and tissues of the elbow caused by repeated strain or violent extension of the wrist against a resisting force.

Epicondylitis NOS
Tennis elbow

Procedure Summary (from ODG Treatment): Activity restrictions; Acupuncture; Arthroplasty (elbow); Augmented soft tissue mobilization (ASTM); Autologous blood injection; Band; Biofeedback; Botulinum toxin injection; Brace; Chiropractic; Cold packs; Corticosteroid injections; Deep transverse friction massage; Diathermy; Education; Electrical stimulation (E-STIM); Exercise; Extracorporeal shockwave therapy (ESWT); Fatty acid supplements; Friction massage; Imaging; Injections; Iontophoresis; Laser doppler imaging (LDI); Light therapy; Laser treatment (LLLT); Manipulation; Massage; MRI's; Neural tension; Night splints; Nonprescription medications; Orthotic devices; Patient education; Phonophoresis; Physical therapy; Pulsed electromagnetic field therapy; Radial shockwave therapy (RSWT); Radiography; Return to work; Shockwave therapy; Soft tissue mobilization; Splinting; Stretching; Surgery for cubital tunnel syndrome; Surgery for epicondylitis; Surgery for pronator syndrome ; Tennis elbow band; Tests for cubital tunnel syndrome; Tests for epicondylitis; Tests for pronator syndrome ; Total elbow replacement (TER); Transcutaneous electrical

726.32 Lateral epicondylitis *(cont'd)*

neurostimulation (TENS); Ulnar motor nerve conduction velocity at the elbow; Ultrasound, diagnostic; Ultrasound, therapeutic; Work
Physical Therapy Guidelines:
Medical treatment: 10 visits over 8 weeks
Post-surgical treatment: 12 visits over 12 weeks

Workers' Comp Costs per Claim (based on 7,444 claims)					
Quartile	25%	50%	75%	Mean	% no cost
Indemnity	$1,733	$3,365	$8,337	$8,251	69%
Medical	$347	$1,145	$3,255	$3,213	3%
Total	$378	$1,460	$4,830	$5,832	3%

RTW Claims Data (Calendar-days away from work by decile)										
10%	20%	30%	40%	**50%**	60%	70%	80%	**90%**	100%	Mean
12	15	20	25	**31**	42	56	83	**125**	365	64.73

RTW Post Surgery (Calendar-days away from work by decile)										
10%	20%	30%	40%	**50%**	60%	70%	80%	**90%**	100%	Mean
Repair of tennis elbow										
25	37	52	60	**72**	92	123	180	**276**	365	112.08
Repair of tennis elbow										
13	31	42	58	**71**	84	106	298	**365**	365	124.26
Revision of tennis elbow										
16	32	47	61	**77**	103	131	202	**299**	365	119.79

Integrated Disability Durations, in days*
Median (mid-point) 14.0 Mean (average) 40.60
Mode (most frequent) 1 Calculated rec. 17

Percent of Cases
(1249 cases)

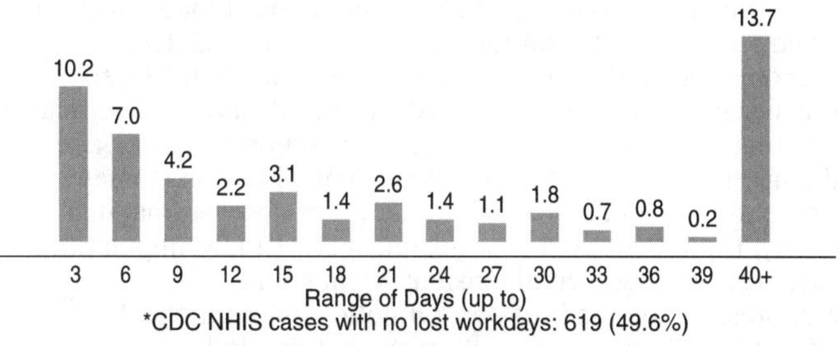

Range of Days (up to)
*CDC NHIS cases with no lost workdays: 619 (49.6%)

Impact on Total Absence: Prevalence 0.0756% of total lost workdays; Incidence 0.79 days per 100 workers

Occupational Disability Durations, in days
Median (mid-point) 14 - Benchmark Indemnity Costs $10,500

Percent of Cases
(2086 cases)

30.0
21.6
17.2
12.9
7.4
5.2
5.6
1 day 2 days 3 to 5 6 to 10 11 to 20 21 to 30 31 or more

Range of Days
Impact on Occupational Absence: Prevalence 0.3312% of occupational lost workdays; Incidence 0.05 days per 100 workers

726.33 Olecranon bursitis

Return-To-Work Summary Guidelines		
Dataset	**Midrange**	**At-Risk**
Claims data	32 days	54 days
All absences	5 days	37 days

726.33 Olecranon bursitis *(cont'd)*

Return-To-Work "Best Practice" Guidelines
Without surgery, modified work: 0 day
Without surgery, regular manual work: 4 days
Without surgery, heavy manual work: 35 days

Capabilities & Activity Modifications:
Modified work: Repetitive motion activities not more than 4 times/hr; single upper extremity work if injured arm is non-dominant arm; lifting and carrying up to 3 lbs not more than 4 times/hr; pulling and pushing up to 5 lbs 3 times/hr; gripping using light tools (pens, scissors, etc) with 5-minute break at least every 20 min; avoid direct pressure on the elbow area; limit repetitive keying up to 15 keystrokes/min not more than 2 hrs/day; driving car up to 2 hrs/day; no full extension activities; possible immobilization by long arm splint or cast, tennis elbow splint, or wrist splint; no climbing ladders.
Regular manual work: Repetitive motion activities not more than 8 times/hr; use of injured dominant arm for moderate work; lifting and carrying up to 20 lbs not more than 15 times/hr; pulling and pushing up to 40 lbs 15 times/hr; gripping using moderate tools (pliers, screwdrivers, etc) full time; driving car or light truck up to 6 hrs/day or heavy truck up to 4 hrs/day; full extension activities up to 12 times/hr with up to 10 lbs of weight; possible immobilization by sling, wrist splint, or tennis elbow splint; climbing ladders up to 50 rungs/hr.
Description: Inflammation of the connective tissue of the elbow due to arthritis, infection, injury, or excessive exercise or effort.
Other names: Miner's elbow
Bursitis of elbow
Procedure Summary (from ODG Treatment): Activity restrictions; Acupuncture; Arthroplasty (elbow); Augmented soft tissue mobilization (ASTM); Autologous blood injection; Band; Biofeedback; Botulinum toxin injection; Brace; Chiropractic; Cold packs; Corticosteroid injections; Deep transverse friction massage; Diathermy; Education; Electrical stimulation (E-STIM); Exercise; Extracorporeal shockwave therapy (ESWT); Fatty acid supplements; Friction massage; Imaging; Injections; Iontophoresis; Laser doppler imaging (LDI); Light therapy; Laser treatment (LLLT); Manipulation; Massage; MRI's; Neural tension; Night splints; Nonprescription medications; Orthotic devices; Patient education; Phonophoresis; Physical therapy; Pulsed electromagnetic field therapy; Radial shockwave therapy (RSWT); Radiography; Return to work; Shockwave therapy; Soft tissue mobilization; Splinting; Stretching; Surgery for cubital tunnel syndrome; Surgery for epicondylitis; Surgery for pronator syndrome ; Tennis elbow band; Tests for cubital tunnel syndrome; Tests for epicondylitis; Tests for pronator syndrome ; Total elbow replacement (TER); Transcutaneous electrical neurostimulation (TENS); Ulnar motor nerve conduction velocity at the elbow; Ultrasound, diagnostic; Ultrasound, therapeutic; Work
Physical Therapy Guidelines:
Medical treatment: 9 visits over 8 weeks

Workers' Comp Costs per Claim (based on 1,765 claims)					
Quartile	25%	50%	75%	Mean	% no cost
Indemnity	$903	$2,363	$3,896	$3,779	83%
Medical	$263	$473	$987	$1,367	4%
Total	$263	$494	$1,313	$2,048	4%

RTW Claims Data (Calendar-days away from work by decile)										
10%	20%	30%	40%	**50%**	60%	70%	80%	**90%**	100%	Mean
11	15	19	25	**32**	35	37	42	**54**	68	30.69

726.33 Olecranon bursitis *(cont'd)*

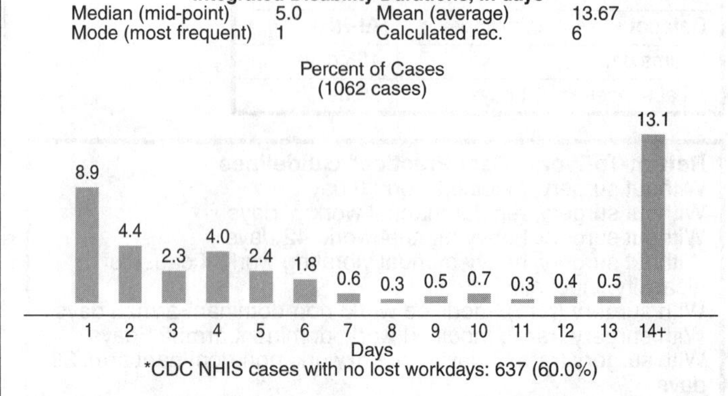

Impact on Total Absence: Prevalence 0.0171% of total lost workdays; Incidence 0.18 days per 100 workers

726.6 Enthesopathy of knee

Return-To-Work Summary Guidelines		
Dataset	**Midrange**	**At-Risk**
Claims data	22 days	48 days
All absences	13 days	43 days

Return-To-Work "Best Practice" Guidelines
Without surgery, clerical/modified work: 0 days
Without surgery, manual/standing work: 7 days
With surgery, clerical/modified work: 14 days
With surgery, manual/standing work: 42 days

Capabilities & Activity Modifications:
Sedentary/modified work: Standing limited to 5-10 min/hr; walking only on a smooth surface using crutches with limited pressure on the foot; no walking on an irregular surface; no climbing stairs; no climbing ladders or hill climbing requiring frequent knee flexion; no activities requiring balance; no applying strength against bent knee (squatting, kneeling, crouching, stooping, pedaling, etc.); elevate leg half of time; may need immobilization; limited weight bearing.
Manual/standing work: Standing not more than 50 min/hr; walking on a smooth surface up to 1,200 ft/hr carrying up to 25 lbs; walking on an irregular surface up to 900 ft/hr carrying up to 25 lbs; climbing stairs up to 8 flights/hr carrying up to 40 lbs; climbing ladders up to 50 rungs/hr carrying up to 25 lbs; activities requiring balance up to 45 min/hr (if able to work with two hands without assistance for balance); applying strength against bent knee (pedaling, squatting, kneeling, etc.) up to 60 times/hr; may need brace for uneven ground or ladders.
Description: Occurs when tendons in the knee develop microscopic tears and inflammation. Pain, swelling, and inability to use the knee may be sudden or gradual symptoms.
Procedure Summary (from ODG Treatment): ACI; Activity restrictions; Anterior cruciate ligament (ACL) repair; ACL diagnostic tests; ACL injury rehabilitation; Acupuncture; Arthroplasty; Arthroscopy; Autologous cartilage implantation (ACI); Bone-growth stimulators; Braces; Canes; Cetylated fatty acids (CFA) topical cream; Chiropractic; Chondroplasty; Cold/heat packs; Cold lasers; Continuous-flow cryotherapy; Continuous passive motion (CPM); Corticosteroid injections; Crutches; Deep transverse friction massage (DTFM); Diagnostic arthroscopy; Education for knee replacement; Electromyographic biofeedback treatment; Exercise; Glucosamine; Hyaluronic acid injections; Imaging; Immobilization; Injections; Insoles; Interferential current therapy (IFC); Knee brace; Knee joint replacement; KT 1000

726.6 Enthesopathy of knee *(cont'd)*

arthrometer; Lachman test; Lateral pull test and patellar tilt test; Lateral retinacular release; Low level laser therapy (LLLT); Magnet therapy; Manipulation; Meniscal allograft transplantation; Meniscectomy; Microprocessor-controlled knee prostheses; Modified duty; Mosaicplasty; MRI's (magnetic resonance imaging); Non-surgical intervention for PFPS (patellofemoral pain syndrome); Occupational therapy; Orthoses; Osteochondral autograft transplant system (OATS); Osteotomy; Pharmacotherapy; Physical therapy; Pivot shift test (MacIntosh test) ; Posterior cruciate ligament (PCL) repair; Post-op ambulatory infusion pumps (local anesthetic); Prolotherapy; Prostheses (artificial limb); Pulsed magnetic field therapy (PMFT); Radiography; Return to work; SAMe (S-adenosylmethionine); Single photon emission computed tomography (SPECT); Static progressive stretch (SPS) therapy; Stretching and flexibility; Surgery; SynviscÒ; Therapeutic knee splint; Therapeutic ultrasound; Transcutaneous electrical neurostimulation (TENS); Ultrasound, diagnostic; Ultrasound, therapeutic; Ultrasound fracture healing (bone-growth stimulators); Viscosupplementation; Walkers; Walking aids (canes, crutches, braces, orthoses, & walkers); Work

Workers' Comp Costs per Claim (based on 2,018 claims)

Quartile	25%	50%	75%	Mean	% no cost
Indemnity	$1,386	$2,515	$4,263	$4,359	81%
Medical	$273	$525	$1,449	$1,533	5%
Total	$284	$588	$2,058	$2,406	4%

RTW Claims Data (Calendar-days away from work by decile)

10%	20%	30%	40%	**50%**	60%	70%	80%	**90%**	100%	Mean
11	14	14	16	**22**	34	42	43	**48**	365	31.52

Integrated Disability Durations, in days*

Median (mid-point)	13.0	Mean (average)	19.96
Mode (most frequent)	1	Calculated rec.	12

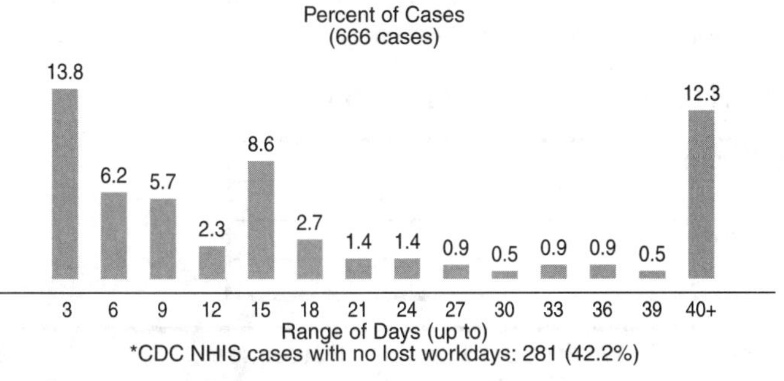

*CDC NHIS cases with no lost workdays: 281 (42.2%)

Impact on Total Absence: Prevalence 0.0227% of total lost workdays; Incidence 0.24 days per 100 workers

726.7 Enthesopathy of ankle and tarsus

Return-To-Work Summary Guidelines

Dataset	Midrange	At-Risk
Claims data	41 days	58 days
All absences	15 days	50 days

Return-To-Work "Best Practice" Guidelines
Without surgery, clerical/modified work: 0 days
Without surgery, manual/standing work: 5-7 days
With surgery, clerical/modified work: 7-10 days
With surgery, manual/standing work: 42-49 days

Capabilities & Activity Modifications:
Sedentary/modified work: Standing limited to 5-10 min/hr; walking only on a smooth surface using crutches with limited pressure on the foot; no walking on an irregular surface; no climbing stairs; no climbing ladders or hill climbing requiring frequent knee flexion; no activities requiring balance; no applying strength against bent knee (squatting, kneeling, crouching, stooping, pedaling, etc.); elevate leg half of time; may need immobilization; limited weight bearing.
Manual/standing work: Standing not more than 50 min/hr; walking on a smooth surface up to 1,200 ft/hr carrying up to 25 lbs; walking on an irregular surface up to 900 ft/hr carrying up to 25 lbs; climbing stairs up to 8 flights/hr carrying up to 40 lbs; climbing ladders up to 50 rungs/hr carrying up to 25 lbs; activities requiring balance up to 45 min/hr (if able to work with two hands without assistance for balance); applying strength against bent knee (pedaling, squatting, kneeling, etc.) up to 60 times/hr; may need brace for uneven ground or ladders.

Description: Occurs when tendons in the ankle or instep develop microscopic tears and inflammation. Pain, swelling, and inability to use the foot or ankle may be sudden or gradual symptoms.

Procedure Summary (from ODG Treatment):
Accommodative modalities; Achilles tendon ruptures (treatment); Activity restrictions; Actovegin; Ankle prostheses (total ankle replacement); Anterior drawer test; Anti-inflammatory medications (NSAIDs); Arthrodesis (fusion); Arthroplasty (total ankle replacement); Autologous conditioned serum (ACS); Bed rest; Biofeedback; Bone scan (imaging); Bracing (immobilization); Cast (immobilization); Causality; Chiropractic; Cold packs; Computed tomography (CT); Continuous-flow cryotherapy; Corticosteroids (topical); Diathermy; Dorsiflexion night splints; Education (patient); Elastic bandage (immobilization); Electron generating device; Exercise; Extracorporeal shock wave therapy (ESWT); Functional treatment; Fusion; Heat therapy (ice/heat); Heparin; Heel pads; Ice packs; Imaging; Immobilization; Ingrown toenail surgery; Injections; Insoles with magnetic foil; Inversion stress test; Iontophoresis; Lace-up ankle support; Laser therapy (LLLT); Lateral ligament ankle reconstruction (surgery); Lineal tomography; Low-intensity laser therapy (LLLT); Magnets; Magnetic resonance imaging (MRI); Manipulation; Massage; Mechanical treatment (taping/orthoses); Modified duty; Narcotics; Night splints; Nonprescription medications; Orthotic devices; Osteotomy; Ottawa ankle rules (OAR); Patient education; Phonophoresis; Physical therapy (PT); Prolotherapy (sclerotherapy); Radiography; Rest (RICE); Return to work; Sclerotherapy (prolotherapy); Semi-rigid ankle support; Shock wave therapy, extracorporeal (ESWT); Steroids (injection); Stretching (flexibility); Supports; Surgery; Surgery for achilles tendon ruptures; Surgery for ankle sprains; Surgery for calcaneal fractures; Surgery for hallux valgus; Surgery for plantar fasciitis; Surgery for tarsal tunnel syndrome; Talar tilt test; Tai Chi; Taping; Tension night splints (TNS); Therapeutic exercise; Thompson test; Total ankle replacement (arthroplasty); Transcutaneous electrical neurostimulation (TENS); Ultrasound, diagnostic; Ultrasound, therapeutic; Work

Physical Therapy Guidelines:
Allow for fading of treatment frequency (from up to 3 visits per week to 1 or less), plus active self-directed home PT
Medical treatment: 9 visits over 8 weeks
Post-surgical treatment: 9 visits over 8 weeks

Workers' Comp Costs per Claim (based on 1,096 claims)

Quartile	25%	50%	75%	Mean	% no cost
Indemnity	$2,720	$5,565	$16,412	$14,168	57%
Medical	$462	$1,890	$7,161	$6,177	2%
Total	$515	$2,751	$12,201	$12,398	2%

726.7 Enthesopathy of ankle and tarsus *(cont'd)*

RTW Claims Data (Calendar-days away from work by decile)										
10%	20%	30%	40%	**50%**	60%	70%	80%	**90%**	100%	Mean
10	12	17	32	**41**	42	44	49	**58**	365	40.24

Integrated Disability Durations, in days*

Median (mid-point)	15.0	Mean (average)	28.66
Mode (most frequent)	1	Calculated rec.	15

Percent of Cases (1542 cases)

Range of Days (up to)	3	6	9	12	15	18	21	24	27	30	33	36	39	40+
Percent	8.8	5.5	5.9	4.7	3.0	1.2	1.2	0.6	0.7	0.5	0.5	0.5	0.7	21.0

*CDC NHIS cases with no lost workdays: 696 (45.1%)

Impact on Total Absence: Prevalence 0.0716% of total lost workdays; Incidence 0.75 days per 100 workers

726.70 Enthesopathy of ankle and tarsus, unspecified

Return-To-Work Summary Guidelines		
Dataset	**Midrange**	**At-Risk**
Claims data	41 days	58 days
All absences	15 days	50 days

Return-To-Work "Best Practice" Guidelines
Sedentary work: 1 day
Manual/standing work: 10 days
Heavy manual/standing work: 28 days

Capabilities & Activity Modifications:
Sedentary/modified work: Standing limited to 5-10 min/hr; walking only on a smooth surface using crutches with limited pressure on the foot; no walking on an irregular surface; no climbing stairs; no climbing ladders or hill climbing requiring frequent knee flexion; no activities requiring balance; no applying strength against bent knee (squatting, kneeling, crouching, stooping, pedaling, etc.); elevate leg half of time; may need immobilization; limited weight bearing.
Manual/standing work: Standing not more than 50 min/hr; walking on a smooth surface up to 1,200 ft/hr carrying up to 25 lbs; walking on an irregular surface up to 900 ft/hr carrying up to 25 lbs; climbing stairs up to 8 flights/hr carrying up to 40 lbs; climbing ladders up to 50 rungs/hr carrying up to 25 lbs; activities requiring balance up to 45 min/hr (if able to work with two hands without assistance for balance); applying strength against bent knee (pedaling, squatting, kneeling, etc.) up to 60 times/hr; may need brace for uneven ground or ladders.
Description: Occurs when tendons in the ankle or instep develop microscopic tears and inflammation. Pain, swelling, and inability to use the foot or ankle may be sudden or gradual symptoms.

Metatarsalgia NOS

Excludes:
Morton's metatarsalgia (355.6)

Procedure Summary (from ODG Treatment):
Accommodative modalities; Achilles tendon ruptures (treatment); Activity restrictions; Actovegin; Ankle prostheses (total ankle replacement); Anterior drawer test; Anti-inflammatory medications (NSAIDs); Arthrodesis (fusion); Arthroplasty (total ankle replacement); Autologous conditioned serum (ACS); Bed rest; Biofeedback; Bone scan (imaging); Bracing (immobilization); Cast (immobilization); Causality; Chiropractic; Cold packs; Computed tomography (CT); Continuous-flow cryotherapy; Corticosteroids (topical); Diathermy; Dorsiflexion night splints; Education (patient); Elastic bandage (immobilization); Electron generating device; Exercise; Extracorporeal shock wave therapy (ESWT); Functional treatment; Fusion; Heat therapy (ice/heat); Heparin; Heel pads; Ice packs; Imaging; Immobilization; Ingrown toenail surgery; Injections; Insoles with magnetic foil; Inversion stress test; Iontophoresis; Lace-up ankle support; Laser therapy (LLLT); Lateral ligament ankle reconstruction (surgery); Lineal tomography; Low-intensity laser therapy (LLLT); Magnets; Magnetic resonance imaging (MRI); Manipulation; Massage; Mechanical treatment (taping/orthoses); Modified duty; Narcotics; Night splints; Nonprescription medications; Orthotic devices; Osteotomy; Ottawa ankle rules (OAR); Patient education; Phonophoresis; Physical therapy (PT); Prolotherapy (sclerotherapy); Radiography; Rest (RICE); Return to work; Sclerotherapy (prolotherapy); Semi-rigid ankle support; Shock wave therapy, extracorporeal (ESWT); Steroids (injection); Stretching (flexibility); Supports; Surgery; Surgery for achilles tendon ruptures; Surgery for ankle sprains; Surgery for calcaneal fractures; Surgery for hallux valgus; Surgery for plantar fasciitis; Surgery for tarsal tunnel syndrome; Talar tilt test; Tai Chi; Taping; Tension night splints (TNS); Therapeutic exercise; Thompson test; Total ankle replacement (arthroplasty); Transcutaneous electrical neurostimulation (TENS); Ultrasound, diagnostic; Ultrasound, therapeutic; Work

Workers' Comp Costs per Claim (based on 67 claims)					
Quartile	25%	50%	75%	Mean	% no cost
Medical	$252	$803	$4,137	$3,404	3%
Total	$252	$840	$5,019	$5,405	0%

Impact on Total Absence: Prevalence 0.0002% of total lost workdays

726.71 Achilles bursitis or tendinitis

Return-To-Work Summary Guidelines		
Dataset	**Midrange**	**At-Risk**
Claims data	25 days	58 days
All absences	8 days	45 days

Return-To-Work "Best Practice" Guidelines
Mild, sedentary/modified work: 0 days
Mild, regular/standing work: 4 days
Severe, with cast, sedentary/modified work: 14 days
Severe, with cast, regular/standing work: 42 days

Capabilities & Activity Modifications:
Sedentary/modified work: Standing limited to 5-10 min/hr; walking only on a smooth surface using crutches with limited pressure on the foot; no walking on an irregular surface; no climbing stairs; no climbing ladders or hill climbing requiring frequent knee flexion; no activities requiring balance; no applying strength against bent knee (squatting, kneeling, crouching, stooping, pedaling, etc.); elevate leg half of time; may need immobilization; limited weight bearing.
Manual/standing work: Standing not more than 50 min/hr; walking on a smooth surface up to 1,200 ft/hr carrying up to 25 lbs; walking on an irregular surface up to 900 ft/hr carrying up to 25 lbs; climbing stairs up to 8 flights/hr carrying up to 40 lbs; climbing ladders up to 50 rungs/hr carrying up to 25 lbs; activities requiring balance up to 45 min/hr (if able to work with

726.71 Achilles bursitis or tendinitis *(cont'd)*

two hands without assistance for balance); applying strength against bent knee (pedaling, squatting, kneeling, etc.) up to 60 times/hr; may need brace for uneven ground or ladders.

Description: Inflammation of the connective tissue of the ankle or instep due to arthritis, infection, injury, or excessive exercise or effort.

Procedure Summary (from ODG Treatment):
Accommodative modalities; Achilles tendon ruptures (treatment); Activity restrictions; Actovegin; Ankle prostheses (total ankle replacement); Anterior drawer test; Anti-inflammatory medications (NSAIDs); Arthrodesis (fusion); Arthroplasty (total ankle replacement); Autologous conditioned serum (ACS); Bed rest; Biofeedback; Bone scan (imaging); Bracing (immobilization); Cast (immobilization); Causality; Chiropractic; Cold packs; Computed tomography (CT); Continuous-flow cryotherapy; Corticosteroids (topical); Diathermy; Dorsiflexion night splints; Education (patient); Elastic bandage (immobilization); Electron generating device; Exercise; Extracorporeal shock wave therapy (ESWT); Functional treatment; Fusion; Heat therapy (ice/heat); Heparin; Heel pads; Ice packs; Imaging; Immobilization; Ingrown toenail surgery; Injections; Insoles with magnetic foil; Inversion stress test; Iontophoresis; Lace-up ankle support; Laser therapy (LLLT); Lateral ligament ankle reconstruction (surgery); Lineal tomography; Low-intensity laser therapy (LLLT); Magnets; Magnetic resonance imaging (MRI); Manipulation; Massage; Mechanical treatment (taping/orthoses); Modified duty; Narcotics; Night splints; Nonprescription medications; Orthotic devices; Osteotomy; Ottawa ankle rules (OAR); Patient education; Phonophoresis; Physical therapy (PT); Prolotherapy (sclerotherapy); Radiography; Rest (RICE); Return to work; Sclerotherapy (prolotherapy); Semi-rigid ankle support; Shock wave therapy, extracorporeal (ESWT); Steroids (injection); Stretching (flexibility); Supports; Surgery; Surgery for achilles tendon ruptures; Surgery for ankle sprains; Surgery for calcaneal fractures; Surgery for hallux valgus; Surgery for plantar fasciitis; Surgery for tarsal tunnel syndrome; Talar tilt test; Tai Chi; Taping; Tension night splints (TNS); Therapeutic exercise; Thompson test; Total ankle replacement (arthroplasty); Transcutaneous electrical neurostimulation (TENS); Ultrasound, diagnostic; Ultrasound, therapeutic; Work

Physical Therapy Guidelines:
Medical treatment: 9 visits over 8 weeks

Workers' Comp Costs per Claim (based on 435 claims)					
Quartile	25%	50%	75%	Mean	% no cost
Indemnity	$1,239	$3,455	$7,928	$12,906	70%
Medical	$305	$861	$2,951	$3,481	2%
Total	$326	$1,176	$4,316	$7,382	2%

RTW Claims Data (Calendar-days away from work by decile)										
10%	20%	30%	40%	**50%**	60%	70%	80%	**90%**	100%	Mean
10	13	14	19	**25**	37	41	45	**58**	72	29.92

726.71 Achilles bursitis or tendinitis *(cont'd)*

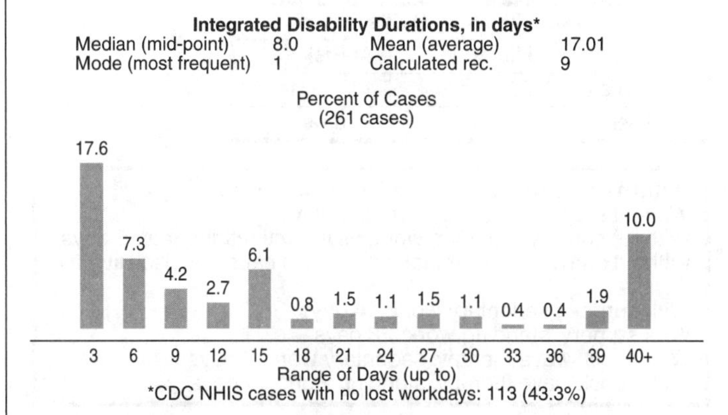

Impact on Total Absence: Prevalence 0.0074% of total lost workdays; Incidence 0.08 days per 100 workers

726.72 Tibialis tendinitis

Return-To-Work Summary Guidelines		
Dataset	**Midrange**	**At-Risk**
Claims data	35 days	71 days
All absences	22 days	67 days

Return-To-Work "Best Practice" Guidelines
Sedentary/modified work: 3 days
Manual/standing work: 21 days
Heavy manual/standing work: 35 days

Description: Inflammatory condition of one of the muscles of the leg.

Tibialis (anterior) (posterior) tendinitis

Physical Therapy Guidelines:
Medical treatment: 9 visits over 8 weeks
Post-surgical treatment: 12 visits over 12 weeks

Workers' Comp Costs per Claim (based on 296 claims)					
Quartile	25%	50%	75%	Mean	% no cost
Indemnity	$3,518	$7,203	$23,930	$17,156	42%
Medical	$1,239	$4,284	$12,884	$9,457	2%
Total	$1,796	$8,516	$20,601	$19,661	2%

RTW Claims Data (Calendar-days away from work by decile)										
10%	20%	30%	40%	**50%**	60%	70%	80%	**90%**	100%	Mean
14	21	22	27	**35**	39	48	62	**71**	77	38.43

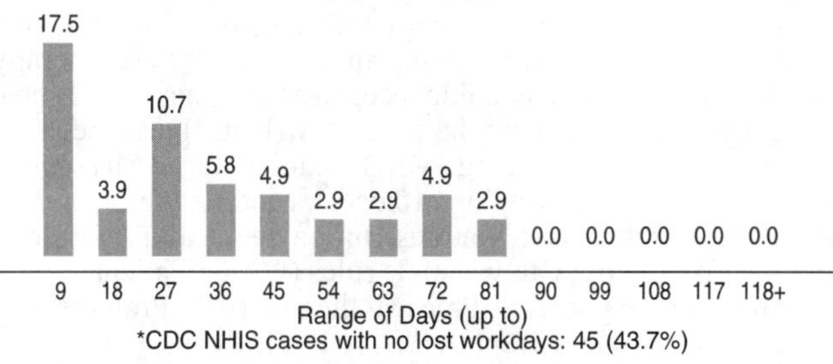

Impact on Total Absence: Prevalence 0.0049% of total lost workdays; Incidence 0.05 days per 100 workers

726.73 Calcaneal spur

Return-To-Work Summary Guidelines		
Dataset	**Midrange**	**At-Risk**
Claims data	20 days	103 days
All absences	13 days	71 days

Return-To-Work "Best Practice" Guidelines
Without surgery, sedentary work: 0 days
Without surgery, standing work, using anti-fatigue mat: 5 days
Without surgery, regular standing work if cause of disability: 21 days
With surgery, sedentary work: 14 days
With surgery, standing work: 28 days
With shock wave therapy, sedentary work: 7 days
With shock wave therapy, standing work: 14 days

Capabilities & Activity Modifications:
Sedentary/modified work: Standing limited to 5-10 min/hr; walking only on a smooth surface using crutches with limited pressure on the foot; no walking on an irregular surface; no climbing stairs; no climbing ladders or hill climbing requiring frequent knee flexion; no activities requiring balance; no applying strength against bent knee (squatting, kneeling, crouching, stooping, pedaling, etc.); elevate leg half of time; may need immobilization; limited weight bearing.
Manual/standing work: Standing not more than 50 min/hr; walking on a smooth surface up to 1,200 ft/hr carrying up to 25 lbs; walking on an irregular surface up to 900 ft/hr carrying up to 25 lbs; climbing stairs up to 8 flights/hr carrying up to 40 lbs; climbing ladders up to 50 rungs/hr carrying up to 25 lbs; activities requiring balance up to 45 min/hr (if able to work with two hands without assistance for balance); applying strength against bent knee (pedaling, squatting, kneeling, etc.) up to 60 times/hr; may need brace for uneven ground or ladders.
Description: Growths of extra bone on the heel caused by excessive pulling on the heel bone by tendons or connective tissue. They are usually painful, especially when walking and may become inflamed, causing a throbbing pain.
Other names: Heel spur, Jogger's heel
Procedure Summary (from ODG Treatment):
Accommodative modalities; Achilles tendon ruptures (treatment); Activity restrictions; Actovegin; Ankle prostheses (total ankle replacement); Anterior drawer test; Anti-inflammatory medications (NSAIDs); Arthrodesis (fusion); Arthroplasty (total ankle replacement); Autologous conditioned serum (ACS); Bed rest; Biofeedback; Bone scan (imaging); Bracing (immobilization); Cast (immobilization); Causality; Chiropractic; Cold packs; Computed tomography (CT); Continuous-flow cryotherapy; Corticosteroids (topical); Diathermy; Dorsiflexion night splints; Education (patient); Elastic bandage (immobilization); Electron generating device; Exercise; Extracorporeal shock wave therapy (ESWT); Functional treatment; Fusion; Heat therapy (ice/heat); Heparin; Heel pads; Ice packs; Imaging; Immobilization; Ingrown toenail surgery; Injections; Insoles with magnetic foil; Inversion stress test; Iontophoresis; Lace-up ankle support; Laser therapy (LLLT); Lateral ligament ankle reconstruction (surgery); Lineal tomography; Low-intensity laser therapy (LLLT); Magnets; Magnetic resonance imaging (MRI); Manipulation; Massage; Mechanical treatment (taping/orthoses); Modified duty; Narcotics; Night splints; Nonprescription medications; Orthotic devices; Osteotomy; Ottawa ankle rules (OAR); Patient education; Phonophoresis; Physical therapy (PT); Prolotherapy (sclerotherapy); Radiography; Rest (RICE); Return to work; Sclerotherapy (prolotherapy); Semi-rigid ankle support; Shock wave therapy, extracorporeal (ESWT); Steroids (injection); Stretching (flexibility); Supports; Surgery; Surgery for achilles tendon ruptures; Surgery for ankle sprains; Surgery for

726.73 Calcaneal spur *(cont'd)*

calcaneal fractures; Surgery for hallux valgus; Surgery for plantar fasciitis; Surgery for tarsal tunnel syndrome; Talar tilt test; Tai Chi; Taping; Tension night splints (TNS); Therapeutic exercise; Thompson test; Total ankle replacement (arthroplasty); Transcutaneous electrical neurostimulation (TENS); Ultrasound, diagnostic; Ultrasound, therapeutic; Work

Workers' Comp Costs per Claim (based on 32 claims)					
Quartile	25%	50%	75%	Mean	% no cost
Medical	$441	$625	$672	$991	6%
Total	$441	$646	$1,008	$1,163	6%

RTW Claims Data (Calendar-days away from work by decile)										
10%	20%	30%	40%	**50%**	60%	70%	80%	**90%**	100%	Mean
10	12	14	14	**20**	25	30	55	**103**	365	40.05

Integrated Disability Durations, in days*

Median (mid-point)	13.0	Mean (average)	27.63
Mode (most frequent)	14	Calculated rec.	17

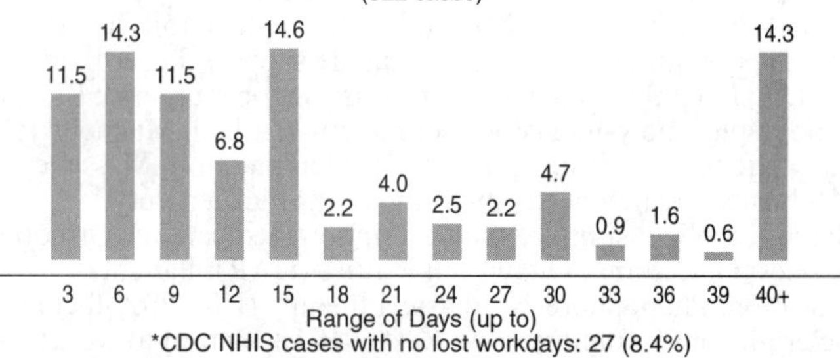

*CDC NHIS cases with no lost workdays: 27 (8.4%)

Impact on Total Absence: Prevalence 0.0240% of total lost workdays; Incidence 0.25 days per 100 workers

726.79 Other

Return-To-Work Summary Guidelines		
Dataset	**Midrange**	**At-Risk**
Claims data	29 days	69 days
All absences	12 days	57 days

Return-To-Work "Best Practice" Guidelines
Sedentary/modified work: 3 days
Manual/standing work: 21 days
Heavy manual/standing work: 35 days

Description: Inflammatory condition of one of the outer muscles of the leg.
Other names: Sinus tarsi syndrome
Peroneal tendinitis

Workers' Comp Costs per Claim (based on 266 claims)					
Quartile	25%	50%	75%	Mean	% no cost
Indemnity	$2,856	$8,295	$16,349	$13,151	45%
Medical	$1,092	$4,011	$12,128	$8,235	2%
Total	$1,334	$6,279	$21,441	$15,627	2%

RTW Claims Data (Calendar-days away from work by decile)										
10%	20%	30%	40%	**50%**	60%	70%	80%	**90%**	100%	Mean
11	14	21	24	**29**	35	40	52	**69**	75	33.88

726.79 Other *(cont'd)*

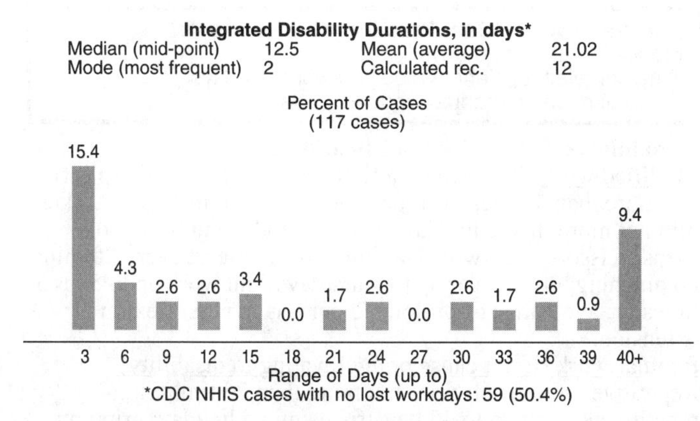

Impact on Total Absence: Prevalence 0.0036% of total lost workdays; Incidence 0.04 days per 100 workers

726.9 Unspecified enthesopathy

Return-To-Work Summary Guidelines		
Dataset	**Midrange**	**At-Risk**
Claims data	15 days	25 days
All absences	11 days	23 days

Return-To-Work "Best Practice" Guidelines
Medical treatment, clerical/modified work: 0 days
Medical treatment, manual work: 10 days
With surgery (for more specific diagnosis), clerical/modified work: 5 days
With surgery (for more specific diagnosis), manual work: 21 days

Description: Inflammatory process involving the area where a ligament or tendon is inserted into bone. Pain and other symptoms depend on where the inflammation occurs.

Workers' Comp Costs per Claim (based on 614 claims)

Quartile	25%	50%	75%	Mean	% no cost
Indemnity	$1,859	$5,912	$21,588	$17,578	68%
Medical	$221	$704	$4,053	$5,594	4%
Total	$231	$824	$6,783	$11,435	4%

RTW Claims Data (Calendar-days away from work by decile)

10%	20%	30%	40%	**50%**	60%	70%	80%	**90%**	100%	Mean
9	10	11	13	**15**	20	21	22	**25**	365	22.53

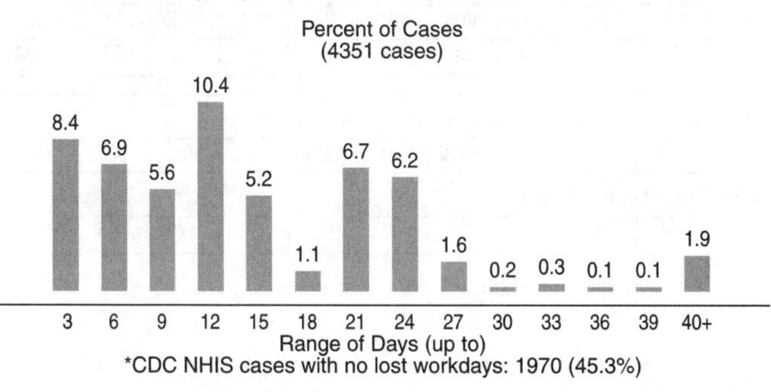

Impact on Total Absence: Prevalence 0.1174% of total lost workdays; Incidence 1.23 days per 100 workers

727 Other disorders of synovium, tendon, and bursa

Return-To-Work Summary Guidelines		
Dataset	**Midrange**	**At-Risk**
Claims data	23 days	62 days
All absences	13 days	47 days

Return-To-Work "Best Practice" Guidelines
See more specific diagnoses under 727

Workers' Comp Costs per Claim (based on 18,618 claims)

Quartile	25%	50%	75%	Mean	% no cost
Indemnity	$1,596	$3,423	$7,959	$7,333	72%
Medical	$294	$704	$2,678	$2,945	3%
Total	$305	$872	$4,211	$5,079	3%

RTW Claims Data (Calendar-days away from work by decile)

10%	20%	30%	40%	**50%**	60%	70%	80%	**90%**	100%	Mean
12	14	18	21	**23**	30	35	40	**62**	365	34.72

RTW Post Surgery (Calendar-days away from work by decile)

	10%	20%	30%	40%	**50%**	60%	70%	80%	**90%**	100%	Mean
Repair of ruptured tendon	5	15	29	39	**52**	76	103	131	**180**	349	79.95
Incision of tendon sheath	16	26	33	44	**49**	61	76	106	**238**	365	85.09
Incise finger tendon sheath	10	14	19	25	**32**	41	54	67	**116**	365	54.72

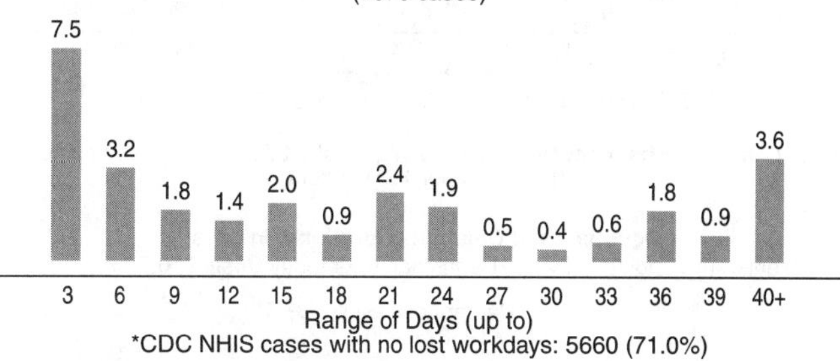

Impact on Total Absence: Prevalence 0.1504% of total lost workdays; Incidence 1.58 days per 100 workers

727.0 Synovitis and tenosynovitis

Return-To-Work Summary Guidelines		
Dataset	**Midrange**	**At-Risk**
Claims data	23 days	54 days
All absences	10 days	39 days

Return-To-Work "Best Practice" Guidelines
Medical treatment, clerical/modified work: 0 days
Medical treatment, manual work: 21 days
Medical treatment, heavy manual work: 35 days
Surgical treatment, clerical/modified work: 7 days
Surgical treatment, manual work: 21 days

Description: Inflammation of a tendon accompanied by an inflammation of the sheath around the tendon that provides nourishment and protection. This occurs most often in the

727.0 Synovitis and tenosynovitis *(cont'd)*

tendons of the hand or fingers. Symptoms include pain with movement or touch, visibly swollen tendon sheaths, or a grating sensation when the joint is moved.

Physical Therapy Guidelines:
Medical treatment: 9 visits over 8 weeks

Workers' Comp Costs per Claim (based on 15,282 claims)					
Quartile	25%	50%	75%	Mean	% no cost
Indemnity	$1,355	$2,657	$6,027	$5,812	76%
Medical	$273	$588	$1,890	$2,028	3%
Total	$273	$672	$2,709	$3,481	3%

RTW Claims Data (Calendar-days away from work by decile)										
10%	20%	30%	40%	**50%**	60%	70%	80%	**90%**	100%	Mean
10	14	19	21	**23**	32	35	38	**54**	365	30.93

RTW Post Surgery (Calendar-days away from work by decile)										
10%	20%	30%	40%	**50%**	60%	70%	80%	**90%**	100%	Mean
Incision of tendon sheath										
16	26	33	44	**48**	61	76	107	**238**	365	85.13
Incise finger tendon sheath										
10	14	19	25	**32**	41	54	67	**116**	365	54.72

Integrated Disability Durations, in days*

Median (mid-point)	10.0	Mean (average)	18.48
Mode (most frequent)	1	Calculated rec.	10

Percent of Cases
(2901 cases)

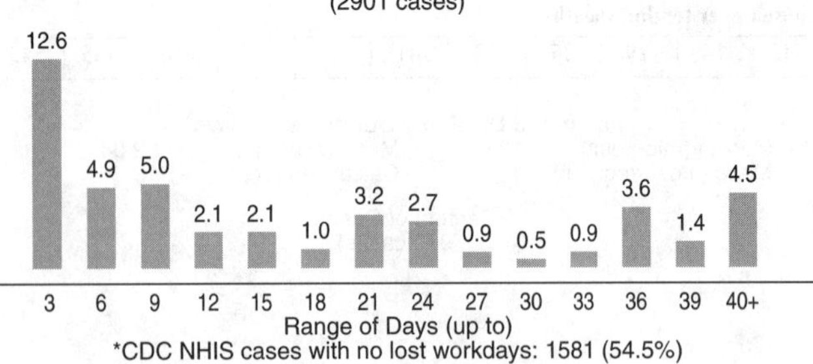

*CDC NHIS cases with no lost workdays: 1581 (54.5%)

Impact on Total Absence: Prevalence 0.0721% of total lost workdays; Incidence 0.76 days per 100 workers

Occupational Disability Durations, in days
Median (mid-point) 14 - Benchmark Indemnity Costs $10,500

Percent of Cases
(750 cases)

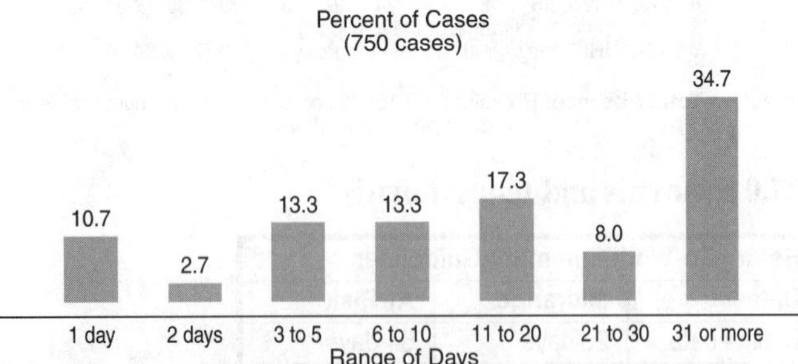

Impact on Occupational Absence: Prevalence 0.1191% of occupational lost workdays; Incidence 0.02 days per 100 workers

727.03 Trigger finger (acquired)

Return-To-Work Summary Guidelines		
Dataset	**Midrange**	**At-Risk**
Claims data	26 days	64 days
All absences	13 days	58 days

727.03 Trigger finger (acquired) *(cont'd)*

Return-To-Work "Best Practice" Guidelines
Medical treatment: 0 days
Surgical release, clerical/modified work: 14 days
Surgical release, manual work: 28 days

Capabilities & Activity Modifications:
Modified work: Repetitive motion activities (w or w/o splint) not more than 4 times/hr; repetitive keying up to 15 keystrokes/min not more than 2 hrs/day; gripping and using light tools (pens, scissors, etc.) with 5-minute break at least every 20 min; no pinching; driving car up to 2 hrs/day; light work up to 5 lbs 3 times/hr; avoidance of prolonged periods in wrist flexion or extension.
Regular work (if not cause or aggravating to disability): Repetitive motion activities not more than 25 times/hr; repetitive keying up to 45 keystrokes/min 8 hrs/day; gripping and using moderate tools (pliers, screwdrivers, etc.) fulltime; pinching up to 5 times/min; driving car or light truck up to 6 hrs/day or heavy truck up to 3 hrs/day; moderate to heavy work up to 35 lbs not more than 7 times/hr.
Description: A condition in which the finger becomes locked in a bent position because of an inflamed and swollen tendon. Straightening the finger or thumb produces a popping sound. Other symptoms include pain and swelling over the palm.
Procedure Summary (from ODG Treatment): Activity restrictions; Acupuncture; Arthrodesis (fusion); Arthroplasty (joint replacement); Casting versus splints; Chiropractic (manipulation); Cold packs; Computed tomography (CT); Continuous passive motion (CPM); de Quervain's tenosynovitis surgery; Dupuytren's release (fasciectomy); Ergonomic interventions; Exercises; Fasciotomy; Fusion; Imaging; Immobilization (treatment); Injection; Joint replacement; Mallet finger injuries (treatment); Manipulation; Modified duty; MRI's (magnetic resonance imaging); Nonprescription medications; Occupational therapy (OT); Physical therapy (PT); Plaster casting; Radiography (x-rays); Rest; Return to work; Splints; Surgery for broken wrist; TENS (transcutaneous electrical neurostimulation); Trapeziectomy; Triangular fibrocartilage complex (TFCC) reconstruction ; Trigger finger surgery; Vitamin C; Work; X-rays; Yoga
Physical Therapy Guidelines:
Post-surgical treatment: 9 visits over 8 weeks

Workers' Comp Costs per Claim (based on 1,199 claims)					
Quartile	25%	50%	75%	Mean	% no cost
Indemnity	$1,355	$2,646	$6,101	$5,416	53%
Medical	$672	$1,785	$3,696	$3,137	1%
Total	$756	$2,615	$6,479	$5,714	1%

RTW Claims Data (Calendar-days away from work by decile)										
10%	20%	30%	40%	**50%**	60%	70%	80%	**90%**	100%	Mean
11	13	14	20	**26**	28	40	49	**64**	77	30.94

RTW Post Surgery (Calendar-days away from work by decile)										
10%	20%	30%	40%	**50%**	60%	70%	80%	**90%**	100%	Mean
Incise finger tendon sheath										
11	14	19	24	**31**	42	53	67	**119**	365	55.31

727.03 Trigger finger (acquired) *(cont'd)*

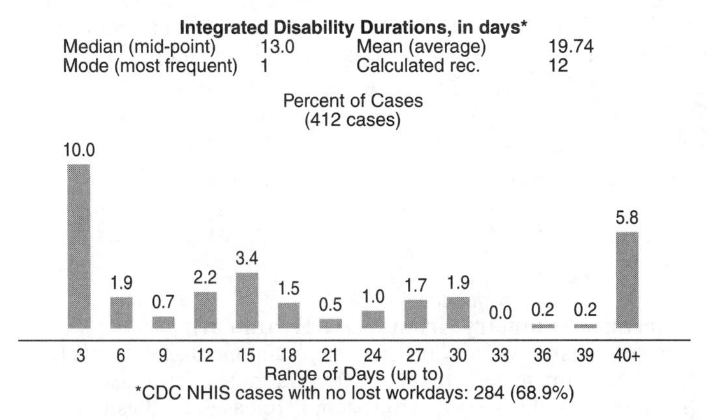

Impact on Total Absence: Prevalence 0.0074% of total lost workdays; Incidence 0.08 days per 100 workers

727.04 Radial styloid tenosynovitis

Return-To-Work Summary Guidelines		
Dataset	**Midrange**	**At-Risk**
Claims data	30 days	65 days
All absences	10 days	57 days

Return-To-Work "Best Practice" Guidelines
Medical treatment, clerical/modified work: 0-1 days
Medical treatment, manual work: 10 days
Medical treatment, regular work if cause of disability: 42 days
Medical treatment, heavy manual work: 56 days
Surgical release, clerical/modified work: 14 days
Surgical release, manual work: 42 days

Capabilities & Activity Modifications:
Modified work: Repetitive motion activities (w or w/o splint) not more than 4 times/hr; repetitive keying up to 15 keystrokes/min not more than 2 hrs/day; gripping and using light tools (pens, scissors, etc.) with 5-minute break at least every 20 min; no pinching; driving car up to 2 hrs/day; light work up to 5 lbs 3 times/hr; avoidance of prolonged periods in wrist flexion or extension.
Regular work (if not cause or aggravating to disability) : Repetitive motion activities not more than 25 times/hr; repetitive keying up to 45 keystrokes/min 8 hrs/day; gripping and using moderate tools (pliers, screwdrivers, etc.) fulltime; pinching up to 5 times/min; driving car or light truck up to 6 hrs/day or heavy truck up to 3 hrs/day; moderate to heavy work up to 35 lbs not more than 7 times/hr.
Description: Inflammation of the tendons that control the thumb causing pain with thumb motion, swelling over the wrist, and a popping sensation.
Other names: DeQuervains, De Quervains
de Quervain's disease
Procedure Summary (from ODG Treatment): Activity restrictions; Acupuncture; Arthrodesis (fusion); Arthroplasty (joint replacement); Casting versus splints; Chiropractic (manipulation); Cold packs; Computed tomography (CT); Continuous passive motion (CPM); de Quervain's tenosynovitis surgery; Dupuytren's release (fasciectomy); Ergonomic interventions; Exercises; Fasciotomy; Fusion; Imaging; Immobilization (treatment); Injection; Joint replacement; Mallet finger injuries (treatment); Manipulation; Modified duty; MRI's (magnetic resonance imaging); Nonprescription medications; Occupational therapy (OT); Physical therapy (PT); Plaster casting; Radiography (x-rays); Rest; Return to work; Splints; Surgery for broken wrist; TENS (transcutaneous

727.04 Radial styloid tenosynovitis *(cont'd)*

electrical neurostimulation); Trapeziectomy; Triangular fibrocartilage complex (TFCC) reconstruction ; Trigger finger surgery; Vitamin C; Work; X-rays; Yoga
Physical Therapy Guidelines:
Allow for fading of treatment frequency (from up to 3 visits per week to 1 or less), plus active self-directed home PT
Medical treatment: 12 visits over 8 weeks
Post-surgical treatment: 14 visits over 12 weeks

Workers' Comp Costs per Claim (based on 1,849 claims)					
Quartile	25%	50%	75%	Mean	% no cost
Indemnity	$1,701	$3,465	$8,484	$7,062	65%
Medical	$441	$1,271	$3,434	$3,105	2%
Total	$462	$1,722	$5,324	$5,642	1%

RTW Claims Data (Calendar-days away from work by decile)										
10%	20%	30%	40%	**50%**	60%	70%	80%	**90%**	100%	Mean
10	13	15	22	**30**	41	44	56	**65**	84	34.39

RTW Post Surgery (Calendar-days away from work by decile)										
10%	20%	30%	40%	**50%**	60%	70%	80%	**90%**	100%	Mean
Incision of tendon sheath										
14	25	32	44	**48**	60	76	106	**228**	365	79.62

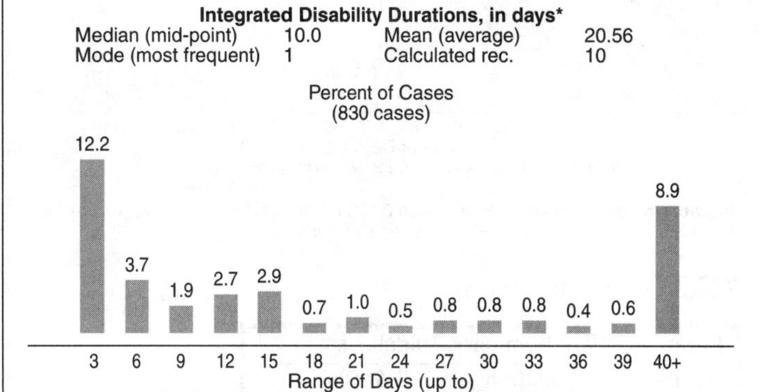

Impact on Total Absence: Prevalence 0.0191% of total lost workdays; Incidence 0.20 days per 100 workers

727.1 Bunion

Return-To-Work Summary Guidelines		
Dataset	**Midrange**	**At-Risk**
Claims data	40 days	86 days
All absences	34 days	85 days

Return-To-Work "Best Practice" Guidelines
Without surgery: 0-1 days
With bunionectomy, sedentary work: 10-35 days
With bunionectomy, standing work: 42-84 days

Capabilities & Activity Modifications:
Sedentary/modified work: Standing limited to 5-10 min/hr; walking only on a smooth surface using crutches with limited pressure on the foot; no walking on an irregular surface; no climbing stairs; no climbing ladders or hill climbing requiring frequent knee flexion; no activities requiring balance; no applying strength against bent knee (squatting, kneeling, crouching, stooping, pedaling, etc.); elevate leg half of time; may need immobilization; limited weight bearing.
Manual/standing work: Standing not more than 50 min/hr; walking on a smooth surface up to 1,200 ft/hr carrying up to 25 lbs; walking on an irregular surface up to 900 ft/hr carrying up

727.1 Bunion *(cont'd)*

to 25 lbs; climbing stairs up to 8 flights/hr carrying up to 40 lbs; climbing ladders up to 50 rungs/hr carrying up to 25 lbs; activities requiring balance up to 45 min/hr (if able to work with two hands without assistance for balance); applying strength against bent knee (pedaling, squatting, kneeling, etc.) up to 60 times/hr; may need brace for uneven ground or ladders.
Description: Inflammation and thickening of the fluid-filled sac (bursa) at the base of the big toe causing the big toe to turn toward the other toes. There could be a painful, bony enlargement on the inside edge of the toe and the toe may grow over one of the other toes. This condition sometimes occurs on the fifth toe.

RTW Claims Data (Calendar-days away from work by decile)										
10%	20%	30%	40%	**50%**	60%	70%	80%	**90%**	100%	Mean
10	11	14	34	**40**	42	44	69	**86**	365	45.37

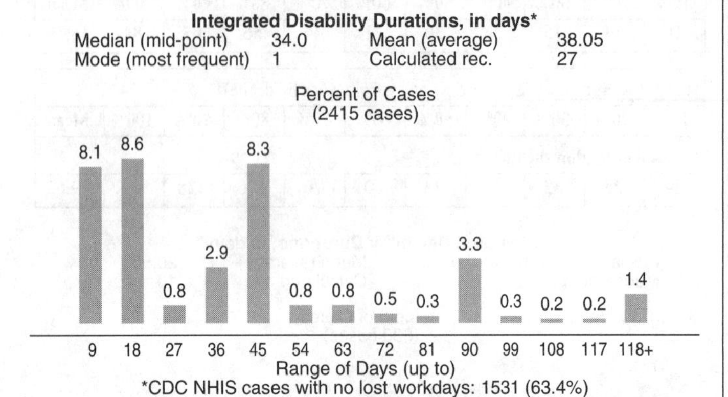

Impact on Total Absence: Prevalence 0.0994% of total lost workdays; Incidence 1.04 days per 100 workers

727.3 Other bursitis

Return-To-Work Summary Guidelines		
Dataset	**Midrange**	**At-Risk**
Claims data	23 days	31 days
All absences	19 days	30 days

Return-To-Work "Best Practice" Guidelines
Medical treatment, clerical/modified work: 0 days
Medical treatment, manual work: 7 days
Bursectomy, clerical/modified work: 21 days
Bursectomy, manual work: 28 days

Capabilities & Activity Modifications:
Modified work: No overhead work (reaching above shoulder) plus no reaching to shoulder level (90 degree position); no holding arm in abduction or flexion; pulling and pushing not more than 8 lbs up to 4 times/hr; lifting and carrying up to 5 lbs 3 times/hr; single arm upper extremity work using injured arm for light work only; possible immobilization by abduction brace, sling, or clavicle brace; no climbing ladders.
Manual work: Reaching above shoulder not more than 12 times/hr with up to 15 lbs of weight; reaching to shoulder up to 15 times/hr with up to 25 lbs of weight; holding arm in abduction or flexion up to 12 times/hr with up to 15 lbs of weight; pulling and pushing up to 60 lbs 20 times/hr; lifting and carrying up to 40 lbs 15 times/hr; single upper extremity work using injured arm for moderate work only (full use of non-injured arm); possible immobilization by abduction brace, sling, or clavicle brace; climbing ladders up to 50 rungs/hr.

727.3 Other bursitis *(cont'd)*

Description: Inflammation of the bursae (fluid-filled sacs that are located at sites of friction and facilitate normal movement). Inflammation causes localized pain, swelling, and limits.

Bursitis NOS

Excludes:
bursitis:
gonococcal (098.52)
subacromial (726.19)
subcoracoid (726.19)
subdeltoid (726.19)
syphilitic (095.7)
"frozen shoulder" (726.0)

Procedure Summary (from ODG Treatment):
Acromioplasty; Activity restrictions; Acupuncture; Adson's test (AT); Anterior scalene block; Arthrography; Arthroplasty (shoulder); Arthroscopy; Arthroscopic release of adhesions; Bipolar interferential electrotherapy; Biofeedback; Biopsychosocial rehab; Cardiovascular functional testing; Chiropractic; Cold lasers; Continuous-flow cryotherapy; Continuous passive motion (CPM); Corticosteroid injections; Costoclavicular maneuver (CCM); Cutaneous laser treatment; Deep friction massage; Diagnostic arthroscopy; Diathermy; Distension arthrography; Electrical stimulation; Electrodiagnostic testing for TOS (thoracic outlet syndrome); Elevated arm stress test (EAST); Ergonomic interventions; Exercises; Extracorporeal shock wave therapy (ESWT); Hydroplasty/ hydrodilation; Imaging; Immobilization; Impingement test; Injections; Interferential therapy; Laser therapy; Low level laser therapy (LLLT); Magnetic resonance imaging (MRI); Manipulation; Manipulation under anesthesia (MUA); Massage; Mechanical traction; Modified duty; Multidisciplinary biopsychosocial rehab; Nerve blocks; Osteochondral autologous transplantation (OATS); Physical therapy; Porcine small intestinal submucosa (SIS); Pulsed electromagnetic field; Radiography; Return to work; Rotator cuff repair; Rotator cuff porcine graft repair; Shock wave therapy; Shoulder repair; Steroid injections; Supraclavicular pressure (SCP); Surgery for AC joint separation; Surgery for adhesive capsulitis; Surgery for impingement syndrome; Surgery for rotator cuff repair; Surgery for ruptured biceps tendon; Surgery for shoulder dislocation; Surgery for Thoracic Outlet Syndrome; Thermal capsulorrhaphy; Thermotherapy; Transcutaneous electrical neurostimulation (TENS); Transdermal nitroglycerin; Ultrasound, diagnostic; Ultrasound, therapeutic; Work
Physical Therapy Guidelines:
9 visits over 8 weeks

Workers' Comp Costs per Claim (based on 72 claims)					
Quartile	25%	50%	75%	Mean	% no cost
Medical	$179	$441	$1,281	$1,861	3%
Total	$179	$504	$2,216	$4,038	3%

RTW Claims Data (Calendar-days away from work by decile)										
10%	20%	30%	40%	**50%**	60%	70%	80%	**90%**	100%	Mean
10	14	20	21	**23**	26	28	29	**31**	365	28.63

727.3 Other bursitis *(cont'd)*

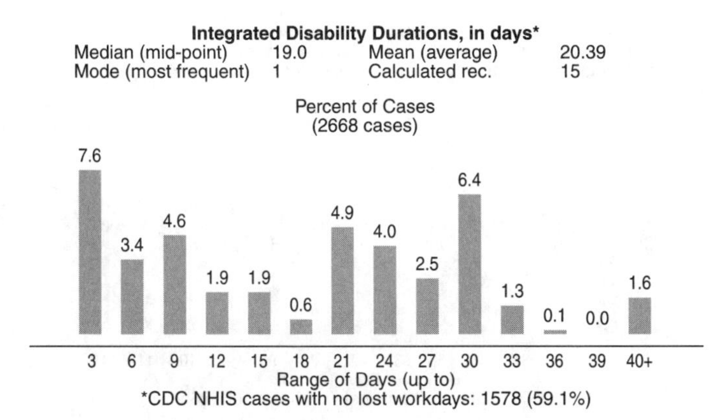

Impact on Total Absence: Prevalence 0.0657% of total lost workdays; Incidence 0.69 days per 100 workers

Occupational Disability Durations, in days
Median (mid-point) 7 - Benchmark Indemnity Costs $5,250

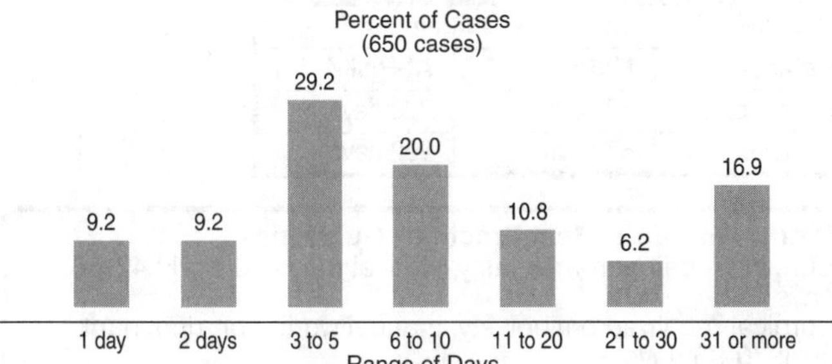

Impact on Occupational Absence: Prevalence 0.0516% of occupational lost workdays; Incidence 0.01 days per 100 workers

727.4 Ganglion and cyst of synovium, tendon, and bursa

Return-To-Work Summary Guidelines		
Dataset	**Midrange**	**At-Risk**
Claims data	22 days	56 days
All absences	14 days	45 days

Return-To-Work "Best Practice" Guidelines
Asymptomatic: 0 days
Aspiration, clerical/modified work: 0 days
Aspiration, manual work: 3 days
Excision of wrist ganglion, clerical/modified work: 7 days
Excision of wrist ganglion, manual work: 14 days
Excision of wrist ganglion, manual work, dominant arm: 14-21 days

Capabilities & Activity Modifications:
Modified work: Repetitive motion activities (w or w/o splint) not more than 4 times/hr; repetitive keying up to 15 keystrokes/min not more than 2 hrs/day; gripping and using light tools (pens, scissors, etc.) with 5-minute break at least every 20 min; no pinching; driving car up to 2 hrs/day; light work up to 5 lbs 3 times/hr; avoidance of prolonged periods in wrist flexion or extension.
Regular work (if not cause or aggravating to disability) : Repetitive motion activities not more than 25 times/hr; repetitive keying up to 45 keystrokes/min 8 hrs/day; gripping and using moderate tools (pliers, screwdrivers, etc.) fulltime; pinching up to 5 times/min; driving car or light truck up to 6 hrs/day or heavy truck up to 3 hrs/day; moderate to heavy work up to 35 lbs not more than 7 times/hr.

727.4 Ganglion and cyst of synovium, tendon, and bursa *(cont'd)*

Description: A fluid-filled sac which develops over a tendon or joint, commonly at the wrist, fingers, and ankle, causing pain and swelling and a mass that can be felt through the skin. It is usually soft, but sometimes hardens with time.
Procedure Summary (from ODG Treatment): Activity restrictions; Acupuncture; Arthrodesis (fusion); Arthroplasty (joint replacement); Casting versus splints; Chiropractic (manipulation); Cold packs; Computed tomography (CT); Continuous passive motion (CPM); de Quervain's tenosynovitis surgery; Dupuytren's release (fasciectomy); Ergonomic interventions; Exercises; Fasciotomy; Fusion; Imaging; Immobilization (treatment); Injection; Joint replacement; Mallet finger injuries (treatment); Manipulation; Modified duty; MRI's (magnetic resonance imaging); Nonprescription medications; Occupational therapy (OT); Physical therapy (PT); Plaster casting; Radiography (x-rays); Rest; Return to work; Splints; Surgery for broken wrist; TENS (transcutaneous electrical neurostimulation); Trapeziectomy; Triangular fibrocartilage complex (TFCC) reconstruction ; Trigger finger surgery; Vitamin C; Work; X-rays; Yoga
Physical Therapy Guidelines:
Post-surgical treatment: 18 visits over 6 weeks

Workers' Comp Costs per Claim (based on 1,431 claims)					
Quartile	25%	50%	75%	Mean	% no cost
Indemnity	$1,428	$3,171	$7,697	$7,109	68%
Medical	$284	$893	$3,465	$3,094	2%
Total	$284	$1,208	$4,851	$5,419	2%

RTW Claims Data (Calendar-days away from work by decile)										
10%	20%	30%	40%	**50%**	60%	70%	80%	**90%**	100%	Mean
12	14	16	20	**22**	27	33	41	**56**	321	29.27

Integrated Disability Durations, in days*
Median (mid-point) 14.0 Mean (average) 19.60
Mode (most frequent) 1 Calculated rec. 12

Percent of Cases
(1211 cases)

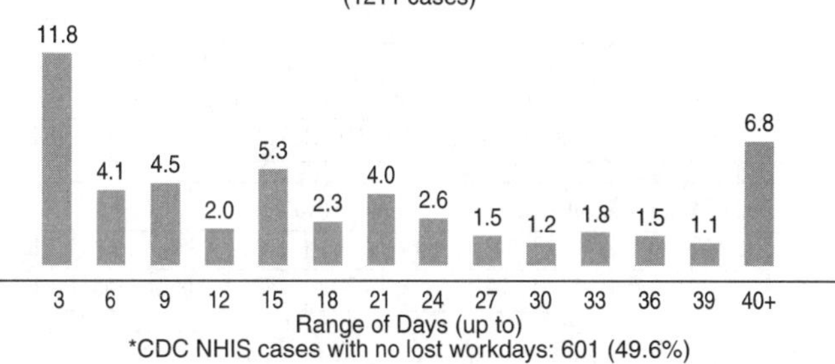

Impact on Total Absence: Prevalence 0.0353% of total lost workdays; Incidence 0.37 days per 100 workers

Occupational Disability Durations, in days
Median (mid-point) 13 - Benchmark Indemnity Costs $9,750

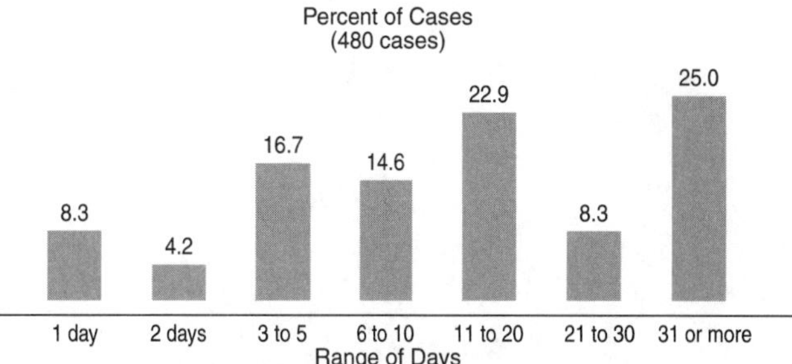

Impact on Occupational Absence: Prevalence 0.0707% of occupational lost workdays; Incidence 0.01 days per 100 workers

727.6 Rupture of tendon, nontraumatic

Return-To-Work Summary Guidelines		
Dataset	**Midrange**	**At-Risk**
Claims data	52 days	166 days
All absences	46 days	127 days

Return-To-Work "Best Practice" Guidelines
Surgery/rotator cuff repair/acromioplasty, clerical/modified work: 21 days
Surgery/rotator cuff repair/acromioplasty, manual work, non-dominant arm: 48 days
Surgery/rotator cuff repair/acromioplasty, manual work, dominant arm: 84 days
Surgery/rotator cuff repair/acromioplasty, heavy manual work: indefinite

Capabilities & Activity Modifications:
Modified work: No overhead work (reaching above shoulder) plus no reaching to shoulder level (90 degree position); no holding arm in abduction or flexion; pulling and pushing not more than 8 lbs up to 4 times/hr; lifting and carrying up to 5 lbs 3 times/hr; single arm upper extremity work using injured arm for light work only; possible immobilization by abduction brace, sling, or clavicle brace; no climbing ladders.
Manual work: Reaching above shoulder not more than 12 times/hr with up to 15 lbs of weight; reaching to shoulder up to 15 times/hr with up to 25 lbs of weight; holding arm in abduction or flexion up to 12 times/hr with up to 15 lbs of weight; pulling and pushing up to 60 lbs 20 times/hr; lifting and carrying up to 40 lbs 15 times/hr; single upper extremity work using injured arm for moderate work only (full use of non-injured arm); possible immobilization by abduction brace, sling, or clavicle brace; climbing ladders up to 50 rungs/hr.
Description: A rupture or tear of a tendon causing increasing pain with activity and localized weakness.
Physical Therapy Guidelines:
Post-surgical treatment: 34 visits over 16 weeks

Workers' Comp Costs per Claim (based on 1,391 claims)

Quartile	25%	50%	75%	Mean	% no cost
Indemnity	$3,717	$7,550	$14,396	$12,969	42%
Medical	$1,817	$7,004	$12,968	$10,124	0%
Total	$2,783	$10,259	$21,042	$17,614	0%

RTW Claims Data (Calendar-days away from work by decile)

10%	20%	30%	40%	**50%**	60%	70%	80%	**90%**	100%	Mean
18	22	34	47	**52**	67	84	97	**166**	365	81.33

RTW Post Surgery (Calendar-days away from work by decile)

10%	20%	30%	40%	**50%**	60%	70%	80%	**90%**	100%	Mean
Repair of ruptured tendon										
5	16	29	39	**52**	76	107	131	**180**	349	80.84

727.6 Rupture of tendon, nontraumatic *(cont'd)*

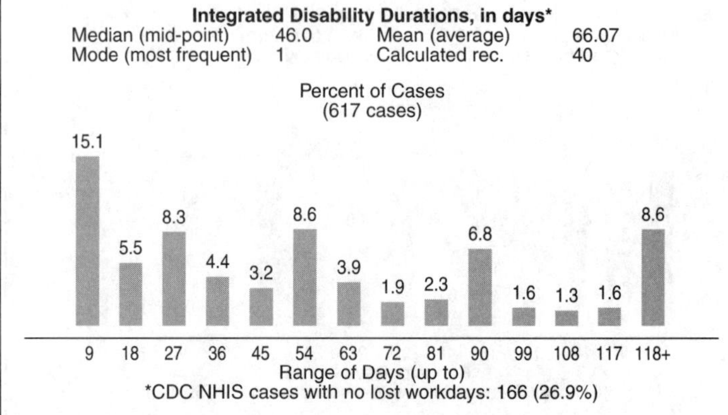

Impact on Total Absence: Prevalence 0.0880% of total lost workdays; Incidence 0.92 days per 100 workers

727.61 Complete rupture of rotator cuff

Return-To-Work Summary Guidelines		
Dataset	**Midrange**	**At-Risk**
Claims data	72 days	222 days
All absences	57 days	202 days

Return-To-Work "Best Practice" Guidelines
Surgical repair/acromioplasty, clerical/modified work: 42-56 days
Surgical repair/acromioplasty, manual work, non-dominant arm: 70-90 days
Surgical repair/acromioplasty, manual work, dominant arm: 106-180 days
Surgical repair/acromioplasty, heavy manual work: indefinite

Capabilities & Activity Modifications:
Modified work: No overhead work (reaching above shoulder) plus no reaching to shoulder level (90 degree position); no holding arm in abduction or flexion; pulling and pushing not more than 8 lbs up to 4 times/hr; lifting and carrying up to 5 lbs 3 times/hr; single arm upper extremity work using injured arm for light work only; possible immobilization by abduction brace, sling, or clavicle brace; no climbing ladders.
Manual work: Reaching above shoulder not more than 12 times/hr with up to 15 lbs of weight; reaching to shoulder up to 15 times/hr with up to 25 lbs of weight; holding arm in abduction or flexion up to 12 times/hr with up to 15 lbs of weight; pulling and pushing up to 60 lbs 20 times/hr; lifting and carrying up to 40 lbs 15 times/hr; single upper extremity work using injured arm for moderate work only (full use of non-injured arm); possible immobilization by abduction brace, sling, or clavicle brace; climbing ladders up to 50 rungs/hr.
Description: A rupture or tear of the rotator cuff, causing pain that increases with activity and localized weakness.
Procedure Summary (from ODG Treatment):
Acromioplasty; Activity restrictions; Acupuncture; Adson's test (AT); Anterior scalene block; Arthrography; Arthroplasty (shoulder); Arthroscopy; Arthroscopic release of adhesions; Bipolar interferential electrotherapy; Biofeedback; Biopsychosocial rehab; Cardiovascular functional testing; Chiropractic; Cold lasers; Continuous-flow cryotherapy; Continuous passive motion (CPM); Corticosteroid injections; Costoclavicular maneuver (CCM); Cutaneous laser treatment; Deep friction massage; Diagnostic arthroscopy; Diathermy; Distension arthrography; Electrical stimulation; Electrodiagnostic testing for TOS (thoracic outlet syndrome); Elevated arm stress test (EAST); Ergonomic interventions; Exercises; Extracorporeal shock wave therapy (ESWT);

727.61 Complete rupture of rotator cuff *(cont'd)*

Hydroplasty/ hydrodilation; Imaging; Immobilization; Impingement test; Injections; Interferential therapy; Laser therapy; Low level laser therapy (LLLT); Magnetic resonance imaging (MRI); Manipulation; Manipulation under anesthesia (MUA); Massage; Mechanical traction; Modified duty; Multidisciplinary biopsychosocial rehab; Nerve blocks; Osteochondral autologous transplantation (OATS); Physical therapy; Porcine small intestinal submucosa (SIS); Pulsed electromagnetic field; Radiography; Return to work; Rotator cuff repair; Rotator cuff porcine graft repair; Shock wave therapy; Shoulder repair; Steroid injections; Supraclavicular pressure (SCP); Surgery for AC joint separation; Surgery for adhesive capsulitis; Surgery for impingement syndrome; Surgery for rotator cuff repair; Surgery for ruptured biceps tendon; Surgery for shoulder dislocation; Surgery for Thoracic Outlet Syndrome; Thermal capsulorrhaphy; Thermotherapy; Transcutaneous electrical neurostimulation (TENS); Transdermal nitroglycerin; Ultrasound, diagnostic; Ultrasound, therapeutic; Work

Physical Therapy Guidelines:
Post-surgical treatment: 40 visits over 16 weeks

Workers' Comp Costs per Claim (based on 72 claims)

Quartile	25%	50%	75%	Mean	% no cost
Indemnity	$3,528	$9,093	$18,134	$18,145	45%
Medical	$3,843	$10,327	$18,869	$12,808	0%
Total	$5,156	$15,372	$27,615	$22,835	0%

RTW Claims Data (Calendar-days away from work by decile)

10%	20%	30%	40%	**50%**	60%	70%	80%	**90%**	100%	Mean
14	21	43	49	**72**	86	102	146	**222**	365	99.54

Integrated Disability Durations, in days*
Median (mid-point) 57.0 Mean (average) 88.93
Mode (most frequent) 21 Calculated rec. 56

Percent of Cases
(310 cases)

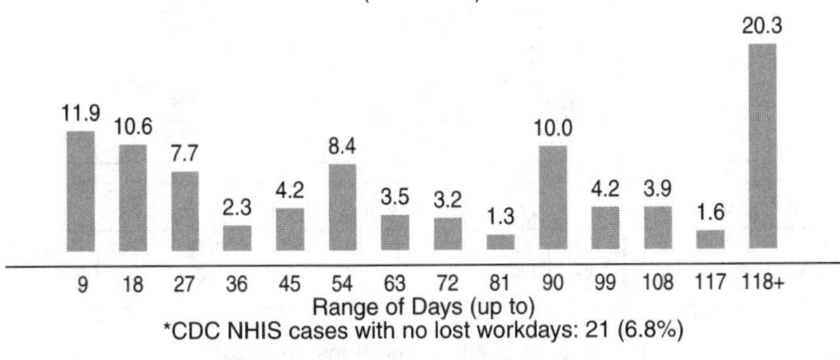

Range of Days (up to)
*CDC NHIS cases with no lost workdays: 21 (6.8%)

Impact on Total Absence: Prevalence 0.0759% of total lost workdays; Incidence 0.80 days per 100 workers

Occupational Disability Durations, in days
Median (mid-point) 26 - Benchmark Indemnity Costs $19,500

Percent of Cases
(45 cases)

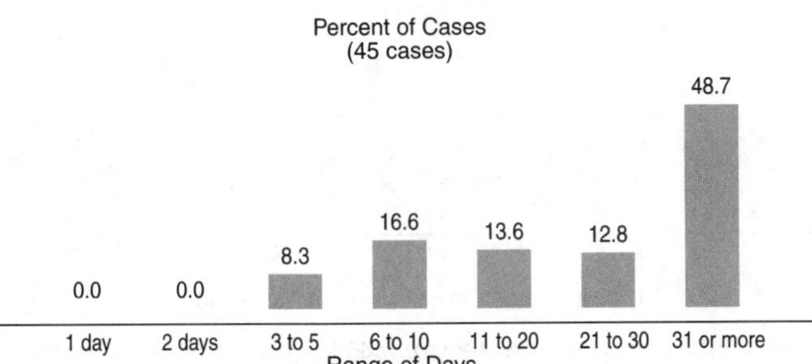

Range of Days
Impact on Occupational Absence: Prevalence 0.0132% of occupational lost workdays

727.62 Tendons of biceps (long head)

Return-To-Work Summary Guidelines		
Dataset	**Midrange**	**At-Risk**
Claims data	41 days	67 days
All absences	29 days	60 days

Return-To-Work "Best Practice" Guidelines
Surgical repair, clerical/modified work: 28 days
Surgical repair, manual work, non-dominant arm: 42 days
Surgical repair, manual work, dominant arm: 56 days

Description: A rupture or tear of the biceps, causing pain that increases with activity and localized weakness.

Physical Therapy Guidelines:
Post-surgical treatment: 24 visits over 16 weeks

Workers' Comp Costs per Claim (based on 718 claims)

Quartile	25%	50%	75%	Mean	% no cost
Indemnity	$3,591	$7,765	$13,923	$12,117	44%
Medical	$1,502	$6,846	$11,204	$8,647	1%
Total	$2,111	$9,907	$18,459	$15,414	1%

RTW Claims Data (Calendar-days away from work by decile)

10%	20%	30%	40%	**50%**	60%	70%	80%	**90%**	100%	Mean
18	25	29	32	**41**	44	54	57	**67**	85	40.83

Integrated Disability Durations, in days*
Median (mid-point) 29.0 Mean (average) 30.37
Mode (most frequent) 1 Calculated rec. 22

Percent of Cases
(275 cases)

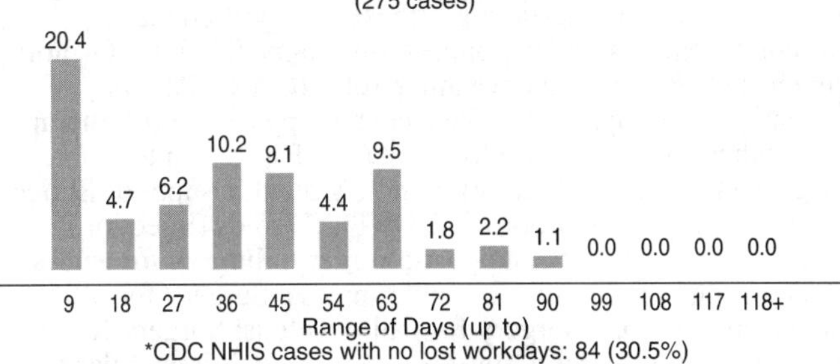

Range of Days (up to)
*CDC NHIS cases with no lost workdays: 84 (30.5%)

Impact on Total Absence: Prevalence 0.0171% of total lost workdays; Incidence 0.18 days per 100 workers

727.67 Achilles tendon

Return-To-Work Summary Guidelines		
Dataset	**Midrange**	**At-Risk**
Claims data	94 days	176 days
All absences	74 days	175 days

Return-To-Work "Best Practice" Guidelines
Surgical repair, sedentary/modified work: 21 days
Surgical repair, manual/standing work: 70 days
Surgical repair, heavy manual/standing work: 112-175 days

Capabilities & Activity Modifications:
Sedentary/modified work: Standing limited to 5-10 min/hr; walking only on a smooth surface using crutches with limited pressure on the foot; no walking on an irregular surface; no climbing stairs; no climbing ladders or hill climbing requiring frequent knee flexion; no activities requiring balance; no applying strength against bent knee (squatting, kneeling, crouching, stooping, pedaling, etc.); elevate leg half of time; may need immobilization; limited weight bearing.

727.67 Achilles tendon *(cont'd)*

Manual/standing work: Standing not more than 50 min/hr; walking on a smooth surface up to 1,200 ft/hr carrying up to 25 lbs; walking on an irregular surface up to 900 ft/hr carrying up to 25 lbs; climbing stairs up to 8 flights/hr carrying up to 40 lbs; climbing ladders up to 50 rungs/hr carrying up to 25 lbs; activities requiring balance up to 45 min/hr (if able to work with two hands without assistance for balance); applying strength against bent knee (pedaling, squatting, kneeling, etc.) up to 60 times/hr; may need brace for uneven ground or ladders.

Description: A rupture or tear of the Achilles tendon, causing pain that increases with activity and localized weakness.

Procedure Summary (from ODG Treatment):
Accommodative modalities; Achilles tendon ruptures (treatment); Activity restrictions; Actovegin; Ankle prostheses (total ankle replacement); Anterior drawer test; Anti-inflammatory medications (NSAIDs); Arthrodesis (fusion); Arthroplasty (total ankle replacement); Autologous conditioned serum (ACS); Bed rest; Biofeedback; Bone scan (imaging); Bracing (immobilization); Cast (immobilization); Causality; Chiropractic; Cold packs; Computed tomography (CT); Continuous-flow cryotherapy; Corticosteroids (topical); Diathermy; Dorsiflexion night splints; Education (patient); Elastic bandage (immobilization); Electron generating device; Exercise; Extracorporeal shock wave therapy (ESWT); Functional treatment; Fusion; Heat therapy (ice/heat); Heparin; Heel pads; Ice packs; Imaging; Immobilization; Ingrown toenail surgery; Injections; Insoles with magnetic foil; Inversion stress test; Iontophoresis; Lace-up ankle support; Laser therapy (LLLT); Lateral ligament ankle reconstruction (surgery); Lineal tomography; Low-intensity laser therapy (LLLT); Magnets; Magnetic resonance imaging (MRI); Manipulation; Massage; Mechanical treatment (taping/orthoses); Modified duty; Narcotics; Night splints; Nonprescription medications; Orthotic devices; Osteotomy; Ottawa ankle rules (OAR); Patient education; Phonophoresis; Physical therapy (PT); Prolotherapy (sclerotherapy); Radiography; Rest (RICE); Return to work; Sclerotherapy (prolotherapy); Semi-rigid ankle support; Shock wave therapy, extracorporeal (ESWT); Steroids (injection); Stretching (flexibility); Supports; Surgery; Surgery for achilles tendon ruptures; Surgery for ankle sprains; Surgery for calcaneal fractures; Surgery for hallux valgus; Surgery for plantar fasciitis; Surgery for tarsal tunnel syndrome; Talar tilt test; Tai Chi; Taping; Tension night splints (TNS); Therapeutic exercise; Thompson test; Total ankle replacement (arthroplasty); Transcutaneous electrical neurostimulation (TENS); Ultrasound, diagnostic; Ultrasound, therapeutic; Work

Physical Therapy Guidelines:
Post-surgical treatment: 48 visits over 16 weeks

Workers' Comp Costs per Claim (based on 184 claims)

Quartile	25%	50%	75%	Mean	% no cost
Indemnity	$4,515	$6,846	$13,398	$11,459	43%
Medical	$2,961	$6,610	$13,335	$9,535	1%
Total	$5,670	$10,427	$18,407	$16,100	1%

RTW Claims Data (Calendar-days away from work by decile)

10%	20%	30%	40%	**50%**	60%	70%	80%	**90%**	100%	Mean
22	44	58	73	**94**	110	124	148	**176**	215	96.54

727.67 Achilles tendon *(cont'd)*

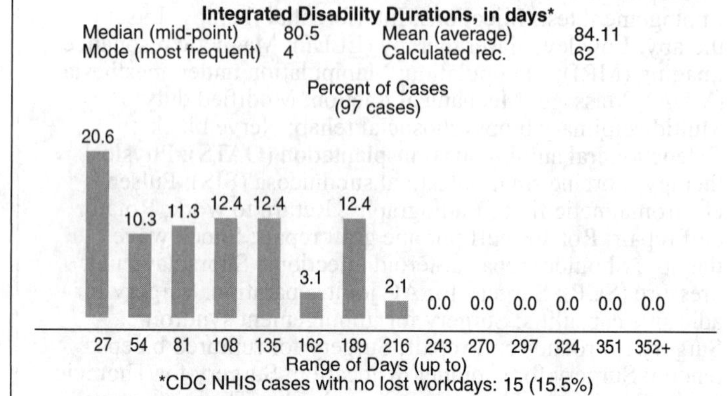

Impact on Total Absence: Prevalence 0.0203% of total lost workdays; Incidence 0.21 days per 100 workers

728 Disorders of muscle, ligament, and fascia

Return-To-Work Summary Guidelines		
Dataset	**Midrange**	**At-Risk**
Claims data	23 days	48 days
All absences	21 days	29 days

Return-To-Work "Best Practice" Guidelines
See 728.9

Excludes:
enthesopathies (726.0-726.9)
muscular dystrophies (359.0-359.1)
myoneural disorders (358.0-358.9)
myopathies (359.2-359.9)
old disruption of ligaments of knee (717.81-717.89)

Workers' Comp Costs per Claim (based on 1,108 claims)

Quartile	25%	50%	75%	Mean	% no cost
Indemnity	$2,058	$4,337	$12,863	$11,608	56%
Medical	$347	$1,397	$4,935	$6,991	3%
Total	$410	$2,363	$8,883	$12,184	3%

RTW Claims Data (Calendar-days away from work by decile)

10%	20%	30%	40%	**50%**	60%	70%	80%	**90%**	100%	Mean
14	20	22	23	**23**	24	25	27	**48**	365	29.40

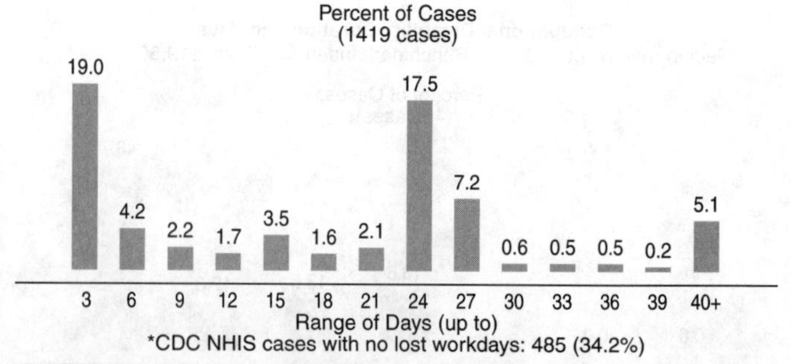

Impact on Total Absence: Prevalence 0.0536% of total lost workdays; Incidence 0.56 days per 100 workers

728 Disorders of muscle, ligament, and fascia

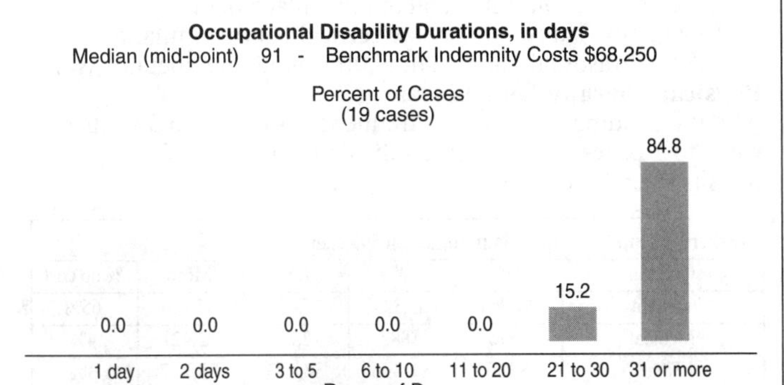

Impact on Occupational Absence: Prevalence 0.0196% of occupational lost workdays

728.6 Contracture of palmar fascia

Return-To-Work Summary Guidelines		
Dataset	**Midrange**	**At-Risk**
Claims data	27 days	45 days
All absences	16 days	43 days

Return-To-Work "Best Practice" Guidelines
Medical treatment: 0 days
Dupuytren's release/fasciectomy, non-dominant hand, clerical work: 10 days
Dupuytren's release/fasciectomy, non-dominant hand, manual work: 28 days
Dupuytren's release/fasciectomy, dominant hand, clerical work: 14 days
Dupuytren's release/fasciectomy, dominant hand, manual work: 42 days

Description: Inherited deformity of the hand and/or foot causing the fingers or toes to eventually become fixed in a bent position. The condition is not painful but it causes difficulty with gripping or grasping large objects.

Dupuytren's contracture

Physical Therapy Guidelines:
Post-surgical treatment: 12 visits over 8 weeks

Workers' Comp Costs per Claim (based on 46 claims)

Quartile	25%	50%	75%	Mean	% no cost
Indemnity	$4,421	$8,358	$12,968	$11,832	17%
Medical	$4,547	$8,395	$10,889	$9,265	0%
Total	$5,114	$14,060	$25,001	$19,125	0%

RTW Claims Data (Calendar-days away from work by decile)

10%	20%	30%	40%	**50%**	60%	70%	80%	**90%**	100%	Mean
10	13	14	15	**27**	29	36	42	**45**	365	34.31

728.6 Contracture of palmar fascia *(cont'd)*

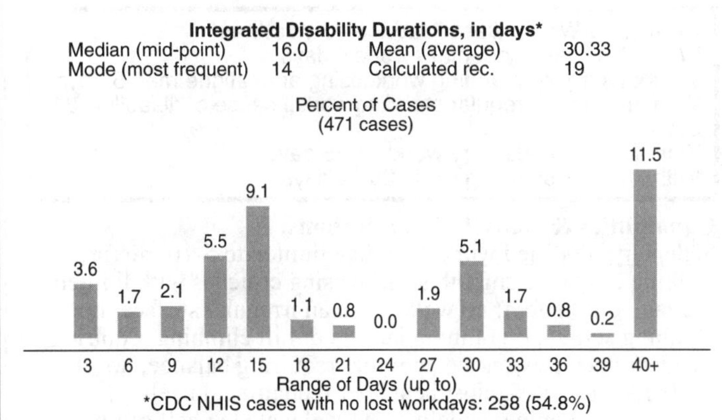

Impact on Total Absence: Prevalence 0.0190% of total lost workdays; Incidence 0.20 days per 100 workers

728.7 Other fibromatoses

Return-To-Work Summary Guidelines		
Dataset	**Midrange**	**At-Risk**
Claims data	26 days	103 days
All absences	10 days	75 days

Return-To-Work "Best Practice" Guidelines
See 728.9

Workers' Comp Costs per Claim (based on 606 claims)

Quartile	25%	50%	75%	Mean	% no cost
Indemnity	$1,764	$3,413	$7,844	$8,040	64%
Medical	$315	$893	$2,825	$2,579	4%
Total	$347	$1,580	$4,862	$5,546	3%

RTW Claims Data (Calendar-days away from work by decile)

10%	20%	30%	40%	**50%**	60%	70%	80%	**90%**	100%	Mean
14	20	23	24	**26**	35	51	72	**103**	138	43.64

Integrated Disability Durations, in days*
Median (mid-point) 10.5 Mean (average) 23.90
Mode (most frequent) 1 Calculated rec. 11

Percent of Cases
(426 cases)

19.2 4.5 0.7 1.9 1.4 1.2 1.4 5.6 1.9 0.7 0.5 1.4 0.2 10.1

3 6 9 12 15 18 21 24 27 30 33 36 39 40+
Range of Days (up to)
*CDC NHIS cases with no lost workdays: 210 (49.3%)

Impact on Total Absence: Prevalence 0.0152% of total lost workdays; Incidence 0.16 days per 100 workers

728.71 Plantar fascial fibromatosis

Return-To-Work Summary Guidelines		
Dataset	**Midrange**	**At-Risk**
Claims data	32 days	88 days
All absences	15 days	85 days

728.71 Plantar fascial fibromatosis *(cont'd)*

Return-To-Work "Best Practice" Guidelines
Without surgery, sedentary work: 0 days
Without surgery, standing work, using anti-fatigue mat: 5 days
Without surgery, regular standing work if cause of disability: 21 days
With surgery, sedentary work: 21-35 days
With surgery, standing work: 35-84 days

Capabilities & Activity Modifications:
Sedentary/modified work: Standing limited to 5-10 min/hr; walking only on a smooth surface using crutches with limited pressure on the foot; no walking on an irregular surface; no climbing stairs; no climbing ladders or hill climbing requiring frequent knee flexion; no activities requiring balance; no applying strength against bent knee (squatting, kneeling, crouching, stooping, pedaling, etc.); elevate leg half of time; may need immobilization; limited weight bearing.
Manual/standing work: Standing not more than 50 min/hr; walking on a smooth surface up to 1,200 ft/hr carrying up to 25 lbs; walking on an irregular surface up to 900 ft/hr carrying up to 25 lbs; climbing stairs up to 8 flights/hr carrying up to 40 lbs; climbing ladders up to 50 rungs/hr carrying up to 25 lbs; activities requiring balance up to 45 min/hr (if able to work with two hands without assistance for balance); applying strength against bent knee (pedaling, squatting, kneeling, etc.) up to 60 times/hr; may need brace for uneven ground or ladders.
Description: Inflammation of the plantar fascia (fibrous tissue in the sole of the foot), causing pain in the heel.

Contracture of plantar fascia
Plantar fasciitis (traumatic)

Procedure Summary (from ODG Treatment):
Accommodative modalities; Achilles tendon ruptures (treatment); Activity restrictions; Actovegin; Ankle prostheses (total ankle replacement); Anterior drawer test; Anti-inflammatory medications (NSAIDs); Arthrodesis (fusion); Arthroplasty (total ankle replacement); Autologous conditioned serum (ACS); Bed rest; Biofeedback; Bone scan (imaging); Bracing (immobilization); Cast (immobilization); Causality; Chiropractic; Cold packs; Computed tomography (CT); Continuous-flow cryotherapy; Corticosteroids (topical); Diathermy; Dorsiflexion night splints; Education (patient); Elastic bandage (immobilization); Electron generating device; Exercise; Extracorporeal shock wave therapy (ESWT); Functional treatment; Fusion; Heat therapy (ice/heat); Heparin; Heel pads; Ice packs; Imaging; Immobilization; Ingrown toenail surgery; Injections; Insoles with magnetic foil; Inversion stress test; Iontophoresis; Lace-up ankle support; Laser therapy (LLLT); Lateral ligament ankle reconstruction (surgery); Lineal tomography; Low-intensity laser therapy (LLLT); Magnets; Magnetic resonance imaging (MRI); Manipulation; Massage; Mechanical treatment (taping/orthoses); Modified duty; Narcotics; Night splints; Nonprescription medications; Orthotic devices; Osteotomy; Ottawa ankle rules (OAR); Patient education; Phonophoresis; Physical therapy (PT); Prolotherapy (sclerotherapy); Radiography; Rest (RICE); Return to work; Sclerotherapy (prolotherapy); Semi-rigid ankle support; Shock wave therapy, extracorporeal (ESWT); Steroids (injection); Stretching (flexibility); Supports; Surgery; Surgery for achilles tendon ruptures; Surgery for ankle sprains; Surgery for calcaneal fractures; Surgery for hallux valgus; Surgery for plantar fasciitis; Surgery for tarsal tunnel syndrome; Talar tilt test; Tai Chi; Taping; Tension night splints (TNS); Therapeutic exercise; Thompson test; Total ankle replacement (arthroplasty); Transcutaneous electrical neurostimulation (TENS); Ultrasound, diagnostic; Ultrasound, therapeutic; Work
Physical Therapy Guidelines:
Allow for fading of treatment frequency (from up to 3 visits per week to 1 or less), plus active self-directed home PT
6 visits over 4 weeks

Workers' Comp Costs per Claim (based on 599 claims)

Quartile	25%	50%	75%	Mean	% no cost
Indemnity	$1,764	$3,334	$7,424	$7,720	65%
Medical	$315	$882	$2,762	$2,421	4%
Total	$336	$1,496	$4,473	$5,207	3%

RTW Claims Data (Calendar-days away from work by decile)

10%	20%	30%	40%	**50%**	60%	70%	80%	**90%**	100%	Mean
11	13	20	22	**32**	36	58	83	**88**	323	45.76

Integrated Disability Durations, in days*
Median (mid-point) 15.5 Mean (average) 31.85
Mode (most frequent) 1 Calculated rec. 16

Percent of Cases
(966 cases)

Range of Days (up to)	3	6	9	12	15	18	21	24	27	30	33	36	39	40+
Percent of Cases	13.1	11.2	5.3	5.4	5.2	1.7	5.3	3.3	1.2	1.1	0.9	5.2	1.8	19.7

*CDC NHIS cases with no lost workdays: 190 (19.7%)

Impact on Total Absence: Prevalence 0.0730% of total lost workdays; Incidence 0.77 days per 100 workers

728.9 Unspecified disorder of muscle, ligament, and fascia

Return-To-Work Summary Guidelines

Dataset	Midrange	At-Risk
Claims data	23 days	27 days
All absences	23 days	26 days

Return-To-Work "Best Practice" Guidelines
Limited duty work: 0 days
Regular work: 23 days

RTW Claims Data (Calendar-days away from work by decile)

10%	20%	30%	40%	**50%**	60%	70%	80%	**90%**	100%	Mean
14	21	22	23	**23**	24	24	25	**27**	230	25.29

728.9 Unspecified disorder of muscle, ligament, and fascia *(cont'd)*

Integrated Disability Durations, in days*

Median (mid-point)	23.0	Mean (average)	20.12
Mode (most frequent)	23	Calculated rec.	22

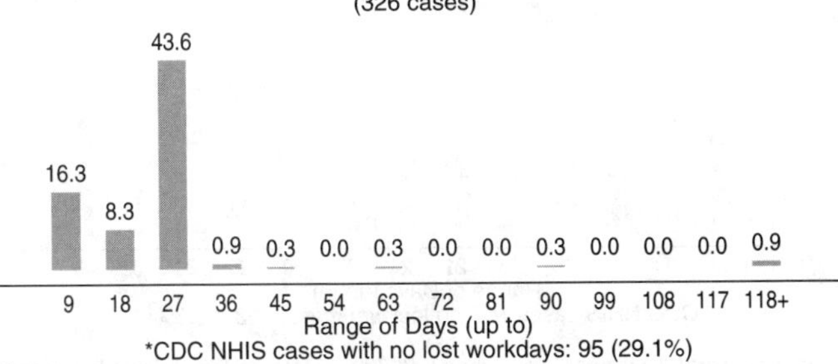

*CDC NHIS cases with no lost workdays: 95 (29.1%)

Impact on Total Absence: Prevalence 0.0137% of total lost workdays; Incidence 0.14 days per 100 workers

729 Other disorders of soft tissues

Return-To-Work Summary Guidelines		
Dataset	**Midrange**	**At-Risk**
Claims data	14 days	17 days
All absences	7 days	15 days

Return-To-Work "Best Practice" Guidelines
See 729.0

Excludes:
acroparesthesia (443.89)
carpal tunnel syndrome (354.0)
disorders of the back (720.0-724.9)
entrapment syndromes (354.0-355.9)
palindromic rheumatism (719.3)
periarthritis (726.0-726.9)
psychogenic rheumatism (306.0)

Workers' Comp Costs per Claim (based on 1,364 claims)

Quartile	25%	50%	75%	Mean	% no cost
Indemnity	$2,174	$4,841	$12,989	$11,765	62%
Medical	$431	$1,722	$5,639	$5,478	3%
Total	$473	$2,268	$9,450	$10,058	3%

Occupational Disability Durations, in days
Median (mid-point) 30 - Benchmark Indemnity Costs $22,500
(160 cases)
Impact on Occupational Absence: Prevalence 0.0544% of occupational lost workdays; Incidence 0.01 days per 100 workers

729.0 Rheumatism, unspecified and fibrositis

Return-To-Work Summary Guidelines		
Dataset	**Midrange**	**At-Risk**
Claims data	15 days	18 days
All absences	14 days	18 days

Return-To-Work "Best Practice" Guidelines
Moderate pain: 0 days
Debilitating pain, with hospitalization: 14 days

Description: Inflammation of the connective tissues, especially the muscles and joints.

729.0 Rheumatism, unspecified and fibrositis

RTW Claims Data (Calendar-days away from work by decile)

10%	20%	30%	40%	**50%**	60%	70%	80%	**90%**	100%	Mean
13	13	14	14	**15**	15	16	17	**18**	365	20.70

Integrated Disability Durations, in days*

Median (mid-point)	14.0	Mean (average)	16.34
Mode (most frequent)	14	Calculated rec.	15

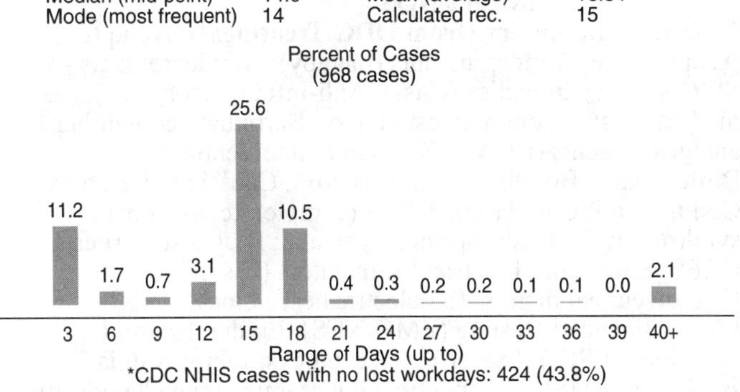

*CDC NHIS cases with no lost workdays: 424 (43.8%)

Impact on Total Absence: Prevalence 0.0262% of total lost workdays; Incidence 0.28 days per 100 workers

Occupational Disability Durations, in days
Median (mid-point) 14 - Benchmark Indemnity Costs $10,500

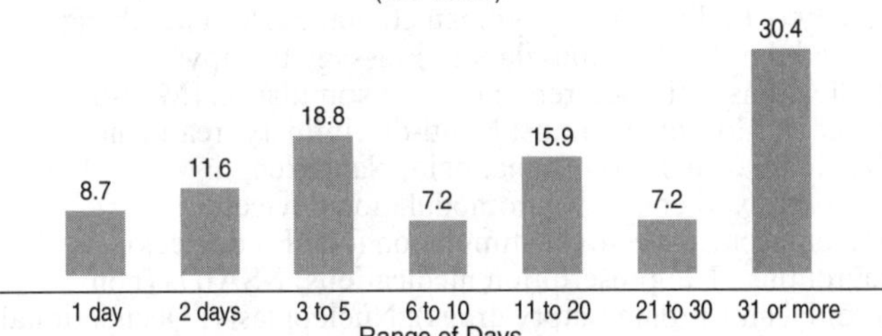

Impact on Occupational Absence: Prevalence 0.1095% of occupational lost workdays; Incidence 0.02 days per 100 workers

729.1 Myalgia and myositis, unspecified

Return-To-Work Summary Guidelines		
Dataset	**Midrange**	**At-Risk**
Claims data	21 days	363 days
All absences	14 days	114 days

Return-To-Work "Best Practice" Guidelines
Moderate pain: 0 days
Debilitating pain, with hospitalization, modified work: 14 days
Debilitating pain, with hospitalization, regular work: 42 days
Myofascial pain syndrome, trigger point injection: 1-7 days
Myofascial pain syndrome, acupuncture: 7-21 days
Myofascial pain syndrome, physical therapy: 14-21 days
Fibromyalgia: Controversial & self-perpetuating diagnosis - see related conditions & return to regular activities as soon as possible

Capabilities & Activity Modifications:
Clerical/modified work: Lifting with knees (with a straight back, no stooping) not more than 5 lbs up to 3 times/hr; squatting up to 4 times/hr; standing or walking with a 5-minute break at least every 20 minutes; sitting with a 5-minute break every 30 minutes; no extremes of extension or flexion; no extremes of twisting; no climbing ladders; driving car only up to 2 hrs/day.
Manual work: Lifting with knees (with a straight back) not more than 25 lbs up to 15 times/hr; squatting up to 16 times/hr; standing or walking with a 10-minute break at least every 1-2 hours; sitting with a 10-minute break every 1-2 hours; extremes

729.1 Myalgia and myositis, unspecified *(cont'd)*

of flexion or extension allowed up to 12 times/hr; extremes of twisting allowed up to 16 times/hr; climbing ladders allowed up to 25 rungs 6 times/hr; driving car or light truck up to a full work day; driving heavy truck up to 4 hrs/day.

Description: Muscle pain (myalgia) or inflammation (myositis).

Fibromyositis NOS

Procedure Summary (from ODG Treatment): Actiq®; Acupuncture; Antidepressants (therapy); Antidepressants - SSRI's versus tricyclics (class); Anti-inflammatory medications; Autonomic test battery; Barbituate-containing analgesic agents (BCAs); Behavioral interventions; Biofeedback; Botulinum toxin (Botox); Capsaicin; Celebrex®; Cod liver oil; Cold lasers; CRPS (complex regional pain syndrome); Cyclobenzaprine; Cymbalta; Diagnostic criteria for CRPS; Education; Electrical stimulators (E-stim); Electroceutical therapy (bioelectric nerve block); Electrodiagnostic testing (EMG/NCS); Epidural steroid injections (ESI's); Exercise; Facet blocks; Fibromyalgia syndrome (FMS); Gabapentin; Glucosamine (and Chondroitin Sulfate); H-wave stimulation (devices); Ibuprofen; Implantable pumps for narcotics; Implantable spinal cord stimulators; Injection with anaesthetics and/or steroids; Interdisciplinary rehabilitation programs; Interferential current stimulation (ICS); Intrathecal pumps; Intravenous regional sympathetic blocks (for RSD, nerve blocks); Ketamine; Low level laser therapy (LLLT); Lumbar sympathetic block; Magnet therapy; Manual therapy & manipulation; Massage therapy; Medications; Microcurrent electrical stimulation (MENS devices); Morphine pumps; Multi-disciplinary treatment; Muscle relaxants; Myofascial pain; Naproxen; Neuroreflexotherapy; Neuromodulation devices; Neuromuscular electrical stimulation (NMES devices); Neurontin®; Nonprescription medications; NSAIDs (non steroidal anti-inflammatory drugs); Nucleoplasty; Occupational therapy (OT); Oral morphine; Opioids; Oxycontin®; Pain management programs; Percutaneous electrical nerve stimulation (PENS); Percutaneous neuromodulation therapy (PNT); Phentolamine infusion test; Physical therapy (PT); Prolotherapy; Psychological evaluations; Return to work; RSD (reflex sympathetic dystrophy); Salicylate topicals; Sclerotherapy (prolotherapy); Spinal cord stimulators (SCS); Stellate ganglion block; Stress infrared telethermography; Sympathectomy; Sympathetic therapy; Thermography (infrared stress thermography); Transcutaneous electrical nerve stimulation (TENS); Treatment for CRPS; Trigger point injections; Vicodin®; Vioxx®; Yoga

Physical Therapy Guidelines:
Allow for fading of treatment frequency (from up to 3 visits per week to 1 or less), plus active self-directed home PT
9-10 visits over 8 weeks

Chiropractic Guidelines:
Allow for fading of treatment frequency (from up to 3 visits per week to 1 or less), plus active self-directed home therapy
9 visits over 8 weeks

Workers' Comp Costs per Claim (based on 511 claims)

Quartile	25%	50%	75%	Mean	% no cost
Indemnity	$2,111	$5,366	$12,548	$13,222	42%
Medical	$714	$3,071	$9,765	$7,639	1%
Total	$1,250	$5,859	$17,094	$15,286	1%

RTW Claims Data (Calendar-days away from work by decile)

10%	20%	30%	40%	**50%**	60%	70%	80%	**90%**	100%	Mean
10	13	14	16	**21**	31	42	52	**363**	365	67.44

729.1 Myalgia and myositis, unspecified *(cont'd)*

Integrated Disability Durations, in days*

Median (mid-point)	14.0	Mean (average)	47.94
Mode (most frequent)	1	Calculated rec.	19

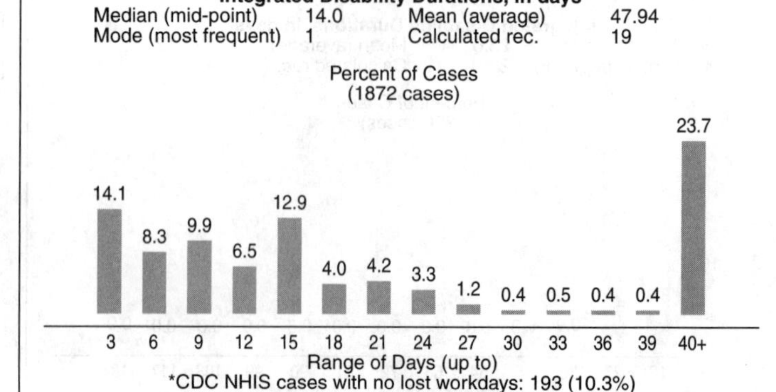

*CDC NHIS cases with no lost workdays: 193 (10.3%)

Impact on Total Absence: Prevalence 0.2379% of total lost workdays; Incidence 2.50 days per 100 workers

729.2 Neuralgia, neuritis, and radiculitis, unspecified

Return-To-Work Summary Guidelines

Dataset	Midrange	At-Risk
Claims data	14 days	67 days
All absences	12 days	42 days

Return-To-Work "Best Practice" Guidelines
Diagnostic testing: 0 days
Treatment, clerical/modified work: 7 days
Treatment, manual work: 14 days

Description: Disease of a nerve (neuralgia) or disease of a spinal nerve root (radiculitis) causing burning, sharp shooting pain along the nerve pathway, which is sometimes combined with a change or loss of sensation.

Excludes:
brachia radiculitis (723.4)
cervical radiculitis (723.4)
lumbosacral radiculitis (724.4)
mononeuritis (354.0-355.9)
radiculitis due to intervertebral disc involvement (722.0-722.2,722.7)
sciatica (724.3)

Physical Therapy Guidelines:
Allow for fading of treatment frequency (from up to 3 visits per week to 1 or less), plus active self-directed home PT
8-10 visits over 4 weeks

Chiropractic Guidelines:
Allow for fading of treatment frequency (from up to 3 visits per week to 1 or less), plus active self-directed home therapy
8 visits over 6 weeks

Workers' Comp Costs per Claim (based on 323 claims)

Quartile	25%	50%	75%	Mean	% no cost
Indemnity	$3,213	$5,418	$16,664	$11,992	52%
Medical	$830	$3,056	$9,188	$7,195	4%
Total	$1,082	$4,704	$14,343	$13,227	4%

RTW Claims Data (Calendar-days away from work by decile)

10%	20%	30%	40%	**50%**	60%	70%	80%	**90%**	100%	Mean
9	11	13	14	**14**	15	17	28	**67**	365	31.65

729.2 Neuralgia, neuritis, and radiculitis, unspecified *(cont'd)*

Integrated Disability Durations, in days*

Median (mid-point)	12.0	Mean (average)	22.12
Mode (most frequent)	1	Calculated rec.	12

Percent of Cases
(1531 cases)

12.2 7.3 11.6 7.4 16.7 6.1 0.7 0.3 0.5 0.7 0.7 0.4 0.5 7.4
3 6 9 12 15 18 21 24 27 30 33 36 39 40+
Range of Days (up to)

*CDC NHIS cases with no lost workdays: 424 (27.7%)

Impact on Total Absence: Prevalence 0.0723% of total lost workdays; Incidence 0.76 days per 100 workers

729.5 Pain in limb

Return-To-Work Summary Guidelines		
Dataset	**Midrange**	**At-Risk**
Claims data	12 days	58 days
All absences	6 days	14 days

Return-To-Work "Best Practice" Guidelines
Diagnostic testing: 0 days
Treatment, clerical/modified work: 2 days
Treatment, manual work: 7 days

Description: Pain in one or more limbs that may originate from skin, nerves, muscle, bone, joint, or brain.

RTW Claims Data (Calendar-days away from work by decile)										
10%	20%	30%	40%	**50%**	60%	70%	80%	**90%**	100%	Mean
8	9	10	11	**12**	13	14	16	**58**	365	27.24

Integrated Disability Durations, in days*

Median (mid-point)	6.0	Mean (average)	12.10
Mode (most frequent)	2	Calculated rec.	7

Percent of Cases
(1093 cases)

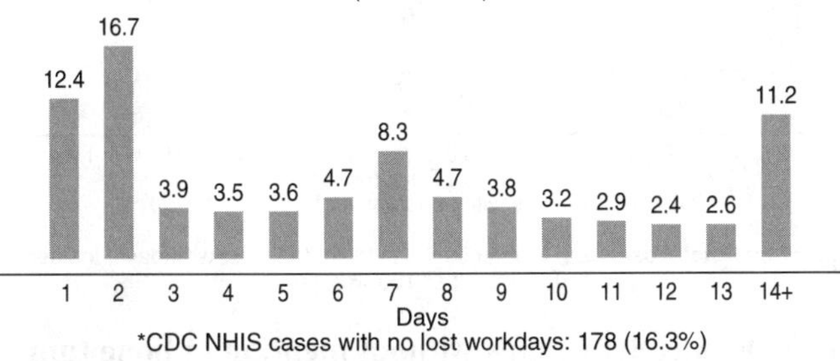

*CDC NHIS cases with no lost workdays: 178 (16.3%)

Impact on Total Absence: Prevalence 0.0327% of total lost workdays; Incidence 0.34 days per 100 workers

729.8 Other musculoskeletal symptoms referable to limbs

Return-To-Work Summary Guidelines		
Dataset	**Midrange**	**At-Risk**
Claims data	11 days	14 days
All absences	8 days	14 days

729.8 Other musculoskeletal symptoms referable to limbs *(cont'd)*

Return-To-Work "Best Practice" Guidelines
Diagnostic testing: 0 days
Treatment, clerical/modified work: 3 days
Treatment, manual work: 10 days

Workers' Comp Costs per Claim (based on 55 claims)					
Quartile	25%	50%	75%	Mean	% no cost
Medical	$378	$1,040	$2,930	$1,850	14%
Total	$378	$1,145	$3,812	$2,433	14%

RTW Claims Data (Calendar-days away from work by decile)										
10%	20%	30%	40%	**50%**	60%	70%	80%	**90%**	100%	Mean
9	10	10	10	**11**	11	12	13	**14**	342	13.55

Integrated Disability Durations, in days*

Median (mid-point)	8.0	Mean (average)	8.47
Mode (most frequent)	1	Calculated rec.	6

Percent of Cases
(630 cases)

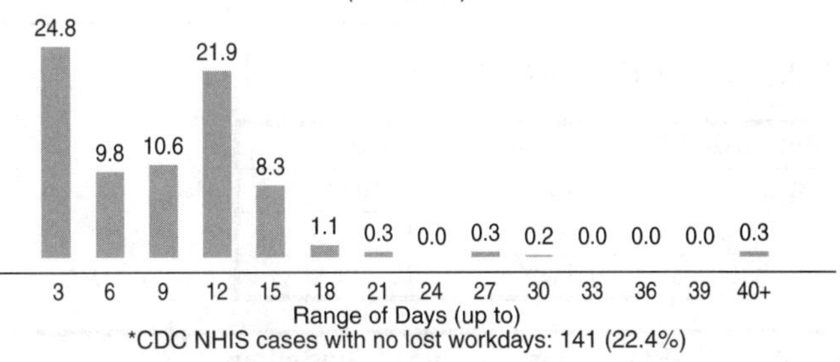

*CDC NHIS cases with no lost workdays: 141 (22.4%)

Impact on Total Absence: Prevalence 0.0122% of total lost workdays; Incidence 0.13 days per 100 workers

OSTEOPATHIES, CHONDROPATHIES, AND ACQUIRED MUSCULOSKELETAL DEFORMITIES (730-739)

RTW Claims Data (Calendar-days away from work by decile)										
10%	20%	30%	40%	**50%**	60%	70%	80%	**90%**	100%	Mean
12	14	15	20	**38**	41	50	71	**108**	365	53.17

Impact on Total Absence: Prevalence 1.1990% of total lost workdays; Incidence 12.59 days per 100 workers

Occupational Disability Durations, in days
Median (mid-point) 18 - Benchmark Indemnity Costs $13,500 (20 cases)
Impact on Occupational Absence: Prevalence 0.0040% of occupational lost workdays

730 Osteomyelitis, periostitis, and other infections involving bone

Return-To-Work Summary Guidelines		
Dataset	**Midrange**	**At-Risk**
Claims data	17 days	115 days
All absences	14 days	115 days

Description: Osteomyelitis is the inflammation of bone and periostitis is the inflammation of the connective tissue that covers the bone.

Excludes:
jaw (526.4-526.5)
petrous bone (383.2)
Use additional code to identify organism, such as Staphylococcus (041.1)

730 Osteomyelitis, periostitis, and other infections involving bone *(cont'd)*

The following fifth-digit subclassification is for use with category 730; valid digits are in [brackets] under each code. See list at beginning of chapter for definitions:

0 site unspecified
1 shoulder region
2 upper arm
3 forearm
4 hand
5 pelvic region and thigh
6 lower leg
7 ankle and foot
8 other specified sites
9 multiple sites

Workers' Comp Costs per Claim (based on 213 claims)					
Quartile	25%	50%	75%	Mean	% no cost
Indemnity	$4,893	$11,004	$22,376	$25,629	22%
Medical	$5,187	$15,771	$36,876	$46,264	2%
Total	$8,526	$24,434	$53,256	$65,347	0%

730.2 Unspecified osteomyelitis

Return-To-Work Summary Guidelines		
Dataset	**Midrange**	**At-Risk**
Claims data	50 days	116 days
All absences	40 days	101 days

Return-To-Work "Best Practice" Guidelines
Diagnosis: 0 days
Hospitalization, clerical/modified work: 14 days
Hospitalization, manual work (depending on body site): 50 days

Description: A severe bone infection usually caused by bacteria but sometimes by fungus, with symptoms of bone pain, redness, loss of appetite, fever, and/or fatigue.

[0-9] Osteitis or osteomyelitis NOS, with or without mention of periostitis

Workers' Comp Costs per Claim (based on 72 claims)					
Quartile	25%	50%	75%	Mean	% no cost
Indemnity	$5,271	$10,385	$15,477	$16,118	24%
Medical	$4,116	$16,727	$40,163	$42,543	3%
Total	$6,363	$25,856	$50,894	$53,723	0%

RTW Claims Data (Calendar-days away from work by decile)										
10%	20%	30%	40%	**50%**	60%	70%	80%	**90%**	100%	Mean
14	14	15	40	**50**	51	52	68	**116**	365	56.66

730.2 Unspecified osteomyelitis *(cont'd)*

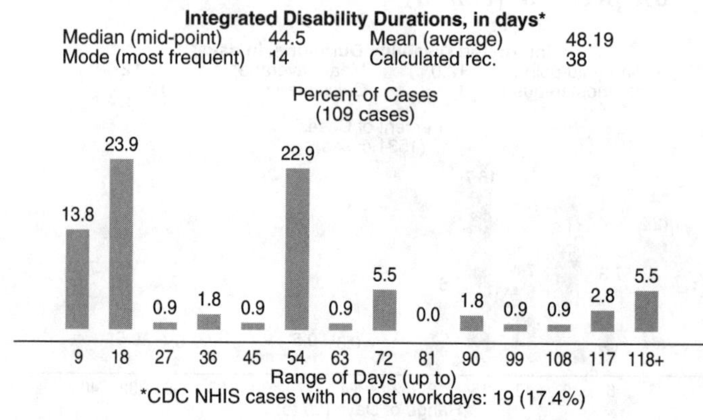

Impact on Total Absence: Prevalence 0.0128% of total lost workdays; Incidence 0.13 days per 100 workers

731 Osteitis deformans and osteopathies associated with other disorders classified elsewhere

Return-To-Work Summary Guidelines		
Dataset	**Midrange**	**At-Risk**
Claims data	50 days	72 days
All absences	42 days	71 days

Return-To-Work "Best Practice" Guidelines
See 731.0

RTW Claims Data (Calendar-days away from work by decile)										
10%	20%	30%	40%	**50%**	60%	70%	80%	**90%**	100%	Mean
14	14	15	42	**50**	51	69	70	**72**	365	59.43

Integrated Disability Durations, in days*
Median (mid-point) 45.5 Mean (average) 51.01
Mode (most frequent) 14 Calculated rec. 39

Percent of Cases
(129 cases)

Range of Days (up to)	9	18	27	36	45	54	63	72	81	90	99	108	117	118+
Percent	9.3	16.3	1.6	0.0	1.6	12.4	0.0	11.6	0.8	0.0	0.0	0.0	0.8	3.1

*CDC NHIS cases with no lost workdays: 55 (42.6%)

Impact on Total Absence: Prevalence 0.0111% of total lost workdays; Incidence 0.12 days per 100 workers

731.0 Osteitis deformans without mention of bone tumor

Return-To-Work Summary Guidelines		
Dataset	**Midrange**	**At-Risk**
Claims data	50 days	72 days
All absences	49 days	71 days

Return-To-Work "Best Practice" Guidelines
Asymptomatic: 0 days
Medical treatment, clerical/modified work: 0 days
Medical treatment, manual work: 50 days
Orthopedic surgery, clerical/modified work: 14 days
Orthopedic surgery, manual work: 70 days

731.0 Osteitis deformans without mention of bone tumor *(cont'd)*

Description: Chronic skeletal disease in which areas of bone grow abnormally, enlarging and becoming soft. There are usually no symptoms but when there are they include deep, aching bone pain that may worsen at night, changes in skull shape or size, hearing loss, loss of height, and/or arthritis of the hips.

Paget's disease of bone

RTW Claims Data (Calendar-days away from work by decile)										
10%	20%	30%	40%	**50%**	60%	70%	80%	**90%**	100%	Mean
14	14	15	44	**50**	51	69	70	**72**	365	55.53

Integrated Disability Durations, in days*

Median (mid-point)	49.0	Mean (average)	48.22
Mode (most frequent)	14	Calculated rec.	40

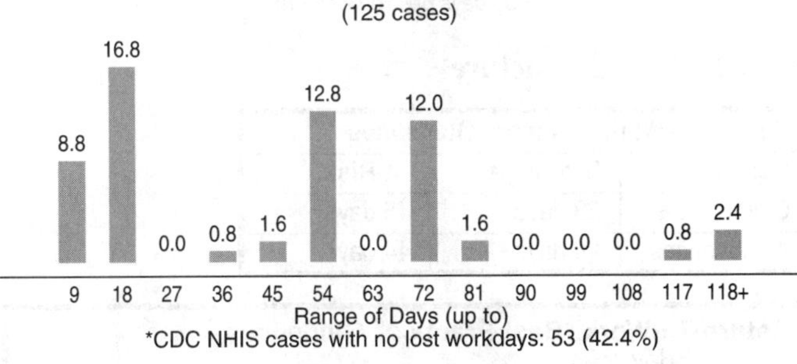

*CDC NHIS cases with no lost workdays: 53 (42.4%)

Impact on Total Absence: Prevalence 0.0102% of total lost workdays; Incidence 0.11 days per 100 workers

732 Osteochondropathies

Return-To-Work Summary Guidelines		
Dataset	**Midrange**	**At-Risk**
Claims data	38 days	108 days
All absences	16 days	79 days

Workers' Comp Costs per Claim (based on 310 claims)					
Quartile	25%	50%	75%	Mean	% no cost
Indemnity	$4,358	$9,083	$24,570	$16,732	17%
Medical	$5,639	$10,553	$19,415	$14,780	0%
Total	$9,240	$19,268	$36,551	$28,740	0%

732.3 Juvenile osteochondrosis of upper extremity

Return-To-Work Summary Guidelines		
Dataset	**Midrange**	**At-Risk**
Claims data	110 days	120 days
All absences	103 days	120 days

Return-To-Work "Best Practice" Guidelines
Kienbock's disorder, wrist fusion, clerical/modified work: 21 days
Kienbock's disorder, wrist fusion, manual work: 84 days

Description: Tissue death and fragmentation, followed by repair and regeneration, within the bone-forming centers of the upper extremities.

732.3 Juvenile osteochondrosis of upper extremity *(cont'd)*

Osteochondrosis (juvenile) of:
- capitulum of humerus (of Panner)
- carpal lunate (of Kienbock)
- hand NOS
- head of humerus (of Haas)
- heads of metacarpas (of Mauclaire)
- lower ulna (of Burns)
- radial head (of Brailsford)
- upper extremity NOS

RTW Claims Data (Calendar-days away from work by decile)										
10%	20%	30%	40%	**50%**	60%	70%	80%	**90%**	100%	Mean
13	13	103	103	**110**	110	115	115	**120**	120	92.20

Impact on Total Absence: Prevalence 0.0013% of total lost workdays; Incidence 0.01 days per 100 workers

732.7 Osteochondritis dissecans

Return-To-Work Summary Guidelines		
Dataset	**Midrange**	**At-Risk**
Claims data	42 days	181 days
All absences	29 days	159 days

Return-To-Work "Best Practice" Guidelines
Arthroscopic surgery, clerical/modified work: 7 days
Arthroscopic surgery, manual work: 28 days
Hip arthroscopy for loose bodies/labral tear, sedentary work: 7 days
Hip arthroscopy for loose bodies/labral tear, standing work: 28 days
Open surgery, clerical/modified work: 14 days
Open surgery, manual work: 42 days

Description: A condition in which a fragment of cartilage and underlying bone becomes dislodged from the bone surface of a joint causing a catching feeling upon bending or straightening the joint, a sensation of grating or popping and pain with movement, and/or aching discomfort over several months.

Workers' Comp Costs per Claim (based on 188 claims)					
Quartile	25%	50%	75%	Mean	% no cost
Indemnity	$3,980	$6,920	$17,031	$14,682	19%
Medical	$4,767	$9,009	$18,218	$13,043	0%
Total	$7,623	$16,821	$32,130	$24,907	0%

RTW Claims Data (Calendar-days away from work by decile)										
10%	20%	30%	40%	**50%**	60%	70%	80%	**90%**	100%	Mean
11	14	23	31	**42**	60	72	114	**181**	365	70.79

Integrated Disability Durations, in days*

Median (mid-point)	29.0	Mean (average)	56.69
Mode (most frequent)	3	Calculated rec.	29

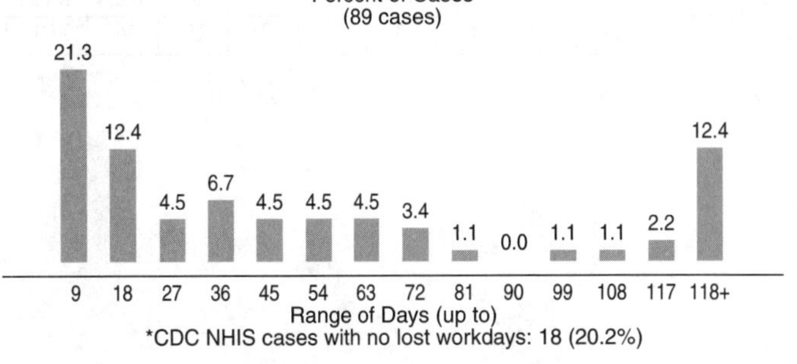

*CDC NHIS cases with no lost workdays: 18 (20.2%)

Impact on Total Absence: Prevalence 0.0118% of total lost workdays; Incidence 0.12 days per 100 workers

733 Other disorders of bone and cartilage

Return-To-Work Summary Guidelines		
Dataset	**Midrange**	**At-Risk**
Claims data	18 days	43 days
All absences	16 days	42 days

Return-To-Work "Best Practice" Guidelines
See 733.9

Excludes:
bone spur (726.91)
cartilage of, or loose body in, joint (717.0-717.9, 718.0-718.9)
giant cell granuloma of jaw (526.3)
osteitis fibrosa cystica generalisata (252.0)
osteomalacia (268.2)
polyostotic fibrous dysplasia of bone (756.54)
prognathism, retrognathism (524.1)
xanthomatosis localized to bone (272.7)

Workers' Comp Costs per Claim (based on 2,827 claims)					
Quartile	25%	50%	75%	Mean	% no cost
Indemnity	$4,725	$12,112	$29,201	$21,921	29%
Medical	$3,633	$11,162	$27,426	$21,723	1%
Total	$5,828	$19,929	$49,980	$37,425	1%

733.0 Osteoporosis

Return-To-Work Summary Guidelines		
Dataset	**Midrange**	**At-Risk**
Claims data	41 days	210 days
All absences	40 days	76 days

Return-To-Work "Best Practice" Guidelines
Medical treatment, clerical/modified work: 0 days
Medical treatment, manual work: 0-14 days
Medical treatment, heavy manual work: 70 days to indefinite
Compression fracture, clerical/modified work: 40 days
Compression fracture, manual work (after evaluation): 72 days

Description: A progressive decrease in bone density causing bones to weaken and fracture. There could be no symptoms until the bones collapse or break spontaneously or after a slight injury. There could also be bone pain and deformities such as a curvature of the spine.

Physical Therapy Guidelines:
8 visits over 10 weeks

Disability Duration Adjustment Factors by Age						
Age Group	18-24	25-34	35-44	45-54	55-64	65-74
Adjustment Factor	NA	NA	1.23	0.75	0.88	1.72

RTW Claims Data (Calendar-days away from work by decile)										
10%	20%	30%	40%	**50%**	60%	70%	80%	**90%**	100%	Mean
14	15	17	39	**41**	70	72	73	**210**	365	75.18

733.0 Osteoporosis *(cont'd)*

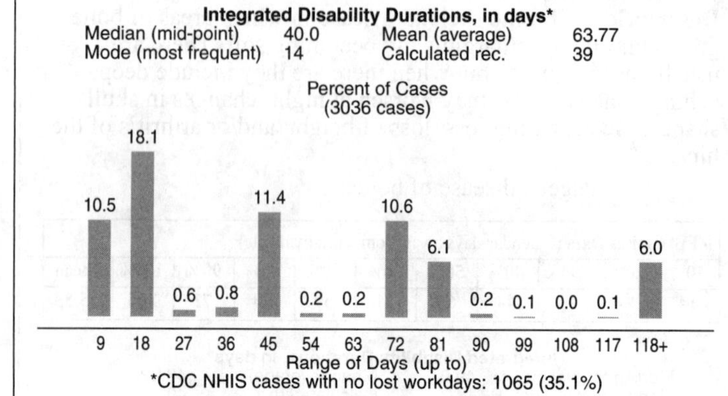

Impact on Total Absence: Prevalence 0.3714% of total lost workdays; Incidence 3.90 days per 100 workers

733.1 Pathologic fracture

Return-To-Work Summary Guidelines		
Dataset	**Midrange**	**At-Risk**
Claims data	23 days	45 days
All absences	16 days	44 days

Return-To-Work "Best Practice" Guidelines
Stable: 1 day
Unstable, clerical/modified work: 14 days
Unstable, manual work: 42 days

Description: A break in an area of bone which as been weakened by a pre-existing disease. The fracture happens without warning or trauma and therefore seemingly spontaneously. Sudden onset of pain is the main symptom.

Spontaneous fracture

Excludes:
traumatic fractures (800-829)

Workers' Comp Costs per Claim (based on 131 claims)					
Quartile	25%	50%	75%	Mean	% no cost
Indemnity	$3,287	$7,035	$18,585	$17,212	38%
Medical	$1,197	$3,764	$14,270	$10,698	4%
Total	$1,439	$5,297	$23,636	$21,268	1%

RTW Claims Data (Calendar-days away from work by decile)										
10%	20%	30%	40%	**50%**	60%	70%	80%	**90%**	100%	Mean
13	14	15	16	**23**	41	42	43	**45**	365	31.35

Integrated Disability Durations, in days*
Median (mid-point) 16.0 Mean (average) 25.56
Mode (most frequent) 1 Calculated rec. 15

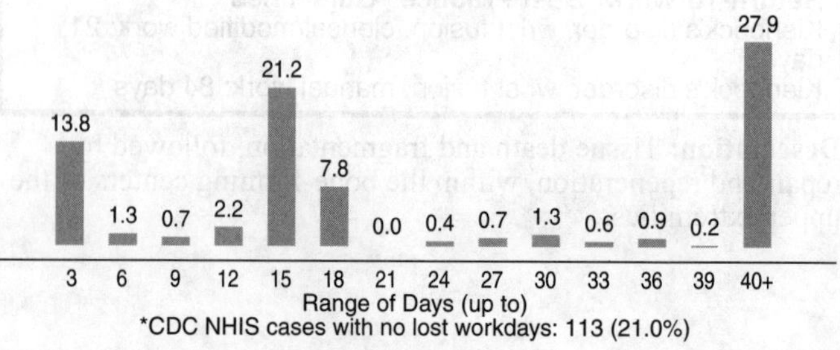

Impact on Total Absence: Prevalence 0.0321% of total lost workdays; Incidence 0.34 days per 100 workers

733.13 Pathologic fracture of vertebrae

Return-To-Work Summary Guidelines		
Dataset	Midrange	At-Risk
Claims data	23 days	49 days
All absences	16 days	44 days

Return-To-Work "Best Practice" Guidelines
Clerical/modified work: 21-28 days
Manual work: 49 days to indefinite

Capabilities & Activity Modifications:
Clerical/modified work: No lifting over shoulder; lifting to level of shoulder not more than 5 lbs up to 2 times/hr; standing or walking with a 5-minute break at least every 20 minutes; sitting with a 5-minute break every 30 minutes (using an operator head set if extended phone operations); no extremes of motion including extension or flexion; no extremes of twisting or lateral rotation; no climbing ladders; driving car only up to 2 hrs/day; possible use of cervical collar with change of position and stretching every 30 min; modify workstation or position to eliminate lifting away from body or using twisting motion.
Manual work: Lifting over shoulder not more than 25 lbs up to 15 times/hr; lifting to level of shoulder up to 30 lbs of weight not more than 15 times/hr; standing or walking with a 10-minute break at least every 1-2 hours; sitting with a 10-minute break every 1-2 hours; extremes of flexion or extension allowed up to 20 times/hr; extremes of twisting allowed up to 16 times/hr; climbing ladders allowed up to 40 rungs 8 times/hr; driving car or light truck up to a full work day; driving heavy truck up to 4 hrs/day.
Description: Breakage of the vertebrae when a pre-existing disease has weakened it. The fracture happens without warning or trauma and therefore seemingly spontaneously. The main symptom is a sudden onset of back pain.
Other names: Compression fracture of spine
Collapse of vertebra NOS
Procedure Summary (from ODG Treatment): Activity restrictions; Acupuncture; Arthrodesis (fusion); Arthroplasty; Back schools; Bed rest; Biofeedback; Bone scan; Botulinum toxin (injection); Cervical orthosis; Chiropractic care; Chymopapain (injection); Cognitive behavioral rehabilitation; Cold packs; Collars (cervical); Computed tomography (CT); Computerized range of motion (ROM); Corticosteroid injection; Decompression; Diathermy; Discography; Disc prosthesis; Discectomy/laminectomy; Education (patient); Electromyography (EMG); Electrotherapies; Electromagnetic therapy (PEMT); Epidural steroid injection (ESI); Ergonomics; Exercise; Facet-joint injections; Facet rhizotomy; Flexibility; Fluoroscopy (for ESI's); Fusion (spinal); H-Reflex tests; Heat/cold applications; High-dose methylprednisolone; Imaging; Immobilization (collars); Injections; Laminectomy; Laminoplasty; Laser therapy; Magnetic resonance imaging (MRI); Manipulation; Manipulation under anesthesia (MUA) ; Massage; Methylprednisolone; Multidisciplinary biopsychosocial (rehabilitation); Myelography; Nonprescription medications; Occupational therapy (OT); Opioids; Oral corticosteroids; Patient education; Percutaneous electrical nerve stimulation (PENS); Percutaneous neuromodulation therapy (PNT); Percutaneous radio-frequency neurotomy; Physical therapy (PT); Prolotherapy (also known as sclerotherapy); Pulsed electromagnetic therapy (PEMT); Radiofrequency neurotomy; Radiography (x-rays); Range of motion (ROM); Rest; Return to work; Sensory evoked potentials (SEPs); Soft collars; Steroids; Stretching; Surface EMG (electromyography); Surgery; Therapeutic exercises; Thermography (diagnostic); Traction; Transcutaneous electrical neurostimulation (TENS); Trigger point injections; Ultrasound, diagnostic (imaging); Ultrasound, therapeutic; Videofluoroscopy (for range of motion); Work

Workers' Comp Costs per Claim (based on 29 claims)					
Quartile	25%	50%	75%	Mean	% no cost
Medical	$5,261	$10,574	$19,425	$16,878	0%
Total	$8,621	$22,701	$36,761	$29,991	0%

Impact on Total Absence: Prevalence 0.0003% of total lost workdays

733.9 Other and unspecified disorders of bone and cartilage

Return-To-Work Summary Guidelines		
Dataset	Midrange	At-Risk
Claims data	18 days	43 days
All absences	16 days	42 days

Return-To-Work "Best Practice" Guidelines
Medical treatment, clerical/modified work: 0 days
Medical treatment, manual work: 14 days
Medical treatment, heavy manual work: 40 days

Workers' Comp Costs per Claim (based on 1,220 claims)					
Quartile	25%	50%	75%	Mean	% no cost
Indemnity	$4,242	$9,345	$22,334	$17,366	19%
Medical	$6,342	$10,658	$21,284	$17,379	0%
Total	$9,408	$18,879	$39,134	$31,520	0%

RTW Claims Data (Calendar-days away from work by decile)										
10%	20%	30%	40%	**50%**	60%	70%	80%	**90%**	100%	Mean
13	14	15	16	**18**	39	40	41	**43**	365	31.84

RTW Post Surgery (Calendar-days away from work by decile)										
10%	20%	30%	40%	**50%**	60%	70%	80%	**90%**	100%	Mean
Knee arthroscopy/surgery										
19	26	37	44	**50**	65	97	145	**269**	365	96.47

Integrated Disability Durations, in days*

Median (mid-point)	16.0	Mean (average)	26.70
Mode (most frequent)	40	Calculated rec.	25

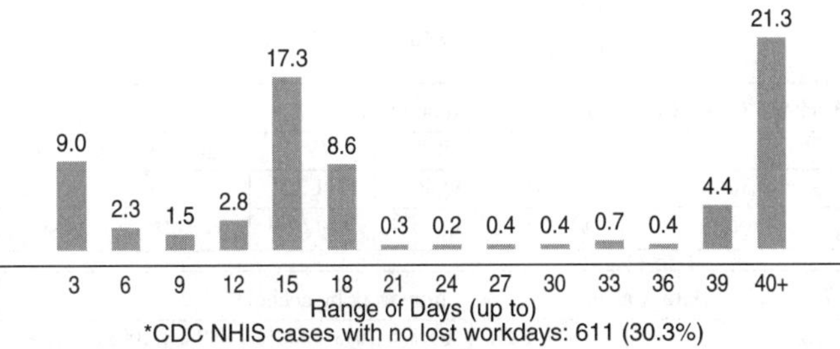

*CDC NHIS cases with no lost workdays: 611 (30.3%)

Impact on Total Absence: Prevalence 0.1110% of total lost workdays; Incidence 1.17 days per 100 workers

734 Flat foot

Return-To-Work Summary Guidelines		
Dataset	Midrange	At-Risk
Claims data	13 days	30 days
All absences	4 days	16 days

734 Flat foot *(cont'd)*

Return-To-Work "Best Practice" Guidelines
0 days

Description: Abnormal but fairly common deformity in which the arch of the foot is flat.

Pes planus (acquired)
Talipes planus (acquired)

Excludes:
congenital (754.61)
rigid flat foot (754.61)
spastic (everted) flat foot (754.61)

RTW Claims Data (Calendar-days away from work by decile)										
10%	20%	30%	40%	**50%**	60%	70%	80%	**90%**	100%	Mean
9	11	11	12	**13**	14	15	17	**30**	365	30.73

Integrated Disability Durations, in days*

Median (mid-point)	4.0	Mean (average)	13.24
Mode (most frequent)	1	Calculated rec.	6

Percent of Cases
(867 cases)

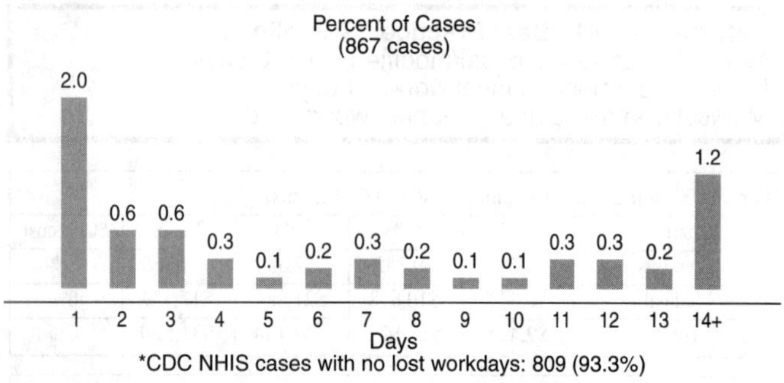

*CDC NHIS cases with no lost workdays: 809 (93.3%)

Impact on Total Absence: Prevalence 0.0022% of total lost workdays; Incidence 0.02 days per 100 workers

735 Acquired deformities of toe

Return-To-Work Summary Guidelines		
Dataset	**Midrange**	**At-Risk**
Claims data	15 days	63 days
All absences	12 days	53 days

Return-To-Work "Best Practice" Guidelines
See 735.0

Excludes:
congenital (754.60-754.69, 755.65-755.66)

Workers' Comp Costs per Claim (based on 51 claims)					
Quartile	25%	50%	75%	Mean	% no cost
Medical	$1,187	$3,407	$11,204	$11,547	4%
Total	$1,491	$4,757	$14,900	$19,809	4%

RTW Claims Data (Calendar-days away from work by decile)										
10%	20%	30%	40%	**50%**	60%	70%	80%	**90%**	100%	Mean
9	10	11	13	**15**	41	43	45	**63**	365	36.50

735 Acquired deformities of toe *(cont'd)*

Integrated Disability Durations, in days*

Median (mid-point)	12.0	Mean (average)	28.37
Mode (most frequent)	1	Calculated rec.	13

Percent of Cases
(1453 cases)

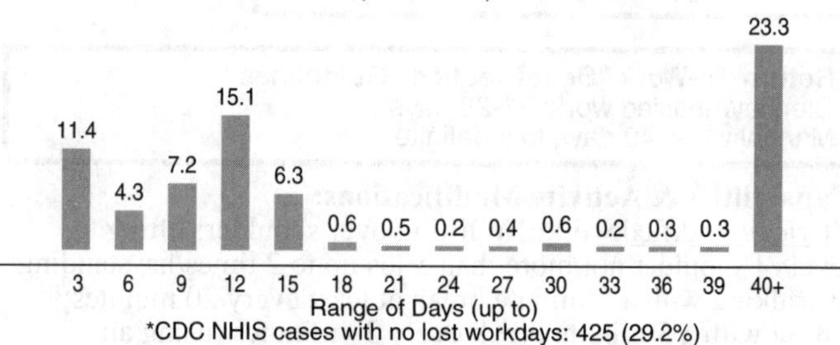

*CDC NHIS cases with no lost workdays: 425 (29.2%)

Impact on Total Absence: Prevalence 0.0861% of total lost workdays; Incidence 0.91 days per 100 workers

735.0 Hallux valgus (acquired)

Return-To-Work Summary Guidelines		
Dataset	**Midrange**	**At-Risk**
Claims data	46 days	94 days
All absences	34 days	94 days

Return-To-Work "Best Practice" Guidelines
Without surgery, sedentary work: 0 days
Without surgery, standing work: 10 days
With bunionectomy, sedentary work: 10 days
With bunionectomy, standing work: 42 days

Capabilities & Activity Modifications:
Sedentary/modified work: Standing limited to 5-10 min/hr; walking only on a smooth surface using crutches with limited pressure on the foot; no walking on an irregular surface; no climbing stairs; no climbing ladders or hill climbing requiring frequent knee flexion; no activities requiring balance; no applying strength against bent knee (squatting, kneeling, crouching, stooping, pedaling, etc.); elevate leg half of time; may need immobilization; limited weight bearing.
Manual/standing work: Standing not more than 50 min/hr; walking on a smooth surface up to 1,200 ft/hr carrying up to 25 lbs; walking on an irregular surface up to 900 ft/hr carrying up to 25 lbs; climbing stairs up to 8 flights/hr carrying up to 40 lbs; climbing ladders up to 50 rungs/hr carrying up to 25 lbs; activities requiring balance up to 45 min/hr (if able to work with two hands without assistance for balance); applying strength against bent knee (pedaling, squatting, kneeling, etc.) up to 60 times/hr; may need brace for uneven ground or ladders.
Description: Deformity of the foot causing the big toe to angle toward the other toes of that foot, leading to pain with walking.
Procedure Summary (from ODG Treatment):
Accommodative modalities; Achilles tendon ruptures (treatment); Activity restrictions; Actovegin; Ankle prostheses (total ankle replacement); Anterior drawer test; Anti-inflammatory medications (NSAIDs); Arthrodesis (fusion); Arthroplasty (total ankle replacement); Autologous conditioned serum (ACS); Bed rest; Biofeedback; Bone scan (imaging); Bracing (immobilization); Cast (immobilization); Causality; Chiropractic; Cold packs; Computed tomography (CT); Continuous-flow cryotherapy; Corticosteroids (topical); Diathermy; Dorsiflexion night splints; Education (patient); Elastic bandage (immobilization); Electron generating device; Exercise; Extracorporeal shock wave therapy (ESWT); Functional treatment; Fusion; Heat therapy (ice/heat); Heparin; Heel pads; Ice packs; Imaging; Immobilization; Ingrown

735.0 Hallux valgus (acquired) *(cont'd)*

toenail surgery; Injections; Insoles with magnetic foil; Inversion stress test; Iontophoresis; Lace-up ankle support; Laser therapy (LLLT); Lateral ligament ankle reconstruction (surgery); Lineal tomography; Low-intensity laser therapy (LLLT); Magnets; Magnetic resonance imaging (MRI); Manipulation; Massage; Mechanical treatment (taping/orthoses); Modified duty; Narcotics; Night splints; Nonprescription medications; Orthotic devices; Osteotomy; Ottawa ankle rules (OAR); Patient education; Phonophoresis; Physical therapy (PT); Prolotherapy (sclerotherapy); Radiography; Rest (RICE); Return to work; Sclerotherapy (prolotherapy); Semi-rigid ankle support; Shock wave therapy, extracorporeal (ESWT); Steroids (injection); Stretching (flexibility); Supports; Surgery; Surgery for achilles tendon ruptures; Surgery for ankle sprains; Surgery for calcaneal fractures; Surgery for hallux valgus; Surgery for plantar fasciitis; Surgery for tarsal tunnel syndrome; Talar tilt test; Tai Chi; Taping; Tension night splints (TNS); Therapeutic exercise; Thompson test; Total ankle replacement (arthroplasty); Transcutaneous electrical neurostimulation (TENS); Ultrasound, diagnostic; Ultrasound, therapeutic; Work

Physical Therapy Guidelines:
Medical treatment: 9 visits over 8 weeks
Post-surgical treatment: 9 visits over 8 weeks

RTW Claims Data (Calendar-days away from work by decile)										
10%	20%	30%	40%	**50%**	60%	70%	80%	**90%**	100%	Mean
30	30	34	34	**46**	46	47	47	**94**	94	50.20

Impact on Total Absence: Prevalence 0.0007% of total lost workdays; Incidence 0.01 days per 100 workers

735.1 Hallux varus (acquired)

Return-To-Work Summary Guidelines		
Dataset	**Midrange**	**At-Risk**
Claims data	15 days	63 days
All absences	12 days	53 days

Return-To-Work "Best Practice" Guidelines
Without surgery, sedentary work: 0 days
Without surgery, standing work: 10 days
With surgery, sedentary work: 10 days
With surgery, standing work: 42 days

Capabilities & Activity Modifications:
Sedentary/modified work: Standing limited to 5-10 min/hr; walking only on a smooth surface using crutches with limited pressure on the foot; no walking on an irregular surface; no climbing stairs; no climbing ladders or hill climbing requiring frequent knee flexion; no activities requiring balance; no applying strength against bent knee (squatting, kneeling, crouching, stooping, pedaling, etc.); elevate leg half of time; may need immobilization; limited weight bearing.
Manual/standing work: Standing not more than 50 min/hr; walking on a smooth surface up to 1,200 ft/hr carrying up to 25 lbs; walking on an irregular surface up to 900 ft/hr carrying up to 25 lbs; climbing stairs up to 8 flights/hr carrying up to 40 lbs; climbing ladders up to 50 rungs/hr carrying up to 25 lbs; activities requiring balance up to 45 min/hr (if able to work with two hands without assistance for balance); applying strength against bent knee (pedaling, squatting, kneeling, etc.) up to 60 times/hr; may need brace for uneven ground or ladders.
Description: Deformity of the foot causing the big toe to angle away from the other toes of that foot, leading to pain with walking.

735.1 Hallux varus (acquired) *(cont'd)*

Procedure Summary (from ODG Treatment):
Accommodative modalities; Achilles tendon ruptures (treatment); Activity restrictions; Actovegin; Ankle prostheses (total ankle replacement); Anterior drawer test; Anti-inflammatory medications (NSAIDs); Arthrodesis (fusion); Arthroplasty (total ankle replacement); Autologous conditioned serum (ACS); Bed rest; Biofeedback; Bone scan (imaging); Bracing (immobilization); Cast (immobilization); Causality; Chiropractic; Cold packs; Computed tomography (CT); Continuous-flow cryotherapy; Corticosteroids (topical); Diathermy; Dorsiflexion night splints; Education (patient); Elastic bandage (immobilization); Electron generating device; Exercise; Extracorporeal shock wave therapy (ESWT); Functional treatment; Fusion; Heat therapy (ice/heat); Heparin; Heel pads; Ice packs; Imaging; Immobilization; Ingrown toenail surgery; Injections; Insoles with magnetic foil; Inversion stress test; Iontophoresis; Lace-up ankle support; Laser therapy (LLLT); Lateral ligament ankle reconstruction (surgery); Lineal tomography; Low-intensity laser therapy (LLLT); Magnets; Magnetic resonance imaging (MRI); Manipulation; Massage; Mechanical treatment (taping/orthoses); Modified duty; Narcotics; Night splints; Nonprescription medications; Orthotic devices; Osteotomy; Ottawa ankle rules (OAR); Patient education; Phonophoresis; Physical therapy (PT); Prolotherapy (sclerotherapy); Radiography; Rest (RICE); Return to work; Sclerotherapy (prolotherapy); Semi-rigid ankle support; Shock wave therapy, extracorporeal (ESWT); Steroids (injection); Stretching (flexibility); Supports; Surgery; Surgery for achilles tendon ruptures; Surgery for ankle sprains; Surgery for calcaneal fractures; Surgery for hallux valgus; Surgery for plantar fasciitis; Surgery for tarsal tunnel syndrome; Talar tilt test; Tai Chi; Taping; Tension night splints (TNS); Therapeutic exercise; Thompson test; Total ankle replacement (arthroplasty); Transcutaneous electrical neurostimulation (TENS); Ultrasound, diagnostic; Ultrasound, therapeutic; Work

Physical Therapy Guidelines:
Medical treatment: 9 visits over 8 weeks
Post-surgical treatment: 9 visits over 8 weeks

Impact on Total Absence: Prevalence 0.0003% of total lost workdays

735.4 Other hammer toe (acquired)

Return-To-Work Summary Guidelines		
Dataset	**Midrange**	**At-Risk**
Claims data	28 days	80 days
All absences	14 days	65 days

Return-To-Work "Best Practice" Guidelines
Medical treatment: 0 days
Hammertoe operation, one toe, sedentary work: 7-14 days
Hammertoe operation, one toe, stationary standing work: 14-28 days
Hammertoe operation, one toe, standing work, walking: 28-56 days

Capabilities & Activity Modifications:
Sedentary/modified work: Standing limited to 5-10 min/hr; walking only on a smooth surface using crutches with limited pressure on the foot; no walking on an irregular surface; no climbing stairs; no climbing ladders or hill climbing requiring frequent knee flexion; no activities requiring balance; no applying strength against bent knee (squatting, kneeling, crouching, stooping, pedaling, etc.); elevate leg half of time; may need immobilization; limited weight bearing.
Manual/standing work: Standing not more than 50 min/hr; walking on a smooth surface up to 1,200 ft/hr carrying up to 25 lbs; walking on an irregular surface up to 900 ft/hr carrying up

735.4 Other hammer toe (acquired) *(cont'd)*

to 25 lbs; climbing stairs up to 8 flights/hr carrying up to 40 lbs; climbing ladders up to 50 rungs/hr carrying up to 25 lbs; activities requiring balance up to 45 min/hr (if able to work with two hands without assistance for balance); applying strength against bent knee (pedaling, squatting, kneeling, etc.) up to 60 times/hr; may need brace for uneven ground or ladders.

Description: Deformity of the toe (usually the second or the fifth) causing it to bend upward like a claw resulting in a painful corn on the top of the joint and deformed nail growth.

Procedure Summary (from ODG Treatment): Accommodative modalities; Achilles tendon ruptures (treatment); Activity restrictions; Actovegin; Ankle prostheses (total ankle replacement); Anterior drawer test; Anti-inflammatory medications (NSAIDs); Arthrodesis (fusion); Arthroplasty (total ankle replacement); Autologous conditioned serum (ACS); Bed rest; Biofeedback; Bone scan (imaging); Bracing (immobilization); Cast (immobilization); Causality; Chiropractic; Cold packs; Computed tomography (CT); Continuous-flow cryotherapy; Corticosteroids (topical); Diathermy; Dorsiflexion night splints; Education (patient); Elastic bandage (immobilization); Electron generating device; Exercise; Extracorporeal shock wave therapy (ESWT); Functional treatment; Fusion; Heat therapy (ice/heat); Heparin; Heel pads; Ice packs; Imaging; Immobilization; Ingrown toenail surgery; Injections; Insoles with magnetic foil; Inversion stress test; Iontophoresis; Lace-up ankle support; Laser therapy (LLLT); Lateral ligament ankle reconstruction (surgery); Lineal tomography; Low-intensity laser therapy (LLLT); Magnets; Magnetic resonance imaging (MRI); Manipulation; Massage; Mechanical treatment (taping/orthoses); Modified duty; Narcotics; Night splints; Nonprescription medications; Orthotic devices; Osteotomy; Ottawa ankle rules (OAR); Patient education; Phonophoresis; Physical therapy (PT); Prolotherapy (sclerotherapy); Radiography; Rest (RICE); Return to work; Sclerotherapy (prolotherapy); Semi-rigid ankle support; Shock wave therapy, extracorporeal (ESWT); Steroids (injection); Stretching (flexibility); Supports; Surgery; Surgery for achilles tendon ruptures; Surgery for ankle sprains; Surgery for calcaneal fractures; Surgery for hallux valgus; Surgery for plantar fasciitis; Surgery for tarsal tunnel syndrome; Talar tilt test; Tai Chi; Taping; Tension night splints (TNS); Therapeutic exercise; Thompson test; Total ankle replacement (arthroplasty); Transcutaneous electrical neurostimulation (TENS); Ultrasound, diagnostic; Ultrasound, therapeutic; Work

Physical Therapy Guidelines:
Medical treatment: 9 visits over 8 weeks
Post-surgical treatment: 9 visits over 8 weeks

RTW Claims Data (Calendar-days away from work by decile)

10%	20%	30%	40%	**50%**	60%	70%	80%	**90%**	100%	Mean
9	12	14	16	**28**	35	52	57	**80**	365	38.92

735.4 Other hammer toe (acquired) *(cont'd)*

Integrated Disability Durations, in days*

Median (mid-point)	14.0	Mean (average)	29.64
Mode (most frequent)	1	Calculated rec.	15

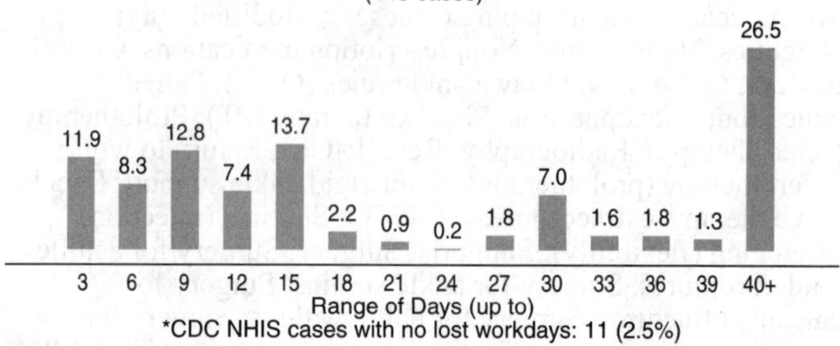

*CDC NHIS cases with no lost workdays: 11 (2.5%)

Impact on Total Absence: Prevalence 0.0380% of total lost workdays; Incidence 0.40 days per 100 workers

736 Other acquired deformities of limbs

Return-To-Work Summary Guidelines

Dataset	Midrange	At-Risk
Claims data	38 days	108 days
All absences	16 days	79 days

Excludes:
congenital (754.3-755.9)

Workers' Comp Costs per Claim (based on 1,036 claims)

Quartile	25%	50%	75%	Mean	% no cost
Indemnity	$3,087	$9,125	$25,599	$22,162	63%
Medical	$515	$1,097	$6,542	$12,511	1%
Total	$536	$1,454	$13,094	$20,873	1%

736.1 Mallet finger

Return-To-Work Summary Guidelines

Dataset	Midrange	At-Risk
Claims data	17 days	70 days
All absences	5 days	48 days

Return-To-Work "Best Practice" Guidelines
Clerical/modified work: 1 day
Manual work: 10 days

Description: A finger that is permanently flexed due to an injury.

Other names: Hammer finger

Physical Therapy Guidelines:
16 visits over 8 weeks

Workers' Comp Costs per Claim (based on 574 claims)

Quartile	25%	50%	75%	Mean	% no cost
Indemnity	$1,334	$1,943	$4,568	$3,835	87%
Medical	$378	$641	$1,040	$1,045	2%
Total	$378	$667	$1,292	$1,550	2%

RTW Claims Data (Calendar-days away from work by decile)

10%	20%	30%	40%	**50%**	60%	70%	80%	**90%**	100%	Mean
10	11	12	14	**17**	23	38	52	**70**	110	31.16

736.1 Mallet finger *(cont'd)*

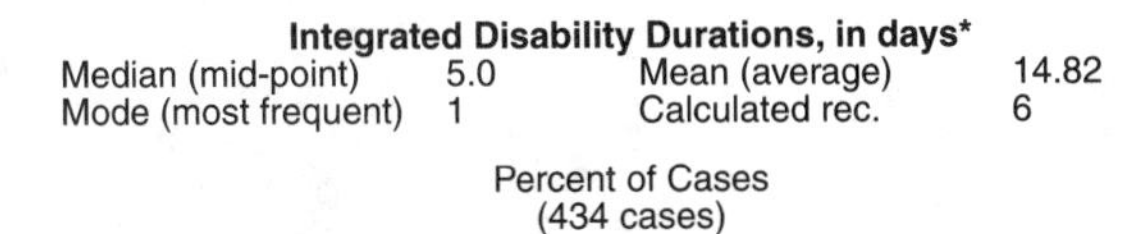

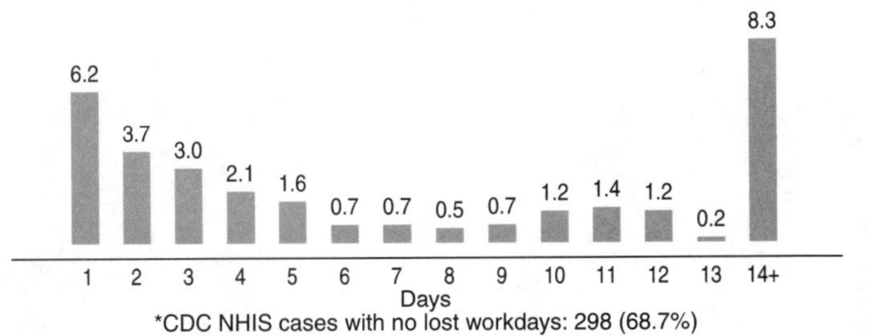

*CDC NHIS cases with no lost workdays: 298 (68.7%)

Impact on Total Absence: Prevalence 0.0059% of total lost workdays; Incidence 0.06 days per 100 workers

736.4 Genu valgum or varum (acquired)

Return-To-Work Summary Guidelines		
Dataset	**Midrange**	**At-Risk**
Claims data	38 days	108 days
All absences	16 days	79 days

Return-To-Work "Best Practice" Guidelines
Osteotomy (e.g., Fulkerson), clerical/modified work: 28 days
Osteotomy, manual work: 70 days

Description: Deformity of the legs in which the knees are abnormally close together while the ankles are abnormally far apart, causing the knees to knock when the person walks.
Other names: Knock-knees

737 Curvature of spine

Return-To-Work Summary Guidelines		
Dataset	**Midrange**	**At-Risk**
Claims data	24 days	58 days
All absences	21 days	58 days

Return-To-Work "Best Practice" Guidelines
Without treatment: 0 days
With surgery, clerical/modified work: 21 days
With surgery, manual work: 56 days

Description: Abnormal curvature of the spine that may cause fatigue in the back after prolonged sitting or standing and eventual muscle pain.

Excludes:
congenital (754.2)

Physical Therapy Guidelines:
12 visits over 10 weeks
See 722.1 for post-surgical visits
Chiropractic Guidelines:
Trial of 6 visits over 3 weeks
With evidence of objective functional improvement, total of up to 12 visits over 10 weeks, avoid chronicity

Workers' Comp Costs per Claim (based on 32 claims)					
Quartile	25%	50%	75%	Mean	% no cost
Medical	$17,273	$33,343	$67,568	$48,490	6%
Total	$17,273	$70,455	$128,121	$88,128	6%

737 Curvature of spine *(cont'd)*

RTW Claims Data (Calendar-days away from work by decile)										
10%	20%	30%	40%	**50%**	60%	70%	80%	**90%**	100%	Mean
14	20	21	22	**24**	55	56	57	**58**	365	41.36

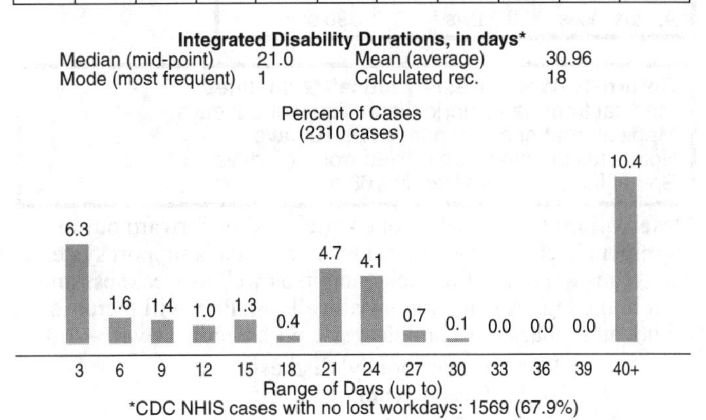

*CDC NHIS cases with no lost workdays: 1569 (67.9%)

Impact on Total Absence: Prevalence 0.0678% of total lost workdays; Incidence 0.71 days per 100 workers

Occupational Disability Durations, in days
Median (mid-point) 47 - Benchmark Indemnity Costs $35,250

Percent of Cases
(178 cases)

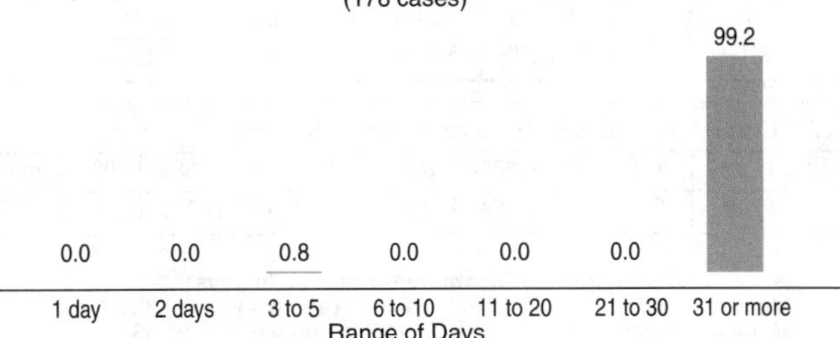

Impact on Occupational Absence: Prevalence 0.0949% of occupational lost workdays; Incidence 0.02 days per 100 workers

738 Other acquired deformity

Return-To-Work Summary Guidelines		
Dataset	**Midrange**	**At-Risk**
Claims data	24 days	107 days
All absences	10 days	71 days

Return-To-Work "Best Practice" Guidelines
See 738.0

Excludes:
congenital (754.0-756.9, 758.0-759.9)
dentofacial anomalies (524.0-524.9)

Workers' Comp Costs per Claim (based on 200 claims)					
Quartile	25%	50%	75%	Mean	% no cost
Indemnity	$5,303	$11,713	$30,272	$21,263	18%
Medical	$7,329	$12,915	$37,916	$27,619	1%
Total	$10,490	$29,012	$64,586	$45,201	1%

Occupational Disability Durations, in days
Median (mid-point) 51 - Benchmark Indemnity Costs $38,250
(40 cases)
Impact on Occupational Absence: Prevalence 0.0231% of occupational lost workdays

738.4 Acquired spondylolisthesis

Return-To-Work Summary Guidelines		
Dataset	**Midrange**	**At-Risk**
Claims data	54 days	227 days
All absences	30 days	198 days

Return-To-Work "Best Practice" Guidelines
Medical treatment, clerical/modified work: 2 days
Medical treatment, manual work: 10 days
Spinal fusion, clerical/modified work: 49 days
Spinal fusion, manual work: 168 days

Description: Occurs when one vertebra slips forward out of alignment because of a failure in the vertebrae's support system. This leads to pain in the back and hip as well as weakness and pain in the leg, causing abnormal walking. Pain will increase with leaning backward and decrease with bending over.

Degenerative spondylolisthesis
Spondylolysis, acquired

Excludes:
congenital (756.12)

Workers' Comp Costs per Claim (based on 122 claims)					
Quartile	25%	50%	75%	Mean	% no cost
Indemnity	\$8,169	\$16,532	\$37,643	\$27,525	16%
Medical	\$8,526	\$24,560	\$59,336	\$36,845	2%
Total	\$17,777	\$39,690	\$94,668	\$60,437	2%

RTW Claims Data (Calendar-days away from work by decile)										
10%	20%	30%	40%	**50%**	60%	70%	80%	**90%**	100%	Mean
19	26	33	40	**54**	102	125	137	**227**	238	87.70

Integrated Disability Durations, in days*
Median (mid-point) 31.5 Mean (average) 63.29
Mode (most frequent) 4 Calculated rec. 33

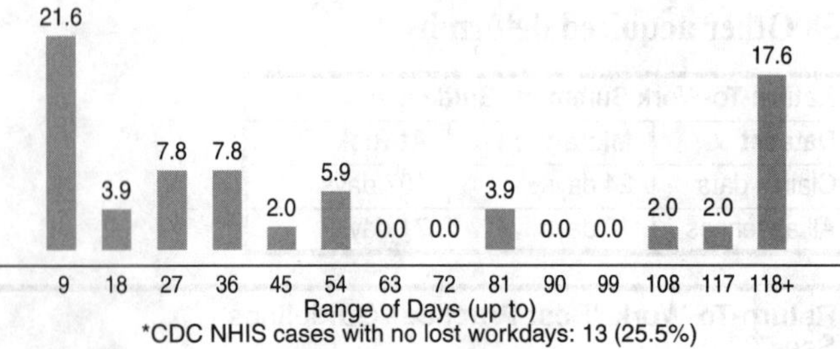

*CDC NHIS cases with no lost workdays: 13 (25.5%)

Impact on Total Absence: Prevalence 0.0071% of total lost workdays; Incidence 0.07 days per 100 workers

16. SYMPTOMS, SIGNS, AND ILL-DEFINED CONDITIONS (780-799)

Impact on Total Absence: Prevalence 1.4090% of total lost workdays; Incidence 14.80 days per 100 workers

RTW Claims Data (Calendar-days away from work by decile)										
10%	20%	30%	40%	**50%**	60%	70%	80%	**90%**	100%	Mean
10	12	13	14	**15**	16	18	29	**63**	365	37.07

This section includes symptoms, signs, abnormal results of laboratory or other investigative procedures, and ill-defined conditions regarding which no diagnosis classifiable elsewhere is recorded.

Signs and symptoms that point rather definitely to a given diagnosis are assigned to some category in the preceding part of the classification. In general, categories 780-796 include the more ill-defined conditions and symptoms that point with perhaps equal suspicion to two or more diseases or to two or more systems of the body, and without the necessary study of the case to make a final diagnosis. Practically all categories in this group could be designated as "not otherwise specified," or as "unknown etiology," or as "transient." The Alphabetic Index should be consulted to determine which symptoms and signs are to be allocated here and which to more specific sections of the classification; the residual subcategories numbered .9 are provided for other relevant symptoms which cannot be allocated elsewhere in the classification.

The conditions and signs or symptoms included in categories 780-796 consist of: (a) cases for which no more specific diagnosis can be made even after all facts bearing on the case have been investigated; (b) signs or symptoms existing at the time of initial encounter that proved to be transient and whose causes could not be determined; (c) provisional diagnoses in a patient who failed to return for further investigation or care; (d) cases referred elsewhere for investigation or treatment before the diagnosis was made; (e) cases in which a more precise diagnosis was not available for any other reason; (f) certain symptoms which represent important problems in medical care and which it might be desired to classify in addition to a known cause.

SYMPTOMS (780-789)

RTW Claims Data (Calendar-days away from work by decile)										
10%	20%	30%	40%	**50%**	60%	70%	80%	**90%**	100%	Mean
10	12	13	14	**15**	17	26	31	**78**	365	41.11

Impact on Total Absence: Prevalence 1.2016% of total lost workdays; Incidence 12.62 days per 100 workers

Occupational Disability Durations, in days
Median (mid-point) 4 - Benchmark Indemnity Costs $3,000

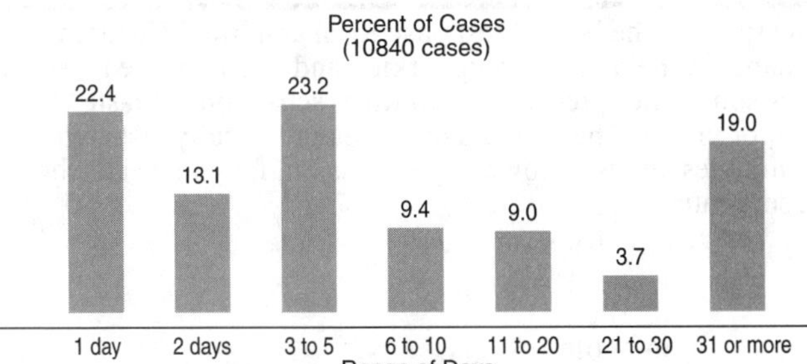

Impact on Occupational Absence: Prevalence 0.4918% of occupational lost workdays; Incidence 0.08 days per 100 workers

780 General symptoms

Return-To-Work Summary Guidelines		
Dataset	**Midrange**	**At-Risk**
Claims data	15 days	30 days
All absences	11 days	28 days

Return-To-Work "Best Practice" Guidelines
See 780.0

Workers' Comp Costs per Claim (based on 230 claims)					
Quartile	25%	50%	75%	Mean	% no cost
Indemnity	$3,822	$8,883	$30,996	$28,011	69%
Medical	$630	$1,202	$6,143	$10,125	4%
Total	$672	$1,365	$10,962	$18,897	3%

Occupational Disability Durations, in days
Median (mid-point) 3 - Benchmark Indemnity Costs $2,250

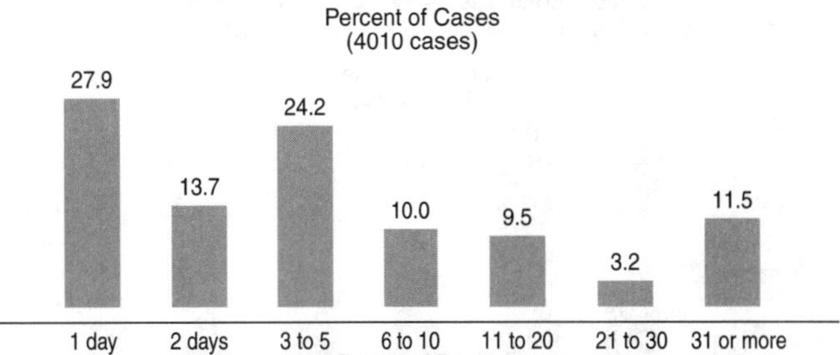

Impact on Occupational Absence: Prevalence 0.1364% of occupational lost workdays; Incidence 0.02 days per 100 workers

780.0 Alteration of consciousness

Return-To-Work Summary Guidelines		
Dataset	**Midrange**	**At-Risk**
Claims data	15 days	66 days
All absences	14 days	41 days

Return-To-Work "Best Practice" Guidelines
With hospitalization and immediate return of consciousness: 3 days
Delayed return of consciousness (seek other diagnosis): 14-28 days

Description: Any alteration in the normal state of consciousness, from dizziness to loss of consciousness altogether.

Excludes:
coma:
diabetic (250.2-250.3)
hepatic (572.2)
originating in the perinatal period (779.2)

Workers' Comp Costs per Claim (based on 34 claims)					
Quartile	25%	50%	75%	Mean	% no cost
Medical	$893	$1,927	$6,584	$11,217	0%
Total	$893	$2,184	$12,170	$20,132	0%

RTW Claims Data (Calendar-days away from work by decile)										
10%	20%	30%	40%	**50%**	60%	70%	80%	**90%**	100%	Mean
11	13	14	14	**15**	17	28	30	**66**	365	40.57

780.0 Alteration of consciousness *(cont'd)*

Integrated Disability Durations, in days*

Median (mid-point)	14.0	Mean (average)	29.24
Mode (most frequent)	14	Calculated rec.	18

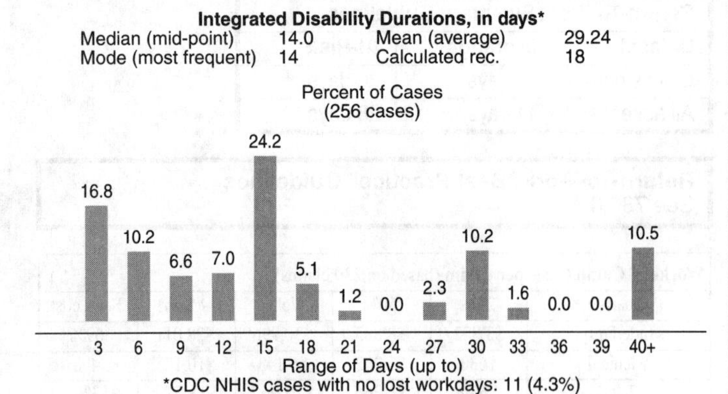

Impact on Total Absence: Prevalence 0.0211% of total lost workdays; Incidence 0.22 days per 100 workers

Occupational Disability Durations, in days
Median (mid-point) 5 - Benchmark Indemnity Costs $3,750

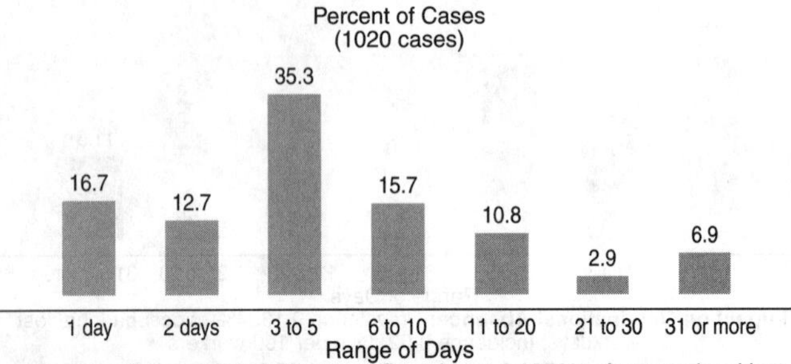

Impact on Occupational Absence: Prevalence 0.0578% of occupational lost workdays; Incidence 0.01 days per 100 workers

780.2 Syncope and collapse

Return-To-Work Summary Guidelines		
Dataset	**Midrange**	**At-Risk**
Claims data	27 days	61 days
All absences	7 days	31 days

Return-To-Work "Best Practice" Guidelines
With hospitalization, rule out arrhythmia, clerical/modified work: 2 days
With hospitalization, rule out arrhythmia, manual work: 4 days
Mobile equipment work, after evaluation & compliance with state/fed rules: 28 days

Description: Temporary loss of consciousness due to inadequate blood flow to the brain. Symptoms that precede fainting often include dizziness, weakness, nausea, sweating, and/or loss of color in the face.

Blackout
Fainting
(Near) (Pre)syncope
Vasovagal attack

Excludes:

carotid sinus syncope (337.0)
heat syncope (992.1)
neurocirculatory asthenia (306.2)
orthostatic hypotension (458.0)
shock NOS (785.50)

Workers' Comp Costs per Claim (based on 131 claims)

Quartile	25%	50%	75%	Mean	% no cost
Medical	$431	$714	$1,239	$1,424	6%
Total	$441	$725	$1,628	$1,746	4%

780.2 Syncope and collapse *(cont'd)*

RTW Claims Data (Calendar-days away from work by decile)

10%	20%	30%	40%	**50%**	60%	70%	80%	**90%**	100%	Mean
10	12	14	24	**27**	28	29	31	**61**	365	36.32

Integrated Disability Durations, in days*

Median (mid-point)	7.0	Mean (average)	19.55
Mode (most frequent)	2	Calculated rec.	9

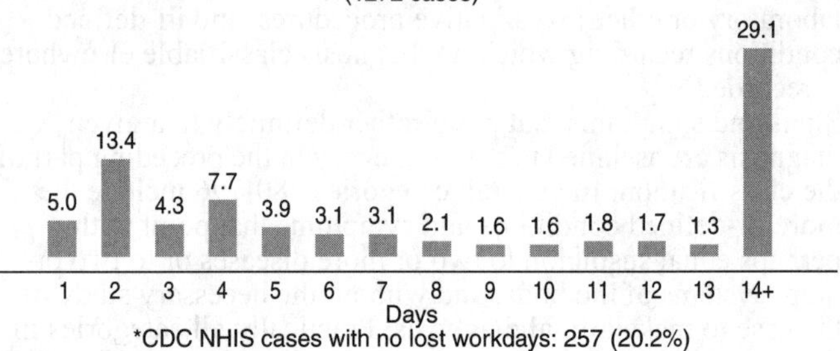

Impact on Total Absence: Prevalence 0.0586% of total lost workdays; Incidence 0.62 days per 100 workers

Occupational Disability Durations, in days
Median (mid-point) 3 - Benchmark Indemnity Costs $2,250

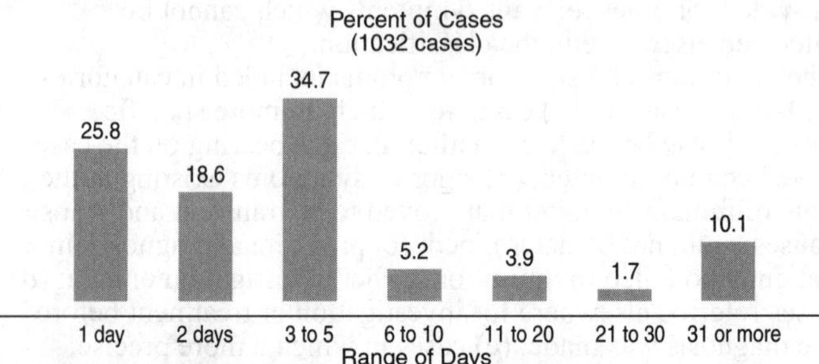

Impact on Occupational Absence: Prevalence 0.0351% of occupational lost workdays; Incidence 0.01 days per 100 workers

780.3 Convulsions

Return-To-Work Summary Guidelines		
Dataset	**Midrange**	**At-Risk**
Claims data	15 days	86 days
All absences	13 days	37 days

Return-To-Work "Best Practice" Guidelines
Medical treatment of recurrent seizures, clerical/modified work: 0 days
Medical treatment of recurrent seizures, dangerous work (after evaluation for full control): 14 days

Description: The body's response to an abnormal electrical discharge in the brain causing jerking and spasm of the muscles that is sometimes preceded by unusual sensations of taste, smell, or vision. The convulsion or seizure usually lasts two to five minutes and is followed by confusion, fatigue, headache, and sore muscles.

Convulsions:
NOS
febrile
infantile
Convulsive:
disorder NOS
seizure NOS
Fit NOS

780.3 Convulsions *(cont'd)*

Excludes:
convulsions:
epileptic (345.10-345.91)
in newborn (779.0)

RTW Claims Data (Calendar-days away from work by decile)

10%	20%	30%	40%	**50%**	60%	70%	80%	**90%**	100%	Mean
11	13	14	14	**15**	15	17	20	**86**	365	36.77

Integrated Disability Durations, in days*
Median (mid-point) 13.0 Mean (average) 24.98
Mode (most frequent) 1 Calculated rec. 13

Percent of Cases
(740 cases)

20.4 7.4 5.4 6.8 24.7 10.0 1.2 0.3 0.1 0.7 0.5 0.0 0.7 8.1

3 6 9 12 15 18 21 24 27 30 33 36 39 40+
Range of Days (up to)

*CDC NHIS cases with no lost workdays: 101 (13.6%)

Impact on Total Absence: Prevalence 0.0471% of total lost workdays; Incidence 0.50 days per 100 workers

Occupational Disability Durations, in days
Median (mid-point) 7 - Benchmark Indemnity Costs $5,250
(190 cases)
Impact on Occupational Absence: Prevalence 0.0150% of occupational lost workdays

780.4 Dizziness and giddiness

Return-To-Work Summary Guidelines		
Dataset	**Midrange**	**At-Risk**
Claims data	13 days	33 days
All absences	2 days	14 days

Return-To-Work "Best Practice" Guidelines
Diagnostic evaluation: 1 day

Description: The feeling of being unsteady or faint which is usually caused by a momentary decrease in blood pressure to the brain or because of disorders of the inner ear. There could also be nausea, vomiting, or fainting in serious cases.

Light-headedness
Vertigo NOS

Excludes:
Meniere's disease and other specified vertiginous syndromes (386.0-386.9)

RTW Claims Data (Calendar-days away from work by decile)

10%	20%	30%	40%	**50%**	60%	70%	80%	**90%**	100%	Mean
9	10	11	12	**13**	13	14	15	**33**	365	25.44

780.4 Dizziness and giddiness *(cont'd)*

Integrated Disability Durations, in days*
Median (mid-point) 2.0 Mean (average) 8.70
Mode (most frequent) 1 Calculated rec. 3

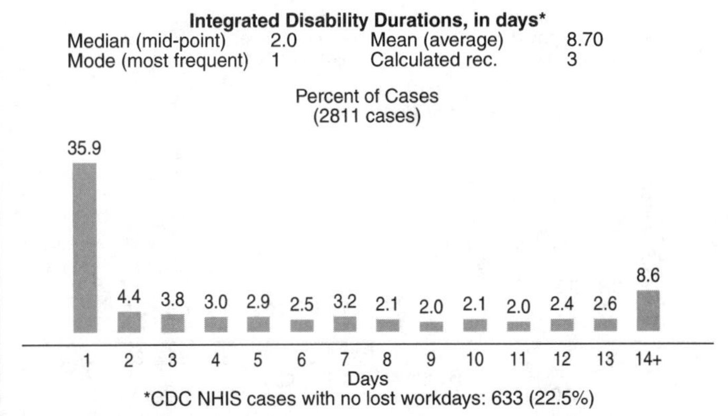

*CDC NHIS cases with no lost workdays: 633 (22.5%)

Impact on Total Absence: Prevalence 0.0559% of total lost workdays; Incidence 0.59 days per 100 workers

Occupational Disability Durations, in days
Median (mid-point) 1 - Benchmark Indemnity Costs $750

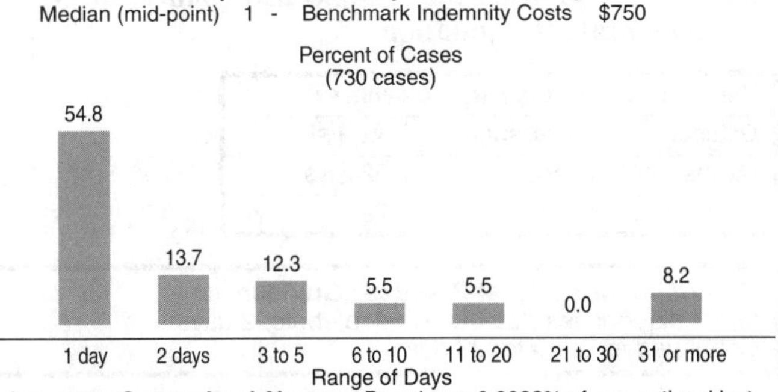

Impact on Occupational Absence: Prevalence 0.0082% of occupational lost workdays

780.5 Sleep disturbances

Return-To-Work Summary Guidelines		
Dataset	**Midrange**	**At-Risk**
Claims data	15 days	31 days
All absences	13 days	20 days

Return-To-Work "Best Practice" Guidelines
Therapy for snoring, somnoplasty: 1 day
Therapy for snoring, surgery (tonsillectomy or uvulopalatopharyngoplasty): 14 days
Obesity comorbidity (BMI >= 30), multiply by: 1.5

Description: Sleep disturbances stemming from the person's body or mind, such as snoring or insomnia.

Excludes:
that of nonorganic origin (307.40-307.49)

RTW Claims Data (Calendar-days away from work by decile)

10%	20%	30%	40%	**50%**	60%	70%	80%	**90%**	100%	Mean
12	13	14	14	**15**	15	16	18	**31**	365	23.85

780.5 Sleep disturbances *(cont'd)*

Integrated Disability Durations, in days*

Median (mid-point)	13.0	Mean (average)	16.10
Mode (most frequent)	1	Calculated rec.	11

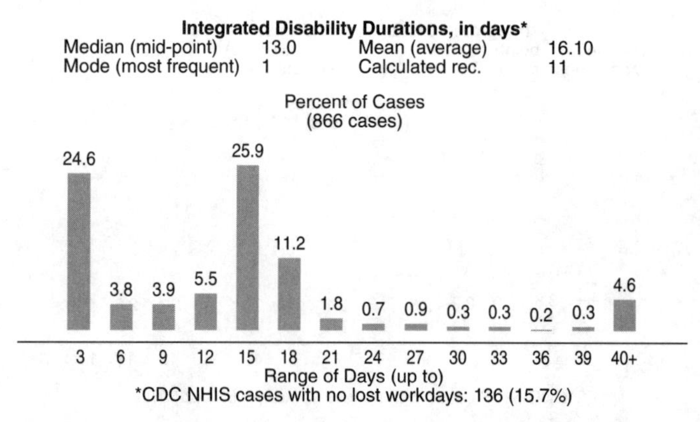

*CDC NHIS cases with no lost workdays: 136 (15.7%)

Impact on Total Absence: Prevalence 0.0347% of total lost workdays; Incidence 0.36 days per 100 workers

780.6 Fever and other physiologic disturbances of temperature regulation

Return-To-Work Summary Guidelines		
Dataset	**Midrange**	**At-Risk**
Claims data	28 days	32 days
All absences	2 days	29 days

Return-To-Work "Best Practice" Guidelines
Other diagnoses ruled out, when afebrile: 2 days
Continued fever up to: 28 days

Description: Elevation of body temperature usually as a result of an infectious disease. A fever is classified as a body temperature over 100.4 degrees Fahrenheit if measured orally and 99.4 degrees if measured rectally.

Chills with fever
Fever NOS
Hyperpyrexia NOS
Pyrexia

Excludes:
pyrexia of unknown origin (during):
in newborn (778.4)
labor (659.2)
the puerperium (672)

RTW Claims Data (Calendar-days away from work by decile)

10%	20%	30%	40%	**50%**	60%	70%	80%	**90%**	100%	Mean
21	27	28	28	**28**	29	29	30	**32**	99	27.75

Integrated Disability Durations, in days*

Median (mid-point)	2.0	Mean (average)	9.69
Mode (most frequent)	2	Calculated rec.	4

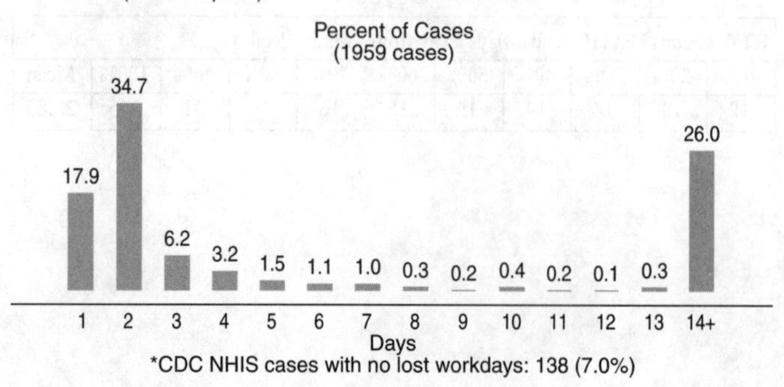

*CDC NHIS cases with no lost workdays: 138 (7.0%)

Impact on Total Absence: Prevalence 0.0521% of total lost workdays; Incidence 0.55 days per 100 workers

780.7 Malaise and fatigue

Return-To-Work Summary Guidelines		
Dataset	**Midrange**	**At-Risk**
Claims data	15 days	365 days
All absences	13 days	365 days

Return-To-Work "Best Practice" Guidelines
Acute: 1 day
Debilitating chronic fatigue: 14 days
Chronic fatigue syndrome: Controversial diagnosis - see related conditions

Description: General weakness, lethargy, and discomfort, often preceding the onset of a disease.

Asthenia NOS
Lethargy
Postviral (asthenic) syndrome
Tiredness

Excludes:
debility, unspecified (799.3)
fatigue (during):
combat (308.0-308.9)
heat (992.6)
pregnancy (646.8)
neurasthenia (300.5)
senile asthenia (797)

RTW Claims Data (Calendar-days away from work by decile)

10%	20%	30%	40%	**50%**	60%	70%	80%	**90%**	100%	Mean
13	14	14	15	**15**	16	18	364	**365**	365	96.38

Integrated Disability Durations, in days*

Median (mid-point)	13.0	Mean (average)	55.39
Mode (most frequent)	1	Calculated rec.	21

Percent of Cases
(2375 cases)

31.7 | 5.2 | 2.1 | 3.7 | 21.9 | 10.5 | 0.1 | 0.0 | 0.1 | 0.0 | 0.1 | 0.2 | 0.1 | 12.1

3 6 9 12 15 18 21 24 27 30 33 36 39 40+
Range of Days (up to)

*CDC NHIS cases with no lost workdays: 290 (12.2%)

Impact on Total Absence: Prevalence 0.3413% of total lost workdays; Incidence 3.58 days per 100 workers

Occupational Disability Durations, in days
Median (mid-point) 1 - Benchmark Indemnity Costs $750

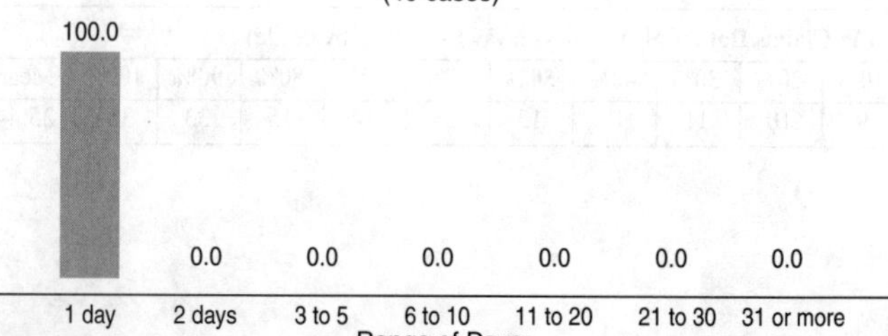

Impact on Occupational Absence: Prevalence 0.0004% of occupational lost workdays

780.71 Chronic fatigue syndrome

Return-To-Work Summary Guidelines		
Dataset	Midrange	At-Risk
Claims data	15 days	365 days
All absences	13 days	365 days

Return-To-Work "Best Practice" Guidelines
Moderate cases, modified duty: 180-365 days
Severe cases: indefinite

Description: Chronic fatigue syndrome is characterized by fatigue that is medically unexplained, of new onset, lasts at least six months, is not the result of ongoing exertion, is not substantially relieved by rest, and causes a substantial reduction in activity levels. CFIDS fatigue must be accompanied by four or more of the following symptoms: impaired memory/ concentration, sore throat, tender neck or armpit lymph nodes, muscle pain, headaches of a new type, pattern or severity, unrefreshing sleep, relapse of symptoms after exercise, and pain in multiple joints.
Other names: Chronic fatigue and immune dysfunction syndrome, CFIDS

780.79 Other malaise and fatigue

Return-To-Work Summary Guidelines		
Dataset	Midrange	At-Risk
Claims data	15 days	365 days
All absences	13 days	365 days

Return-To-Work "Best Practice" Guidelines
Acute: 1 day
Debilitating chronic fatigue: 14 days
Chronic fatigue syndrome: Controversial diagnosis - see related conditions or see below
Moderate cases, modified duty: 180-365 days
Severe cases: indefinite

Description: General weakness, lethargy, and discomfort, often preceding the onset of a disease.

784 Symptoms involving head and neck

Return-To-Work Summary Guidelines		
Dataset	Midrange	At-Risk
Claims data	51 days	119 days
All absences	13 days	119 days

Return-To-Work "Best Practice" Guidelines
See 784.0

Excludes:
encephalopathy NOS (348.3)
specific symptoms involving neck classifiable to 723 (723.0-723.9)

Workers' Comp Costs per Claim (based on 416 claims)					
Quartile	25%	50%	75%	Mean	% no cost
Indemnity	$2,331	$6,111	$12,968	$12,398	53%
Medical	$557	$1,796	$6,027	$6,106	5%
Total	$567	$2,819	$12,978	$12,245	5%

784 Symptoms involving head and neck *(cont'd)*

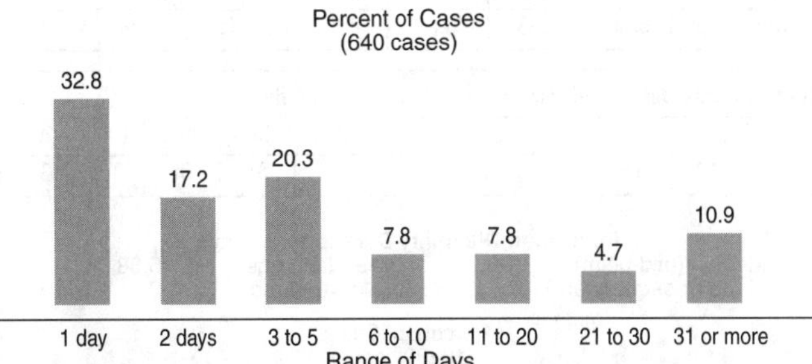

Impact on Occupational Absence: Prevalence 0.0145% of occupational lost workdays

784.0 Headache

Return-To-Work Summary Guidelines		
Dataset	Midrange	At-Risk
Claims data	15 days	88 days
All absences	1 days	12 days

Return-To-Work "Best Practice" Guidelines
Mild (depending on underlying diagnosis): 0 days
Severe (depending on underlying diagnosis): 1 day

Description: A pain in the head from any cause.
Facial pain
Pain in head NOS

Excludes:
atypical face pain (350.2)
migraine (346.0-346.9)
tension headache (307.81)

Procedure Summary (from ODG Treatment): Activity restrictions; Acupuncture; Anticonvulsants; Antidepressants; Antiepilectics; Bed rest; Behavioral therapy; Botulinum toxin type A; Branched-chain amino acids (BCAAs); Cell transplantation therapy ; Complementary and alternative medicine (CAM); Corticosteroids (for acute traumatic brain injury); Cognitive therapy; Craniectomy; Craniotomy; CT (computed tomography); Decompressive surgery; EEG (Electroencephalography); Field of vision testing; Fluid resuscitation; Glasgow Coma Scale (GCS); Greater occipital nerve block (GONB); Hyperventilation; Hypothermia; Imaging; Interdisciplinary rehabilitation programs; Lumbar puncture; Mannitol; Melatonin; Methylphenidate; Modified Ashworth Scale (MAS); MRI (magnetic resonance imaging); Nutrition; Occupational therapy (OT); Oxygen therapy; PET (positron emission tomography); Physical therapy (PT); QEEG (Quantified Electroencephalography); Relaxation treatment (for migraines); Return to work; Sedation; Skull x-rays; Sleep aids; SPECT (single photon emission computed tomography); Steroids; Triptans; Vision evaluation; Wilsonii injecta; Work
Physical Therapy Guidelines:
6 visits over 6 weeks
Chiropractic Guidelines:
12 visits over 6 weeks

Workers' Comp Costs per Claim (based on 298 claims)					
Quartile	25%	50%	75%	Mean	% no cost
Indemnity	$3,224	$6,332	$12,968	$12,536	43%
Medical	$956	$2,835	$7,949	$7,206	4%
Total	$1,292	$5,623	$15,897	$14,728	4%

784.0 Headache *(cont'd)*

Disability Duration Adjustment Factors by Age						
Age Group	18-24	25-34	35-44	45-54	55-64	65-74
Adjustment Factor	0.63	0.82	1.10	1.15	1.90	0.89

RTW Claims Data (Calendar-days away from work by decile)

10%	20%	30%	40%	**50%**	60%	70%	80%	**90%**	100%	Mean
10	12	13	14	**15**	18	22	38	**88**	365	36.71

Integrated Disability Durations, in days*

Median (mid-point) 1.0 Mean (average) 6.38
Mode (most frequent) 1 Calculated rec. 2

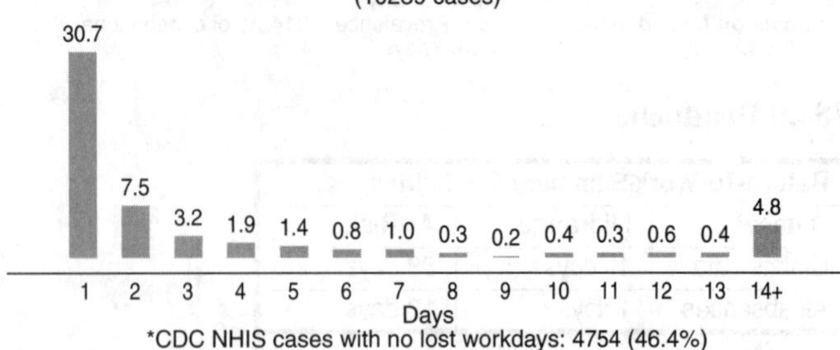

*CDC NHIS cases with no lost workdays: 4754 (46.4%)

Impact on Total Absence: Prevalence 0.1034% of total lost workdays; Incidence 1.09 days per 100 workers

Occupational Disability Durations, in days

Median (mid-point) 2 - Benchmark Indemnity Costs $1,500

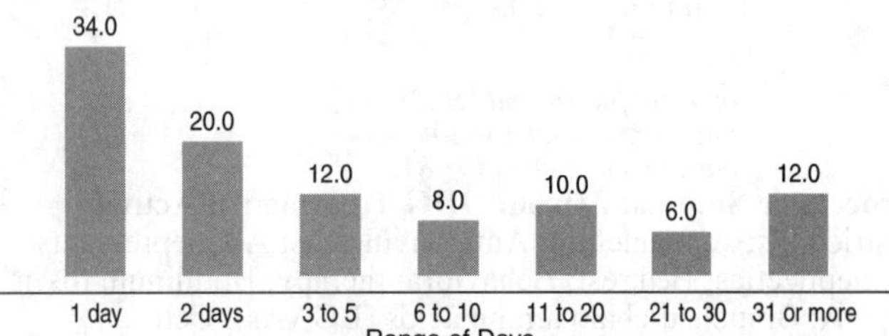

Impact on Occupational Absence: Prevalence 0.0113% of occupational lost workdays

785 Symptoms involving cardiovascular system

Return-To-Work Summary Guidelines		
Dataset	**Midrange**	**At-Risk**
Claims data	14 days	90 days
All absences	7 days	31 days

Excludes:
heart failure NOS (428.9)

Workers' Comp Costs per Claim (based on 91 claims)					
Quartile	25%	50%	75%	Mean	% no cost
Indemnity	$7,592	$17,603	$38,735	$30,003	42%
Medical	$1,607	$5,229	$22,670	$17,132	4%
Total	$1,607	$12,212	$53,907	$35,394	4%

RTW Claims Data (Calendar-days away from work by decile)

10%	20%	30%	40%	**50%**	60%	70%	80%	**90%**	100%	Mean
9	10	12	14	**14**	15	17	31	**90**	365	40.39

785 Symptoms involving cardiovascular system

Integrated Disability Durations, in days*

Median (mid-point) 7.0 Mean (average) 21.47
Mode (most frequent) 2 Calculated rec. 9

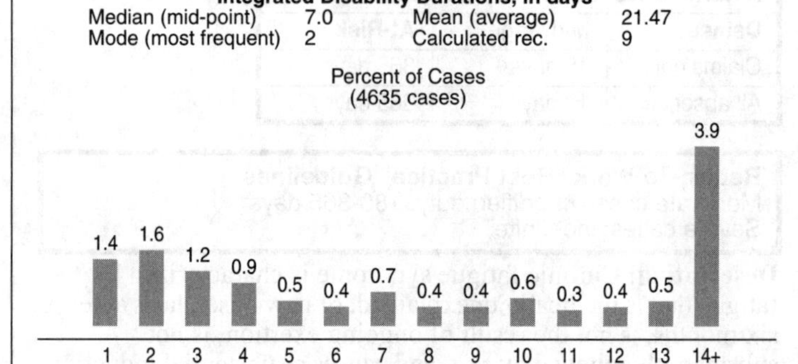

*CDC NHIS cases with no lost workdays: 4028 (86.9%)

Impact on Total Absence: Prevalence 0.0385% of total lost workdays; Incidence 0.40 days per 100 workers

Occupational Disability Durations, in days

Median (mid-point) 7 - Benchmark Indemnity Costs $5,250 (40 cases)

Impact on Occupational Absence: Prevalence 0.0031% of occupational lost workdays

785.1 Palpitations

Return-To-Work Summary Guidelines		
Dataset	**Midrange**	**At-Risk**
Claims data	16 days	180 days
All absences	5 days	26 days

Return-To-Work "Best Practice" Guidelines
Diagnostic evaluation: 1-5 days

Description: Unusually rapid, strong, or irregular heartbeat, usually noticeable by the individual. There may also be shortness of breath, tingling of the hands and mouth, lightheadedness, and weakness.

Awareness of heart beat

Excludes:
specified dysrhythmias (427.0-427.9)

RTW Claims Data (Calendar-days away from work by decile)

10%	20%	30%	40%	**50%**	60%	70%	80%	**90%**	100%	Mean
10	12	13	14	**16**	18	26	63	**180**	365	60.34

Integrated Disability Durations, in days*

Median (mid-point) 5.0 Mean (average) 22.55
Mode (most frequent) 1 Calculated rec. 8

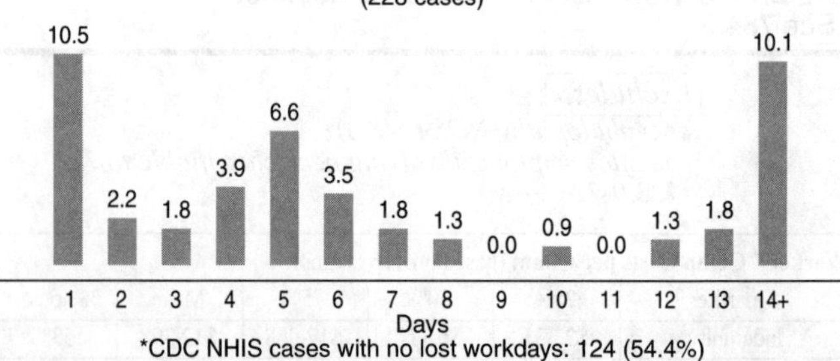

*CDC NHIS cases with no lost workdays: 124 (54.4%)

Impact on Total Absence: Prevalence 0.0069% of total lost workdays; Incidence 0.07 days per 100 workers

785.2 Undiagnosed cardiac murmurs

Return-To-Work Summary Guidelines		
Dataset	**Midrange**	**At-Risk**
Claims data	14 days	18 days
All absences	13 days	17 days

Return-To-Work "Best Practice" Guidelines
Asymptomatic: 0 days
Mild: 7 days
Severe: 14 days

Description: An abnormal sound in the heart originating from the cardiac or vascular region, often resembling a humming or fluttering sound. In more serious cases, the individual could have symptoms of chest pain, palpitations, fainting, change in pulse rate, and/or shortness of breath.

Heart murmur NOS

RTW Claims Data (Calendar-days away from work by decile)										
10%	20%	30%	40%	**50%**	60%	70%	80%	**90%**	100%	Mean
9	12	13	14	**14**	15	15	16	**18**	365	17.05

Integrated Disability Durations, in days*

Median (mid-point)	13.0	Mean (average)	12.91
Mode (most frequent)	14	Calculated rec.	13

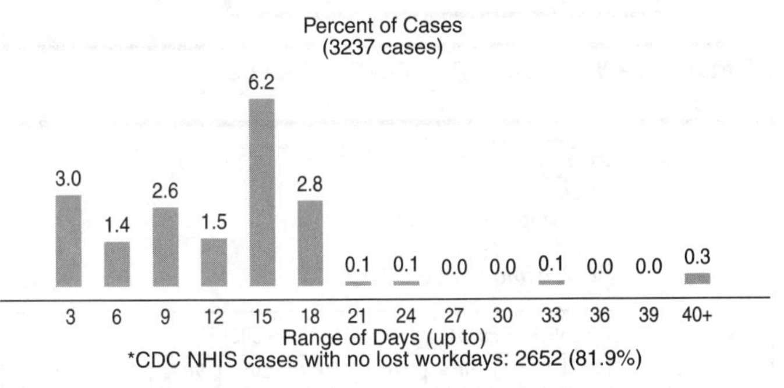

*CDC NHIS cases with no lost workdays: 2652 (81.9%)

Impact on Total Absence: Prevalence 0.0223% of total lost workdays; Incidence 0.23 days per 100 workers

785.4 Gangrene

Return-To-Work Summary Guidelines		
Dataset	**Midrange**	**At-Risk**
Claims data	55 days	132 days
All absences	51 days	132 days

Return-To-Work "Best Practice" Guidelines
Medical treatment: 1 week
Amputation of foot, allowing prosthesis to set, sedentary work: 63-70 days
Amputation of foot, allowing prosthesis to set, manual/standing work: 105 days to indefinite days

Description: The destruction of tissue (as a result of full or partial loss of blood to the area) followed by bacterial invasion. Symptoms include changing skin color from pale to red to green, fluid-filled blisters, warm swollen skin, fever, chills, nausea, and/or an unpleasant odor.

Gangrene:
NOS
spreading cutaneous
Phagedena
Use additional code for any associated condition, as:
diabetes (250.7)
Raynaud's syndrome (443.0)

785.4 Gangrene *(cont'd)*

Excludes:
gangrene of certain sites—*see Alphabetic Index*
gangrene with atherosclerosis of the extremities (440.24)
gas gangrene (040.0)

Workers' Comp Costs per Claim (based on 57 claims)					
Quartile	25%	50%	75%	Mean	% no cost
Indemnity	$10,353	$18,522	$38,735	$32,425	20%
Medical	$4,547	$17,042	$27,668	$25,240	0%
Total	$8,757	$28,418	$62,549	$51,180	0%

RTW Claims Data (Calendar-days away from work by decile)										
10%	20%	30%	40%	**50%**	60%	70%	80%	**90%**	100%	Mean
14	15	32	43	**55**	64	71	105	**132**	365	76.94

Integrated Disability Durations, in days*

Median (mid-point)	52.0	Mean (average)	74.91
Mode (most frequent)	14	Calculated rec.	48

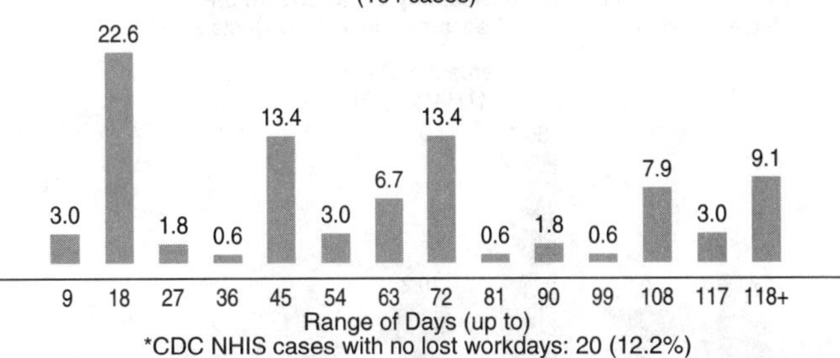

*CDC NHIS cases with no lost workdays: 20 (12.2%)

Impact on Total Absence: Prevalence 0.0318% of total lost workdays; Incidence 0.33 days per 100 workers

786 Symptoms involving respiratory system and other chest symptoms

Return-To-Work Summary Guidelines		
Dataset	**Midrange**	**At-Risk**
Claims data	14 days	20 days
All absences	2 days	14 days

Return-To-Work "Best Practice" Guidelines
See 786.0

Workers' Comp Costs per Claim (based on 179 claims)					
Quartile	25%	50%	75%	Mean	% no cost
Medical	$347	$725	$1,449	$2,034	10%
Total	$347	$735	$2,153	$9,707	9%

RTW Claims Data (Calendar-days away from work by decile)										
10%	20%	30%	40%	**50%**	60%	70%	80%	**90%**	100%	Mean
10	12	13	14	**14**	15	15	16	**20**	365	21.63

786 Symptoms involving respiratory system and other chest symptoms *(cont'd)*

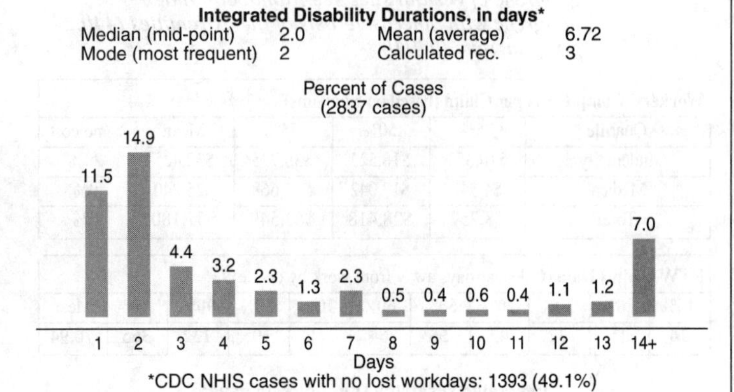

Impact on Total Absence: Prevalence 0.0287% of total lost workdays; Incidence 0.30 days per 100 workers

Occupational Disability Durations, in days
Median (mid-point) 3 - Benchmark Indemnity Costs $2,250

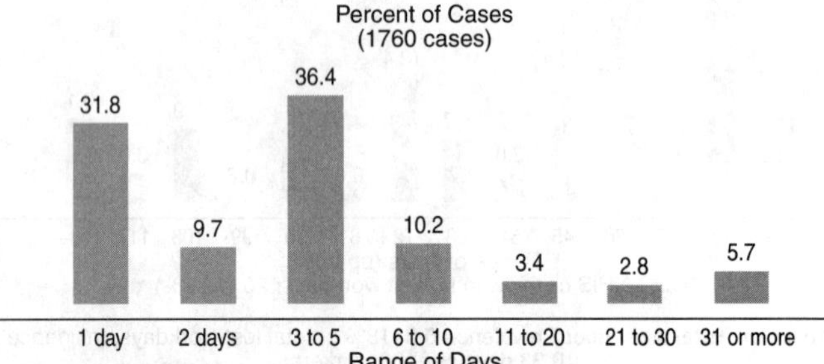

Impact on Occupational Absence: Prevalence 0.0598% of occupational lost workdays; Incidence 0.01 days per 100 workers

786.0 Dyspnea and respiratory abnormalities

Return-To-Work Summary Guidelines		
Dataset	**Midrange**	**At-Risk**
Claims data	16 days	146 days
All absences	3 days	84 days

Return-To-Work "Best Practice" Guidelines
Clerical/modified work: 0 days
Manual work: 2 days

Description: Shortness of breath.

Workers' Comp Costs per Claim (based on 97 claims)					
Quartile	25%	50%	75%	Mean	% no cost
Medical	$357	$735	$1,428	$2,561	10%
Total	$357	$746	$1,617	$16,333	8%

RTW Claims Data (Calendar-days away from work by decile)										
10%	20%	30%	40%	**50%**	60%	70%	80%	**90%**	100%	Mean
9	11	12	15	**16**	33	74	92	**146**	302	55.69

786.0 Dyspnea and respiratory abnormalities

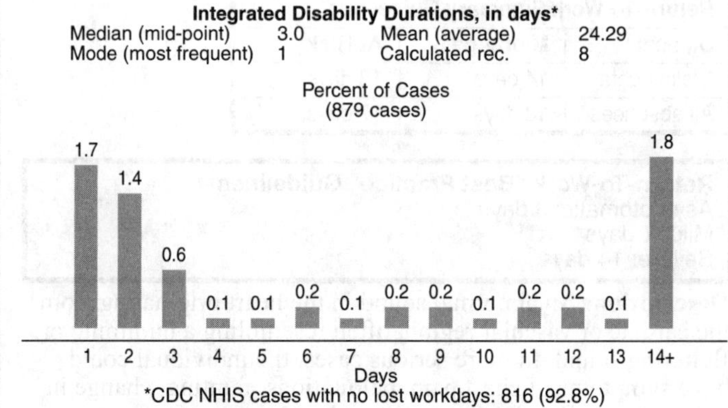

Impact on Total Absence: Prevalence 0.0045% of total lost workdays; Incidence 0.05 days per 100 workers

786.2 Cough

Return-To-Work Summary Guidelines		
Dataset	**Midrange**	**At-Risk**
Claims data	14 days	17 days
All absences	2 days	7 days

Return-To-Work "Best Practice" Guidelines
0 days

Excludes:
cough:
psychogenic (306.1)
smokers' (491.0)
with hemorrhage (786.3)

RTW Claims Data (Calendar-days away from work by decile)										
10%	20%	30%	40%	**50%**	60%	70%	80%	**90%**	100%	Mean
9	10	12	13	**14**	15	15	16	**17**	20	13.39

Integrated Disability Durations, in days*
Median (mid-point) 2.0 Mean (average) 3.12
Mode (most frequent) 1 Calculated rec. 2

Percent of Cases
(561 cases)

27.8, 12.1, 7.1, 3.0, 1.2, 1.2, 2.1, 0.4, 0.4, 0.5, 0.4, 0.4, 0.5, 3.0

1 2 3 4 5 6 7 8 9 10 11 12 13 14+
Days
*CDC NHIS cases with no lost workdays: 223 (39.8%)

Impact on Total Absence: Prevalence 0.0031% of total lost workdays; Incidence 0.03 days per 100 workers

786.5 Chest pain

Return-To-Work Summary Guidelines		
Dataset	**Midrange**	**At-Risk**
Claims data	14 days	68 days
All absences	6 days	26 days

786.5 Chest pain *(cont'd)*

Return-To-Work "Best Practice" Guidelines
Vague symptom, see more specific diagnosis
Diagnostic evaluation: 2 days

Description: Usually a symptom of something else, chest pain can be anywhere from mild to life threatening.

Workers' Comp Costs per Claim (based on 68 claims)

Quartile	25%	50%	75%	Mean	% no cost
Medical	$420	$966	$2,562	$1,609	8%
Total	$420	$966	$2,678	$1,943	8%

RTW Claims Data (Calendar-days away from work by decile)

10%	20%	30%	40%	**50%**	60%	70%	80%	**90%**	100%	Mean
9	10	12	13	**14**	16	21	31	**68**	365	33.05

Integrated Disability Durations, in days*
Median (mid-point) 6.0 Mean (average) 15.88
Mode (most frequent) 2 Calculated rec. 7

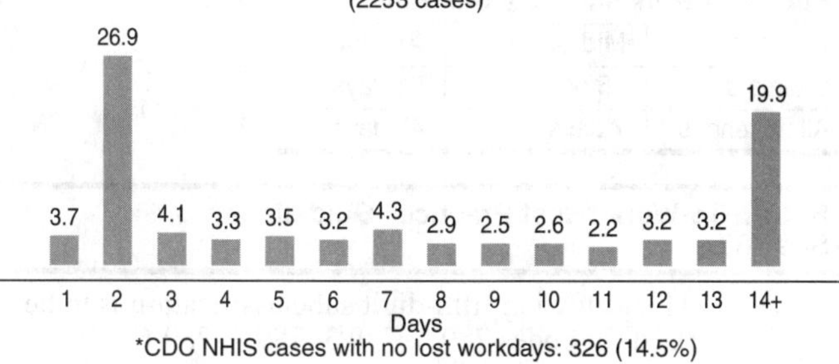

*CDC NHIS cases with no lost workdays: 326 (14.5%)

Impact on Total Absence: Prevalence 0.0904% of total lost workdays; Incidence 0.95 days per 100 workers

Occupational Disability Durations, in days
Median (mid-point) 2 - Benchmark Indemnity Costs $1,500

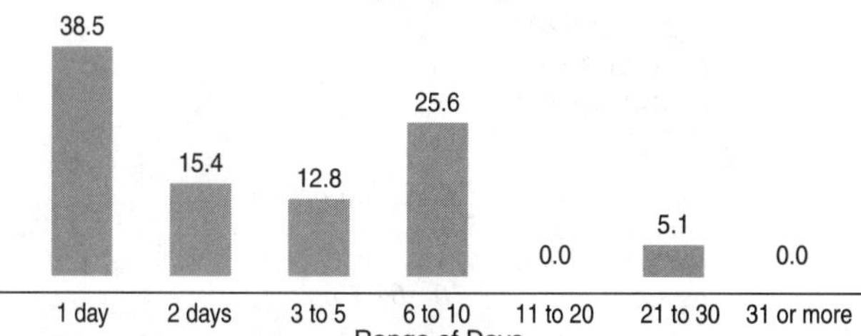

Impact on Occupational Absence: Prevalence 0.0088% of occupational lost workdays

787 Symptoms involving digestive system

Return-To-Work Summary Guidelines		
Dataset	**Midrange**	**At-Risk**
Claims data	17 days	150 days
All absences	6 days	63 days

Return-To-Work "Best Practice" Guidelines
See 787.0

Excludes:
constipation (564.0)
diarrhea NOS (558.9)
pylorospasm (537.81)
congenital (750.5)

787 Symptoms involving digestive system *(cont'd)*

Occupational Disability Durations, in days
Median (mid-point) 5 - Benchmark Indemnity Costs $3,750

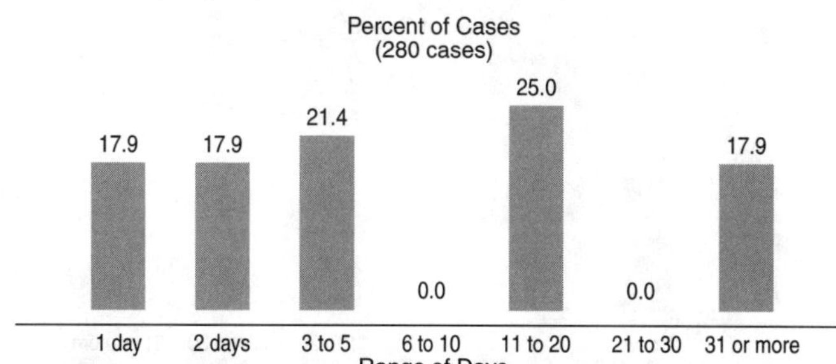

Impact on Occupational Absence: Prevalence 0.0158% of occupational lost workdays

787.0 Nausea and vomiting

Return-To-Work Summary Guidelines		
Dataset	**Midrange**	**At-Risk**
Claims data	12 days	27 days
All absences	1 days	12 days

Return-To-Work "Best Practice" Guidelines
Diagnostic evaluation: 1 day

Description: Nausea is an unpleasant feeling in the stomach that is usually followed by vomiting. Vomiting is the forceful expulsion of stomach contents through the mouth. Both are often symptoms of another condition.

Emesis

Excludes:
hematemesis NOS (578.0)
vomiting:
bilious, following gastrointestinal surgery (564.3)
cyclical (536.2)
psychogenic (306.4)
excessive, in pregnancy (643.0-643.9)
habit (536.2)
of newborn (779.3)
psychogenic NOS (307.54)

RTW Claims Data (Calendar-days away from work by decile)

10%	20%	30%	40%	**50%**	60%	70%	80%	**90%**	100%	Mean
8	9	10	11	**12**	13	14	15	**27**	264	22.15

Integrated Disability Durations, in days*
Median (mid-point) 1.0 Mean (average) 5.65
Mode (most frequent) 1 Calculated rec. 2

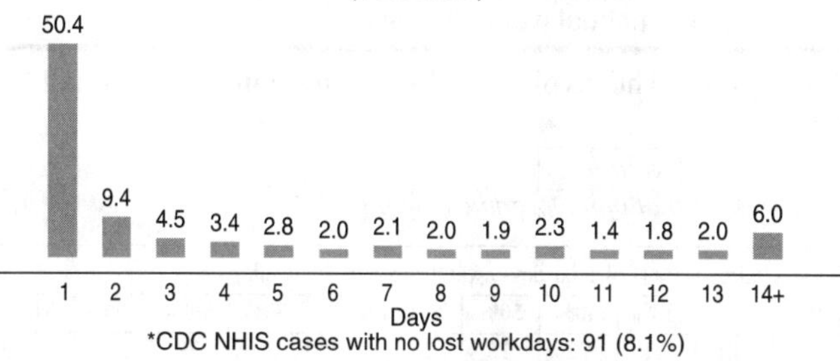

*CDC NHIS cases with no lost workdays: 91 (8.1%)

Impact on Total Absence: Prevalence 0.0172% of total lost workdays; Incidence 0.18 days per 100 workers

787.0 Nausea and vomiting *(cont'd)*

Occupational Disability Durations, in days
Median (mid-point) 3 - Benchmark Indemnity Costs $2,250

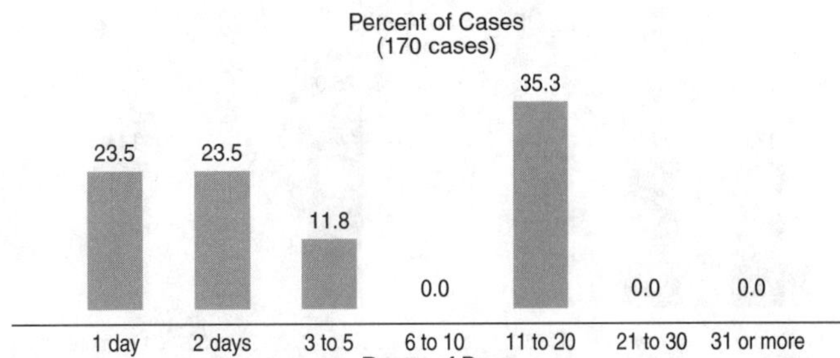

Impact on Occupational Absence: Prevalence 0.0057% of occupational lost workdays

788 Symptoms involving urinary system

Return-To-Work Summary Guidelines		
Dataset	**Midrange**	**At-Risk**
Claims data	20 days	44 days
All absences	7 days	42 days

Return-To-Work "Best Practice" Guidelines
See 788.0

Excludes:
hematuria (599.7)
nonspecific findings on examination of the urine (791.0-791.9)
small kidney of unknown cause (589.0-589.9)
uremia NOS (586)

Workers' Comp Costs per Claim (based on 36 claims)					
Quartile	25%	50%	75%	Mean	% no cost
Indemnity	$5,691	$26,691	$68,534	$49,751	21%
Medical	$10,133	$25,914	$43,880	$49,620	0%
Total	$17,241	$45,854	$126,924	$88,897	0%

788.3 Urinary incontinence

Return-To-Work Summary Guidelines		
Dataset	**Midrange**	**At-Risk**
Claims data	25 days	39 days
All absences	23 days	35 days

Return-To-Work "Best Practice" Guidelines
Medical treatment: 0 days
Urethropexy, clerical/modified work: 21 days
Urethropexy, manual work: 28 days

Description: The involuntary loss of urine in large or small amounts.

Excludes:
that of nonorganic origin (307.6)

RTW Claims Data (Calendar-days away from work by decile)										
10%	20%	30%	40%	**50%**	60%	70%	80%	**90%**	100%	Mean
14	20	21	22	**25**	28	29	30	**39**	365	28.73

788.3 Urinary incontinence *(cont'd)*

Integrated Disability Durations, in days*

Median (mid-point)	23.0	Mean (average)	25.42
Mode (most frequent)	21	Calculated rec.	23

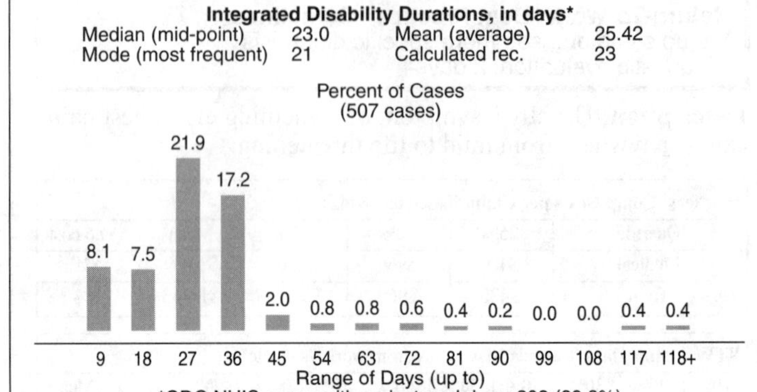

*CDC NHIS cases with no lost workdays: 202 (39.8%)

Impact on Total Absence: Prevalence 0.0229% of total lost workdays; Incidence 0.24 days per 100 workers

789 Other symptoms involving abdomen and pelvis

Return-To-Work Summary Guidelines		
Dataset	**Midrange**	**At-Risk**
Claims data	15 days	91 days
All absences	7 days	47 days

Return-To-Work "Best Practice" Guidelines
See 789.0

The following fifth-digit subclassification is to be used for codes 789.0, 789.3, 789.4, 789.6
- 0 unspecified site
- 1 right upper quadrant
- 2 left upper quadrant
- 3 right lower quadrant
- 4 left lower quadrant
- 5 periumbilic
- 6 epigastric
- 7 generalized
- 9 other specified site
  multiple sites

Excludes:
symptoms referable to genital organs:
female (625.0-625.9)
male (607.0-608.9)
psychogenic (302.70-302.79)

789.0 Abdominal pain

Return-To-Work Summary Guidelines		
Dataset	**Midrange**	**At-Risk**
Claims data	15 days	91 days
All absences	7 days	47 days

Return-To-Work "Best Practice" Guidelines
Without surgery (other diagnoses ruled out): 2 days

Description: Abdominal pain varies in length and location and is a symptom of many other conditions.

Abdominal tenderness
Colic:
NOS
infantile
Cramps, abdominal
Epigastric pain
Umbilical pain

789.0 Abdominal pain *(cont'd)*

Excludes:
renal colic (788.0)

RTW Claims Data (Calendar-days away from work by decile)										
10%	20%	30%	40%	**50%**	60%	70%	80%	**90%**	100%	Mean
9	11	13	14	**15**	21	30	48	**91**	365	39.67

Integrated Disability Durations, in days*
Median (mid-point) 7.0 Mean (average) 20.29
Mode (most frequent) 2 Calculated rec. 9

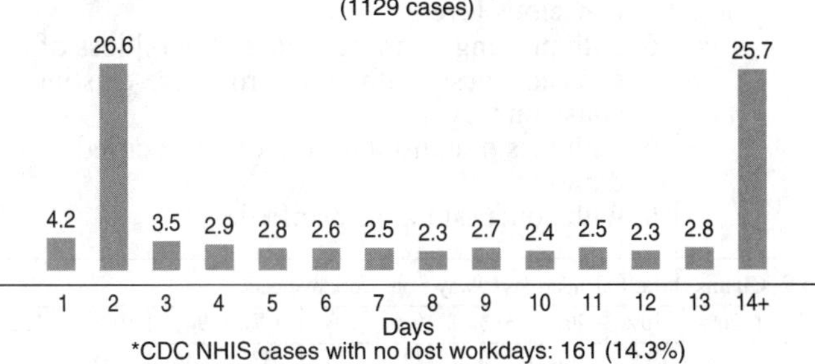

*CDC NHIS cases with no lost workdays: 161 (14.3%)

Impact on Total Absence: Prevalence 0.0580% of total lost workdays; Incidence 0.61 days per 100 workers

Occupational Disability Durations, in days
Median (mid-point) 50 - Benchmark Indemnity Costs $37,500 (60 cases)
Impact on Occupational Absence: Prevalence 0.0340% of occupational lost workdays; Incidence 0.01 days per 100 workers

789.2 Splenomegaly

Return-To-Work Summary Guidelines		
Dataset	**Midrange**	**At-Risk**
Claims data	15 days	73 days
All absences	15 days	67 days

Return-To-Work "Best Practice" Guidelines
"Rule-out" diagnosis: 0 days
Treatment: 14 days

Description: An enlargement of the spleen causing symptoms of upper left abdominal pain and the feeling of being full immediately upon eating.
Other names: Hypersplenism
Enlargement of spleen

RTW Claims Data (Calendar-days away from work by decile)										
10%	20%	30%	40%	**50%**	60%	70%	80%	**90%**	100%	Mean
13	14	14	15	**15**	16	17	25	**73**	365	41.84

789.2 Splenomegaly *(cont'd)*

Integrated Disability Durations, in days*
Median (mid-point) 15.0 Mean (average) 33.98
Mode (most frequent) 14 Calculated rec. 19

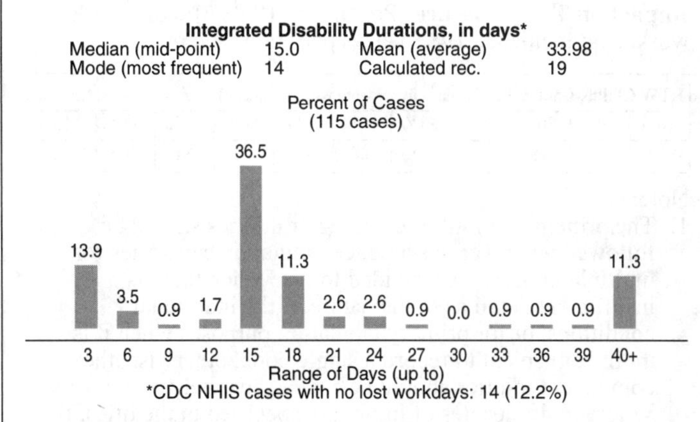

*CDC NHIS cases with no lost workdays: 14 (12.2%)

Impact on Total Absence: Prevalence 0.0101% of total lost workdays; Incidence 0.11 days per 100 workers

17. INJURY AND POISONING (800-999)

Impact on Total Absence: Prevalence 18.8870% of total lost workdays; Incidence 198.31 days per 100 workers

RTW Claims Data (Calendar-days away from work by decile)										
10%	20%	30%	40%	**50%**	60%	70%	80%	**90%**	100%	Mean
10	13	15	17	**21**	29	40	55	**81**	365	37.35

Note:
1. The principle of multiple coding of injuries should be followed wherever possible. Combination categories for multiple injuries are provided for use when there is insufficient detail as to the nature of the individual conditions, or for primary tabulation purposes when it is more convenient to record a single code; otherwise, the component injuries should be coded separately.
   Where multiple sites of injury are specified in the titles, the word "with" indicates involvement of both sites, and the word "and" indicates involvement of either or both sites. The word "finger" includes thumb.
2. Categories for "late effect" of injuries are to be found at 905-909.

FRACTURES (800-829)

Excludes:
malunion (733.81)
nonunion (733.82)
pathologic or spontaneous fracture (733.10-733.19)
The terms "condyle," "coronoid process," "ramus," and "symphysis" indicate the portion of the bone fractured, not the name of the bone involved.
The descriptions "closed" and "open" used in the fourth-digit subdivisions include the following terms:
closed (with or without delayed healing):
comminuted
depressed
elevated
fissured
fracture NOS
greenstick
impacted
linear
march
simple
slipped epiphysis
spiral
open (with or without delayed healing):
compound
infected
missile
puncture
with foreign body
A fracture not indicated as closed or open should be classified as closed.

Occupational Disability Durations, in days
Median (mid-point) 28 - Benchmark Indemnity Costs $21,000

Percent of Cases
(94110 cases)

5.0 | 5.3 | 10.7 | 9.2 | 13.7 | 8.9 | 47.2
1 day | 2 days | 3 to 5 | 6 to 10 | 11 to 20 | 21 to 30 | 31 or more

Range of Days

Impact on Occupational Absence: Prevalence 29.8931% of occupational lost workdays; Incidence 4.78 days per 100 workers

FRACTURE OF SKULL (800-804)

The following fifth-digit subclassification is for use with the appropriate codes in categories 800, 801, 803, and 804:
0 unspecified state of consciousness
1 with no loss of consciousness
2 with brief [less than one hour] loss of consciousness
3 with moderate [1-24 hours] loss of consciousness
4 with prolonged [more than 24 hours] loss of consciousness and return to pre-existing conscious level
5 with prolonged [more than 24 hours] loss of consciousness, without return to pre-existing conscious level
6 with loss of consciousness of unspecified duration
9 with concussion, unspecified

RTW Claims Data (Calendar-days away from work by decile)										
10%	20%	30%	40%	**50%**	60%	70%	80%	**90%**	100%	Mean
11	14	15	17	**20**	22	25	33	**44**	365	24.90

Impact on Total Absence: Prevalence 0.1503% of total lost workdays; Incidence 1.58 days per 100 workers

Occupational Disability Durations, in days
Median (mid-point) 25 - Benchmark Indemnity Costs $18,750

Percent of Cases
(3764 cases)

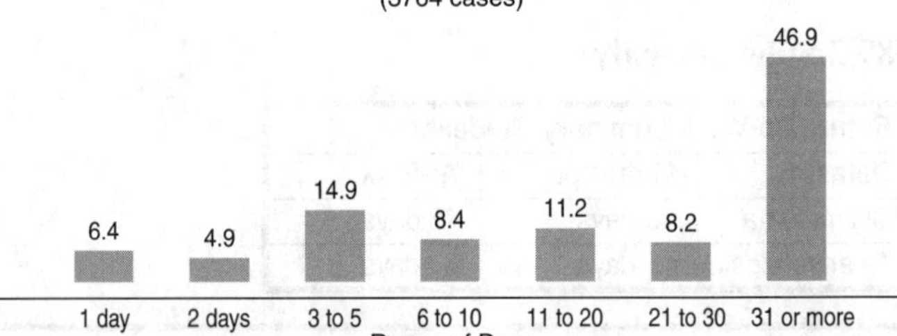

Range of Days

Impact on Occupational Absence: Prevalence 1.0674% of occupational lost workdays; Incidence 0.17 days per 100 workers

802 Fracture of face bones

Return-To-Work Summary Guidelines		
Dataset	**Midrange**	**At-Risk**
Claims data	20 days	38 days
All absences	13 days	30 days

Return-To-Work "Best Practice" Guidelines
Nose, without surgery: 1 day
Rhinoplasty, major septal repair, clerical/modified work: 14 days
Rhinoplasty, major septal repair, manual work: 21 days
Other face bones: 21 days

Description: A break in the bones of the face. Symptoms include swelling, pain, tenderness, temporary or permanent impairment and, sometimes, visible deformity.

Workers' Comp Costs per Claim (based on 2,453 claims)					
Quartile	25%	50%	75%	Mean	% no cost
Indemnity	$977	$2,347	$5,366	$5,612	78%
Medical	$410	$1,008	$3,455	$3,535	2%
Total	$420	$1,113	$4,242	$4,767	2%

802 Fracture of face bones *(cont'd)*

RTW Claims Data (Calendar-days away from work by decile)										
10%	20%	30%	40%	**50%**	60%	70%	80%	**90%**	100%	Mean
11	14	15	16	**20**	21	23	27	**38**	192	21.96

RTW Post Surgery (Calendar-days away from work by decile)										
10%	20%	30%	40%	**50%**	60%	70%	80%	**90%**	100%	Mean
Repair of nasal septum										
6	8	9	11	**13**	17	21	33	**75**	245	27.82

Integrated Disability Durations, in days*
Median (mid-point) 13.0 Mean (average) 14.26
Mode (most frequent) 1 Calculated rec. 10

Percent of Cases
(2155 cases)

20.8 6.0 4.3 3.4 9.6 4.3 7.7 5.1 2.3 1.3 1.2 0.9 0.8 3.9

3 6 9 12 15 18 21 24 27 30 33 36 39 40+
Range of Days (up to)
*CDC NHIS cases with no lost workdays: 608 (28.2%)

Impact on Total Absence: Prevalence 0.0652% of total lost workdays; Incidence 0.68 days per 100 workers

803 Other and unqualified skull fractures

Return-To-Work Summary Guidelines		
Dataset	**Midrange**	**At-Risk**
Claims data	22 days	52 days
All absences	21 days	51 days

Return-To-Work "Best Practice" Guidelines
Without brain injury, clerical/modified work: 7 days
Manual work: 21 days
Heavy manual work: 49 days
With brain injury: See other diagnoses

Description: A break or crack in the skull. Symptoms include swelling, pain, tenderness, temporary or permanent impairment and, sometimes, visible deformity.
Other names: Fractured skull, Cracked skull

Requires fifth digit. See beginning of section 800-804 for codes and definitions.
Includes: skull NOS
skull multiple NOS

Procedure Summary (from ODG Treatment): Activity restrictions; Acupuncture; Anticonvulsants; Antidepressants; Antiepilectics; Bed rest; Behavioral therapy; Botulinum toxin type A; Branched-chain amino acids (BCAAs); Cell transplantation therapy ; Complementary and alternative medicine (CAM); Corticosteroids (for acute traumatic brain injury); Cognitive therapy; Craniectomy; Craniotomy; CT (computed tomography); Decompressive surgery; EEG (Electroencephalography); Field of vision testing; Fluid resuscitation; Glasgow Coma Scale (GCS); Greater occipital nerve block (GONB); Hyperventilation; Hypothermia; Imaging; Interdisciplinary rehabilitation programs; Lumbar puncture; Mannitol; Melatonin; Methylphenidate; Modified Ashworth Scale (MAS); MRI (magnetic resonance imaging); Nutrition; Occupational therapy (OT); Oxygen therapy; PET (positron emission tomography); Physical therapy (PT); QEEG (Quantified Electroencephalography); Relaxation treatment (for

803 Other and unqualified skull fractures *(cont'd)*

migraines); Return to work; Sedation; Skull x-rays; Sleep aids; SPECT (single photon emission computed tomography); Steroids; Triptans; Vision evaluation; Wilsonii injecta; Work

RTW Claims Data (Calendar-days away from work by decile)										
10%	20%	30%	40%	**50%**	60%	70%	80%	**90%**	100%	Mean
13	16	20	21	**22**	33	49	50	**52**	365	40.80

Integrated Disability Durations, in days*
Median (mid-point) 21.0 Mean (average) 33.54
Mode (most frequent) 21 Calculated rec. 24

Percent of Cases
(115 cases)

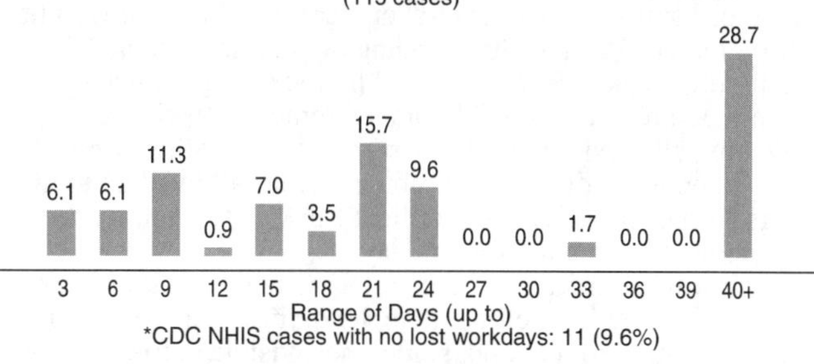

3 6 9 12 15 18 21 24 27 30 33 36 39 40+
Range of Days (up to)
*CDC NHIS cases with no lost workdays: 11 (9.6%)

Impact on Total Absence: Prevalence 0.0103% of total lost workdays; Incidence 0.11 days per 100 workers

FRACTURE OF NECK AND TRUNK (805-809)

RTW Claims Data (Calendar-days away from work by decile)										
10%	20%	30%	40%	**50%**	60%	70%	80%	**90%**	100%	Mean
14	17	26	30	**41**	46	61	92	**137**	365	58.87

Impact on Total Absence: Prevalence 1.1204% of total lost workdays; Incidence 11.77 days per 100 workers

Occupational Disability Durations, in days
Median (mid-point) 21 - Benchmark Indemnity Costs $15,750

Percent of Cases
(11293 cases)

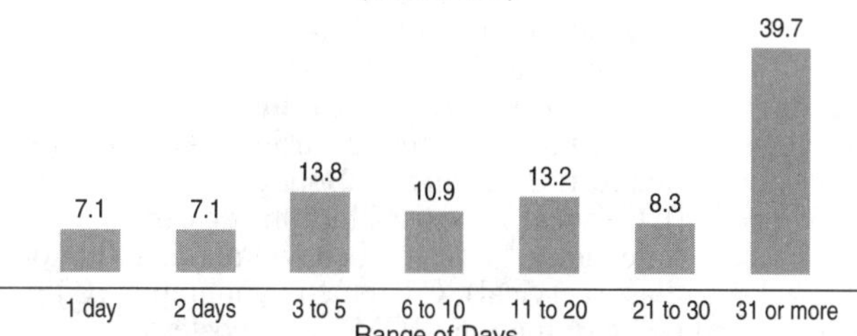

1 day 2 days 3 to 5 6 to 10 11 to 20 21 to 30 31 or more
Range of Days

Impact on Occupational Absence: Prevalence 2.6903% of occupational lost workdays; Incidence 0.43 days per 100 workers

805 Fracture of vertebral column without mention of spinal cord injury

Return-To-Work Summary Guidelines		
Dataset	**Midrange**	**At-Risk**
Claims data	55 days	180 days
All absences	42 days	180 days

Return-To-Work "Best Practice" Guidelines
Stable, clerical/modified work: 0-14 days
Stable, manual work: 28-56 days
Harrington rod placement, clerical/modified work: 120 days
Harrington rod placement, manual work: 180 days
Plus, Harrington rod removal, clerical/modified work: 28 days
Plus, Harrington rod removal, manual work: 42 days

Capabilities & Activity Modifications:

805 Fracture of vertebral column without mention of spinal cord injury *(cont'd)*

Clerical/modified work: No lifting over shoulder; lifting to level of shoulder not more than 5 lbs up to 2 times/hr; standing or walking with a 5-minute break at least every 20 minutes; sitting with a 5-minute break every 30 minutes (using an operator head set if extended phone operations); no extremes of motion including extension or flexion; no extremes of twisting or lateral rotation; no climbing ladders; driving car only up to 2 hrs/day; possible use of cervical collar with change of position and stretching every 30 min; modify workstation or position to eliminate lifting away from body or using twisting motion.
Manual work: Lifting over shoulder not more than 25 lbs up to 15 times/hr; lifting to level of shoulder up to 30 lbs of weight not more than 15 times/hr; standing or walking with a 10-minute break at least every 1-2 hours; sitting with a 10-minute break every 1-2 hours; extremes of flexion or extension allowed up to 20 times/hr; extremes of twisting allowed up to 16 times/hr; climbing ladders allowed up to 40 rungs 8 times/hr; driving car or light truck up to a full work day; driving heavy truck up to 4 hrs/day.
Description: A fracture of the vertebrae in the neck or back. Symptoms include swelling, pain, tenderness, temporary or permanent impairment and, sometimes, visible deformity.
Other names: Broken vertebrae

Includes: neural arch
spine
spinous process
transverse process
vertebra

The following fifth-digit subclassification is for use with codes 805.0-805.1:
0 cervical vertebra, unspecified level
1 first cervical vertebra
2 second cervical vertebra
3 third cervical vertebra
4 fourth cervical vertebra
5 fifth cervical vertebra
6 sixth cervical vertebra
7 seventh cervical vertebra
8 multiple cervical vertebrae

Procedure Summary (from ODG Treatment): Activity restrictions; Acupuncture; Arthrodesis (fusion); Arthroplasty; Back schools; Bed rest; Biofeedback; Bone scan; Botulinum toxin (injection); Cervical orthosis; Chiropractic care; Chymopapain (injection); Cognitive behavioral rehabilitation; Cold packs; Collars (cervical); Computed tomography (CT); Computerized range of motion (ROM); Corticosteroid injection; Decompression; Diathermy; Discography; Disc prosthesis; Discectomy/laminectomy; Education (patient); Electromyography (EMG); Electrotherapies; Electromagnetic therapy (PEMT); Epidural steroid injection (ESI); Ergonomics; Exercise; Facet-joint injections; Facet rhizotomy; Flexibility; Fluoroscopy (for ESI's); Fusion (spinal); H-Reflex tests; Heat/cold applications; High-dose methylprednisolone; Imaging; Immobilization (collars); Injections; Laminectomy; Laminoplasty; Laser therapy; Magnetic resonance imaging (MRI); Manipulation; Manipulation under anesthesia (MUA) ; Massage; Methylprednisolone; Multidisciplinary biopsychosocial (rehabilitation); Myelography; Nonprescription medications; Occupational therapy (OT); Opioids; Oral corticosteroids; Patient education; Percutaneous electrical nerve stimulation (PENS); Percutaneous neuromodulation therapy (PNT); Percutaneous radio-frequency neurotomy; Physical therapy (PT); Prolotherapy (also known as sclerotherapy); Pulsed electromagnetic therapy (PEMT); Radiofrequency neurotomy; Radiography (x-rays); Range of motion (ROM); Rest; Return to work; Sensory evoked potentials (SEPs); Soft collars; Steroids; Stretching; Surface EMG (electromyography); Surgery; Therapeutic exercises; Thermography (diagnostic); Traction; Transcutaneous electrical neurostimulation (TENS); Trigger point injections; Ultrasound, diagnostic (imaging); Ultrasound, therapeutic; Videofluoroscopy (for range of motion); Work
Physical Therapy Guidelines:
Medical treatment: 8 visits over 10 weeks
Post-surgical treatment: 34 visits over 16 weeks

Workers' Comp Costs per Claim (based on 2,508 claims)

Quartile	25%	50%	75%	Mean	% no cost
Indemnity	$3,602	$7,644	$19,058	$17,660	38%
Medical	$1,229	$4,998	$16,758	$16,329	1%
Total	$1,901	$9,303	$26,943	$27,374	1%

RTW Claims Data (Calendar-days away from work by decile)

10%	20%	30%	40%	**50%**	60%	70%	80%	**90%**	100%	Mean
15	25	30	42	**55**	69	110	124	**180**	365	78.49

Integrated Disability Durations, in days*
Median (mid-point) 42.0 Mean (average) 66.38
Mode (most frequent) 1 Calculated rec. 38

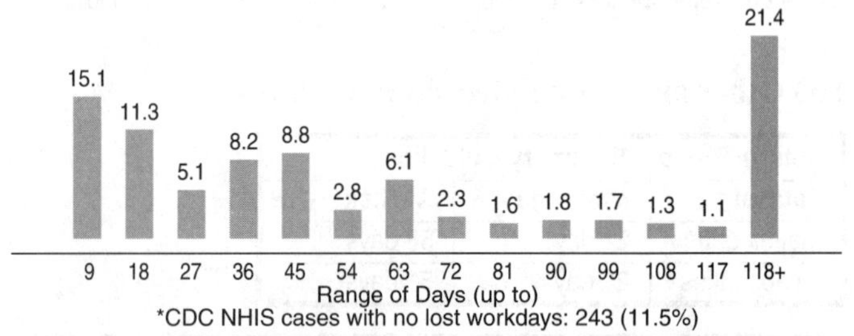

*CDC NHIS cases with no lost workdays: 243 (11.5%)

Impact on Total Absence: Prevalence 0.3675% of total lost workdays; Incidence 3.86 days per 100 workers

806 Fracture of vertebral column with spinal cord injury

Return-To-Work Summary Guidelines		
Dataset	**Midrange**	**At-Risk**
Claims data	123 days	364 days
All absences	116 days	364 days

Return-To-Work "Best Practice" Guidelines
Clerical/modified work: 180 days
Manual work: indefinite

Capabilities & Activity Modifications:
Clerical/modified work: No lifting over shoulder; lifting to level of shoulder not more than 5 lbs up to 2 times/hr; standing or walking with a 5-minute break at least every 20 minutes; sitting with a 5-minute break every 30 minutes (using an operator head set if extended phone operations); no extremes of motion including extension or flexion; no extremes of twisting or lateral rotation; no climbing ladders; driving car only up to 2 hrs/day; possible use of cervical collar with change of position and stretching every 30 min; modify workstation or position to eliminate lifting away from body or using twisting motion.
Manual work: Lifting over shoulder not more than 25 lbs up to 15 times/hr; lifting to level of shoulder up to 30 lbs of weight not more than 15 times/hr; standing or walking with a 10-minute break at least every 1-2 hours; sitting with a 10-minute break every 1-2 hours; extremes of flexion or

806 Fracture of vertebral column with spinal cord injury *(cont'd)*

extension allowed up to 20 times/hr; extremes of twisting allowed up to 16 times/hr; climbing ladders allowed up to 40 rungs 8 times/hr; driving car or light truck up to a full work day; driving heavy truck up to 4 hrs/day.

Includes: any condition classifiable to 805 with:
complete or incomplete transverse lesion (of cord)
hematomyelia
injury to:
cauda equina
nerve
paralysis
paraplegia
quadriplegia
spinal concussion

Procedure Summary (from ODG Treatment): Activity restrictions; Acupuncture; Arthrodesis (fusion); Arthroplasty; Back schools; Bed rest; Biofeedback; Bone scan; Botulinum toxin (injection); Cervical orthosis; Chiropractic care; Chymopapain (injection); Cognitive behavioral rehabilitation; Cold packs; Collars (cervical); Computed tomography (CT); Computerized range of motion (ROM); Corticosteroid injection; Decompression; Diathermy; Discography; Disc prosthesis; Discectomy/laminectomy; Education (patient); Electromyography (EMG); Electrotherapies; Electromagnetic therapy (PEMT); Epidural steroid injection (ESI); Ergonomics; Exercise; Facet-joint injections; Facet rhizotomy; Flexibility; Fluoroscopy (for ESI's); Fusion (spinal); H-Reflex tests; Heat/cold applications; High-dose methylprednisolone; Imaging; Immobilization (collars); Injections; Laminectomy; Laminoplasty; Laser therapy; Magnetic resonance imaging (MRI); Manipulation; Manipulation under anesthesia (MUA) ; Massage; Methylprednisolone; Multidisciplinary biopsychosocial (rehabilitation); Myelography; Nonprescription medications; Occupational therapy (OT); Opioids; Oral corticosteroids; Patient education; Percutaneous electrical nerve stimulation (PENS); Percutaneous neuromodulation therapy (PNT); Percutaneous radio-frequency neurotomy; Physical therapy (PT); Prolotherapy (also known as sclerotherapy); Pulsed electromagnetic therapy (PEMT); Radiofrequency neurotomy; Radiography (x-rays); Range of motion (ROM); Rest; Return to work; Sensory evoked potentials (SEPs); Soft collars; Steroids; Stretching; Surface EMG (electromyography); Surgery; Therapeutic exercises; Thermography (diagnostic); Traction; Transcutaneous electrical neurostimulation (TENS); Trigger point injections; Ultrasound, diagnostic (imaging); Ultrasound, therapeutic; Videofluoroscopy (for range of motion); Work

Physical Therapy Guidelines:
Medical treatment: 8 visits over 10 weeks
Post-surgical treatment: 48 visits over 18 weeks

RTW Claims Data (Calendar-days away from work by decile)

10%	20%	30%	40%	**50%**	60%	70%	80%	**90%**	100%	Mean
21	30	40	53	**123**	179	193	350	**364**	365	156.97

806 Fracture of vertebral column with spinal cord injury *(cont'd)*

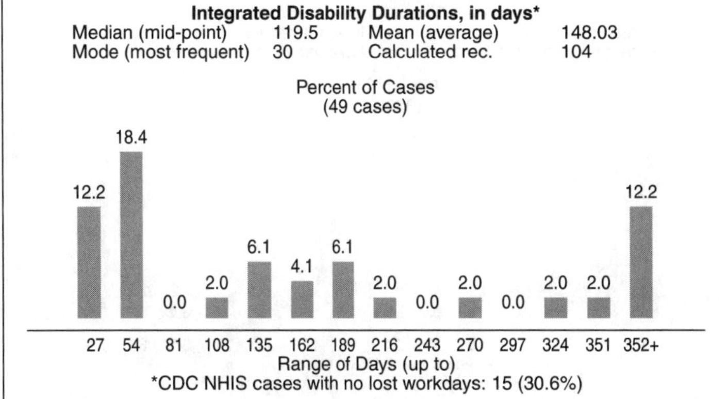

Impact on Total Absence: Prevalence 0.0148% of total lost workdays; Incidence 0.16 days per 100 workers

807 Fracture of rib(s), sternum, larynx, and trachea

Return-To-Work Summary Guidelines		
Dataset	**Midrange**	**At-Risk**
Claims data	28 days	53 days
All absences	15 days	46 days

Return-To-Work "Best Practice" Guidelines
Clerical/modified work: 0-2 days
Manual work: 14 days
Heavy manual work, up to 3 ribs: 28 days
Heavy manual work: 42 days

Description: Broken ribs, larynx, sternum, or trachea. Symptoms include swelling, pain, tenderness, temporary or permanent impairment and, sometimes, visible deformity.
Other names: Broken ribs

The following fifth-digit subclassification is for use with codes 807.0-807.1:
0 rib(s), unspecified
1 one rib
2 two ribs
3 three ribs
4 four ribs
5 five ribs
6 six ribs
7 seven ribs
8 eight or more ribs
9 multiple ribs, unspecified

Physical Therapy Guidelines:
Medical treatment: 8 visits over 10 weeks

Workers' Comp Costs per Claim (based on 3,663 claims)

Quartile	25%	50%	75%	Mean	% no cost
Indemnity	$1,145	$2,200	$4,326	$4,687	70%
Medical	$410	$714	$1,806	$2,149	3%
Total	$431	$945	$3,003	$3,606	3%

RTW Claims Data (Calendar-days away from work by decile)

10%	20%	30%	40%	**50%**	60%	70%	80%	**90%**	100%	Mean
13	14	17	24	**28**	31	41	43	**53**	365	32.49

807 Fracture of rib(s), sternum, larynx, and trachea *(cont'd)*

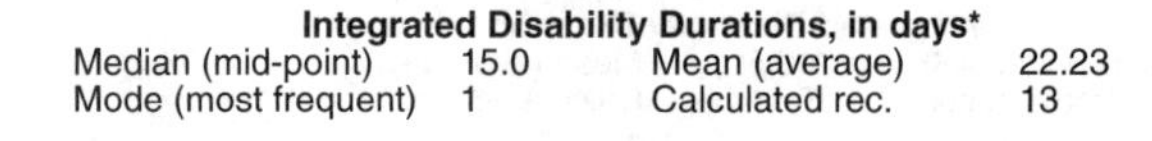

Integrated Disability Durations, in days*
Median (mid-point) 15.0 Mean (average) 22.23
Mode (most frequent) 1 Calculated rec. 13

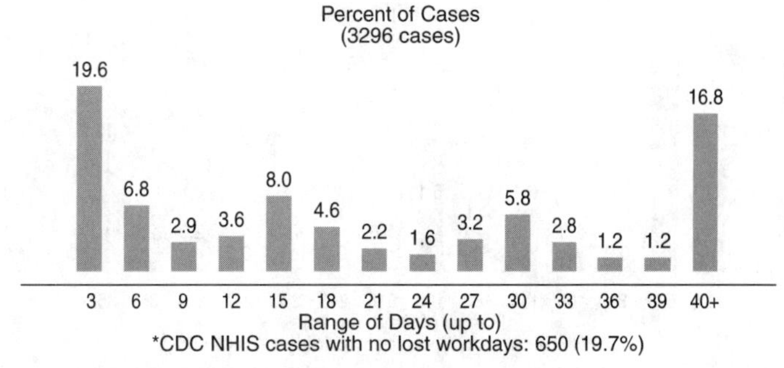

*CDC NHIS cases with no lost workdays: 650 (19.7%)

Impact on Total Absence: Prevalence 0.1738% of total lost workdays; Incidence 1.83 days per 100 workers

808 Fracture of pelvis

Return-To-Work Summary Guidelines		
Dataset	**Midrange**	**At-Risk**
Claims data	61 days	164 days
All absences	59 days	152 days

Return-To-Work "Best Practice" Guidelines
Stress fracture, clerical/modified work: 2 days
Stress fracture, manual work: 14 days
Closed reduction, clerical/modified work: 21 days
Closed reduction, manual work: 28 days
Open reduction, internal fixation, clerical/modified work: 28 days
Open reduction, internal fixation, manual work: 60 days
Arthroplasty, hip, clerical/modified work: 42 days
Arthroplasty, hip, manual work: 84 days

Description: A break in the pelvis bone. Symptoms include swelling, pain, tenderness, temporary or permanent impairment and, sometimes, visible deformity.
Other names: Broken pelvis, Fractured pelvis
Physical Therapy Guidelines:
Medical treatment: 18 visits over 8 weeks
Post-surgical treatment: 24 visits over 10 weeks

Workers' Comp Costs per Claim (based on 749 claims)					
Quartile	25%	50%	75%	Mean	% no cost
Indemnity	$4,515	$9,335	$23,531	$20,365	26%
Medical	$3,486	$11,839	$38,483	$28,509	1%
Total	$5,985	$19,236	$53,571	$43,405	0%

RTW Claims Data (Calendar-days away from work by decile)										
10%	20%	30%	40%	**50%**	60%	70%	80%	**90%**	100%	Mean
16	25	37	48	**61**	82	93	116	**164**	365	76.57

RTW Post Surgery (Calendar-days away from work by decile)										
10%	20%	30%	40%	**50%**	60%	70%	80%	**90%**	100%	Mean
Treat pelvic ring fracture										
20	45	51	66	**83**	100	174	286	**365**	365	134.48

808 Fracture of pelvis *(cont'd)*

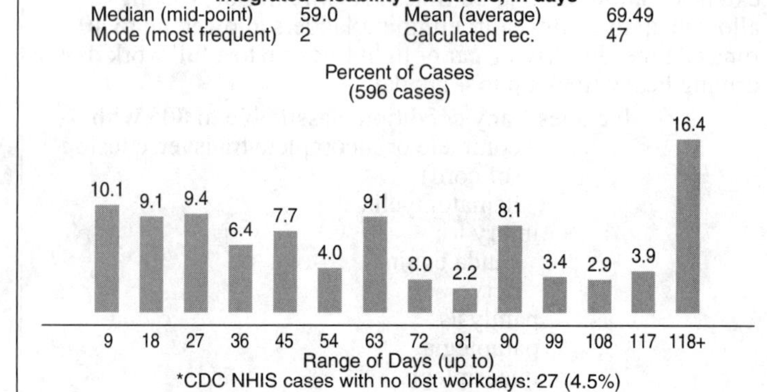

*CDC NHIS cases with no lost workdays: 27 (4.5%)

Impact on Total Absence: Prevalence 0.1168% of total lost workdays; Incidence 1.23 days per 100 workers

FRACTURE OF UPPER LIMB (810-819)

RTW Claims Data (Calendar-days away from work by decile)										
10%	20%	30%	40%	**50%**	60%	70%	80%	**90%**	100%	Mean
13	16	21	25	**33**	42	47	59	**80**	365	41.58

Impact on Total Absence: Prevalence 1.9001% of total lost workdays; Incidence 19.95 days per 100 workers

Occupational Disability Durations, in days
Median (mid-point) 23 - Benchmark Indemnity Costs $17,250

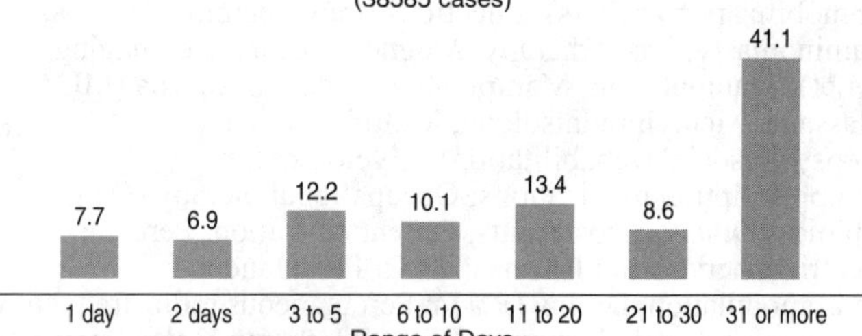

Impact on Occupational Absence: Prevalence 10.0675% of occupational lost workdays; Incidence 1.61 days per 100 workers

810 Fracture of clavicle

Return-To-Work Summary Guidelines		
Dataset	**Midrange**	**At-Risk**
Claims data	41 days	71 days
All absences	31 days	65 days

Return-To-Work "Best Practice" Guidelines
Closed, without manipulation, clerical/modified work: 14 days
Closed, without manipulation, manual work: 42 days

Description: A fracture of the collarbone. Symptoms include swelling, pain, tenderness, temporary or permanent impairment and, sometimes, visible deformity.
Other names: Broken collarbone

Includes: collar bone
interligamentous part of clavicle

The following fifth-digit subclassification is for use with category 810:
0 unspecified part
Clavicle NOS
1 sternal end of clavicle
2 shaft of clavicle
3 acromial end of clavicle

810 Fracture of clavicle *(cont'd)*

Procedure Summary (from ODG Treatment):
Acromioplasty; Activity restrictions; Acupuncture; Adson's test (AT); Anterior scalene block; Arthrography; Arthroplasty (shoulder); Arthroscopy; Arthroscopic release of adhesions; Bipolar interferential electrotherapy; Biofeedback; Biopsychosocial rehab; Cardiovascular functional testing; Chiropractic; Cold lasers; Continuous-flow cryotherapy; Continuous passive motion (CPM); Corticosteroid injections; Costoclavicular maneuver (CCM); Cutaneous laser treatment; Deep friction massage; Diagnostic arthroscopy; Diathermy; Distension arthrography; Electrical stimulation; Electrodiagnostic testing for TOS (thoracic outlet syndrome); Elevated arm stress test (EAST); Ergonomic interventions; Exercises; Extracorporeal shock wave therapy (ESWT); Hydroplasty/ hydrodilation; Imaging; Immobilization; Impingement test; Injections; Interferential therapy; Laser therapy; Low level laser therapy (LLLT); Magnetic resonance imaging (MRI); Manipulation; Manipulation under anesthesia (MUA); Massage; Mechanical traction; Modified duty; Multidisciplinary biopsychosocial rehab; Nerve blocks; Osteochondral autologous transplantation (OATS); Physical therapy; Porcine small intestinal submucosa (SIS); Pulsed electromagnetic field; Radiography; Return to work; Rotator cuff repair; Rotator cuff porcine graft repair; Shock wave therapy; Shoulder repair; Steroid injections; Supraclavicular pressure (SCP); Surgery for AC joint separation; Surgery for adhesive capsulitis; Surgery for impingement syndrome; Surgery for rotator cuff repair; Surgery for ruptured biceps tendon; Surgery for shoulder dislocation; Surgery for Thoracic Outlet Syndrome; Thermal capsulorrhaphy; Thermotherapy; Transcutaneous electrical neurostimulation (TENS); Transdermal nitroglycerin; Ultrasound, diagnostic; Ultrasound, therapeutic; Work

Physical Therapy Guidelines:
8 visits over 10 weeks

Workers' Comp Costs per Claim (based on 574 claims)

Quartile	25%	50%	75%	Mean	% no cost
Indemnity	$2,205	$4,610	$9,072	$8,573	51%
Medical	$872	$1,838	$5,198	$5,250	1%
Total	$998	$3,518	$10,553	$9,479	1%

RTW Claims Data (Calendar-days away from work by decile)

10%	20%	30%	40%	**50%**	60%	70%	80%	**90%**	100%	Mean
13	15	17	28	**41**	42	44	48	**71**	365	40.43

Integrated Disability Durations, in days*

Median (mid-point)	31.0	Mean (average)	35.09
Mode (most frequent)	42	Calculated rec.	35

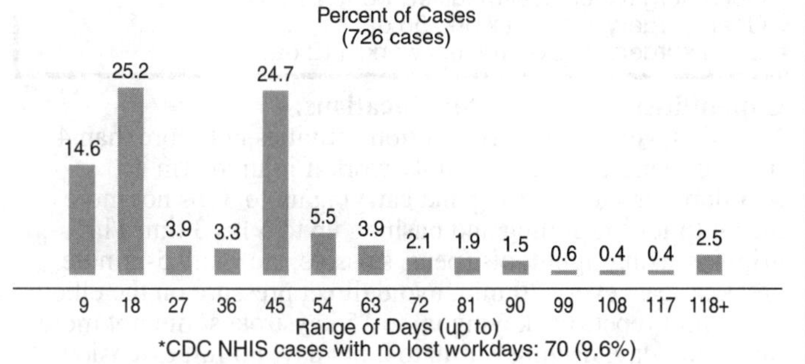

*CDC NHIS cases with no lost workdays: 70 (9.6%)

Impact on Total Absence: Prevalence 0.0680% of total lost workdays; Incidence 0.71 days per 100 workers

811 Fracture of scapula

Return-To-Work Summary Guidelines

Dataset	Midrange	At-Risk
Claims data	42 days	81 days
All absences	27 days	74 days

Return-To-Work "Best Practice" Guidelines
Stable, clerical/modified work: 1 day
Stable, manual work: 21 days
Heavy manual work: 42 days

Description: A fracture of the shoulder blade. Symptoms include swelling, pain, tenderness, temporary or permanent impairment and, sometimes, visible deformity.
Other names: Broken shoulder blade

Includes: shoulder blade
The following fifth-digit subclassification is for use with category 811:
0 unspecified part
1 acromial process
  Acromion (process)
2 coracoid process
3 glenoid cavity and neck of scapula
9 other

Workers' Comp Costs per Claim (based on 367 claims)

Quartile	25%	50%	75%	Mean	% no cost
Indemnity	$2,552	$6,216	$11,739	$11,452	50%
Medical	$1,155	$2,888	$11,204	$8,563	1%
Total	$1,628	$4,646	$16,002	$14,348	1%

RTW Claims Data (Calendar-days away from work by decile)

10%	20%	30%	40%	**50%**	60%	70%	80%	**90%**	100%	Mean
17	21	25	35	**42**	44	53	66	**81**	300	49.30

Integrated Disability Durations, in days*

Median (mid-point)	27.0	Mean (average)	36.34
Mode (most frequent)	1	Calculated rec.	23

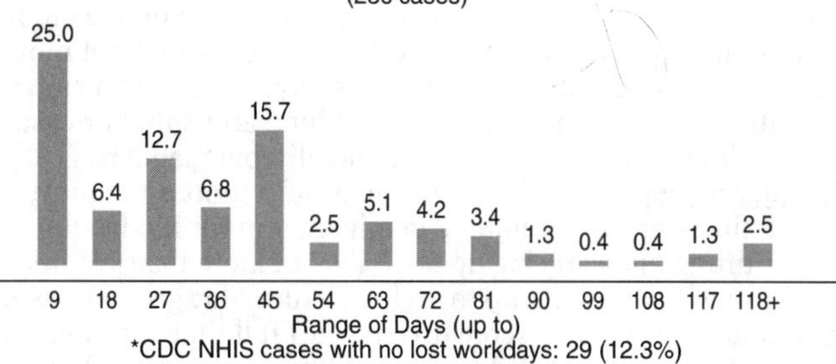

*CDC NHIS cases with no lost workdays: 29 (12.3%)

Impact on Total Absence: Prevalence 0.0222% of total lost workdays; Incidence 0.23 days per 100 workers

811 Fracture of scapula *(cont'd)*

Occupational Disability Durations, in days
Median (mid-point) 15 - Benchmark Indemnity Costs $11,250

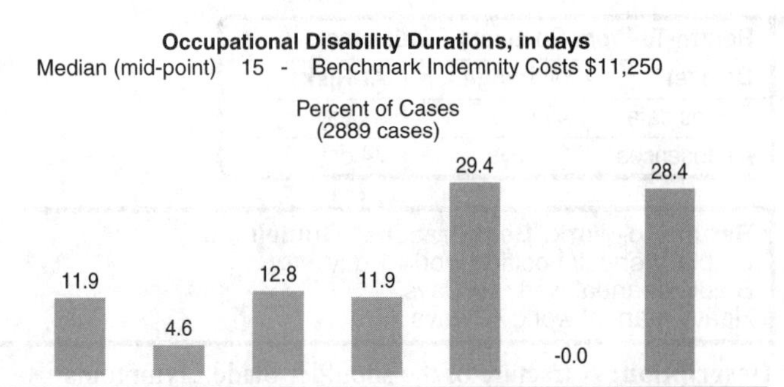

Impact on Occupational Absence: Prevalence 0.4916% of occupational lost workdays; Incidence 0.08 days per 100 workers

812 Fracture of humerus

Return-To-Work Summary Guidelines

Dataset	Midrange	At-Risk
Claims data	24 days	55 days
All absences	16 days	48 days

Return-To-Work "Best Practice" Guidelines
Stress fracture, clerical/modified work: 2 days
Stress fracture, manual work: 14 days
Closed reduction, clerical/modified work, non-dominant hand: 3 days
Closed reduction, clerical/modified work, dominant hand: 7 days
Closed reduction, manual work: 42 days
Open reduction, clerical/modified work: 21 days
Open reduction, manual work: 42 days

Capabilities & Activity Modifications:
Modified work: Repetitive motion activities not more than 4 times/hr; single upper extremity work if injured arm is non-dominant arm; lifting and carrying up to 3 lbs not more than 4 times/hr; pulling and pushing up to 5 lbs 3 times/hr; gripping using light tools (pens, scissors, etc) with 5-minute break at least every 20 min; avoid direct pressure on the elbow area; limit repetitive keying up to 15 keystrokes/min not more than 2 hrs/day; driving car up to 2 hrs/day; no full extension activities; possible immobilization by long arm splint or cast, tennis elbow splint, or wrist splint; no climbing ladders.
Regular manual work: Repetitive motion activities not more than 8 times/hr; use of injured dominant arm for moderate work; lifting and carrying up to 20 lbs not more than 15 times/hr; pulling and pushing up to 40 lbs 15 times/hr; gripping using moderate tools (pliers, screwdrivers, etc) full time; driving car or light truck up to 6 hrs/day or heavy truck up to 4 hrs/day; full extension activities up to 12 times/hr with up to 10 lbs of weight; possible immobilization by sling, wrist splint, or tennis elbow splint; climbing ladders up to 50 rungs/hr.
Description: A fracture of the upper arm bone. Symptoms include swelling, pain, tenderness, temporary or permanent impairment and, sometimes, visible deformity.
Other names: Broken humerus, Broken upper arm
Procedure Summary (from ODG Treatment): Activity restrictions; Arthroplasty (elbow); Chiropractic; Cold packs; Deep transverse friction massage; Education; Electrical stimulation (E-STIM); Exercise; Fractures of humerus; Fractures of radius; Imaging; Iontophoresis; Laser doppler imaging (LDI); Manipulation; MRI's; Neural tension; Night splints; Nonprescription medications; Patient education; Phonophoresis; Physical therapy; Radiography; Return to work;

812 Fracture of humerus *(cont'd)*

Stretching; Surgery; Total elbow replacement (TER); Transcutaneous electrical neurostimulation (TENS); Ultrasound, diagnostic; Ultrasound, therapeutic; Work
Physical Therapy Guidelines:
Medical treatment: 18 visits over 12 weeks
Post-surgical treatment: 24 visits over 14 weeks

Workers' Comp Costs per Claim (based on 2,339 claims)

Quartile	25%	50%	75%	Mean	% no cost
Indemnity	$2,636	$5,061	$10,910	$11,419	42%
Medical	$1,722	$4,211	$11,508	$10,641	1%
Total	$2,436	$6,699	$17,493	$17,285	1%

RTW Claims Data (Calendar-days away from work by decile)

10%	20%	30%	40%	**50%**	60%	70%	80%	**90%**	100%	Mean
12	14	17	21	**24**	34	42	44	**55**	193	30.79

Integrated Disability Durations, in days*
Median (mid-point) 16.0 Mean (average) 22.21
Mode (most frequent) 2 Calculated rec. 14

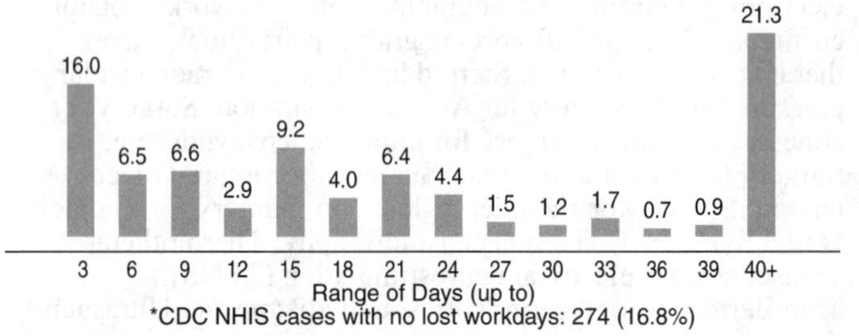

*CDC NHIS cases with no lost workdays: 274 (16.8%)

Impact on Total Absence: Prevalence 0.0890% of total lost workdays; Incidence 0.93 days per 100 workers

813 Fracture of radius and ulna

Return-To-Work Summary Guidelines

Dataset	Midrange	At-Risk
Claims data	42 days	112 days
All absences	29 days	111 days

Return-To-Work "Best Practice" Guidelines
Stable, clerical/modified work: 2 days
Stable, manual work: 14 days
Reduction/manipulation, clerical/modified work: 14 days
Reduction/manipulation, manual work: 28 days
Reduction/manipulation, heavy manual work: 42 days
Open surgery, clerical/modified work: 21 days
Open surgery, manual work: 56 days
Open surgery, heavy manual work: 112 days

Capabilities & Activity Modifications:
Modified work: Repetitive motion activities not more than 4 times/hr; single upper extremity work if injured arm is non-dominant arm; lifting and carrying up to 3 lbs not more than 4 times/hr; pulling and pushing up to 5 lbs 3 times/hr; gripping using light tools (pens, scissors, etc) with 5-minute break at least every 20 min; avoid direct pressure on the elbow area; limit repetitive keying up to 15 keystrokes/min not more than 2 hrs/day; driving car up to 2 hrs/day; no full extension activities; possible immobilization by long arm splint or cast, tennis elbow splint, or wrist splint; no climbing ladders.
Regular manual work: Repetitive motion activities not more than 8 times/hr; use of injured dominant arm for moderate work; lifting and carrying up to 20 lbs not more than 15 times/hr; pulling and pushing up to 40 lbs 15 times/hr; gripping using

813 Fracture of radius and ulna *(cont'd)*

moderate tools (pliers, screwdrivers, etc) full time; driving car or light truck up to 6 hrs/day or heavy truck up to 4 hrs/day; full extension activities up to 12 times/hr with up to 10 lbs of weight; possible immobilization by sling, wrist splint, or tennis elbow splint; climbing ladders up to 50 rungs/hr.
Description: A fracture of one of the two bones in the lower arm. Symptoms include swelling, pain, tenderness, temporary or permanent impairment and, sometimes, visible deformity.
Other names: Broken arm
Procedure Summary (from ODG Treatment): Activity restrictions; Arthroplasty (elbow); Chiropractic; Cold packs; Deep transverse friction massage; Education; Electrical stimulation (E-STIM); Exercise; Fractures of humerus; Fractures of radius; Imaging; Iontophoresis; Laser doppler imaging (LDI); Manipulation; MRI's; Neural tension; Night splints; Nonprescription medications; Patient education; Phonophoresis; Physical therapy; Radiography; Return to work; Stretching; Surgery; Total elbow replacement (TER); Transcutaneous electrical neurostimulation (TENS); Ultrasound, diagnostic; Ultrasound, therapeutic; Work
Physical Therapy Guidelines:
Post-surgical treatment: 16 visits over 8 weeks

Workers' Comp Costs per Claim (based on 9,855 claims)

Quartile	25%	50%	75%	Mean	% no cost
Indemnity	$1,775	$3,612	$7,329	$7,312	55%
Medical	$1,071	$1,969	$6,237	$5,643	1%
Total	$1,229	$3,192	$9,440	$8,985	1%

RTW Claims Data (Calendar-days away from work by decile)

10%	20%	30%	40%	**50%**	60%	70%	80%	**90%**	100%	Mean
14	18	25	31	**42**	53	61	87	**112**	365	53.27

RTW Post Surgery (Calendar-days away from work by decile)

10%	20%	30%	40%	**50%**	60%	70%	80%	**90%**	100%	Mean
Remove bone fixation device										
30	42	51	76	**87**	110	151	220	**305**	365	125.68
Treat radius fracture										
10	17	25	44	**61**	82	115	151	**320**	365	101.48
Treat ulnar fracture										
11	19	38	53	**78**	108	138	195	**249**	365	108.52
Treat fracture radius/ulna										
5	13	31	50	**66**	81	106	140	**212**	365	90.07
7	15	39	54	**66**	83	97	123	**191**	365	87.05
9	20	39	59	**80**	103	129	180	**304**	365	113.07

813 Fracture of radius and ulna *(cont'd)*

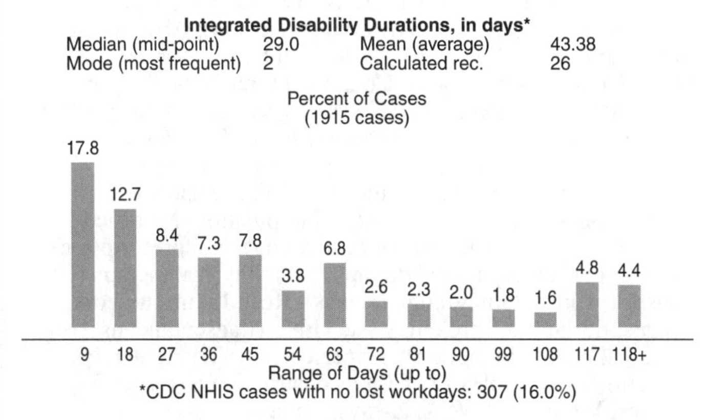

Impact on Total Absence: Prevalence 0.2062% of total lost workdays; Incidence 2.17 days per 100 workers

814 Fracture of carpal bone(s)

Return-To-Work Summary Guidelines		
Dataset	**Midrange**	**At-Risk**
Claims data	27 days	62 days
All absences	18 days	58 days

Return-To-Work "Best Practice" Guidelines
Stable, clerical/modified work: 1 day
Stable, manual work: 7 days
Reduction/manipulation, clerical/modified work: 7 days
Reduction/manipulation, manual work: 21 days
Reduction/manipulation, heavy manual work: 56 days

Capabilities & Activity Modifications:
Modified work: Repetitive motion activities (w or w/o splint) not more than 4 times/hr; repetitive keying up to 15 keystrokes/min not more than 2 hrs/day; gripping and using light tools (pens, scissors, etc.) with 5-minute break at least every 20 min; no pinching; driving car up to 2 hrs/day; light work up to 5 lbs 3 times/hr; avoidance of prolonged periods in wrist flexion or extension.
Regular work (if not cause or aggravating to disability) : Repetitive motion activities not more than 25 times/hr; repetitive keying up to 45 keystrokes/min 8 hrs/day; gripping and using moderate tools (pliers, screwdrivers, etc.) fulltime; pinching up to 5 times/min; driving car or light truck up to 6 hrs/day or heavy truck up to 3 hrs/day; moderate to heavy work up to 35 lbs not more than 7 times/hr.
Description: A fracture in the wrist. Symptoms include swelling, pain, tenderness, temporary or permanent impairment and, sometimes, visible deformity.
Other names: Broken wrist

The following fifth-digit subclassification is for use with category 814:

0 carpal bone, unspecified
  Wrist NOS
1 navicular [scaphoid] of wrist
2 lunate [semilunar] bone of wrist
3 triquetral [cuneiform] bone of wrist
4 pisiform
5 trapezium bone [larger multangular]
6 trapezoid bone [smaller multangular]
7 capitate bone [os magnum]
8 hamate [unciform] bone
9 other

814 Fracture of carpal bone(s) *(cont'd)*

Procedure Summary (from ODG Treatment): Activity restrictions; Acupuncture; Arthrodesis (fusion); Arthroplasty (joint replacement); Casting versus splints; Chiropractic (manipulation); Cold packs; Computed tomography (CT); Continuous passive motion (CPM); de Quervain's tenosynovitis surgery; Dupuytren's release (fasciectomy); Ergonomic interventions; Exercises; Fasciotomy; Fusion; Imaging; Immobilization (treatment); Injection; Joint replacement; Mallet finger injuries (treatment); Manipulation; Modified duty; MRI's (magnetic resonance imaging); Nonprescription medications; Occupational therapy (OT); Physical therapy (PT); Plaster casting; Radiography (x-rays); Rest; Return to work; Splints; Surgery for broken wrist; TENS (transcutaneous electrical neurostimulation); Trapeziectomy; Triangular fibrocartilage complex (TFCC) reconstruction ; Trigger finger surgery; Vitamin C; Work; X-rays; Yoga

Physical Therapy Guidelines:
Medical treatment: 8 visits over 10 weeks
Post-surgical treatment: 16 visits over 10 weeks

Workers' Comp Costs per Claim (based on 2,823 claims)

Quartile	25%	50%	75%	Mean	% no cost
Indemnity	$1,890	$3,817	$7,571	$7,273	67%
Medical	$798	$1,271	$2,436	$3,032	1%
Total	$882	$1,544	$4,872	$5,475	1%

RTW Claims Data (Calendar-days away from work by decile)

10%	20%	30%	40%	**50%**	60%	70%	80%	**90%**	100%	Mean
12	16	21	22	**27**	42	48	57	**62**	282	37.09

Integrated Disability Durations, in days*
Median (mid-point) 18.0 Mean (average) 24.83
Mode (most frequent) 1 Calculated rec. 15

Percent of Cases
(2736 cases)

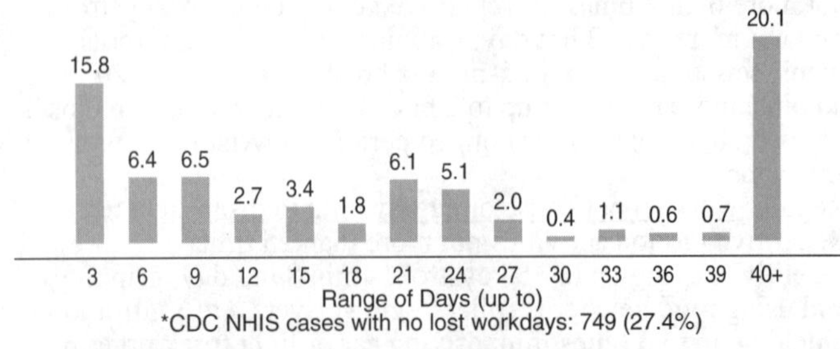

*CDC NHIS cases with no lost workdays: 749 (27.4%)

Impact on Total Absence: Prevalence 0.1458% of total lost workdays; Incidence 1.53 days per 100 workers

815 Fracture of metacarpal bone(s)

Return-To-Work Summary Guidelines

Dataset	Midrange	At-Risk
Claims data	30 days	61 days
All absences	22 days	54 days

Return-To-Work "Best Practice" Guidelines
Single, closed, without reduction, clerical/modified work: 2 days
Single, closed, without reduction, manual work: 21 days
Single, closed, without reduction, regular work if cause of disability: 42 days
Single, open, clerical/modified work: 28 days
Single, open, manual work: 42 days

815 Fracture of metacarpal bone(s) *(cont'd)*

Description: A fracture in the hand (excluding the finger). Symptoms include swelling, pain, tenderness, temporary or permanent impairment and, sometimes, visible deformity.
Other names: Broken hand

Includes: hand [except finger]
metacarpus

The following fifth-digit subclassification is for use with category 815:
0 metacarpal bone(s), site unspecified
1 base of thumb [first] metacarpal
Bennett's fracture
2 base of other metacarpal bone(s)
3 shaft of metacarpal bone(s)
4 neck of metacarpal bone(s)
9 multiple sites of metacarpus

Physical Therapy Guidelines:
Medical treatment: 9 visits over 3 weeks
Post-surgical treatment: 16 visits over 10 weeks

Workers' Comp Costs per Claim (based on 4,609 claims)

Quartile	25%	50%	75%	Mean	% no cost
Indemnity	$1,260	$2,394	$4,683	$5,463	65%
Medical	$683	$1,061	$2,237	$2,804	2%
Total	$756	$1,344	$4,221	$4,763	2%

RTW Claims Data (Calendar-days away from work by decile)

10%	20%	30%	40%	**50%**	60%	70%	80%	**90%**	100%	Mean
14	20	23	27	**30**	39	42	46	**61**	365	36.59

RTW Post Surgery (Calendar-days away from work by decile)

10%	20%	30%	40%	**50%**	60%	70%	80%	**90%**	100%	Mean
Treat metacarpal fracture										
4	17	26	36	**44**	52	70	86	**97**	255	53.56
Treat metacarpal fracture										
6	12	19	33	**41**	56	64	88	**145**	365	66.42

Integrated Disability Durations, in days*
Median (mid-point) 22.0 Mean (average) 26.63
Mode (most frequent) 2 Calculated rec. 18

Percent of Cases
(1888 cases)

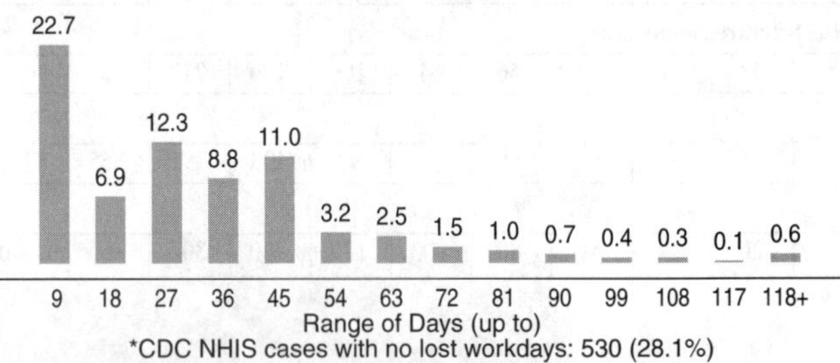

*CDC NHIS cases with no lost workdays: 530 (28.1%)

Impact on Total Absence: Prevalence 0.1068% of total lost workdays; Incidence 1.12 days per 100 workers

816 Fracture of one or more phalanges of hand

Return-To-Work Summary Guidelines

Dataset	Midrange	At-Risk
Claims data	27 days	71 days
All absences	14 days	63 days

816 Fracture of one or more phalanges of hand

Return-To-Work "Best Practice" Guidelines
Tuft fracture: 0 days
Closed, without reduction, clerical/modified work: 2 days
Closed, without reduction, manual work: 21 days
Closed, without reduction, regular work if cause of disability: 42 days
Open, clerical/modified work: 14 days
Open, manual work: 42 days
Open, regular work if cause of disability: 70 days

Capabilities & Activity Modifications:
Modified work: Repetitive motion activities (w or w/o splint) not more than 4 times/hr; repetitive keying up to 15 keystrokes/min not more than 2 hrs/day; gripping and using light tools (pens, scissors, etc.) with 5-minute break at least every 20 min; no pinching; driving car up to 2 hrs/day; light work up to 5 lbs 3 times/hr; avoidance of prolonged periods in wrist flexion or extension.
Regular work (if not cause or aggravating to disability) : Repetitive motion activities not more than 25 times/hr; repetitive keying up to 45 keystrokes/min 8 hrs/day; gripping and using moderate tools (pliers, screwdrivers, etc.) fulltime; pinching up to 5 times/min; driving car or light truck up to 6 hrs/day or heavy truck up to 3 hrs/day; moderate to heavy work up to 35 lbs not more than 7 times/hr.
Description: A fracture in one of the fingers or the thumb. Symptoms include swelling, pain, tenderness, temporary or permanent impairment and, sometimes, visible deformity.
Other names: Broken finger, Broken thumb

Includes: finger(s)
thumb

The following fifth-digit subclassification is for use with category 816:

0 phalanx or phalanges, unspecified
1 middle or proximal phalanx or phalanges
2 distal phalanx or phalanges
3 multiple sites

Procedure Summary (from ODG Treatment): Activity restrictions; Acupuncture; Arthrodesis (fusion); Arthroplasty (joint replacement); Casting versus splints; Chiropractic (manipulation); Cold packs; Computed tomography (CT); Continuous passive motion (CPM); de Quervain's tenosynovitis surgery; Dupuytren's release (fasciectomy); Ergonomic interventions; Exercises; Fasciotomy; Fusion; Imaging; Immobilization (treatment); Injection; Joint replacement; Mallet finger injuries (treatment); Manipulation; Modified duty; MRI's (magnetic resonance imaging); Nonprescription medications; Occupational therapy (OT); Physical therapy (PT); Plaster casting; Radiography (x-rays); Rest; Return to work; Splints; Surgery for broken wrist; TENS (transcutaneous electrical neurostimulation); Trapeziectomy; Triangular fibrocartilage complex (TFCC) reconstruction ; Trigger finger surgery; Vitamin C; Work; X-rays; Yoga
Physical Therapy Guidelines:
Minor, 8 visits over 5 weeks
Post-surgical treatment: Complicated, 16 visits over 10 weeks

Workers' Comp Costs per Claim (based on 25,939 claims)

Quartile	25%	50%	75%	Mean	% no cost
Indemnity	$935	$1,985	$4,127	$4,139	79%
Medical	$431	$725	$1,313	$1,637	3%
Total	$441	$798	$1,838	$2,521	3%

RTW Claims Data (Calendar-days away from work by decile)

10%	20%	30%	40%	**50%**	60%	70%	80%	**90%**	100%	Mean
13	15	19	22	**27**	40	43	54	**71**	365	37.13

816 Fracture of one or more phalanges of hand

RTW Post Surgery (Calendar-days away from work by decile)

10%	20%	30%	40%	**50%**	60%	70%	80%	**90%**	100%	Mean
Debride skin/muscle/bone, fx										
2	5	10	14	**21**	34	55	77	**116**	365	51.56
Repair finger tendon										
4	10	18	22	**40**	54	69	87	**146**	365	63.00
Treat finger fracture, each										
5	9	16	26	**44**	51	67	84	**156**	365	60.66
Treat finger fracture, each										
4	10	17	29	**41**	55	73	96	**159**	365	65.94
Treat finger fracture, each										
4	12	20	30	**40**	59	72	91	**164**	365	65.72
Pin finger fracture, each										
6	11	17	23	**28**	42	51	59	**75**	160	39.00
Treat finger fracture, each										
2	4	7	14	**22**	33	46	61	**89**	365	39.09

Integrated Disability Durations, in days*

Median (mid-point)	14.0	Mean (average)	23.58
Mode (most frequent)	1	Calculated rec.	13

Percent of Cases
(3486 cases)

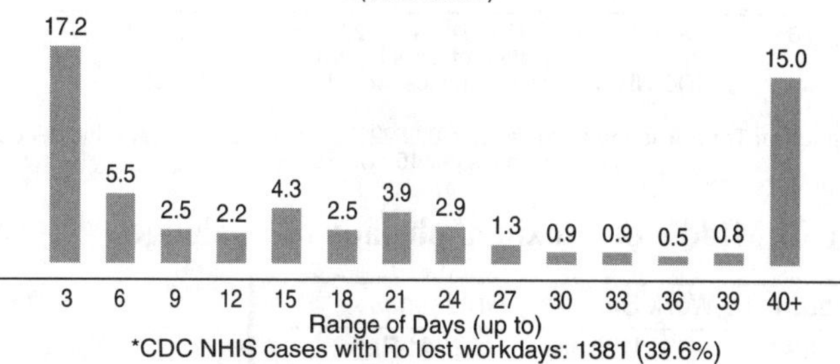

Impact on Total Absence: Prevalence 0.1467% of total lost workdays; Incidence 1.54 days per 100 workers

816.0 Closed

Return-To-Work Summary Guidelines

Dataset	Midrange	At-Risk
Claims data	26 days	71 days
All absences	9 days	56 days

Return-To-Work "Best Practice" Guidelines
See 816

Workers' Comp Costs per Claim (based on 18,858 claims)

Quartile	25%	50%	75%	Mean	% no cost
Indemnity	$872	$1,764	$3,192	$2,850	83%
Medical	$368	$609	$1,019	$1,131	3%
Total	$378	$651	$1,271	$1,616	3%

RTW Claims Data (Calendar-days away from work by decile)

10%	20%	30%	40%	**50%**	60%	70%	80%	**90%**	100%	Mean
12	14	18	21	**26**	36	43	55	**71**	106	34.56

816.0 Closed *(cont'd)*

RTW Post Surgery (Calendar-days away from work by decile)										
10%	20%	30%	40%	**50%**	60%	70%	80%	**90%**	100%	Mean
Treat finger fracture, each										
6	10	16	27	**44**	51	67	90	**156**	365	61.44
Treat finger fracture, each										
6	13	22	33	**42**	53	63	83	**131**	365	59.20
Treat finger fracture, each										
7	13	18	26	**32**	44	62	72	**146**	365	55.66
Treat finger fracture, each										
2	5	8	16	**25**	30	39	59	**94**	365	38.56

Integrated Disability Durations, in days*

Median (mid-point)	9.0	Mean (average)	19.00
Mode (most frequent)	1	Calculated rec.	10

Percent of Cases
(1913 cases)

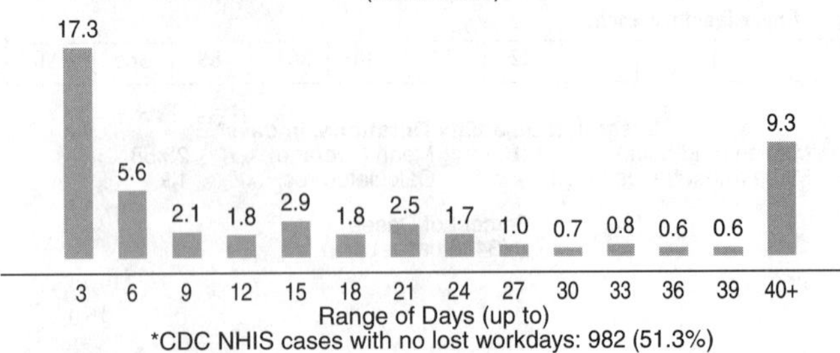

Impact on Total Absence: Prevalence 0.0522% of total lost workdays; Incidence 0.55 days per 100 workers

816.01 Middle or proximal phalanx or phalanges

Return-To-Work Summary Guidelines		
Dataset	**Midrange**	**At-Risk**
Claims data	41 days	76 days
All absences	17 days	60 days

Return-To-Work "Best Practice" Guidelines
Casting/surgery, clerical/modified work: 7 days
Casting/surgery, manual work: 42 days
Casting/surgery, heavy manual work: 56 days

Description: Fracture of the middle or proximal bones in the fingers or toes.
Other names: Broken finger, Broken toe

Workers' Comp Costs per Claim (based on 3,747 claims)					
Quartile	25%	50%	75%	Mean	% no cost
Indemnity	$1,050	$2,258	$4,074	$3,530	74%
Medical	$473	$788	$1,743	$1,887	2%
Total	$494	$893	$3,014	$2,836	2%

RTW Claims Data (Calendar-days away from work by decile)										
10%	20%	30%	40%	**50%**	60%	70%	80%	**90%**	100%	Mean
11	16	22	32	**41**	44	55	57	**76**	102	40.29

RTW Post Surgery (Calendar-days away from work by decile)										
10%	20%	30%	40%	**50%**	60%	70%	80%	**90%**	100%	Mean
Treat finger fracture, each										
5	9	16	23	**44**	51	60	78	**114**	365	54.02
Treat finger fracture, each										
5	10	20	32	**43**	54	65	78	**146**	365	62.46

816.01 Middle or proximal phalanx or phalanges *(cont'd)*

Integrated Disability Durations, in days*

Median (mid-point)	17.0	Mean (average)	27.18
Mode (most frequent)	2	Calculated rec.	16

Percent of Cases
(353 cases)

10.8
6.2 5.9
2.5 2.0 1.7 1.7 1.1 1.7 0.8 0.8 0.8 1.1
19.5
3 6 9 12 15 18 21 24 27 30 33 36 39 40+
Range of Days (up to)
*CDC NHIS cases with no lost workdays: 152 (43.1%)

Impact on Total Absence: Prevalence 0.0161% of total lost workdays; Incidence 0.17 days per 100 workers

816.02 Distal phalanx or phalanges

Return-To-Work Summary Guidelines		
Dataset	**Midrange**	**At-Risk**
Claims data	22 days	60 days
All absences	6 days	41 days

Return-To-Work "Best Practice" Guidelines
Splinting, clerical/modified work: 2 days
Splinting, manual work: 21 days

Description: Fracture of the bones at the top of the fingers or toes.
Other names: Broken finger, Broken toe

Workers' Comp Costs per Claim (based on 7,047 claims)					
Quartile	25%	50%	75%	Mean	% no cost
Indemnity	$830	$1,554	$2,699	$2,286	85%
Medical	$368	$588	$945	$888	2%
Total	$378	$620	$1,134	$1,248	2%

RTW Claims Data (Calendar-days away from work by decile)										
10%	20%	30%	40%	**50%**	60%	70%	80%	**90%**	100%	Mean
11	15	20	21	**22**	24	31	44	**60**	102	29.60

RTW Post Surgery (Calendar-days away from work by decile)										
10%	20%	30%	40%	**50%**	60%	70%	80%	**90%**	100%	Mean
Treat finger fracture, each										
3	6	13	19	**25**	33	39	58	**75**	160	34.94

816.02 Distal phalanx or phalanges *(cont'd)*

Integrated Disability Durations, in days*

Median (mid-point)	6.0	Mean (average)	15.47
Mode (most frequent)	2	Calculated rec.	7

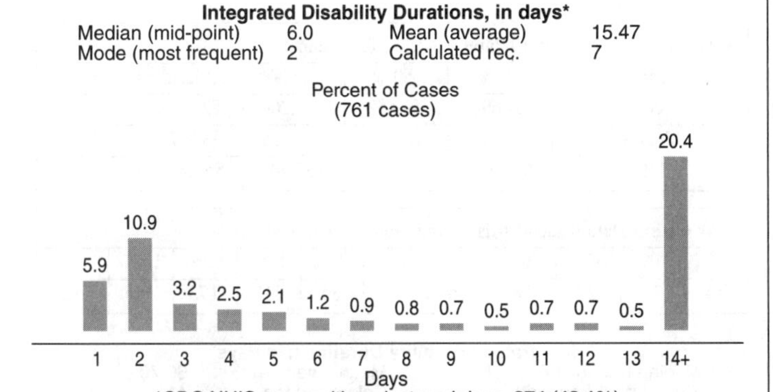

*CDC NHIS cases with no lost workdays: 374 (49.1%)

Impact on Total Absence: Prevalence 0.0176% of total lost workdays; Incidence 0.19 days per 100 workers

818 Ill-defined fractures of upper limb

Return-To-Work Summary Guidelines		
Dataset	**Midrange**	**At-Risk**
Claims data	27 days	43 days
All absences	16 days	43 days

Return-To-Work "Best Practice" Guidelines
Stable, clerical/modified work: 2 days
Stable, manual work: 14 days
Reduction/manipulation, clerical/modified work: 14 days
Reduction/manipulation, manual work: 28 days
Reduction/manipulation, heavy manual work: 42 days

Description: Non-specific fracture of bones in an upper limb such as the arm. Symptoms include swelling, pain, tenderness, temporary or permanent impairment and, sometimes, visible deformity.

Includes: arm NOS
multiple bones of same upper limb

Excludes:
multiple fractures of:
metacarpal bone(s) with phalanx or phalanges (817.0-817.1)
phalanges of hand alone (816.0-816.1)
radius with ulna (813.0-813.9)

Physical Therapy Guidelines:
8 visits over 10 weeks

RTW Claims Data (Calendar-days away from work by decile)										
10%	20%	30%	40%	**50%**	60%	70%	80%	**90%**	100%	Mean
13	14	15	16	**27**	28	30	42	**43**	277	26.39

818 Ill-defined fractures of upper limb *(cont'd)*

Integrated Disability Durations, in days*

Median (mid-point)	16.0	Mean (average)	21.52
Mode (most frequent)	14	Calculated rec.	17

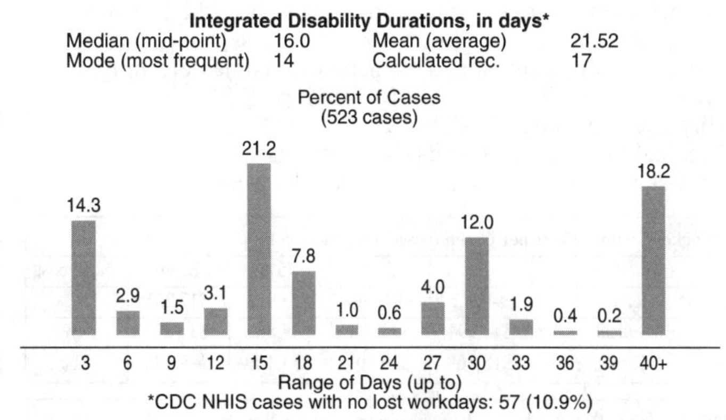

*CDC NHIS cases with no lost workdays: 57 (10.9%)

Impact on Total Absence: Prevalence 0.0296% of total lost workdays; Incidence 0.31 days per 100 workers

FRACTURE OF LOWER LIMB (820-829)

RTW Claims Data (Calendar-days away from work by decile)										
10%	20%	30%	40%	**50%**	60%	70%	80%	**90%**	100%	Mean
13	17	22	33	**42**	54	68	84	**104**	365	53.37

Impact on Total Absence: Prevalence 3.6290% of total lost workdays; Incidence 38.11 days per 100 workers

Occupational Disability Durations, in days
Median (mid-point) 24 - Benchmark Indemnity Costs $18,000

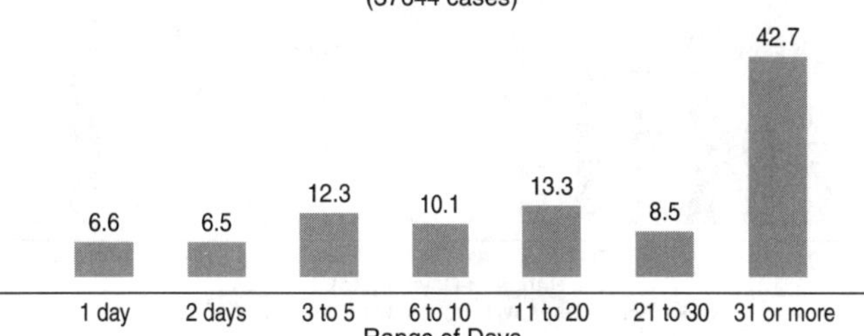

Impact on Occupational Absence: Prevalence 10.2490% of occupational lost workdays; Incidence 1.64 days per 100 workers

820 Fracture of neck of femur

Return-To-Work Summary Guidelines		
Dataset	**Midrange**	**At-Risk**
Claims data	44 days	196 days
All absences	43 days	195 days

Return-To-Work "Best Practice" Guidelines
Closed reduction, clerical/modified work: 28 days
Closed reduction, manual work: 42 days
Open reduction, internal fixation, clerical/modified work: 28 days
Open reduction, internal fixation, manual work: 84 days
Open reduction, internal fixation, heavy manual work: 196 days
Plus, removal of internal fixation, clerical/modified work: 7 days
Plus, removal of internal fixation, manual work: 21 days
Arthroplasty, hip, clerical/modified work: 42 days
Arthroplasty, hip, manual work: 84 days

820 Fracture of neck of femur *(cont'd)*

Description: Fracture of the top of the femur (thigh bone). Symptoms include swelling, pain, tenderness, temporary or permanent impairment and, sometimes, visible deformity.
Other names: Broken thigh, Broken hip
Physical Therapy Guidelines:
Medical treatment: 18 visits over 8 weeks
Post-surgical treatment: 24 visits over 10 weeks

Workers' Comp Costs per Claim (based on 885 claims)

Quartile	25%	50%	75%	Mean	% no cost
Indemnity	$4,242	$8,736	$18,953	$17,261	21%
Medical	$14,994	$23,294	$34,860	$31,877	0%
Total	$18,669	$29,799	$53,109	$45,431	0%

RTW Claims Data (Calendar-days away from work by decile)

10%	20%	30%	40%	**50%**	60%	70%	80%	**90%**	100%	Mean
15	22	28	38	**44**	79	85	116	**196**	365	73.79

RTW Post Surgery (Calendar-days away from work by decile)

10%	20%	30%	40%	**50%**	60%	70%	80%	**90%**	100%	Mean
Treat thigh fracture										
55	71	84	102	**127**	141	174	222	**321**	365	149.29

Integrated Disability Durations, in days*
Median (mid-point) 43.0 Mean (average) 70.49
Mode (most frequent) 28 Calculated rec. 46

Percent of Cases
(1176 cases)

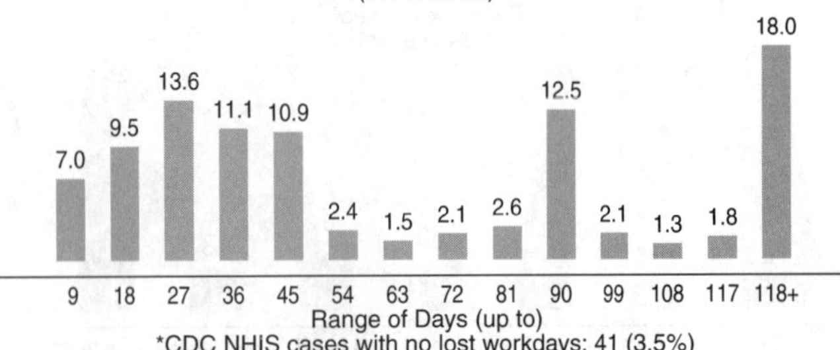

Range of Days (up to)
*CDC NHIS cases with no lost workdays: 41 (3.5%)

Impact on Total Absence: Prevalence 0.2364% of total lost workdays; Incidence 2.48 days per 100 workers

821 Fracture of other and unspecified parts of femur

Return-To-Work Summary Guidelines		
Dataset	**Midrange**	**At-Risk**
Claims data	45 days	173 days
All absences	42 days	161 days

Return-To-Work "Best Practice" Guidelines
Closed reduction, clerical/modified work (accomodating foot elevation): 7 days
Closed reduction, clerical/modified work (after bed rest/ traction): 14 days
Closed reduction, manual work: 42 days
Open reduction, internal fixation, clerical/modified work: 28 days
Open reduction, internal fixation, manual work: 84 days
Plus, removal of internal fixation, clerical/modified work: 7 days
Plus, removal of internal fixation, manual work: 21 days

Description: Fracture of the thighbone. Symptoms include swelling, pain, tenderness, temporary or permanent impairment and, sometimes, visible deformity.
Other names: Broken thigh, Broken upper leg
Physical Therapy Guidelines:
Post-surgical treatment: 30 visits over 12 weeks

821 Fracture of other and unspecified parts of femur *(cont'd)*

Workers' Comp Costs per Claim (based on 635 claims)

Quartile	25%	50%	75%	Mean	% no cost
Indemnity	$4,694	$9,482	$27,206	$21,338	24%
Medical	$7,098	$22,334	$42,935	$35,624	1%
Total	$12,338	$29,516	$65,447	$51,875	1%

RTW Claims Data (Calendar-days away from work by decile)

10%	20%	30%	40%	**50%**	60%	70%	80%	**90%**	100%	Mean
14	20	28	38	**45**	76	85	117	**173**	365	74.24

Integrated Disability Durations, in days*
Median (mid-point) 42.0 Mean (average) 66.70
Mode (most frequent) 14 Calculated rec. 41

Percent of Cases
(452 cases)

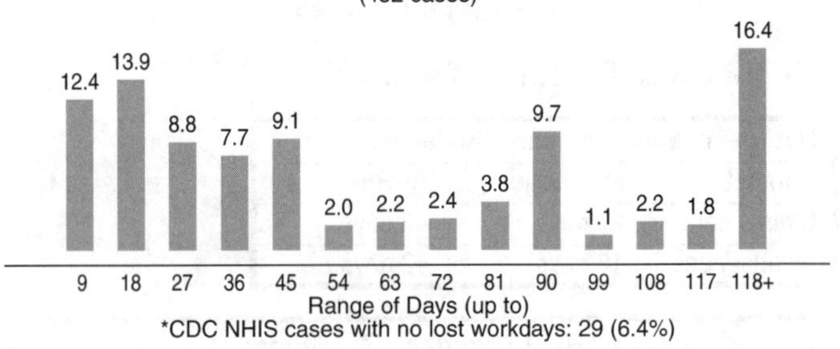

Range of Days (up to)
*CDC NHIS cases with no lost workdays: 29 (6.4%)

Impact on Total Absence: Prevalence 0.0833% of total lost workdays; Incidence 0.88 days per 100 workers

822 Fracture of patella

Return-To-Work Summary Guidelines		
Dataset	**Midrange**	**At-Risk**
Claims data	42 days	88 days
All absences	37 days	86 days

Return-To-Work "Best Practice" Guidelines
Sedentary/modified work: 7 days
Standing work: 21-42 days
Heavy standing work: 42-84 days

Capabilities & Activity Modifications:
Sedentary/modified work: Standing limited to 5-10 min/hr; walking only on a smooth surface using crutches with limited pressure on the foot; no walking on an irregular surface; no climbing stairs; no climbing ladders or hill climbing requiring frequent knee flexion; no activities requiring balance; no applying strength against bent knee (squatting, kneeling, crouching, stooping, pedaling, etc.); elevate leg half of time; may need immobilization; limited weight bearing.
Manual/standing work: Standing not more than 50 min/hr; walking on a smooth surface up to 1,200 ft/hr carrying up to 25 lbs; walking on an irregular surface up to 900 ft/hr carrying up to 25 lbs; climbing stairs up to 8 flights/hr carrying up to 40 lbs; climbing ladders up to 50 rungs/hr carrying up to 25 lbs; activities requiring balance up to 45 min/hr (if able to work with two hands without assistance for balance); applying strength against bent knee (pedaling, squatting, kneeling, etc.) up to 60 times/hr; may need brace for uneven ground or ladders.
Description: Fracture of the knee. Symptoms include swelling, pain, tenderness, temporary or permanent impairment and, sometimes, visible deformity.
Other names: Broken knee
Procedure Summary (from ODG Treatment): ACI; Activity restrictions; Anterior cruciate ligament (ACL) repair; ACL diagnostic tests; ACL injury rehabilitation; Acupuncture;

822 Fracture of patella *(cont'd)*

Arthroplasty; Arthroscopy; Autologous cartilage implantation (ACI); Bone-growth stimulators; Braces; Canes; Cetylated fatty acids (CFA) topical cream; Chiropractic; Chondroplasty; Cold/ heat packs; Cold lasers; Continuous-flow cryotherapy; Continuous passive motion (CPM); Corticosteroid injections; Crutches; Deep transverse friction massage (DTFM); Diagnostic arthroscopy; Education for knee replacement; Electromyographic biofeedback treatment; Exercise; Glucosamine; Hyaluronic acid injections; Imaging; Immobilization; Injections; Insoles; Interferential current therapy (IFC); Knee brace; Knee joint replacement; KT 1000 arthrometer; Lachman test; Lateral pull test and patellar tilt test; Lateral retinacular release; Low level laser therapy (LLLT); Magnet therapy; Manipulation; Meniscal allograft transplantation; Meniscectomy; Microprocessor-controlled knee prostheses; Modified duty; Mosaicplasty; MRI's (magnetic resonance imaging); Non-surgical intervention for PFPS (patellofemoral pain syndrome); Occupational therapy; Orthoses; Osteochondral autograft transplant system (OATS); Osteotomy; Pharmacotherapy; Physical therapy; Pivot shift test (MacIntosh test) ; Posterior cruciate ligament (PCL) repair; Post-op ambulatory infusion pumps (local anesthetic); Prolotherapy; Prostheses (artificial limb); Pulsed magnetic field therapy (PMFT); Radiography; Return to work; SAMe (S-adenosylmethionine); Single photon emission computed tomography (SPECT); Static progressive stretch (SPS) therapy; Stretching and flexibility; Surgery; SynviscÒ; Therapeutic knee splint; Therapeutic ultrasound; Transcutaneous electrical neurostimulation (TENS); Ultrasound, diagnostic; Ultrasound, therapeutic; Ultrasound fracture healing (bone-growth stimulators); Viscosupplementation; Walkers; Walking aids (canes, crutches, braces, orthoses, & walkers); Work

Physical Therapy Guidelines:
Post-surgical treatment: 10 visits over 8 weeks

Workers' Comp Costs per Claim (based on 1,368 claims)

Quartile	25%	50%	75%	Mean	% no cost
Indemnity	$2,205	$4,263	$8,253	$7,520	45%
Medical	$1,250	$2,825	$10,101	$7,623	1%
Total	$1,733	$5,345	$15,089	$11,832	1%

RTW Claims Data (Calendar-days away from work by decile)

10%	20%	30%	40%	**50%**	60%	70%	80%	**90%**	100%	Mean
13	20	23	35	**42**	46	63	83	**88**	365	49.15

RTW Post Surgery (Calendar-days away from work by decile)

10%	20%	30%	40%	**50%**	60%	70%	80%	**90%**	100%	Mean
Treat kneecap fracture										
19	45	54	73	**86**	97	122	170	**253**	365	109.38

Integrated Disability Durations, in days*

Median (mid-point) 37.0 Mean (average) 42.15
Mode (most frequent) 42 Calculated rec. 40

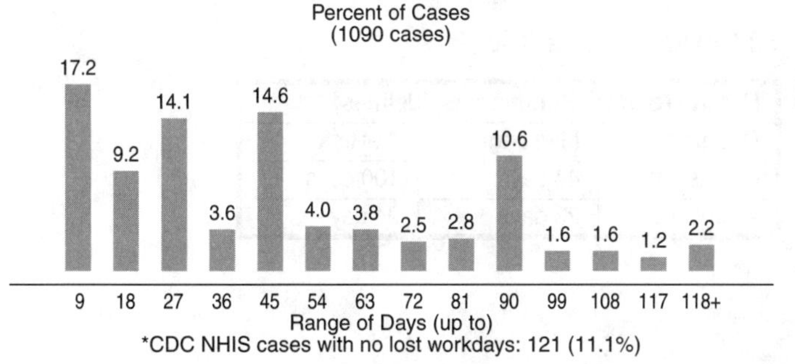

*CDC NHIS cases with no lost workdays: 121 (11.1%)

Impact on Total Absence: Prevalence 0.1207% of total lost workdays; Incidence 1.27 days per 100 workers

823 Fracture of tibia and fibula

Return-To-Work Summary Guidelines		
Dataset	**Midrange**	**At-Risk**
Claims data	45 days	119 days
All absences	40 days	108 days

Return-To-Work "Best Practice" Guidelines
Fibula, closed, clerical/modified work: 7 days
Fibula, closed, manual work: 42 days
Fibula, with surgery, clerical/modified work: 14 days
Fibula, with surgery, manual work: 70 days
Tibia, closed, clerical/modified work: 14 days
Tibia, closed, manual work: 63 days
Tibia, with surgery, clerical/modified work: 21 days
Tibia, with surgery, manual work: 119 days

Capabilities & Activity Modifications:
Sedentary/modified work: Standing limited to 5-10 min/hr; walking only on a smooth surface using crutches with limited pressure on the foot; no walking on an irregular surface; no climbing stairs; no climbing ladders or hill climbing requiring frequent knee flexion; no activities requiring balance; no applying strength against bent knee (squatting, kneeling, crouching, stooping, pedaling, etc.); elevate leg half of time; may need immobilization; limited weight bearing.
Manual/standing work: Standing not more than 50 min/hr; walking on a smooth surface up to 1,200 ft/hr carrying up to 25 lbs; walking on an irregular surface up to 900 ft/hr carrying up to 25 lbs; climbing stairs up to 8 flights/hr carrying up to 40 lbs; climbing ladders up to 50 rungs/hr carrying up to 25 lbs; activities requiring balance up to 45 min/hr (if able to work with two hands without assistance for balance); applying strength against bent knee (pedaling, squatting, kneeling, etc.) up to 60 times/hr; may need brace for uneven ground or ladders.

Description: Fracture of one of the bones in the lower leg. Symptoms include swelling, pain, tenderness, temporary or permanent impairment and, sometimes, visible deformity.

Other names: Broken leg

Excludes:
Dupuytren's fracture (824.4-824.5)
ankle (824.4-824.5)
radius (813.42, 813.52)
Pott's fracture (824.4-824.5)
that involving ankle (824.0-824.9)

The following fifth-digit subclassification is for use with category 823:
0 tibia alone
1 fibula alone
2 fibula with tibia

Procedure Summary (from ODG Treatment): ACI; Activity restrictions; Anterior cruciate ligament (ACL) repair; ACL diagnostic tests; ACL injury rehabilitation; Acupuncture; Arthroplasty; Arthroscopy; Autologous cartilage implantation (ACI); Bone-growth stimulators; Braces; Canes; Cetylated fatty acids (CFA) topical cream; Chiropractic; Chondroplasty; Cold/ heat packs; Cold lasers; Continuous-flow cryotherapy; Continuous passive motion (CPM); Corticosteroid injections; Crutches; Deep transverse friction massage (DTFM); Diagnostic arthroscopy; Education for knee replacement; Electromyographic biofeedback treatment; Exercise; Glucosamine; Hyaluronic acid injections; Imaging; Immobilization; Injections; Insoles; Interferential current therapy (IFC); Knee brace; Knee joint replacement; KT 1000 arthrometer; Lachman test; Lateral pull test and patellar tilt test; Lateral retinacular release; Low level laser therapy (LLLT); Magnet therapy; Manipulation; Meniscal allograft transplantation; Meniscectomy; Microprocessor-controlled knee prostheses; Modified duty; Mosaicplasty; MRI's

823 Fracture of tibia and fibula *(cont'd)*

(magnetic resonance imaging); Non-surgical intervention for PFPS (patellofemoral pain syndrome); Occupational therapy; Orthoses; Osteochondral autograft transplant system (OATS); Osteotomy; Pharmacotherapy; Physical therapy; Pivot shift test (MacIntosh test) ; Posterior cruciate ligament (PCL) repair; Post-op ambulatory infusion pumps (local anesthetic); Prolotherapy; Prostheses (artificial limb); Pulsed magnetic field therapy (PMFT); Radiography; Return to work; SAMe (S-adenosylmethionine); Single photon emission computed tomography (SPECT); Static progressive stretch (SPS) therapy; Stretching and flexibility; Surgery; SynviscÒ; Therapeutic knee splint; Therapeutic ultrasound; Transcutaneous electrical neurostimulation (TENS); Ultrasound, diagnostic; Ultrasound, therapeutic; Ultrasound fracture healing (bone-growth stimulators); Viscosupplementation; Walkers; Walking aids (canes, crutches, braces, orthoses, & walkers); Work

Physical Therapy Guidelines:
Medical treatment: 30 visits over 12 weeks
Post-surgical treatment (ORIF): 30 visits over 12 weeks

Workers' Comp Costs per Claim (based on 3,431 claims)

Quartile	25%	50%	75%	Mean	% no cost
Indemnity	$3,161	$7,072	$16,580	$14,428	36%
Medical	$1,659	$5,014	$19,173	$16,670	1%
Total	$2,573	$9,917	$28,581	$25,930	1%

RTW Claims Data (Calendar-days away from work by decile)

10%	20%	30%	40%	**50%**	60%	70%	80%	**90%**	100%	Mean
14	18	24	40	**45**	61	66	76	**118**	365	55.36

RTW Post Surgery (Calendar-days away from work by decile)

10%	20%	30%	40%	**50%**	60%	70%	80%	**90%**	100%	Mean
Remove bone fixation device										
57	86	117	140	**184**	275	365	365	**365**	365	213.58
Treatment of tibia fracture										
36	71	96	124	**141**	166	214	321	**365**	365	170.62

Integrated Disability Durations, in days*
Median (mid-point) 40.0 Mean (average) 47.05
Mode (most frequent) 7 Calculated rec. 34

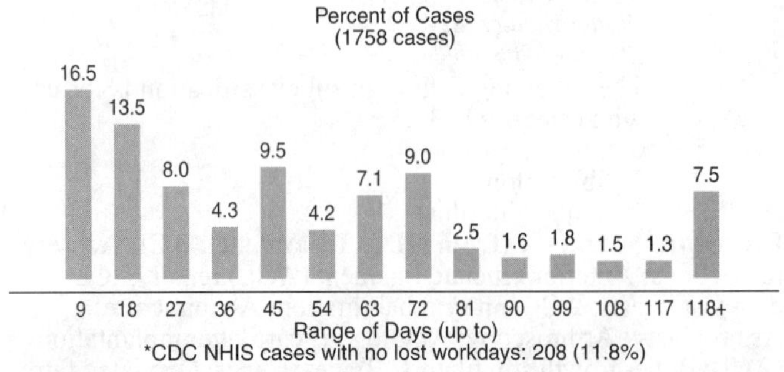

*CDC NHIS cases with no lost workdays: 208 (11.8%)

Impact on Total Absence: Prevalence 0.2155% of total lost workdays; Incidence 2.26 days per 100 workers

823.2 Shaft, closed

Return-To-Work Summary Guidelines		
Dataset	**Midrange**	**At-Risk**
Claims data	46 days	103 days
All absences	42 days	102 days

Return-To-Work "Best Practice" Guidelines
Closed reduction of shaft, clerical/modified work: 14 days
Closed reduction of shaft, manual work: 42-63 days

823.2 Shaft, closed *(cont'd)*

Workers' Comp Costs per Claim (based on 648 claims)

Quartile	25%	50%	75%	Mean	% no cost
Indemnity	$3,896	$7,686	$17,745	$14,466	30%
Medical	$1,701	$8,285	$21,336	$16,352	1%
Total	$3,297	$13,608	$34,220	$26,310	0%

RTW Claims Data (Calendar-days away from work by decile)

10%	20%	30%	40%	**50%**	60%	70%	80%	**90%**	100%	Mean
14	20	32	41	**46**	57	64	82	**103**	173	54.22

Integrated Disability Durations, in days*
Median (mid-point) 42.0 Mean (average) 47.95
Mode (most frequent) 14 Calculated rec. 36

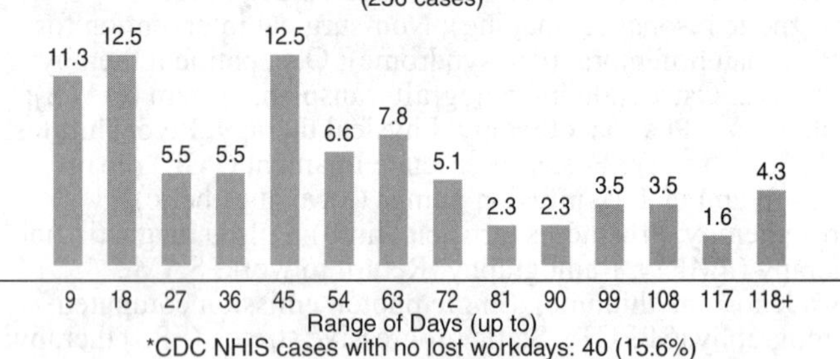

*CDC NHIS cases with no lost workdays: 40 (15.6%)

Impact on Total Absence: Prevalence 0.0306% of total lost workdays; Incidence 0.32 days per 100 workers

823.3 Shaft, open

Return-To-Work Summary Guidelines		
Dataset	**Midrange**	**At-Risk**
Claims data	54 days	124 days
All absences	54 days	124 days

Return-To-Work "Best Practice" Guidelines
Open reduction of shaft, clerical/modified work: 14-28 days
Open reduction of shaft, manual work: 70-119 days

Workers' Comp Costs per Claim (based on 152 claims)

Quartile	25%	50%	75%	Mean	% no cost
Indemnity	$9,965	$21,315	$41,139	$31,462	16%
Medical	$18,407	$39,968	$84,620	$67,866	0%
Total	$24,686	$61,231	$119,847	$94,215	0%

RTW Claims Data (Calendar-days away from work by decile)

10%	20%	30%	40%	**50%**	60%	70%	80%	**90%**	100%	Mean
20	32	32	35	**54**	73	93	101	**124**	142	65.58

Impact on Total Absence: Prevalence 0.0023% of total lost workdays; Incidence 0.02 days per 100 workers

824 Fracture of ankle

Return-To-Work Summary Guidelines		
Dataset	**Midrange**	**At-Risk**
Claims data	44 days	100 days
All absences	23 days	94 days

824 Fracture of ankle *(cont'd)*

Return-To-Work "Best Practice" Guidelines
Closed reduction, sedentary/modified work: 1-7 days
Closed reduction, standing work w/o cast: 21 days
Open reduction, internal fixation, sedentary/modified work: 14 days
Open reduction, internal fixation, standing work w/o cast: 84 days
Comorbidity fracture blister, add: 21 days

Capabilities & Activity Modifications:
Sedentary/modified work: Standing limited to 5-10 min/hr; walking only on a smooth surface using crutches with limited pressure on the foot; no walking on an irregular surface; no climbing stairs; no climbing ladders or hill climbing requiring frequent knee flexion; no activities requiring balance; no applying strength against bent knee (squatting, kneeling, crouching, stooping, pedaling, etc.); elevate leg half of time; may need immobilization; limited weight bearing.
Manual/standing work: Standing not more than 50 min/hr; walking on a smooth surface up to 1,200 ft/hr carrying up to 25 lbs; walking on an irregular surface up to 900 ft/hr carrying up to 25 lbs; climbing stairs up to 8 flights/hr carrying up to 40 lbs; climbing ladders up to 50 rungs/hr carrying up to 25 lbs; activities requiring balance up to 45 min/hr (if able to work with two hands without assistance for balance); applying strength against bent knee (pedaling, squatting, kneeling, etc.) up to 60 times/hr; may need brace for uneven ground or ladders.
Description: Fracture in the ankle. Symptoms include swelling, pain, tenderness, temporary or permanent impairment and, sometimes, visible deformity.
Other names: Broken ankle
Procedure Summary (from ODG Treatment):
Accommodative modalities; Achilles tendon ruptures (treatment); Activity restrictions; Actovegin; Ankle prostheses (total ankle replacement); Anterior drawer test; Anti-inflammatory medications (NSAIDs); Arthrodesis (fusion); Arthroplasty (total ankle replacement); Autologous conditioned serum (ACS); Bed rest; Biofeedback; Bone scan (imaging); Bracing (immobilization); Cast (immobilization); Causality; Chiropractic; Cold packs; Computed tomography (CT); Continuous-flow cryotherapy; Corticosteroids (topical); Diathermy; Dorsiflexion night splints; Education (patient); Elastic bandage (immobilization); Electron generating device; Exercise; Extracorporeal shock wave therapy (ESWT); Functional treatment; Fusion; Heat therapy (ice/heat); Heparin; Heel pads; Ice packs; Imaging; Immobilization; Ingrown toenail surgery; Injections; Insoles with magnetic foil; Inversion stress test; Iontophoresis; Lace-up ankle support; Laser therapy (LLLT); Lateral ligament ankle reconstruction (surgery); Lineal tomography; Low-intensity laser therapy (LLLT); Magnets; Magnetic resonance imaging (MRI); Manipulation; Massage; Mechanical treatment (taping/orthoses); Modified duty; Narcotics; Night splints; Nonprescription medications; Orthotic devices; Osteotomy; Ottawa ankle rules (OAR); Patient education; Phonophoresis; Physical therapy (PT); Prolotherapy (sclerotherapy); Radiography; Rest (RICE); Return to work; Sclerotherapy (prolotherapy); Semi-rigid ankle support; Shock wave therapy, extracorporeal (ESWT); Steroids (injection); Stretching (flexibility); Supports; Surgery; Surgery for achilles tendon ruptures; Surgery for ankle sprains; Surgery for calcaneal fractures; Surgery for hallux valgus; Surgery for plantar fasciitis; Surgery for tarsal tunnel syndrome; Talar tilt test; Tai Chi; Taping; Tension night splints (TNS); Therapeutic exercise; Thompson test; Total ankle replacement (arthroplasty); Transcutaneous electrical neurostimulation (TENS); Ultrasound, diagnostic; Ultrasound, therapeutic; Work
Physical Therapy Guidelines:
Allow for fading of treatment frequency (from up to 3 visits per week to 1 or less), plus active self-directed home PT
Medical treatment: 12 visits over 12 weeks
Post-surgical treatment: 21 visits over 16 weeks

Workers' Comp Costs per Claim (based on 6,287 claims)

Quartile	25%	50%	75%	Mean	% no cost
Indemnity	$2,069	$4,263	$8,337	$7,547	45%
Medical	$1,082	$2,153	$8,033	$6,850	1%
Total	$1,386	$4,389	$12,264	$11,038	1%

RTW Claims Data (Calendar-days away from work by decile)

10%	20%	30%	40%	**50%**	60%	70%	80%	**90%**	100%	Mean
13	16	21	26	**44**	60	79	86	**100**	365	52.74

RTW Post Surgery (Calendar-days away from work by decile)

10%	20%	30%	40%	**50%**	60%	70%	80%	**90%**	100%	Mean
Treatment of ankle fracture										
13	26	47	55	**69**	79	97	116	**184**	365	86.64
Treatment of ankle fracture										
15	29	45	62	**73**	87	103	143	**217**	365	95.94
Treatment of ankle fracture										
25	49	67	77	**89**	103	121	165	**228**	365	112.40
Treatment of ankle fracture										
19	44	62	83	**94**	106	116	129	**173**	365	97.06

Integrated Disability Durations, in days*

Median (mid-point)	23.0	Mean (average)	41.95
Mode (most frequent)	1	Calculated rec.	22

Percent of Cases
(5345 cases)

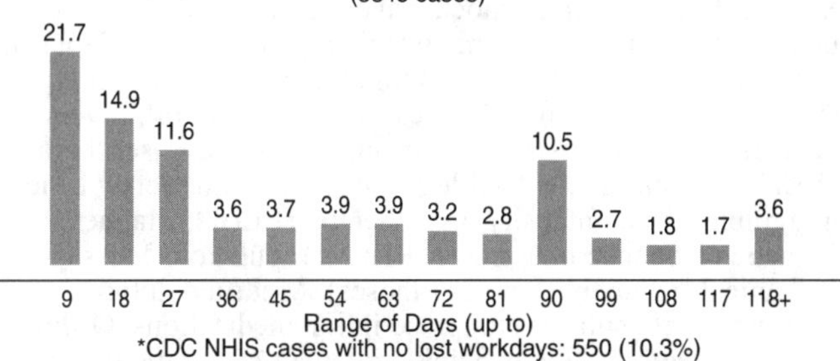

*CDC NHIS cases with no lost workdays: 550 (10.3%)

Impact on Total Absence: Prevalence 0.5946% of total lost workdays; Incidence 6.24 days per 100 workers

825 Fracture of one or more tarsal and metatarsal bones

Return-To-Work Summary Guidelines

Dataset	Midrange	At-Risk
Claims data	42 days	94 days
All absences	34 days	87 days

Return-To-Work "Best Practice" Guidelines
Supportive shoe (stress fracture): 1 day
Closed, without reduction, sedentary work: 7 days
Closed, without reduction, manual work: 35 days
Closed, without reduction, heavy manual work: 42 days
Open, with fixation, sedentary work: 14 days
Open, with fixation, manual work: 56 days
Open, with fixation, heavy manual work: 84 days
Comorbidity fracture blister, add: 21 days

825 Fracture of one or more tarsal and metatarsal bones *(cont'd)*

Capabilities & Activity Modifications:
Sedentary/modified work: Standing limited to 5-10 min/hr; walking only on a smooth surface using crutches with limited pressure on the foot; no walking on an irregular surface; no climbing stairs; no climbing ladders or hill climbing requiring frequent knee flexion; no activities requiring balance; no applying strength against bent knee (squatting, kneeling, crouching, stooping, pedaling, etc.); elevate leg half of time; may need immobilization; limited weight bearing.
Manual/standing work: Standing not more than 50 min/hr; walking on a smooth surface up to 1,200 ft/hr carrying up to 25 lbs; walking on an irregular surface up to 900 ft/hr carrying up to 25 lbs; climbing stairs up to 8 flights/hr carrying up to 40 lbs; climbing ladders up to 50 rungs/hr carrying up to 25 lbs; activities requiring balance up to 45 min/hr (if able to work with two hands without assistance for balance); applying strength against bent knee (pedaling, squatting, kneeling, etc.) up to 60 times/hr; may need brace for uneven ground or ladders.
Description: Broken bone or bones in the instep (tarsus) or space between the instep and the toes (metatarsus). Symptoms include swelling, pain, tenderness, temporary or permanent impairment and, sometimes, visible deformity.
Other names: Broken foot
Procedure Summary (from ODG Treatment):
Accommodative modalities; Achilles tendon ruptures (treatment); Activity restrictions; Actovegin; Ankle prostheses (total ankle replacement); Anterior drawer test; Anti-inflammatory medications (NSAIDs); Arthrodesis (fusion); Arthroplasty (total ankle replacement); Autologous conditioned serum (ACS); Bed rest; Biofeedback; Bone scan (imaging); Bracing (immobilization); Cast (immobilization); Causality; Chiropractic; Cold packs; Computed tomography (CT); Continuous-flow cryotherapy; Corticosteroids (topical); Diathermy; Dorsiflexion night splints; Education (patient); Elastic bandage (immobilization); Electron generating device; Exercise; Extracorporeal shock wave therapy (ESWT); Functional treatment; Fusion; Heat therapy (ice/heat); Heparin; Heel pads; Ice packs; Imaging; Immobilization; Ingrown toenail surgery; Injections; Insoles with magnetic foil; Inversion stress test; Iontophoresis; Lace-up ankle support; Laser therapy (LLLT); Lateral ligament ankle reconstruction (surgery); Lineal tomography; Low-intensity laser therapy (LLLT); Magnets; Magnetic resonance imaging (MRI); Manipulation; Massage; Mechanical treatment (taping/orthoses); Modified duty; Narcotics; Night splints; Nonprescription medications; Orthotic devices; Osteotomy; Ottawa ankle rules (OAR); Patient education; Phonophoresis; Physical therapy (PT); Prolotherapy (sclerotherapy); Radiography; Rest (RICE); Return to work; Sclerotherapy (prolotherapy); Semi-rigid ankle support; Shock wave therapy, extracorporeal (ESWT); Steroids (injection); Stretching (flexibility); Supports; Surgery; Surgery for achilles tendon ruptures; Surgery for ankle sprains; Surgery for calcaneal fractures; Surgery for hallux valgus; Surgery for plantar fasciitis; Surgery for tarsal tunnel syndrome; Talar tilt test; Tai Chi; Taping; Tension night splints (TNS); Therapeutic exercise; Thompson test; Total ankle replacement (arthroplasty); Transcutaneous electrical neurostimulation (TENS); Ultrasound, diagnostic; Ultrasound, therapeutic; Work
Physical Therapy Guidelines:
Medical treatment: 12 visits over 12 weeks
Post-surgical treatment: 21 visits over 16 weeks

825 Fracture of one or more tarsal and metatarsal bones *(cont'd)*

Workers' Comp Costs per Claim (based on 8,518 claims)

Quartile	25%	50%	75%	Mean	% no cost
Indemnity	$1,775	$3,565	$7,487	$6,752	53%
Medical	$756	$1,229	$2,741	$4,286	1%
Total	$903	$2,111	$6,353	$7,464	1%

RTW Claims Data (Calendar-days away from work by decile)

10%	20%	30%	40%	**50%**	60%	70%	80%	**90%**	100%	Mean
14	19	25	36	**42**	53	60	82	**94**	365	50.87

RTW Post Surgery (Calendar-days away from work by decile)

10%	20%	30%	40%	**50%**	60%	70%	80%	**90%**	100%	Mean
Treat heel fracture										
69	94	115	141	**166**	196	301	365	**365**	365	199.36
Treat metatarsal fracture										
24	46	59	66	**80**	100	118	157	**226**	365	107.57

Integrated Disability Durations, in days*
Median (mid-point) 34.0 Mean (average) 40.63
Mode (most frequent) 1 Calculated rec. 27

Percent of Cases
(4114 cases)

Range of Days (up to)	9	18	27	36	45	54	63	72	81	90	99	108	117	118+
Percent of Cases	20.4	11.1	8.5	6.7	8.7	4.6	7.5	2.4	2.3	6.2	2.0	1.5	1.3	2.8

*CDC NHIS cases with no lost workdays: 571 (13.9%)

Impact on Total Absence: Prevalence 0.4254% of total lost workdays; Incidence 4.47 days per 100 workers

826 Fracture of one or more phalanges of foot

Return-To-Work Summary Guidelines

Dataset	Midrange	At-Risk
Claims data	22 days	48 days
All absences	12 days	44 days

Return-To-Work "Best Practice" Guidelines
Clerical/modified work: 0 days
Manual work: 7 days
Heavy manual work: 14 days
Regular work if cause of disability: 42 days

Capabilities & Activity Modifications:
Sedentary/modified work: Standing limited to 5-10 min/hr; walking only on a smooth surface using crutches with limited pressure on the foot; no walking on an irregular surface; no climbing stairs; no climbing ladders or hill climbing requiring frequent knee flexion; no activities requiring balance; no applying strength against bent knee (squatting, kneeling, crouching, stooping, pedaling, etc.); elevate leg half of time; may need immobilization; limited weight bearing.
Manual/standing work: Standing not more than 50 min/hr; walking on a smooth surface up to 1,200 ft/hr carrying up to 25 lbs; walking on an irregular surface up to 900 ft/hr carrying up to 25 lbs; climbing stairs up to 8 flights/hr carrying up to 40 lbs; climbing ladders up to 50 rungs/hr carrying up to 25 lbs; activities requiring balance up to 45 min/hr (if able to work with

826 Fracture of one or more phalanges of foot

two hands without assistance for balance); applying strength against bent knee (pedaling, squatting, kneeling, etc.) up to 60 times/hr; may need brace for uneven ground or ladders.

Description: Fracture of one or more toes. Symptoms include swelling, pain, tenderness, temporary or permanent impairment and, sometimes, visible deformity.

Other names: Broken toe

Includes: toe(s)

Procedure Summary (from ODG Treatment): Accommodative modalities; Achilles tendon ruptures (treatment); Activity restrictions; Actovegin; Ankle prostheses (total ankle replacement); Anterior drawer test; Anti-inflammatory medications (NSAIDs); Arthrodesis (fusion); Arthroplasty (total ankle replacement); Autologous conditioned serum (ACS); Bed rest; Biofeedback; Bone scan (imaging); Bracing (immobilization); Cast (immobilization); Causality; Chiropractic; Cold packs; Computed tomography (CT); Continuous-flow cryotherapy; Corticosteroids (topical); Diathermy; Dorsiflexion night splints; Education (patient); Elastic bandage (immobilization); Electron generating device; Exercise; Extracorporeal shock wave therapy (ESWT); Functional treatment; Fusion; Heat therapy (ice/heat); Heparin; Heel pads; Ice packs; Imaging; Immobilization; Ingrown toenail surgery; Injections; Insoles with magnetic foil; Inversion stress test; Iontophoresis; Lace-up ankle support; Laser therapy (LLLT); Lateral ligament ankle reconstruction (surgery); Lineal tomography; Low-intensity laser therapy (LLLT); Magnets; Magnetic resonance imaging (MRI); Manipulation; Massage; Mechanical treatment (taping/orthoses); Modified duty; Narcotics; Night splints; Nonprescription medications; Orthotic devices; Osteotomy; Ottawa ankle rules (OAR); Patient education; Phonophoresis; Physical therapy (PT); Prolotherapy (sclerotherapy); Radiography; Rest (RICE); Return to work; Sclerotherapy (prolotherapy); Semi-rigid ankle support; Shock wave therapy, extracorporeal (ESWT); Steroids (injection); Stretching (flexibility); Supports; Surgery; Surgery for achilles tendon ruptures; Surgery for ankle sprains; Surgery for calcaneal fractures; Surgery for hallux valgus; Surgery for plantar fasciitis; Surgery for tarsal tunnel syndrome; Talar tilt test; Tai Chi; Taping; Tension night splints (TNS); Therapeutic exercise; Thompson test; Total ankle replacement (arthroplasty); Transcutaneous electrical neurostimulation (TENS); Ultrasound, diagnostic; Ultrasound, therapeutic; Work

Physical Therapy Guidelines:
Medical treatment: 12 visits over 12 weeks
Post-surgical treatment: 12 visits over 12 weeks

Workers' Comp Costs per Claim (based on 6,228 claims)					
Quartile	25%	50%	75%	Mean	% no cost
Indemnity	$819	$1,565	$2,751	$2,444	78%
Medical	$326	$515	$819	$854	3%
Total	$347	$567	$1,229	$1,418	3%

RTW Claims Data (Calendar-days away from work by decile)										
10%	20%	30%	40%	**50%**	60%	70%	80%	**90%**	100%	Mean
10	13	14	17	**22**	31	41	43	**48**	365	29.45

826 Fracture of one or more phalanges of foot

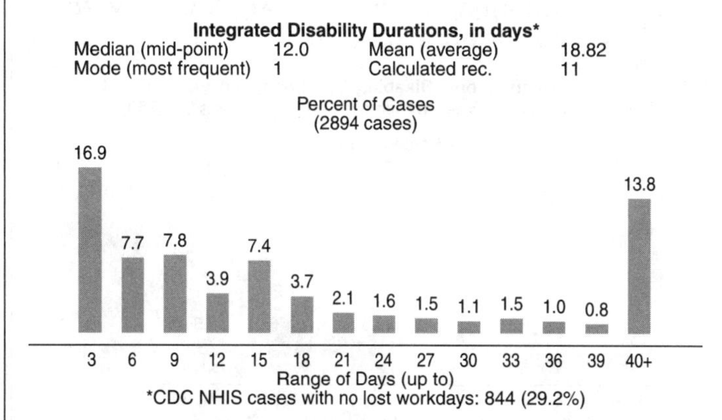

Impact on Total Absence: Prevalence 0.1140% of total lost workdays; Incidence 1.20 days per 100 workers

828 Multiple fractures involving both lower limbs, lower with upper limb, and lower limb(s) with rib(s) and sternum

Return-To-Work Summary Guidelines		
Dataset	**Midrange**	**At-Risk**
Claims data	15 days	65 days
All absences	14 days	65 days

Includes: arm(s) with leg(s) [any bones]
both legs [any bones]
leg(s) with rib(s) or sternum

RTW Claims Data (Calendar-days away from work by decile)										
10%	20%	30%	40%	**50%**	60%	70%	80%	**90%**	100%	Mean
12	13	14	14	**15**	15	32	41	**65**	180	31.75

Integrated Disability Durations, in days*
Median (mid-point) 14.5 Mean (average) 29.32
Mode (most frequent) 14 Calculated rec. 18

Percent of Cases
(46 cases)

2.2 4.3 4.3 8.7 41.3 6.5 0.0 0.0 0.0 0.0 2.2 4.3 0.0 21.7

3 6 9 12 15 18 21 24 27 30 33 36 39 40+
Range of Days (up to)
*CDC NHIS cases with no lost workdays: 2 (4.3%)

Impact on Total Absence: Prevalence 0.0038% of total lost workdays; Incidence 0.04 days per 100 workers

828 Multiple fractures involving both lower limbs, lower with upper limb, and lower limb(s) with rib(s) and sternum *(cont'd)*

Occupational Disability Durations, in days
Median (mid-point) 25 - Benchmark Indemnity Costs $18,750

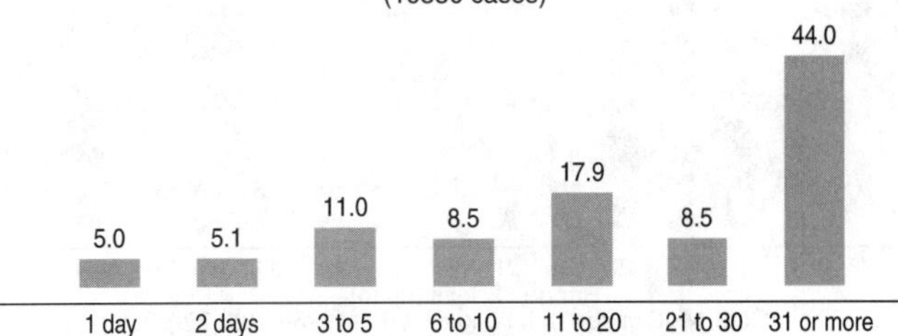

Impact on Occupational Absence: Prevalence 2.9920% of occupational lost workdays; Incidence 0.48 days per 100 workers

DISLOCATION (830-839)

Includes: displacement
subluxation

Excludes:
congenital dislocation (754.0-755.8)
pathological dislocation (718.2)

The following descriptions "closed" and "open," used in the fourth-digit subdivisions, include the terms:
closed:
complete
dislocation NOS
partial
simple
uncomplicated
open:
compound
infected
with foreign body
A dislocation not indicated as closed or open should be classified as closed.

RTW Claims Data (Calendar-days away from work by decile)										
10%	20%	30%	40%	**50%**	60%	70%	80%	**90%**	100%	Mean
12	15	20	24	**32**	41	46	63	**89**	365	43.85

Impact on Total Absence: Prevalence 0.8145% of total lost workdays; Incidence 8.55 days per 100 workers

Occupational Disability Durations, in days
Median (mid-point) 34 - Benchmark Indemnity Costs $25,500

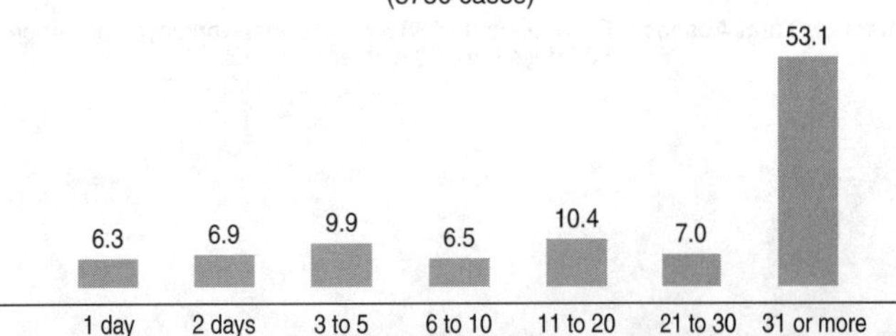

Impact on Occupational Absence: Prevalence 3.3749% of occupational lost workdays; Incidence 0.54 days per 100 workers

830 Dislocation of jaw

Return-To-Work Summary Guidelines		
Dataset	**Midrange**	**At-Risk**
Claims data	41 days	127 days
All absences	6 days	119 days

Return-To-Work "Best Practice" Guidelines
Spontaneous reduction: 0 days
Closed reduction: 5 days

Description: Displacement of the jawbones from their normal position. A dislocation is usually accompanied by torn joint ligaments and damage to the joint capsule. Symptoms usually include pain, swelling, deformity, a bruise-like color, and limitation of movement. There is often a tearing sensation when the injury occurs.

Other names: Dislocated jaw

Includes: jaw (cartilage) (meniscus)
mandible
maxilla (inferior)
temporomandibular (joint)

Workers' Comp Costs per Claim (based on 30 claims)					
Quartile	25%	50%	75%	Mean	% no cost
Medical	$452	$1,549	$3,696	$2,605	0%
Total	$452	$2,399	$6,468	$3,905	0%

RTW Claims Data (Calendar-days away from work by decile)										
10%	20%	30%	40%	**50%**	60%	70%	80%	**90%**	100%	Mean
14	20	24	30	**41**	69	77	119	**127**	156	60.92

Integrated Disability Durations, in days*
Median (mid-point) 6.0 Mean (average) 29.92
Mode (most frequent) 1 Calculated rec. 11

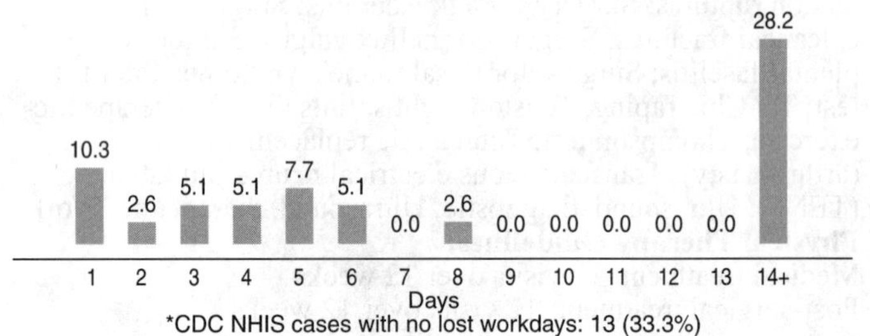

*CDC NHIS cases with no lost workdays: 13 (33.3%)

Impact on Total Absence: Prevalence 0.0022% of total lost workdays; Incidence 0.02 days per 100 workers

831 Dislocation of shoulder

Return-To-Work Summary Guidelines		
Dataset	**Midrange**	**At-Risk**
Claims data	34 days	85 days
All absences	16 days	83 days

831 Dislocation of shoulder *(cont'd)*

Return-To-Work "Best Practice" Guidelines
Recurrent, non-dominant arm, clerical/modified work: 0 days
Recurrent, non-dominant arm, manual work: 7 days
Recurrent, dominant arm, clerical/modified work: 7 days
Recurrent, dominant arm, manual work: 14 days
Acute, non-dominant arm, clerical/modified work: 7 days
Acute, non-dominant arm, manual work: 14 days
Acute, dominant arm, clerical/modified work: 14 days
Acute, dominant arm, manual work: 35 days
Recurrent, surgical treatment, non-dominant arm, clerical/modified work: 14 days
Recurrent, surgical treatment, non-dominant arm, manual work: 42 days
Recurrent, surgical treatment, dominant arm, clerical/modified work: 21 days
Recurrent, surgical treatment, dominant arm, manual work: 84 days

Capabilities & Activity Modifications:
Modified work: No overhead work (reaching above shoulder) plus no reaching to shoulder level (90 degree position); no holding arm in abduction or flexion; pulling and pushing not more than 8 lbs up to 4 times/hr; lifting and carrying up to 5 lbs 3 times/hr; single arm upper extremity work using injured arm for light work only; possible immobilization by abduction brace, sling, or clavicle brace; no climbing ladders.
Manual work: Reaching above shoulder not more than 12 times/hr with up to 15 lbs of weight; reaching to shoulder up to 15 times/hr with up to 25 lbs of weight; holding arm in abduction or flexion up to 12 times/hr with up to 15 lbs of weight; pulling and pushing up to 60 lbs 20 times/hr; lifting and carrying up to 40 lbs 15 times/hr; single upper extremity work using injured arm for moderate work only (full use of non-injured arm); possible immobilization by abduction brace, sling, or clavicle brace; climbing ladders up to 50 rungs/hr.
Description: The separation of the shoulder from the arm. A dislocation is usually accompanied by torn joint ligaments and damage to the joint capsule. Symptoms usually include pain, swelling, deformity, a bruise-like color, and limitation of movement. There is often a tearing sensation when the injury occurs.
Other names: Dislocated shoulder

Excludes:
sternoclavicular joint (839.61, 839.71)
sternum (839.61, 839.71)

The following fifth-digit subclassification is for use with category 831:
0 shoulder, unspecified
Humerus NOS
1 anterior dislocation of humerus
2 posterior dislocation of humerus
3 inferior dislocation of humerus
4 acromioclavicular (joint)
Clavicle
9 other
Scapula

Procedure Summary (from ODG Treatment):
Acromioplasty; Activity restrictions; Acupuncture; Adson's test (AT); Anterior scalene block; Arthrography; Arthroplasty (shoulder); Arthroscopy; Arthroscopic release of adhesions; Bipolar interferential electrotherapy; Biofeedback; Biopsychosocial rehab; Cardiovascular functional testing; Chiropractic; Cold lasers; Continuous-flow cryotherapy; Continuous passive motion (CPM); Corticosteroid injections; Costoclavicular maneuver (CCM); Cutaneous laser treatment; Deep friction massage; Diagnostic arthroscopy; Diathermy; Distension arthrography; Electrical stimulation; Electrodiagnostic testing for TOS (thoracic outlet syndrome); Elevated arm stress test (EAST); Ergonomic interventions; Exercises; Extracorporeal shock wave therapy (ESWT); Hydroplasty/ hydrodilation; Imaging; Immobilization; Impingement test; Injections; Interferential therapy; Laser therapy; Low level laser therapy (LLLT); Magnetic resonance imaging (MRI); Manipulation; Manipulation under anesthesia (MUA); Massage; Mechanical traction; Modified duty; Multidisciplinary biopsychosocial rehab; Nerve blocks; Osteochondral autologous transplantation (OATS); Physical therapy; Porcine small intestinal submucosa (SIS); Pulsed electromagnetic field; Radiography; Return to work; Rotator cuff repair; Rotator cuff porcine graft repair; Shock wave therapy; Shoulder repair; Steroid injections; Supraclavicular pressure (SCP); Surgery for AC joint separation; Surgery for adhesive capsulitis; Surgery for impingement syndrome; Surgery for rotator cuff repair; Surgery for ruptured biceps tendon; Surgery for shoulder dislocation; Surgery for Thoracic Outlet Syndrome; Thermal capsulorrhaphy; Thermotherapy; Transcutaneous electrical neurostimulation (TENS); Transdermal nitroglycerin; Ultrasound, diagnostic; Ultrasound, therapeutic; Work

Physical Therapy Guidelines:
Allow for fading of treatment frequency (from up to 3 visits per week to 1 or less), plus active self-directed home PT
Medical treatment: 12 visits over 12 weeks
Post-surgical treatment (Bankart): 24 visits over 14 weeks

Workers' Comp Costs per Claim (based on 2,352 claims)

Quartile	25%	50%	75%	Mean	% no cost
Indemnity	$1,743	$3,686	$8,957	$8,232	60%
Medical	$735	$1,848	$5,030	$4,790	2%
Total	$882	$2,499	$8,379	$8,114	2%

RTW Claims Data (Calendar-days away from work by decile)

10%	20%	30%	40%	**50%**	60%	70%	80%	**90%**	100%	Mean
12	15	19	23	**34**	39	44	62	**85**	363	42.06

Integrated Disability Durations, in days*
Median (mid-point) 16.0 Mean (average) 29.25
Mode (most frequent) 1 Calculated rec. 16

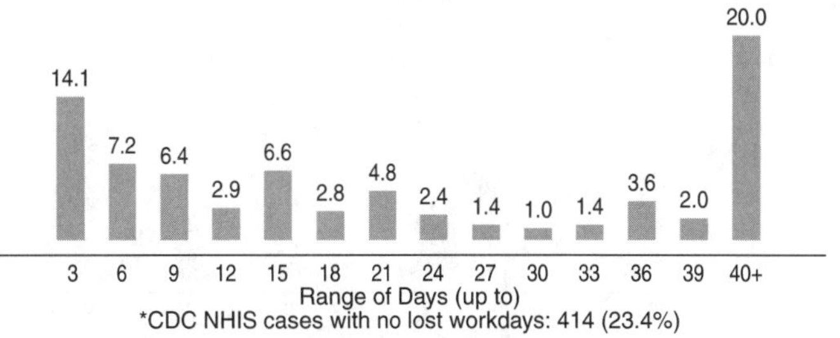

*CDC NHIS cases with no lost workdays: 414 (23.4%)

Impact on Total Absence: Prevalence 0.1171% of total lost workdays; Incidence 1.23 days per 100 workers

831 Dislocation of shoulder *(cont'd)*

Occupational Disability Durations, in days
Median (mid-point) 29 - Benchmark Indemnity Costs $21,750

Percent of Cases
(2100 cases)

Range of Days	1 day	2 days	3 to 5	6 to 10	11 to 20	21 to 30	31 or more
Percent	7.0	7.1	11.3	7.8	11.1	6.8	49.0

Impact on Occupational Absence: Prevalence 0.6908% of occupational lost workdays; Incidence 0.11 days per 100 workers

831.0 Closed dislocation

Return-To-Work Summary Guidelines		
Dataset	**Midrange**	**At-Risk**
Claims data	34 days	84 days
All absences	14 days	65 days

Return-To-Work "Best Practice" Guidelines
See 831

Workers' Comp Costs per Claim (based on 2,301 claims)					
Quartile	25%	50%	75%	Mean	% no cost
Indemnity	$1,701	$3,686	$9,093	$8,287	60%
Medical	$746	$1,880	$5,051	$4,776	2%
Total	$893	$2,552	$8,610	$8,156	2%

RTW Claims Data (Calendar-days away from work by decile)										
10%	20%	30%	40%	**50%**	60%	70%	80%	**90%**	100%	Mean
12	15	20	24	**34**	39	46	58	**84**	233	39.57

Integrated Disability Durations, in days*
Median (mid-point) 14.0 Mean (average) 24.95
Mode (most frequent) 1 Calculated rec. 13

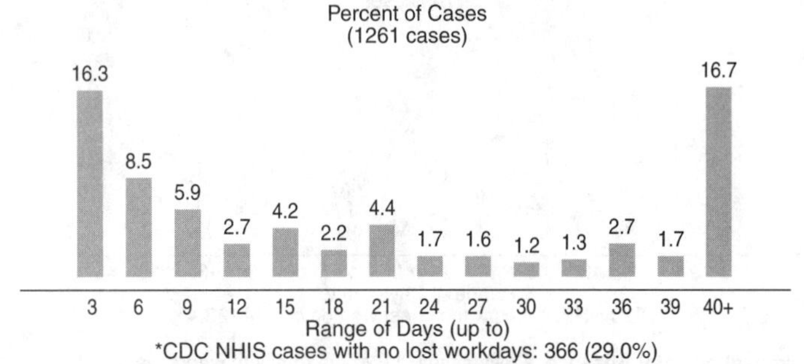

*CDC NHIS cases with no lost workdays: 366 (29.0%)

Impact on Total Absence: Prevalence 0.0660% of total lost workdays; Incidence 0.69 days per 100 workers

831.04 Acromioclavicular joint dislocation

Return-To-Work Summary Guidelines		
Dataset	**Midrange**	**At-Risk**
Claims data	34 days	80 days
All absences	20 days	58 days

831.04 Acromioclavicular joint dislocation *(cont'd)*

Return-To-Work "Best Practice" Guidelines
AC separation, type I-II, non-dominant arm, clerical/modified work: 0 days
AC separation, type I-II, non-dominant arm, manual work: 21 days
AC separation, type I-II, dominant arm, clerical/modified work: 7 days
AC separation, type I-II, dominant arm, manual work: 35 days
AC separation, type III+, non-dominant arm, clerical/modified work: 21 days
AC separation, type III+, non-dominant arm, manual work: 49 days
AC separation, type III+, dominant arm, clerical/modified work: 28 days
AC separation, type III+, dominant arm, manual work: 56 days

Capabilities & Activity Modifications:
Modified work: No overhead work (reaching above shoulder) plus no reaching to shoulder level (90 degree position); no holding arm in abduction or flexion; pulling and pushing not more than 8 lbs up to 4 times/hr; lifting and carrying up to 5 lbs 3 times/hr; single arm upper extremity work using injured arm for light work only; possible immobilization by abduction brace, sling, or clavicle brace; no climbing ladders.
Manual work: Reaching above shoulder not more than 12 times/hr with up to 15 lbs of weight; reaching to shoulder up to 15 times/hr with up to 25 lbs of weight; holding arm in abduction or flexion up to 12 times/hr with up to 15 lbs of weight; pulling and pushing up to 60 lbs 20 times/hr; lifting and carrying up to 40 lbs 15 times/hr; single upper extremity work using injured arm for moderate work only (full use of non-injured arm); possible immobilization by abduction brace, sling, or clavicle brace; climbing ladders up to 50 rungs/hr.
Description: The separation of the joint between the shoulder blade and the collarbone. A dislocation is usually accompanied by torn joint ligaments and damage to the joint capsule. Symptoms usually include pain, swelling, deformity, a bruise-like color, and limitation of movement. There is often a tearing sensation when the injury occurs.
Other names: AC separation
Procedure Summary (from ODG Treatment):
Acromioplasty; Activity restrictions; Acupuncture; Adson's test (AT); Anterior scalene block; Arthrography; Arthroplasty (shoulder); Arthroscopy; Arthroscopic release of adhesions; Bipolar interferential electrotherapy; Biofeedback; Biopsychosocial rehab; Cardiovascular functional testing; Chiropractic; Cold lasers; Continuous-flow cryotherapy; Continuous passive motion (CPM); Corticosteroid injections; Costoclavicular maneuver (CCM); Cutaneous laser treatment; Deep friction massage; Diagnostic arthroscopy; Diathermy; Distension arthrography; Electrical stimulation; Electrodiagnostic testing for TOS (thoracic outlet syndrome); Elevated arm stress test (EAST); Ergonomic interventions; Exercises; Extracorporeal shock wave therapy (ESWT); Hydroplasty/ hydrodilation; Imaging; Immobilization; Impingement test; Injections; Interferential therapy; Laser therapy; Low level laser therapy (LLLT); Magnetic resonance imaging (MRI); Manipulation; Manipulation under anesthesia (MUA); Massage; Mechanical traction; Modified duty; Multidisciplinary biopsychosocial rehab; Nerve blocks; Osteochondral autologous transplantation (OATS); Physical therapy; Porcine small intestinal submucosa (SIS); Pulsed electromagnetic field; Radiography; Return to work; Rotator cuff repair; Rotator cuff porcine graft repair; Shock wave therapy; Shoulder repair; Steroid injections; Supraclavicular pressure (SCP); Surgery for AC joint separation; Surgery for adhesive capsulitis; Surgery for impingement syndrome; Surgery for rotator cuff repair; Surgery for ruptured biceps

831.04 Acromioclavicular joint dislocation *(cont'd)*

tendon; Surgery for shoulder dislocation; Surgery for Thoracic Outlet Syndrome; Thermal capsulorrhaphy; Thermotherapy; Transcutaneous electrical neurostimulation (TENS); Transdermal nitroglycerin; Ultrasound, diagnostic; Ultrasound, therapeutic; Work

Physical Therapy Guidelines:

Allow for fading of treatment frequency (from up to 3 visits per week to 1 or less), plus active self-directed home PT

AC separation, type III+: 8 visits over 8 weeks

Workers' Comp Costs per Claim (based on 823 claims)					
Quartile	25%	50%	75%	Mean	% no cost
Indemnity	$1,764	$3,644	$9,093	$9,094	53%
Medical	$536	$1,444	$4,442	$4,087	2%
Total	$620	$2,121	$8,085	$8,463	2%

RTW Claims Data (Calendar-days away from work by decile)										
10%	20%	30%	40%	**50%**	60%	70%	80%	**90%**	100%	Mean
11	18	22	28	**34**	41	49	56	**80**	134	40.05

Integrated Disability Durations, in days*

Median (mid-point) 20.5 Mean (average) 27.69
Mode (most frequent) 1 Calculated rec. 17

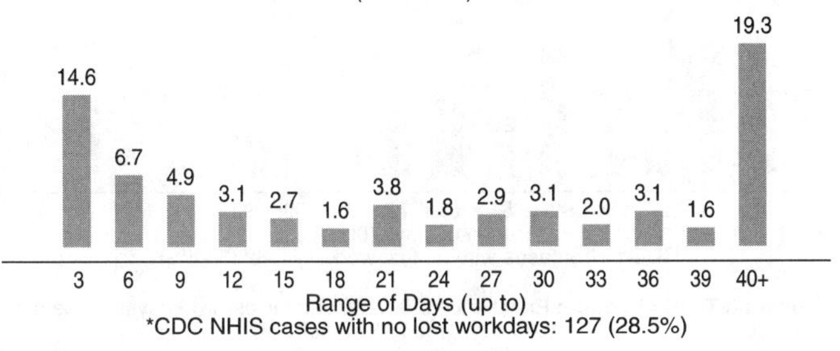

*CDC NHIS cases with no lost workdays: 127 (28.5%)

Impact on Total Absence: Prevalence 0.0260% of total lost workdays; Incidence 0.27 days per 100 workers

832 Dislocation of elbow

Return-To-Work Summary Guidelines		
Dataset	**Midrange**	**At-Risk**
Claims data	27 days	65 days
All absences	21 days	59 days

Return-To-Work "Best Practice" Guidelines
Non-dominant arm, clerical/modified work: 0 days
Non-dominant arm, manual work: 10 days
Non-dominant arm, heavy manual work: 21 days
Dominant arm, clerical/modified work: 7 days
Dominant arm, manual work: 21 days
Dominant arm, heavy manual work: 42 days

Capabilities & Activity Modifications:

Modified work: Repetitive motion activities not more than 4 times/hr; single upper extremity work if injured arm is non-dominant arm; lifting and carrying up to 3 lbs not more than 4 times/hr; pulling and pushing up to 5 lbs 3 times/hr; gripping using light tools (pens, scissors, etc) with 5-minute break at least every 20 min; avoid direct pressure on the elbow area; limit repetitive keying up to 15 keystrokes/min not more than 2 hrs/day; driving car up to 2 hrs/day; no full extension activities; possible immobilization by long arm splint or cast, tennis elbow splint, or wrist splint; no climbing ladders.

Regular manual work: Repetitive motion activities not more than 8 times/hr; use of injured dominant arm for moderate work; lifting and carrying up to 20 lbs not more than 15 times/

832 Dislocation of elbow *(cont'd)*

hr; pulling and pushing up to 40 lbs 15 times/hr; gripping using moderate tools (pliers, screwdrivers, etc) full time; driving car or light truck up to 6 hrs/day or heavy truck up to 4 hrs/day; full extension activities up to 12 times/hr with up to 10 lbs of weight; possible immobilization by sling, wrist splint, or tennis elbow splint; climbing ladders up to 50 rungs/hr.

Description: Displacement of the bones in the elbow joint. A dislocation is usually accompanied by torn joint ligaments and damage to the joint capsule. Symptoms usually include pain, swelling, deformity, a bruise-like color, and limitation of movement. There is often a tearing sensation when the injury occurs.

Other names: Dislocated elbow

The following fifth-digit subclassification is for use with category 832:

0 elbow unspecified
1 anterior dislocation of elbow
2 posterior dislocation of elbow
3 medial dislocation of elbow
4 lateral dislocation of elbow
9 other

Procedure Summary (from ODG Treatment): Activity restrictions; Arthroplasty (elbow); Chiropractic; Cold packs; Deep transverse friction massage; Education; Electrical stimulation (E-STIM); Exercise; Fractures of humerus; Fractures of radius; Imaging; Iontophoresis; Laser doppler imaging (LDI); Manipulation; MRI's; Neural tension; Night splints; Nonprescription medications; Patient education; Phonophoresis; Physical therapy; Radiography; Return to work; Stretching; Surgery; Total elbow replacement (TER); Transcutaneous electrical neurostimulation (TENS); Ultrasound, diagnostic; Ultrasound, therapeutic; Work

Physical Therapy Guidelines:

Stable dislocation: 6 visits over 2 weeks
Unstable dislocation: 20 visits over 9 weeks

Workers' Comp Costs per Claim (based on 272 claims)					
Quartile	25%	50%	75%	Mean	% no cost
Indemnity	$1,817	$4,473	$9,492	$8,495	43%
Medical	$2,268	$4,646	$11,130	$12,985	1%
Total	$3,287	$6,710	$14,112	$17,890	1%

RTW Claims Data (Calendar-days away from work by decile)										
10%	20%	30%	40%	**50%**	60%	70%	80%	**90%**	100%	Mean
10	14	20	23	**27**	37	42	48	**65**	173	34.66

Integrated Disability Durations, in days*

Median (mid-point) 21.0 Mean (average) 26.24
Mode (most frequent) 1 Calculated rec. 17

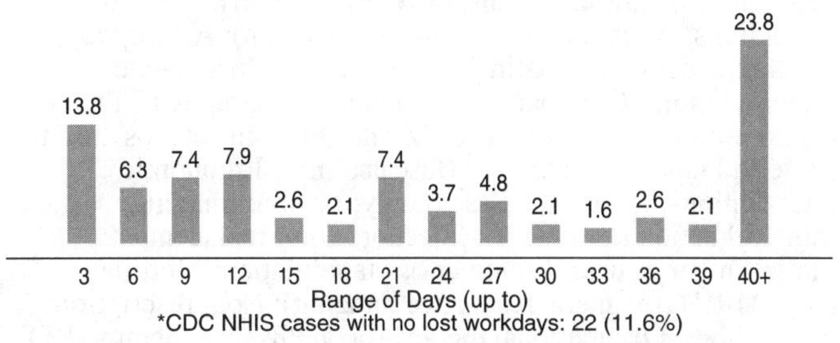

*CDC NHIS cases with no lost workdays: 22 (11.6%)

Impact on Total Absence: Prevalence 0.0129% of total lost workdays; Incidence 0.14 days per 100 workers

833 Dislocation of wrist

Return-To-Work Summary Guidelines

Dataset	Midrange	At-Risk
Claims data	35 days	180 days
All absences	27 days	91 days

Return-To-Work "Best Practice" Guidelines
Non-dominant arm, clerical/modified work: 0 days
Non-dominant arm, manual work: 14 days
Non-dominant arm, heavy manual work: 35 days
Dominant arm, clerical/modified work: 7 days
Dominant arm, manual work: 42 days
Dominant arm, heavy manual work: 63 days
Triangular fibrocartilage complex (TFCC) reconstruction, clerical/modified work: 42 days
TFCC reconstruction, heavy manual work: 180 days

Capabilities & Activity Modifications:
Modified work: Repetitive motion activities (w or w/o splint) not more than 4 times/hr; repetitive keying up to 15 keystrokes/min not more than 2 hrs/day; gripping and using light tools (pens, scissors, etc.) with 5-minute break at least every 20 min; no pinching; driving car up to 2 hrs/day; light work up to 5 lbs 3 times/hr; avoidance of prolonged periods in wrist flexion or extension.
Regular work (if not cause or aggravating to disability) : Repetitive motion activities not more than 25 times/hr; repetitive keying up to 45 keystrokes/min 8 hrs/day; gripping and using moderate tools (pliers, screwdrivers, etc.) fulltime; pinching up to 5 times/min; driving car or light truck up to 6 hrs/day or heavy truck up to 3 hrs/day; moderate to heavy work up to 35 lbs not more than 7 times/hr.
Description: Displacement of the bones in the wrist joint. A dislocation is usually accompanied by torn joint ligaments and damage to the joint capsule. Symptoms usually include pain, swelling, deformity, a bruise-like color, and limitation of movement. There is often a tearing sensation when the injury occurs.
Other names: Dislocated wrist

The following fifth-digit subclassification is for use with category 833:
0 wrist, unspecified part
  Carpal (bone)
  Radius, distal end
1 radioulnar (joint), distal
2 radiocarpal (joint)
3 midcarpal (joint)
4 carpometacarpal (joint)
5 metacarpal (bone), proximal end
9 other
  Ulna, distal end

Procedure Summary (from ODG Treatment): Activity restrictions; Acupuncture; Arthrodesis (fusion); Arthroplasty (joint replacement); Casting versus splints; Chiropractic (manipulation); Cold packs; Computed tomography (CT); Continuous passive motion (CPM); de Quervain's tenosynovitis surgery; Dupuytren's release (fasciectomy); Ergonomic interventions; Exercises; Fasciotomy; Fusion; Imaging; Immobilization (treatment); Injection; Joint replacement; Mallet finger injuries (treatment); Manipulation; Modified duty; MRI's (magnetic resonance imaging); Nonprescription medications; Occupational therapy (OT); Physical therapy (PT); Plaster casting; Radiography (x-rays); Rest; Return to work; Splints; Surgery for broken wrist; TENS (transcutaneous electrical neurostimulation); Trapeziectomy; Triangular fibrocartilage complex (TFCC) reconstruction ; Trigger finger surgery; Vitamin C; Work; X-rays; Yoga
Physical Therapy Guidelines:
Medical treatment: 9 visits over 8 weeks
Post-surgical treatment (TFCC reconstruction): 16 visits over 10 weeks

Workers' Comp Costs per Claim (based on 270 claims)

Quartile	25%	50%	75%	Mean	% no cost
Indemnity	$3,686	$11,477	$35,522	$24,524	32%
Medical	$2,237	$8,542	$27,353	$21,205	0%
Total	$3,245	$14,233	$50,180	$37,784	0%

RTW Claims Data (Calendar-days away from work by decile)

10%	20%	30%	40%	**50%**	60%	70%	80%	**90%**	100%	Mean
13	17	21	27	**35**	42	61	70	**105**	192	50.18

Integrated Disability Durations, in days*
Median (mid-point) 27.0 Mean (average) 41.69
Mode (most frequent) 1 Calculated rec. 24

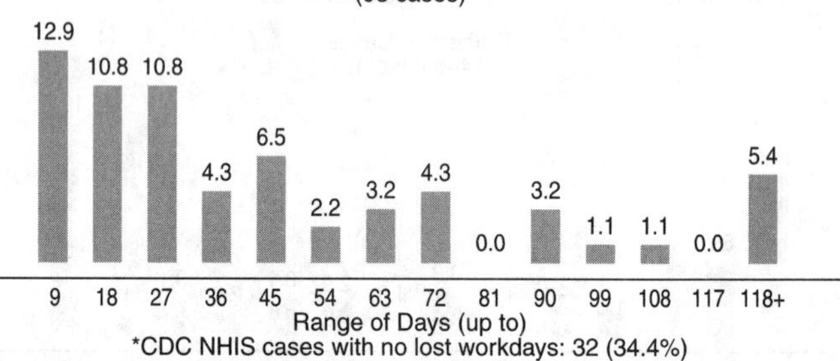

*CDC NHIS cases with no lost workdays: 32 (34.4%)

Impact on Total Absence: Prevalence 0.0075% of total lost workdays; Incidence 0.08 days per 100 workers

834 Dislocation of finger

Return-To-Work Summary Guidelines

Dataset	Midrange	At-Risk
Claims data	19 days	61 days
All absences	6 days	41 days

Return-To-Work "Best Practice" Guidelines
Non-dominant hand, clerical/modified work: 0 days
Non-dominant hand, manual work: 4 days
Dominant hand, clerical/modified work: 7 days
Dominant hand, manual work: 14 days

Description: Displacement of the bones in a finger joint. A dislocation is usually accompanied by torn joint ligaments and damage to the joint capsule. Symptoms usually include pain, swelling, deformity, a bruise-like color, and limitation of movement. There is often a tearing sensation when the injury occurs.
Other names: Dislocated finger

Includes: finger(s)
  phalanx of hand
  thumb

The following fifth-digit subclassification is for use with category 834:
0 finger, unspecified part
1 metacarpophalangeal (joint)
  Metacarpal (bone), distal end
2 interphalangeal (joint), hand

834 Dislocation of finger *(cont'd)*

Physical Therapy Guidelines:
9 visits over 8 weeks
Post-surgical treatment: 16 visits over 10 weeks

Workers' Comp Costs per Claim (based on 1,425 claims)					
Quartile	25%	50%	75%	Mean	% no cost
Indemnity	$1,040	$2,142	$4,956	$4,878	82%
Medical	$420	$793	$1,533	$2,036	3%
Total	$452	$840	$1,890	$2,954	3%

RTW Claims Data (Calendar-days away from work by decile)										
10%	20%	30%	40%	**50%**	60%	70%	80%	**90%**	100%	Mean
11	13	14	16	**19**	24	37	47	**61**	364	30.55

Integrated Disability Durations, in days*

Median (mid-point)	6.0	Mean (average)	14.39
Mode (most frequent)	1	Calculated rec.	7

Percent of Cases
(969 cases)

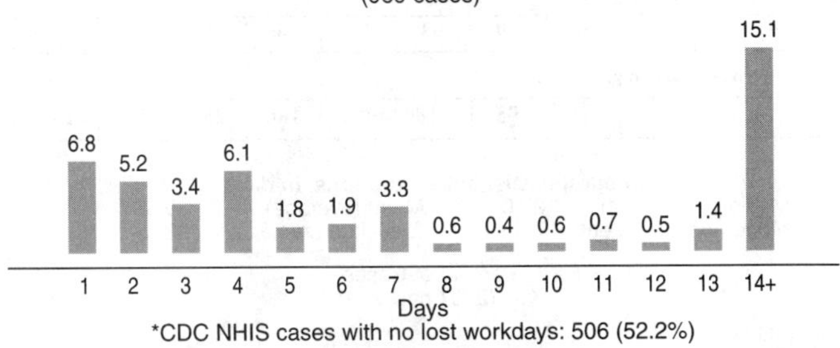

*CDC NHIS cases with no lost workdays: 506 (52.2%)

Impact on Total Absence: Prevalence 0.0196% of total lost workdays; Incidence 0.21 days per 100 workers

835 Dislocation of hip

Return-To-Work Summary Guidelines		
Dataset	**Midrange**	**At-Risk**
Claims data	22 days	50 days
All absences	20 days	48 days

Return-To-Work "Best Practice" Guidelines
Spontaneous reduction, clerical/modified work: 2 days
Spontaneous reduction, manual work: 10 days
Closed reduction, clerical/modified work: 21 days
Closed reduction, manual work: 28 days

Description: Displacement of the bones in the hip joint. A dislocation is usually accompanied by torn joint ligaments and damage to the joint capsule. Symptoms usually include pain, swelling, deformity, a bruise-like color, and limitation of movement. There is often a tearing sensation when the injury occurs.

Other names: Dislocated hip

The following fifth-digit subclassification is for use with category 835:
0 dislocation of hip, unspecified
1 posterior dislocation
2 obturator dislocation
3 other anterior dislocation

Physical Therapy Guidelines:
9 visits over 8 weeks

Workers' Comp Costs per Claim (based on 40 claims)					
Quartile	25%	50%	75%	Mean	% no cost
Medical	$2,730	$7,728	$24,875	$19,543	0%
Total	$4,095	$13,440	$32,456	$29,374	0%

835 Dislocation of hip *(cont'd)*

RTW Claims Data (Calendar-days away from work by decile)										
10%	20%	30%	40%	**50%**	60%	70%	80%	**90%**	100%	Mean
10	12	15	20	**22**	27	28	30	**50**	304	32.35

Integrated Disability Durations, in days*

Median (mid-point)	20.0	Mean (average)	27.25
Mode (most frequent)	28	Calculated rec.	24

Percent of Cases
(102 cases)

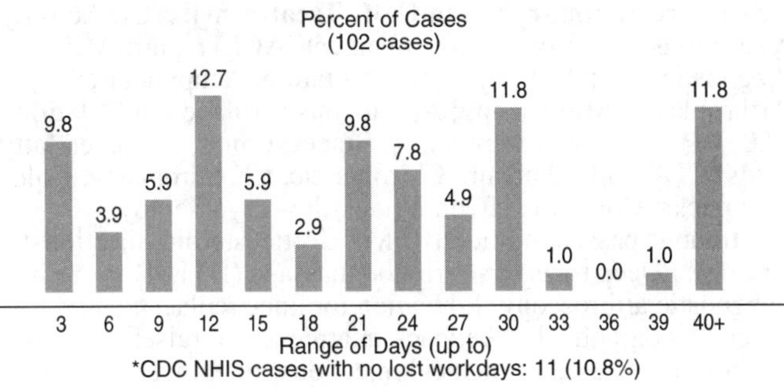

*CDC NHIS cases with no lost workdays: 11 (10.8%)

Impact on Total Absence: Prevalence 0.0073% of total lost workdays; Incidence 0.08 days per 100 workers

836 Dislocation of knee

Return-To-Work Summary Guidelines		
Dataset	**Midrange**	**At-Risk**
Claims data	32 days	88 days
All absences	22 days	80 days

Return-To-Work "Best Practice" Guidelines
Without surgery, without any associated neurovascular injury, clerical/modified work: 7 days
Without surgery, manual/standing work: 21 days
With surgery, clerical/modified work: 14 days
With surgery, manual/standing work: 42 days

Capabilities & Activity Modifications:
Sedentary/modified work: Standing limited to 5-10 min/hr; walking only on a smooth surface using crutches with limited pressure on the foot; no walking on an irregular surface; no climbing stairs; no climbing ladders or hill climbing requiring frequent knee flexion; no activities requiring balance; no applying strength against bent knee (squatting, kneeling, crouching, stooping, pedaling, etc.); elevate leg half of time; may need immobilization; limited weight bearing.
Manual/standing work: Standing not more than 50 min/hr; walking on a smooth surface up to 1,200 ft/hr carrying up to 25 lbs; walking on an irregular surface up to 900 ft/hr carrying up to 25 lbs; climbing stairs up to 8 flights/hr carrying up to 40 lbs; climbing ladders up to 50 rungs/hr carrying up to 25 lbs; activities requiring balance up to 45 min/hr (if able to work with two hands without assistance for balance); applying strength against bent knee (pedaling, squatting, kneeling, etc.) up to 60 times/hr; may need brace for uneven ground or ladders.

Description: Displacement of the bones in the knee joint. A dislocation is usually accompanied by torn joint ligaments and damage to the joint capsule. Symptoms usually include pain, swelling, deformity, a bruise-like color, and limitation of movement. There is often a tearing sensation when the injury occurs.

Other names: Dislocated knee

836 Dislocation of knee *(cont'd)*

Excludes:

dislocation of knee:
old or pathological (718.2)
recurrent (718.3)
internal derangement of knee joint (717.0-717.5, 717.8-717.9)
old tear of cartilage or meniscus of knee (717.0-717.5, 717.8-717.9)

Procedure Summary (from ODG Treatment): ACI; Activity restrictions; Anterior cruciate ligament (ACL) repair; ACL diagnostic tests; ACL injury rehabilitation; Acupuncture; Arthroplasty; Arthroscopy; Autologous cartilage implantation (ACI); Bone-growth stimulators; Braces; Canes; Cetylated fatty acids (CFA) topical cream; Chiropractic; Chondroplasty; Cold/heat packs; Cold lasers; Continuous-flow cryotherapy; Continuous passive motion (CPM); Corticosteroid injections; Crutches; Deep transverse friction massage (DTFM); Diagnostic arthroscopy; Education for knee replacement; Electromyographic biofeedback treatment; Exercise; Glucosamine; Hyaluronic acid injections; Imaging; Immobilization; Injections; Insoles; Interferential current therapy (IFC); Knee brace; Knee joint replacement; KT 1000 arthrometer; Lachman test; Lateral pull test and patellar tilt test; Lateral retinacular release; Low level laser therapy (LLLT); Magnet therapy; Manipulation; Meniscal allograft transplantation; Meniscectomy; Microprocessor-controlled knee prostheses; Modified duty; Mosaicplasty; MRI's (magnetic resonance imaging); Non-surgical intervention for PFPS (patellofemoral pain syndrome); Occupational therapy; Orthoses; Osteochondral autograft transplant system (OATS); Osteotomy; Pharmacotherapy; Physical therapy; Pivot shift test (MacIntosh test) ; Posterior cruciate ligament (PCL) repair; Post-op ambulatory infusion pumps (local anesthetic); Prolotherapy; Prostheses (artificial limb); Pulsed magnetic field therapy (PMFT); Radiography; Return to work; SAMe (S-adenosylmethionine); Single photon emission computed tomography (SPECT); Static progressive stretch (SPS) therapy; Stretching and flexibility; Surgery; SynviscÒ; Therapeutic knee splint; Therapeutic ultrasound; Transcutaneous electrical neurostimulation (TENS); Ultrasound, diagnostic; Ultrasound, therapeutic; Ultrasound fracture healing (bone-growth stimulators); Viscosupplementation; Walkers; Walking aids (canes, crutches, braces, orthoses, & walkers); Work

Physical Therapy Guidelines:
Allow for fading of treatment frequency (from up to 3 visits per week to 1 or less), plus active self-directed home PT
Medical treatment: 9 visits over 8 weeks
Post-surgical treatment: 12 visits over 12 weeks

Workers' Comp Costs per Claim (based on 10,992 claims)

Quartile	25%	50%	75%	Mean	% no cost
Indemnity	$2,741	$5,576	$11,204	$9,813	36%
Medical	$4,284	$6,983	$10,794	$9,044	0%
Total	$5,660	$10,064	$17,724	$15,331	0%

RTW Claims Data (Calendar-days away from work by decile)

10%	20%	30%	40%	**50%**	60%	70%	80%	**90%**	100%	Mean
12	15	20	23	**32**	41	44	57	**88**	365	43.33

836 Dislocation of knee *(cont'd)*

RTW Post Surgery (Calendar-days away from work by decile)

	10%	20%	30%	40%	**50%**	60%	70%	80%	**90%**	100%	Mean
Knee arthroscopy/surgery	19	26	31	41	**51**	55	74	151	**248**	365	89.93
Knee arthroscopy/surgery	12	27	36	47	**55**	72	87	138	**256**	365	94.00
Knee arthroscopy/surgery	16	25	31	39	**46**	58	73	102	**197**	365	78.84
Knee arthroscopy/surgery	12	25	37	45	**58**	73	89	151	**365**	365	99.71
Knee arthroscopy/surgery	16	25	34	41	**52**	62	84	123	**208**	365	84.59
Knee arthroscopy/surgery	13	21	30	37	**44**	53	66	94	**170**	365	72.07
Knee arthroscopy/surgery	22	35	46	59	**69**	93	110	146	**301**	365	107.65
Knee arthroscopy/surgery	27	44	68	81	**95**	118	151	186	**253**	365	124.48

Integrated Disability Durations, in days*
Median (mid-point) 22.0 Mean (average) 35.58
Mode (most frequent) 7 Calculated rec. 22

Percent of Cases
(2901 cases)

18.8 14.2 12.0 5.5 11.2 4.1 2.1 2.2 1.4 1.5 1.0 0.7 0.5 3.9

9 18 27 36 45 54 63 72 81 90 99 108 117 118+
Range of Days (up to)
*CDC NHIS cases with no lost workdays: 605 (20.9%)

Impact on Total Absence: Prevalence 0.2414% of total lost workdays; Incidence 2.54 days per 100 workers

Occupational Disability Durations, in days
Median (mid-point) 27 - Benchmark Indemnity Costs $20,250

Percent of Cases
(1575 cases)

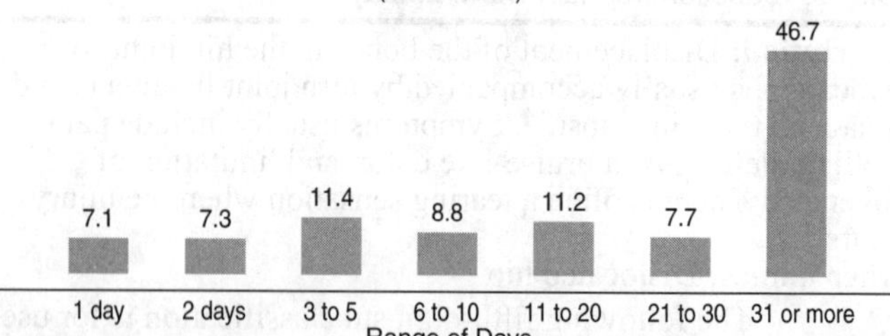

Range of Days

Impact on Occupational Absence: Prevalence 0.4824% of occupational lost workdays; Incidence 0.08 days per 100 workers

836.0 Tear of medial cartilage or meniscus of knee, current

Return-To-Work Summary Guidelines

Dataset	Midrange	At-Risk
Claims data	37 days	94 days
All absences	20 days	85 days

836.0 Tear of medial cartilage or meniscus of knee, current *(cont'd)*

Return-To-Work "Best Practice" Guidelines
Without surgery, clerical/modified work: 0-2 days
Without surgery, manual/standing work: 21 days
With arthroscopy, clerical/modified work: 14 days
With arthroscopy, manual/standing work: 42 days
With arthrotomy, clerical/modified work: 28 days
With arthrotomy, manual/standing work: 56 days
With arthrotomy, heavy manual/standing work: 84 days

Capabilities & Activity Modifications:
Sedentary/modified work: Standing limited to 5-10 min/hr; walking only on a smooth surface using crutches with limited pressure on the foot; no walking on an irregular surface; no climbing stairs; no climbing ladders or hill climbing requiring frequent knee flexion; no activities requiring balance; no applying strength against bent knee (squatting, kneeling, crouching, stooping, pedaling, etc.); elevate leg half of time; may need immobilization; limited weight bearing.
Manual/standing work: Standing not more than 50 min/hr; walking on a smooth surface up to 1,200 ft/hr carrying up to 25 lbs; walking on an irregular surface up to 900 ft/hr carrying up to 25 lbs; climbing stairs up to 8 flights/hr carrying up to 40 lbs; climbing ladders up to 50 rungs/hr carrying up to 25 lbs; activities requiring balance up to 45 min/hr (if able to work with two hands without assistance for balance); applying strength against bent knee (pedaling, squatting, kneeling, etc.) up to 60 times/hr; may need brace for uneven ground or ladders.
Description: Injury or tear of the cartilage in the knee either by trauma or degeneration through aging. Symptoms include tenderness, pain, swelling, limitation of motion, inability to straighten the knee, and/or buckling of the knee.
Other names: Injured knee cartilage, Torn knee cartilage

Bucket handle tear:
NOS current injury
medial meniscus current injury

Procedure Summary (from ODG Treatment): ACI; Activity restrictions; Anterior cruciate ligament (ACL) repair; ACL diagnostic tests; ACL injury rehabilitation; Acupuncture; Arthroplasty; Arthroscopy; Autologous cartilage implantation (ACI); Bone-growth stimulators; Braces; Canes; Cetylated fatty acids (CFA) topical cream; Chiropractic; Chondroplasty; Cold/heat packs; Cold lasers; Continuous-flow cryotherapy; Continuous passive motion (CPM); Corticosteroid injections; Crutches; Deep transverse friction massage (DTFM); Diagnostic arthroscopy; Education for knee replacement; Electromyographic biofeedback treatment; Exercise; Glucosamine; Hyaluronic acid injections; Imaging; Immobilization; Injections; Insoles; Interferential current therapy (IFC); Knee brace; Knee joint replacement; KT 1000 arthrometer; Lachman test; Lateral pull test and patellar tilt test; Lateral retinacular release; Low level laser therapy (LLLT); Magnet therapy; Manipulation; Meniscal allograft transplantation; Meniscectomy; Microprocessor-controlled knee prostheses; Modified duty; Mosaicplasty; MRI's (magnetic resonance imaging); Non-surgical intervention for PFPS (patellofemoral pain syndrome); Occupational therapy; Orthoses; Osteochondral autograft transplant system (OATS); Osteotomy; Pharmacotherapy; Physical therapy; Pivot shift test (MacIntosh test) ; Posterior cruciate ligament (PCL) repair; Post-op ambulatory infusion pumps (local anesthetic); Prolotherapy; Prostheses (artificial limb); Pulsed magnetic field therapy (PMFT); Radiography; Return to work; SAMe (S-adenosylmethionine); Single photon emission computed tomography (SPECT); Static progressive stretch (SPS) therapy; Stretching and flexibility; Surgery; SynviscÒ; Therapeutic knee splint; Therapeutic ultrasound; Transcutaneous electrical neurostimulation (TENS); Ultrasound, diagnostic; Ultrasound, therapeutic; Ultrasound fracture healing (bone-growth stimulators); Viscosupplementation; Walkers; Walking aids (canes, crutches, braces, orthoses, & walkers); Work
Physical Therapy Guidelines:
Medical treatment: 9 visits over 8 weeks
Post-surgical treatment: 12 visits over 12 weeks

Workers' Comp Costs per Claim (based on 6,730 claims)

Quartile	25%	50%	75%	Mean	% no cost
Indemnity	$2,625	$5,124	$9,503	$8,568	38%
Medical	$4,421	$6,657	$9,450	$8,002	0%
Total	$5,765	$9,377	$15,414	$13,355	0%

RTW Claims Data (Calendar-days away from work by decile)

10%	20%	30%	40%	**50%**	60%	70%	80%	**90%**	100%	Mean
13	19	24	29	**37**	44	56	76	**94**	150	47.00

RTW Post Surgery (Calendar-days away from work by decile)

	10%	20%	30%	40%	**50%**	60%	70%	80%	**90%**	100%	Mean
Knee arthroscopy/surgery	19	26	33	41	**51**	55	73	153	**289**	365	92.14
Knee arthroscopy/surgery	12	27	36	48	**58**	72	89	166	**365**	365	100.32
Knee arthroscopy/surgery	16	25	32	39	**47**	59	74	101	**195**	365	78.70
Knee arthroscopy/surgery	10	19	33	42	**58**	67	87	130	**349**	365	92.32
Knee arthroscopy/surgery	16	25	34	41	**52**	61	83	122	**209**	365	84.23
Knee arthroscopy/surgery	13	20	29	35	**44**	52	63	90	**159**	365	70.18
Knee arthroscopy/surgery	24	35	47	59	**66**	81	109	156	**318**	365	108.19
Knee arthroscopy/surgery	25	44	65	78	**88**	108	146	189	**237**	365	119.37

Integrated Disability Durations, in days*

Median (mid-point) 20.0 Mean (average) 31.19
Mode (most frequent) 1 Calculated rec. 18

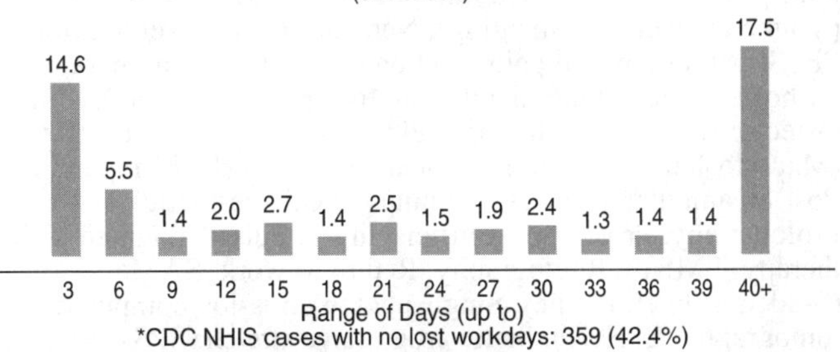

*CDC NHIS cases with no lost workdays: 359 (42.4%)

Impact on Total Absence: Prevalence 0.0449% of total lost workdays; Incidence 0.47 days per 100 workers

836.3 Dislocation of patella, closed

Return-To-Work Summary Guidelines		
Dataset	**Midrange**	**At-Risk**
Claims data	35 days	75 days
All absences	16 days	62 days

836.3 Dislocation of patella, closed *(cont'd)*

Return-To-Work "Best Practice" Guidelines
Without surgery, clerical/modified work: 7 days
Without surgery, manual work: 35 days
With surgery, clerical/modified work: 14 days
With surgery, manual work: 42 days

Capabilities & Activity Modifications:
Sedentary/modified work: Standing limited to 5-10 min/hr; walking only on a smooth surface using crutches with limited pressure on the foot; no walking on an irregular surface; no climbing stairs; no climbing ladders or hill climbing requiring frequent knee flexion; no activities requiring balance; no applying strength against bent knee (squatting, kneeling, crouching, stooping, pedaling, etc.); elevate leg half of time; may need immobilization; limited weight bearing.
Manual/standing work: Standing not more than 50 min/hr; walking on a smooth surface up to 1,200 ft/hr carrying up to 25 lbs; walking on an irregular surface up to 900 ft/hr carrying up to 25 lbs; climbing stairs up to 8 flights/hr carrying up to 40 lbs; climbing ladders up to 50 rungs/hr carrying up to 25 lbs; activities requiring balance up to 45 min/hr (if able to work with two hands without assistance for balance); applying strength against bent knee (pedaling, squatting, kneeling, etc.) up to 60 times/hr; may need brace for uneven ground or ladders.
Description: Displacement of the kneecap (patella). Extreme pain and swelling, a popping noise, and limitation of movement are among the symptoms.
Other names: Kneecap subluxation
Procedure Summary (from ODG Treatment): ACI; Activity restrictions; Anterior cruciate ligament (ACL) repair; ACL diagnostic tests; ACL injury rehabilitation; Acupuncture; Arthroplasty; Arthroscopy; Autologous cartilage implantation (ACI); Bone-growth stimulators; Braces; Canes; Cetylated fatty acids (CFA) topical cream; Chiropractic; Chondroplasty; Cold/heat packs; Cold lasers; Continuous-flow cryotherapy; Continuous passive motion (CPM); Corticosteroid injections; Crutches; Deep transverse friction massage (DTFM); Diagnostic arthroscopy; Education for knee replacement; Electromyographic biofeedback treatment; Exercise; Glucosamine; Hyaluronic acid injections; Imaging; Immobilization; Injections; Insoles; Interferential current therapy (IFC); Knee brace; Knee joint replacement; KT 1000 arthrometer; Lachman test; Lateral pull test and patellar tilt test; Lateral retinacular release; Low level laser therapy (LLLT); Magnet therapy; Manipulation; Meniscal allograft transplantation; Meniscectomy; Microprocessor-controlled knee prostheses; Modified duty; Mosaicplasty; MRI's (magnetic resonance imaging); Non-surgical intervention for PFPS (patellofemoral pain syndrome); Occupational therapy; Orthoses; Osteochondral autograft transplant system (OATS); Osteotomy; Pharmacotherapy; Physical therapy; Pivot shift test (MacIntosh test) ; Posterior cruciate ligament (PCL) repair; Post-op ambulatory infusion pumps (local anesthetic); Prolotherapy; Prostheses (artificial limb); Pulsed magnetic field therapy (PMFT); Radiography; Return to work; SAMe (S-adenosylmethionine); Single photon emission computed tomography (SPECT); Static progressive stretch (SPS) therapy; Stretching and flexibility; Surgery; SynviscÒ; Therapeutic knee splint; Therapeutic ultrasound; Transcutaneous electrical neurostimulation (TENS); Ultrasound, diagnostic; Ultrasound, therapeutic; Ultrasound fracture healing (bone-growth stimulators); Viscosupplementation; Walkers; Walking aids (canes, crutches, braces, orthoses, & walkers); Work
Physical Therapy Guidelines:
Medical treatment: 9 visits over 8 weeks

836.3 Dislocation of patella, closed *(cont'd)*

Workers' Comp Costs per Claim (based on 678 claims)

Quartile	25%	50%	75%	Mean	% no cost
Indemnity	$1,040	$2,709	$6,311	$6,293	54%
Medical	$767	$1,843	$4,421	$4,524	1%
Total	$945	$2,363	$6,804	$7,456	1%

RTW Claims Data (Calendar-days away from work by decile)

10%	20%	30%	40%	**50%**	60%	70%	80%	**90%**	100%	Mean
11	15	23	31	**35**	39	43	53	**75**	146	38.61

Integrated Disability Durations, in days*
Median (mid-point) 16.5 Mean (average) 27.20
Mode (most frequent) 2 Calculated rec. 16

Percent of Cases
(366 cases)

Range of Days (up to)	3	6	9	12	15	18	21	24	27	30	33	36	39	40+
Percent	13.1	7.4	7.1	3.0	6.3	2.2	0.8	1.1	1.9	2.2	2.2	6.3	2.7	19.7

*CDC NHIS cases with no lost workdays: 88 (24.0%)

Impact on Total Absence: Prevalence 0.0223% of total lost workdays; Incidence 0.23 days per 100 workers

836.5 Other dislocation of knee, closed

Return-To-Work Summary Guidelines

Dataset	Midrange	At-Risk
Claims data	38 days	84 days
All absences	7 days	59 days

Return-To-Work "Best Practice" Guidelines
Closed reduction, clerical/modified work: 9 days
Closed reduction, manual work: 28 days
Open reduction, clerical/modified work: 28 days
Open reduction, manual work: 56 days
Open reduction, heavy manual work: 84 days

Capabilities & Activity Modifications:
Sedentary/modified work: Standing limited to 5-10 min/hr; walking only on a smooth surface using crutches with limited pressure on the foot; no walking on an irregular surface; no climbing stairs; no climbing ladders or hill climbing requiring frequent knee flexion; no activities requiring balance; no applying strength against bent knee (squatting, kneeling, crouching, stooping, pedaling, etc.); elevate leg half of time; may need immobilization; limited weight bearing.
Manual/standing work: Standing not more than 50 min/hr; walking on a smooth surface up to 1,200 ft/hr carrying up to 25 lbs; walking on an irregular surface up to 900 ft/hr carrying up to 25 lbs; climbing stairs up to 8 flights/hr carrying up to 40 lbs; climbing ladders up to 50 rungs/hr carrying up to 25 lbs; activities requiring balance up to 45 min/hr (if able to work with two hands without assistance for balance); applying strength against bent knee (pedaling, squatting, kneeling, etc.) up to 60 times/hr; may need brace for uneven ground or ladders.
Description: Displacement of the knee. Symptoms include tenderness, pain, swelling, limitation of motion, inability to straighten the knee, and/or buckling of the knee.
Other names: Injured knee cartilage, Torn knee cartilage

836.5 Other dislocation of knee, closed *(cont'd)*

Procedure Summary (from ODG Treatment): ACI; Activity restrictions; Anterior cruciate ligament (ACL) repair; ACL diagnostic tests; ACL injury rehabilitation; Acupuncture; Arthroplasty; Arthroscopy; Autologous cartilage implantation (ACI); Bone-growth stimulators; Braces; Canes; Cetylated fatty acids (CFA) topical cream; Chiropractic; Chondroplasty; Cold/heat packs; Cold lasers; Continuous-flow cryotherapy; Continuous passive motion (CPM); Corticosteroid injections; Crutches; Deep transverse friction massage (DTFM); Diagnostic arthroscopy; Education for knee replacement; Electromyographic biofeedback treatment; Exercise; Glucosamine; Hyaluronic acid injections; Imaging; Immobilization; Injections; Insoles; Interferential current therapy (IFC); Knee brace; Knee joint replacement; KT 1000 arthrometer; Lachman test; Lateral pull test and patellar tilt test; Lateral retinacular release; Low level laser therapy (LLLT); Magnet therapy; Manipulation; Meniscal allograft transplantation; Meniscectomy; Microprocessor-controlled knee prostheses; Modified duty; Mosaicplasty; MRI's (magnetic resonance imaging); Non-surgical intervention for PFPS (patellofemoral pain syndrome); Occupational therapy; Orthoses; Osteochondral autograft transplant system (OATS); Osteotomy; Pharmacotherapy; Physical therapy; Pivot shift test (MacIntosh test) ; Posterior cruciate ligament (PCL) repair; Post-op ambulatory infusion pumps (local anesthetic); Prolotherapy; Prostheses (artificial limb); Pulsed magnetic field therapy (PMFT); Radiography; Return to work; SAMe (S-adenosylmethionine); Single photon emission computed tomography (SPECT); Static progressive stretch (SPS) therapy; Stretching and flexibility; Surgery; SynviscÒ; Therapeutic knee splint; Therapeutic ultrasound; Transcutaneous electrical neurostimulation (TENS); Ultrasound, diagnostic; Ultrasound, therapeutic; Ultrasound fracture healing (bone-growth stimulators); Viscosupplementation; Walkers; Walking aids (canes, crutches, braces, orthoses, & walkers); Work

Physical Therapy Guidelines:
Medical treatment: 9 visits over 8 weeks

Workers' Comp Costs per Claim (based on 95 claims)

Quartile	25%	50%	75%	Mean	% no cost
Medical	$389	$956	$1,995	$2,909	2%
Total	$389	$1,050	$2,457	$4,930	2%

RTW Claims Data (Calendar-days away from work by decile)

10%	20%	30%	40%	**50%**	60%	70%	80%	**90%**	100%	Mean
10	11	23	31	**38**	41	52	59	**79**	120	41.80

Integrated Disability Durations, in days*

Median (mid-point)	8.0	Mean (average)	22.37
Mode (most frequent)	1	Calculated rec.	10

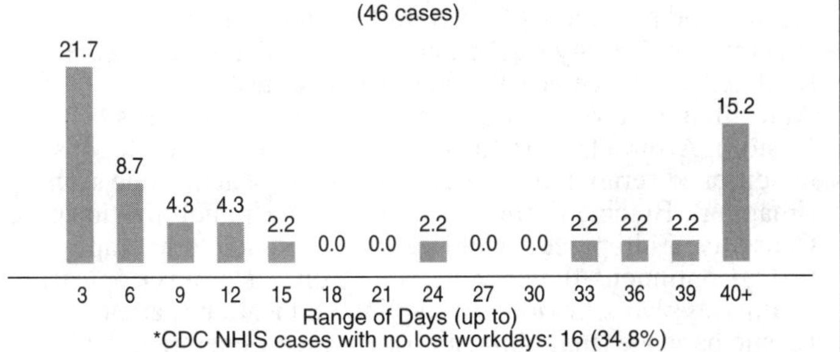

*CDC NHIS cases with no lost workdays: 16 (34.8%)

Impact on Total Absence: Prevalence 0.0019% of total lost workdays; Incidence 0.02 days per 100 workers

837 Dislocation of ankle

Return-To-Work Summary Guidelines		
Dataset	**Midrange**	**At-Risk**
Claims data	53 days	128 days
All absences	37 days	124 days

Return-To-Work "Best Practice" Guidelines
See 837.0

Includes: astragalus
fibula, distal end
navicular, foot
scaphoid, foot
tibia, distal end

Physical Therapy Guidelines:
9 visits over 8 weeks

Workers' Comp Costs per Claim (based on 262 claims)

Quartile	25%	50%	75%	Mean	% no cost
Indemnity	$4,725	$7,980	$14,175	$16,889	18%
Medical	$8,421	$13,556	$23,699	$20,645	0%
Total	$12,443	$20,286	$36,803	$34,474	0%

RTW Claims Data (Calendar-days away from work by decile)

10%	20%	30%	40%	**50%**	60%	70%	80%	**90%**	100%	Mean
12	27	29	31	**53**	71	86	103	**128**	180	62.00

Integrated Disability Durations, in days*

Median (mid-point)	37.0	Mean (average)	56.23
Mode (most frequent)	29	Calculated rec.	40

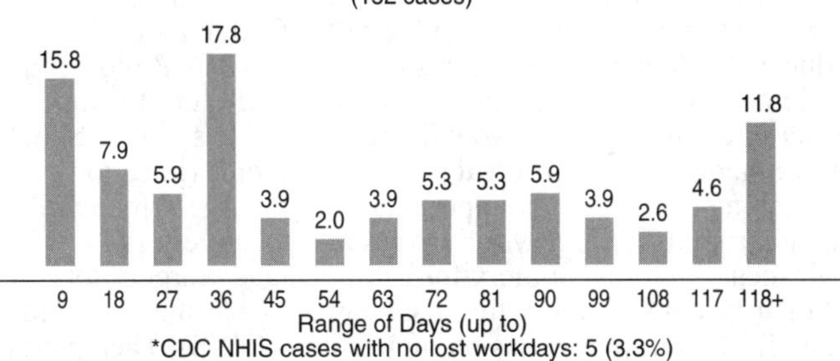

*CDC NHIS cases with no lost workdays: 5 (3.3%)

Impact on Total Absence: Prevalence 0.0244% of total lost workdays; Incidence 0.26 days per 100 workers

837.0 Closed dislocation

Return-To-Work Summary Guidelines		
Dataset	**Midrange**	**At-Risk**
Claims data	67 days	131 days
All absences	60 days	129 days

Return-To-Work "Best Practice" Guidelines
Closed reduction, clerical/modified work: 7 days
Closed reduction, manual work (w/o cast): 28 days

Capabilities & Activity Modifications:
Sedentary/modified work: Standing limited to 5-10 min/hr; walking only on a smooth surface using crutches with limited pressure on the foot; no walking on an irregular surface; no climbing stairs; no climbing ladders or hill climbing requiring frequent knee flexion; no activities requiring balance; no applying strength against bent knee (squatting, kneeling, crouching, stooping, pedaling, etc.); elevate leg half of time; may need immobilization; limited weight bearing.

837.0 Closed dislocation *(cont'd)*

Manual/standing work: Standing not more than 50 min/hr; walking on a smooth surface up to 1,200 ft/hr carrying up to 25 lbs; walking on an irregular surface up to 900 ft/hr carrying up to 25 lbs; climbing stairs up to 8 flights/hr carrying up to 40 lbs; climbing ladders up to 50 rungs/hr carrying up to 25 lbs; activities requiring balance up to 45 min/hr (if able to work with two hands without assistance for balance); applying strength against bent knee (pedaling, squatting, kneeling, etc.) up to 60 times/hr; may need brace for uneven ground or ladders.

Description: A simple dislocation (not complicated by an external wound).

Procedure Summary (from ODG Treatment):
Accommodative modalities; Achilles tendon ruptures (treatment); Activity restrictions; Actovegin; Ankle prostheses (total ankle replacement); Anterior drawer test; Anti-inflammatory medications (NSAIDs); Arthrodesis (fusion); Arthroplasty (total ankle replacement); Autologous conditioned serum (ACS); Bed rest; Biofeedback; Bone scan (imaging); Bracing (immobilization); Cast (immobilization); Causality; Chiropractic; Cold packs; Computed tomography (CT); Continuous-flow cryotherapy; Corticosteroids (topical); Diathermy; Dorsiflexion night splints; Education (patient); Elastic bandage (immobilization); Electron generating device; Exercise; Extracorporeal shock wave therapy (ESWT); Functional treatment; Fusion; Heat therapy (ice/heat); Heparin; Heel pads; Ice packs; Imaging; Immobilization; Ingrown toenail surgery; Injections; Insoles with magnetic foil; Inversion stress test; Iontophoresis; Lace-up ankle support; Laser therapy (LLLT); Lateral ligament ankle reconstruction (surgery); Lineal tomography; Low-intensity laser therapy (LLLT); Magnets; Magnetic resonance imaging (MRI); Manipulation; Massage; Mechanical treatment (taping/orthoses); Modified duty; Narcotics; Night splints; Nonprescription medications; Orthotic devices; Osteotomy; Ottawa ankle rules (OAR); Patient education; Phonophoresis; Physical therapy (PT); Prolotherapy (sclerotherapy); Radiography; Rest (RICE); Return to work; Sclerotherapy (prolotherapy); Semi-rigid ankle support; Shock wave therapy, extracorporeal (ESWT); Steroids (injection); Stretching (flexibility); Supports; Surgery; Surgery for achilles tendon ruptures; Surgery for ankle sprains; Surgery for calcaneal fractures; Surgery for hallux valgus; Surgery for plantar fasciitis; Surgery for tarsal tunnel syndrome; Talar tilt test; Tai Chi; Taping; Tension night splints (TNS); Therapeutic exercise; Thompson test; Total ankle replacement (arthroplasty); Transcutaneous electrical neurostimulation (TENS); Ultrasound, diagnostic; Ultrasound, therapeutic; Work

Physical Therapy Guidelines:
9 visits over 8 weeks

Workers' Comp Costs per Claim (based on 253 claims)					
Quartile	25%	50%	75%	Mean	% no cost
Indemnity	$4,547	$7,665	$13,913	$16,065	18%
Medical	$8,411	$13,167	$22,565	$18,782	0%
Total	$12,285	$19,982	$35,858	$31,949	0%

RTW Claims Data (Calendar-days away from work by decile)										
10%	20%	30%	40%	**50%**	60%	70%	80%	**90%**	100%	Mean
12	27	30	51	**67**	82	92	114	**131**	150	68.36

837.0 Closed dislocation *(cont'd)*

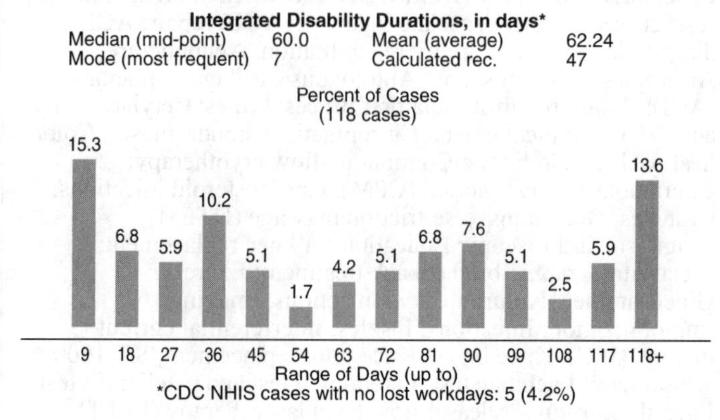

Impact on Total Absence: Prevalence 0.0207% of total lost workdays; Incidence 0.22 days per 100 workers

837.1 Open dislocation

Return-To-Work Summary Guidelines		
Dataset	**Midrange**	**At-Risk**
Claims data	53 days	128 days
All absences	37 days	124 days

Return-To-Work "Best Practice" Guidelines
Open reduction, clerical/modified work: 14 days
Open reduction, manual work: 56 days

Capabilities & Activity Modifications:
Sedentary/modified work: Standing limited to 5-10 min/hr; walking only on a smooth surface using crutches with limited pressure on the foot; no walking on an irregular surface; no climbing stairs; no climbing ladders or hill climbing requiring frequent knee flexion; no activities requiring balance; no applying strength against bent knee (squatting, kneeling, crouching, stooping, pedaling, etc.); elevate leg half of time; may need immobilization; limited weight bearing.
Manual/standing work: Standing not more than 50 min/hr; walking on a smooth surface up to 1,200 ft/hr carrying up to 25 lbs; walking on an irregular surface up to 900 ft/hr carrying up to 25 lbs; climbing stairs up to 8 flights/hr carrying up to 40 lbs; climbing ladders up to 50 rungs/hr carrying up to 25 lbs; activities requiring balance up to 45 min/hr (if able to work with two hands without assistance for balance); applying strength against bent knee (pedaling, squatting, kneeling, etc.) up to 60 times/hr; may need brace for uneven ground or ladders.

Description: A dislocation that is complicated by a wound opening from the surface to the affected joint.

Procedure Summary (from ODG Treatment):
Accommodative modalities; Achilles tendon ruptures (treatment); Activity restrictions; Actovegin; Ankle prostheses (total ankle replacement); Anterior drawer test; Anti-inflammatory medications (NSAIDs); Arthrodesis (fusion); Arthroplasty (total ankle replacement); Autologous conditioned serum (ACS); Bed rest; Biofeedback; Bone scan (imaging); Bracing (immobilization); Cast (immobilization); Causality; Chiropractic; Cold packs; Computed tomography (CT); Continuous-flow cryotherapy; Corticosteroids (topical); Diathermy; Dorsiflexion night splints; Education (patient); Elastic bandage (immobilization); Electron generating device; Exercise; Extracorporeal shock wave therapy (ESWT); Functional treatment; Fusion; Heat therapy (ice/heat); Heparin; Heel pads; Ice packs; Imaging; Immobilization; Ingrown toenail surgery; Injections; Insoles with magnetic foil; Inversion stress test; Iontophoresis; Lace-up ankle support; Laser therapy

837.1 Open dislocation *(cont'd)*

(LLLT); Lateral ligament ankle reconstruction (surgery); Lineal tomography; Low-intensity laser therapy (LLLT); Magnets; Magnetic resonance imaging (MRI); Manipulation; Massage; Mechanical treatment (taping/orthoses); Modified duty; Narcotics; Night splints; Nonprescription medications; Orthotic devices; Osteotomy; Ottawa ankle rules (OAR); Patient education; Phonophoresis; Physical therapy (PT); Prolotherapy (sclerotherapy); Radiography; Rest (RICE); Return to work; Sclerotherapy (prolotherapy); Semi-rigid ankle support; Shock wave therapy, extracorporeal (ESWT); Steroids (injection); Stretching (flexibility); Supports; Surgery; Surgery for achilles tendon ruptures; Surgery for ankle sprains; Surgery for calcaneal fractures; Surgery for hallux valgus; Surgery for plantar fasciitis; Surgery for tarsal tunnel syndrome; Talar tilt test; Tai Chi; Taping; Tension night splints (TNS); Therapeutic exercise; Thompson test; Total ankle replacement (arthroplasty); Transcutaneous electrical neurostimulation (TENS); Ultrasound, diagnostic; Ultrasound, therapeutic; Work

Impact on Total Absence: Prevalence 0.0003% of total lost workdays

838 Dislocation of foot

Return-To-Work Summary Guidelines		
Dataset	**Midrange**	**At-Risk**
Claims data	42 days	116 days
All absences	30 days	94 days

Return-To-Work "Best Practice" Guidelines
Clerical/modified work: 0 days
Manual/standing work: 21 days
Heavy manual/standing work: 42 days

Capabilities & Activity Modifications:
Sedentary/modified work: Standing limited to 5-10 min/hr; walking only on a smooth surface using crutches with limited pressure on the foot; no walking on an irregular surface; no climbing stairs; no climbing ladders or hill climbing requiring frequent knee flexion; no activities requiring balance; no applying strength against bent knee (squatting, kneeling, crouching, stooping, pedaling, etc.); elevate leg half of time; may need immobilization; limited weight bearing.
Manual/standing work: Standing not more than 50 min/hr; walking on a smooth surface up to 1,200 ft/hr carrying up to 25 lbs; walking on an irregular surface up to 900 ft/hr carrying up to 25 lbs; climbing stairs up to 8 flights/hr carrying up to 40 lbs; climbing ladders up to 50 rungs/hr carrying up to 25 lbs; activities requiring balance up to 45 min/hr (if able to work with two hands without assistance for balance); applying strength against bent knee (pedaling, squatting, kneeling, etc.) up to 60 times/hr; may need brace for uneven ground or ladders.
Description: Displacement of bones in the foot. A dislocation is usually accompanied by torn joint ligaments and damage to the joint capsule. Symptoms usually include pain, swelling, deformity, a bruise-like color, and limitation of movement. There is often a tearing sensation when the injury occurs.

838 Dislocation of foot *(cont'd)*

The following fifth-digit subclassification is for use with category 838:
0 foot, unspecified
1 tarsal (bone), joint unspecified
2 midtarsal (joint)
3 tarsometatarsal (joint)
4 metatarsal (bone), joint unspecified
5 metatarsophalangeal (joint)
6 interphalangeal (joint), foot
9 other
Phalanx of foot
Toe(s)

Procedure Summary (from ODG Treatment):
Accommodative modalities; Achilles tendon ruptures (treatment); Activity restrictions; Actovegin; Ankle prostheses (total ankle replacement); Anterior drawer test; Anti-inflammatory medications (NSAIDs); Arthrodesis (fusion); Arthroplasty (total ankle replacement); Autologous conditioned serum (ACS); Bed rest; Biofeedback; Bone scan (imaging); Bracing (immobilization); Cast (immobilization); Causality; Chiropractic; Cold packs; Computed tomography (CT); Continuous-flow cryotherapy; Corticosteroids (topical); Diathermy; Dorsiflexion night splints; Education (patient); Elastic bandage (immobilization); Electron generating device; Exercise; Extracorporeal shock wave therapy (ESWT); Functional treatment; Fusion; Heat therapy (ice/heat); Heparin; Heel pads; Ice packs; Imaging; Immobilization; Ingrown toenail surgery; Injections; Insoles with magnetic foil; Inversion stress test; Iontophoresis; Lace-up ankle support; Laser therapy (LLLT); Lateral ligament ankle reconstruction (surgery); Lineal tomography; Low-intensity laser therapy (LLLT); Magnets; Magnetic resonance imaging (MRI); Manipulation; Massage; Mechanical treatment (taping/orthoses); Modified duty; Narcotics; Night splints; Nonprescription medications; Orthotic devices; Osteotomy; Ottawa ankle rules (OAR); Patient education; Phonophoresis; Physical therapy (PT); Prolotherapy (sclerotherapy); Radiography; Rest (RICE); Return to work; Sclerotherapy (prolotherapy); Semi-rigid ankle support; Shock wave therapy, extracorporeal (ESWT); Steroids (injection); Stretching (flexibility); Supports; Surgery; Surgery for achilles tendon ruptures; Surgery for ankle sprains; Surgery for calcaneal fractures; Surgery for hallux valgus; Surgery for plantar fasciitis; Surgery for tarsal tunnel syndrome; Talar tilt test; Tai Chi; Taping; Tension night splints (TNS); Therapeutic exercise; Thompson test; Total ankle replacement (arthroplasty); Transcutaneous electrical neurostimulation (TENS); Ultrasound, diagnostic; Ultrasound, therapeutic; Work

Workers' Comp Costs per Claim (based on 272 claims)					
Quartile	25%	50%	75%	Mean	% no cost
Indemnity	$3,087	$7,571	$17,651	$15,303	32%
Medical	$1,050	$6,400	$16,517	$14,407	1%
Total	$1,449	$10,689	$29,138	$24,861	1%

RTW Claims Data (Calendar-days away from work by decile)										
10%	20%	30%	40%	**50%**	60%	70%	80%	**90%**	100%	Mean
18	21	25	31	**42**	44	53	77	**116**	199	52.00

838 Dislocation of foot *(cont'd)*

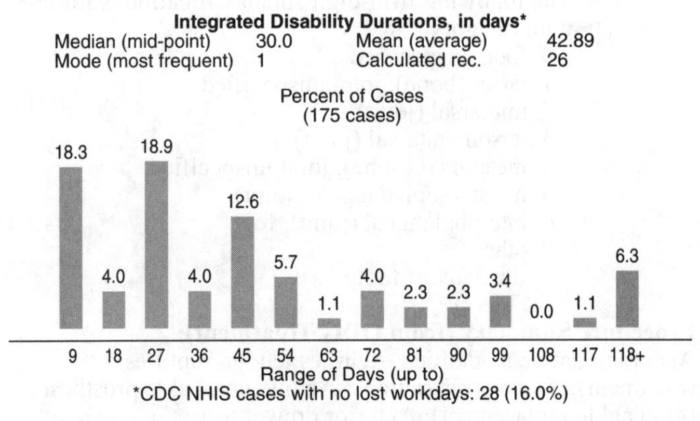

Impact on Total Absence: Prevalence 0.0186% of total lost workdays; Incidence 0.20 days per 100 workers

SPRAINS AND STRAINS OF JOINTS AND ADJACENT MUSCLES (840-848)

Description: A sprain is the rupture of supporting ligament fibers in a joint; a strain is the overexertion of a muscle.

Includes: avulsion of joint capsule, legament, muscle, tendon
hemarthrosis of joint capsule, legament, muscle, tendon
laceration of joint capsule, legament, muscle, tendon
rupture of joint capsule, legament, muscle, tendon
sprain of joint capsule, legament, muscle, tendon
strain of joint capsule, legament, muscle, tendon
tear of joint capsule, legament, muscle, tendon

Excludes:
laceration of tendon in open wounds (880-884 and 890-894 with .2)

RTW Claims Data (Calendar-days away from work by decile)										
10%	20%	30%	40%	**50%**	60%	70%	80%	**90%**	100%	Mean
10	12	14	16	**20**	25	35	42	**63**	365	32.29

Impact on Total Absence: Prevalence 4.7668% of total lost workdays; Incidence 50.05 days per 100 workers

Occupational Disability Durations, in days
Median (mid-point) 8 - Benchmark Indemnity Costs $6,000

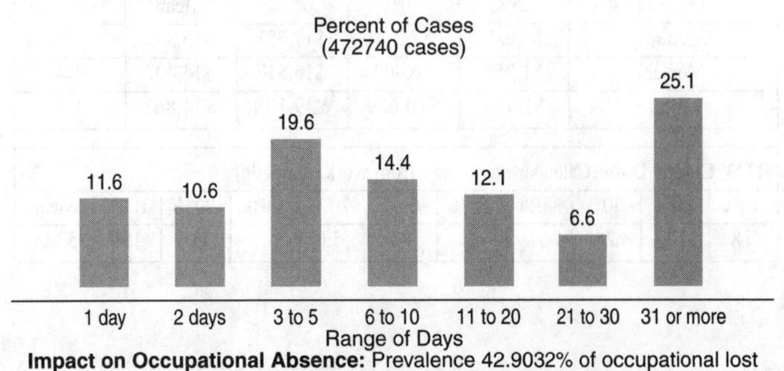

Impact on Occupational Absence: Prevalence 42.9032% of occupational lost workdays; Incidence 6.86 days per 100 workers

840 Sprains and strains of shoulder and upper arm

Return-To-Work Summary Guidelines		
Dataset	**Midrange**	**At-Risk**
Claims data	20 days	52 days
All absences	9 days	43 days

Return-To-Work "Best Practice" Guidelines
Mild (grade I), clerical/modified work: 0 days
Mild, manual work: 14 days
Moderate (grade II), clerical/modified work: 5-7 days
Moderate, manual work: 21 days
Severe (grade III), clerical/modified work: 7-10 days
Severe, manual work: 42 days

Capabilities & Activity Modifications:
Modified work: No overhead work (reaching above shoulder) plus no reaching to shoulder level (90 degree position); no holding arm in abduction or flexion; pulling and pushing not more than 8 lbs up to 4 times/hr; lifting and carrying up to 5 lbs 3 times/hr; single arm upper extremity work using injured arm for light work only; possible immobilization by abduction brace, sling, or clavicle brace; no climbing ladders.
Manual work: Reaching above shoulder not more than 12 times/hr with up to 15 lbs of weight; reaching to shoulder up to 15 times/hr with up to 25 lbs of weight; holding arm in abduction or flexion up to 12 times/hr with up to 15 lbs of weight; pulling and pushing up to 60 lbs 20 times/hr; lifting and carrying up to 40 lbs 15 times/hr; single upper extremity work using injured arm for moderate work only (full use of non-injured arm); possible immobilization by abduction brace, sling, or clavicle brace; climbing ladders up to 50 rungs/hr.
Description: Injury to the ligament (sprain) or to the muscle (strain) of the shoulder or upper arm. Sprains and strains are usually accompanied by a tearing of the tissue as well as symptoms of pain, limited motion, swelling, bruising, and/or a change in sensation.
Other names: Sprained shoulder, Strained shoulder
Procedure Summary (from ODG Treatment):
Acromioplasty; Activity restrictions; Acupuncture; Adson's test (AT); Anterior scalene block; Arthrography; Arthroplasty (shoulder); Arthroscopy; Arthroscopic release of adhesions; Bipolar interferential electrotherapy; Biofeedback; Biopsychosocial rehab; Cardiovascular functional testing; Chiropractic; Cold lasers; Continuous-flow cryotherapy; Continuous passive motion (CPM); Corticosteroid injections; Costoclavicular maneuver (CCM); Cutaneous laser treatment; Deep friction massage; Diagnostic arthroscopy; Diathermy; Distension arthrography; Electrical stimulation; Electrodiagnostic testing for TOS (thoracic outlet syndrome); Elevated arm stress test (EAST); Ergonomic interventions; Exercises; Extracorporeal shock wave therapy (ESWT); Hydroplasty/ hydrodilation; Imaging; Immobilization; Impingement test; Injections; Interferential therapy; Laser therapy; Low level laser therapy (LLLT); Magnetic resonance imaging (MRI); Manipulation; Manipulation under anesthesia (MUA); Massage; Mechanical traction; Modified duty; Multidisciplinary biopsychosocial rehab; Nerve blocks; Osteochondral autologous transplantation (OATS); Physical therapy; Porcine small intestinal submucosa (SIS); Pulsed electromagnetic field; Radiography; Return to work; Rotator cuff repair; Rotator cuff porcine graft repair; Shock wave therapy; Shoulder repair; Steroid injections; Supraclavicular pressure (SCP); Surgery for AC joint separation; Surgery for adhesive capsulitis; Surgery for impingement syndrome; Surgery for rotator cuff repair; Surgery for ruptured biceps tendon; Surgery for shoulder dislocation; Surgery for Thoracic Outlet Syndrome; Thermal capsulorrhaphy; Thermotherapy;

840 Sprains and strains of shoulder and upper arm *(cont'd)*

Transcutaneous electrical neurostimulation (TENS); Transdermal nitroglycerin; Ultrasound, diagnostic; Ultrasound, therapeutic; Work

Physical Therapy Guidelines:
Allow for fading of treatment frequency (from up to 3 visits per week to 1 or less), plus active self-directed home PT
Medical treatment: 9 visits over 8 weeks
Post-surgical treatment (RC repair/acromioplasty): 24 visits over 14 weeks

Chiropractic Guidelines:
Allow for fading of treatment frequency (from up to 3 visits per week to 1 or less), plus active self-directed home therapy
9 visits over 8 weeks

Workers' Comp Costs per Claim (based on 75,457 claims)

Quartile	25%	50%	75%	Mean	% no cost
Indemnity	$1,764	$3,675	$8,516	$7,821	76%
Medical	$263	$641	$2,289	$2,852	4%
Total	$273	$756	$3,402	$4,769	4%

Disability Duration Adjustment Factors by Age

Age Group	18-24	25-34	35-44	45-54	55-64	65-74
Adjustment Factor	0.80	0.84	0.93	1.08	1.28	1.36

RTW Claims Data (Calendar-days away from work by decile)

10%	20%	30%	40%	**50%**	60%	70%	80%	**90%**	100%	Mean
10	12	14	16	**20**	23	34	43	**52**	365	29.55

RTW Post Surgery (Calendar-days away from work by decile)

	10%	20%	30%	40%	**50%**	60%	70%	80%	**90%**	100%	Mean
Partial removal, collar bone	35	54	75	94	**114**	145	174	220	**365**	365	144.67
Remove shoulder bone, part	33	53	66	90	**101**	117	157	218	**329**	365	135.09
Repair rotator cuff, acute	33	52	75	95	**110**	137	164	209	**296**	365	137.20
Repair rotator cuff, chronic	37	59	82	101	**123**	151	184	226	**351**	365	148.77
Release of shoulder ligament	41	60	80	101	**121**	146	180	268	**365**	365	155.42
Repair of shoulder	35	60	82	99	**121**	146	177	231	**338**	365	147.37
Repair biceps tendon	21	58	73	93	**108**	131	170	212	**321**	365	136.07
Repair of ruptured tendon	7	17	41	58	**82**	94	103	136	**202**	365	93.68
Shoulder arthroscopy/surgery	34	52	72	89	**104**	129	166	209	**313**	365	133.51
Shoulder arthroscopy/surgery	31	45	63	77	**90**	117	150	193	**329**	365	127.09
Shoulder arthroscopy/surgery	34	48	67	87	**114**	139	175	234	**365**	365	142.94
Shoulder arthroscopy/surgery	28	41	67	77	**94**	117	158	209	**317**	365	128.85
Shoulder arthroscopy/surgery	26	45	62	80	**97**	125	163	209	**333**	365	132.03

840 Sprains and strains of shoulder and upper arm *(cont'd)*

Integrated Disability Durations, in days*

Median (mid-point)	9.0	Mean (average)	17.04
Mode (most frequent)	1	Calculated rec.	9

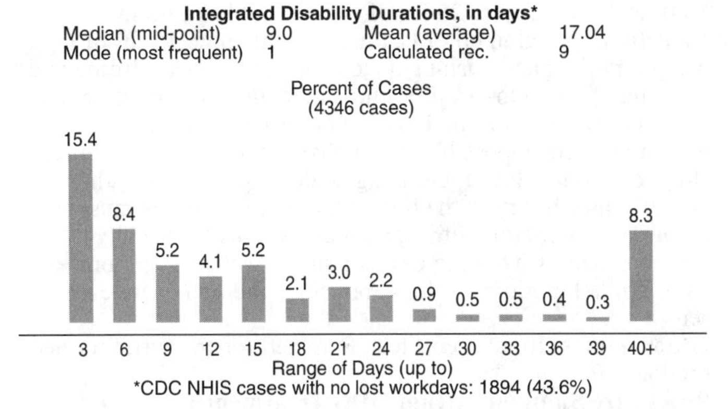

*CDC NHIS cases with no lost workdays: 1894 (43.6%)

Impact on Total Absence: Prevalence 0.1235% of total lost workdays; Incidence 1.30 days per 100 workers

Occupational Disability Durations, in days
Median (mid-point) 15 - Benchmark Indemnity Costs $11,250

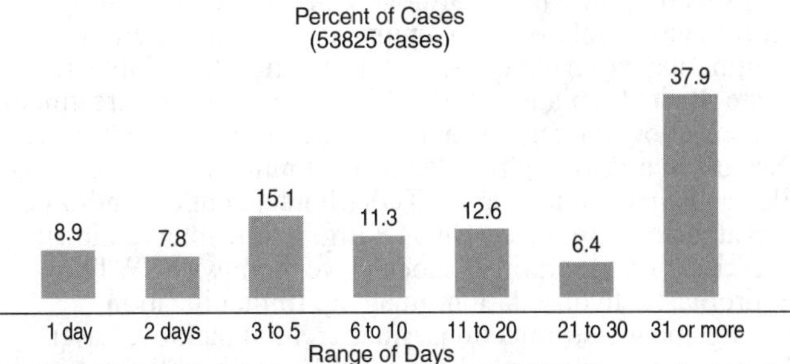

Impact on Occupational Absence: Prevalence 9.1591% of occupational lost workdays; Incidence 1.47 days per 100 workers

840.4 Rotator cuff (capsule)

Return-To-Work Summary Guidelines

Dataset	Midrange	At-Risk
Claims data	45 days	180 days
All absences	23 days	125 days

Return-To-Work "Best Practice" Guidelines
Medical treatment, modified work: 0 days
Medical treatment, manual work: 7 days
Medical treatment, manual overhead work: 28 days
Medical treatment, heavy manual work: 56 days
Arthroscopic surgical repair/acromioplasty, clerical/modified work: 28 days
Arthroscopic surgical repair/acromioplasty, manual work, non-dominant arm: 56 days
Arthroscopic surgical repair/acromioplasty, manual work, dominant arm: 70 days
Open surgery, clerical/modified work: 42-56 days
Open surgery, manual work, non-dominant arm: 70-90 days
Open surgery, manual work, dominant arm: 106-180 days
Open surgery, heavy manual work if cause of disability: indefinite

Capabilities & Activity Modifications:
Modified work: No overhead work (reaching above shoulder) plus no reaching to shoulder level (90 degree position); no holding arm in abduction or flexion; pulling and pushing not more than 8 lbs up to 4 times/hr; lifting and carrying up to 5 lbs 3 times/hr; single arm upper extremity work using injured arm for light work only; possible immobilization by abduction brace, sling, or clavicle brace; no climbing ladders.

840.4 Rotator cuff (capsule) *(cont'd)*

Manual work: Reaching above shoulder not more than 12 times/hr with up to 15 lbs of weight; reaching to shoulder up to 15 times/hr with up to 25 lbs of weight; holding arm in abduction or flexion up to 12 times/hr with up to 15 lbs of weight; pulling and pushing up to 60 lbs 20 times/hr; lifting and carrying up to 40 lbs 15 times/hr; single upper extremity work using injured arm for moderate work only (full use of non-injured arm); possible immobilization by abduction brace, sling, or clavicle brace; climbing ladders up to 50 rungs/hr.

Description: Injury to the ligament (sprain) or to the muscle (strain) of the rotator cuff. Sprains and strains are usually accompanied by a tearing of the tissue as well as symptoms of pain, limited motion, swelling, bruising, and/or a change in sensation.

Other names: Rotator cuff tear, Sprained rotator cuff, Strained rotator cuff

Procedure Summary (from ODG Treatment):
Acromioplasty; Activity restrictions; Acupuncture; Adson's test (AT); Anterior scalene block; Arthrography; Arthroplasty (shoulder); Arthroscopy; Arthroscopic release of adhesions; Bipolar interferential electrotherapy; Biofeedback; Biopsychosocial rehab; Cardiovascular functional testing; Chiropractic; Cold lasers; Continuous-flow cryotherapy; Continuous passive motion (CPM); Corticosteroid injections; Costoclavicular maneuver (CCM); Cutaneous laser treatment; Deep friction massage; Diagnostic arthroscopy; Diathermy; Distension arthrography; Electrical stimulation; Electrodiagnostic testing for TOS (thoracic outlet syndrome); Elevated arm stress test (EAST); Ergonomic interventions; Exercises; Extracorporeal shock wave therapy (ESWT); Hydroplasty/ hydrodilation; Imaging; Immobilization; Impingement test; Injections; Interferential therapy; Laser therapy; Low level laser therapy (LLLT); Magnetic resonance imaging (MRI); Manipulation; Manipulation under anesthesia (MUA); Massage; Mechanical traction; Modified duty; Multidisciplinary biopsychosocial rehab; Nerve blocks; Osteochondral autologous transplantation (OATS); Physical therapy; Porcine small intestinal submucosa (SIS); Pulsed electromagnetic field; Radiography; Return to work; Rotator cuff repair; Rotator cuff porcine graft repair; Shock wave therapy; Shoulder repair; Steroid injections; Supraclavicular pressure (SCP); Surgery for AC joint separation; Surgery for adhesive capsulitis; Surgery for impingement syndrome; Surgery for rotator cuff repair; Surgery for ruptured biceps tendon; Surgery for shoulder dislocation; Surgery for Thoracic Outlet Syndrome; Thermal capsulorrhaphy; Thermotherapy; Transcutaneous electrical neurostimulation (TENS); Transdermal nitroglycerin; Ultrasound, diagnostic; Ultrasound, therapeutic; Work

Physical Therapy Guidelines:
Post-surgical treatment: 24 visits over 14 weeks

Workers' Comp Costs per Claim (based on 7,167 claims)					
Quartile	25%	50%	75%	Mean	% no cost
Indemnity	$3,969	$8,909	$18,438	$14,466	48%
Medical	$1,250	$7,172	$16,002	$10,571	1%
Total	$1,544	$10,437	$25,400	$18,256	1%

RTW Claims Data (Calendar-days away from work by decile)										
10%	20%	30%	40%	**50%**	60%	70%	80%	**90%**	100%	Mean
13	17	26	38	**45**	59	77	106	**175**	365	75.94

840.4 Rotator cuff (capsule) *(cont'd)*

RTW Post Surgery (Calendar-days away from work by decile)										
10%	20%	30%	40%	**50%**	60%	70%	80%	**90%**	100%	Mean
Partial removal, collar bone										
35	52	76	95	**111**	148	173	218	**365**	365	145.13
Remove shoulder bone, part										
33	47	61	82	**95**	114	153	205	**297**	365	128.46
Repair rotator cuff, acute										
33	54	79	95	**107**	137	167	213	**314**	365	139.10
Repair rotator cuff, chronic										
37	55	85	101	**124**	149	185	234	**347**	365	148.55
Release of shoulder ligament										
37	51	77	95	**117**	138	193	284	**365**	365	153.47
Repair of shoulder										
33	58	82	99	**120**	146	174	230	**339**	365	146.89
Shoulder arthroscopy/surgery										
32	52	66	82	**96**	123	152	224	**329**	365	132.86
Shoulder arthroscopy/surgery										
31	46	62	80	**109**	126	163	215	**304**	365	133.64
Shoulder arthroscopy/surgery										
36	47	69	88	**106**	126	184	237	**334**	365	142.11
Shoulder arthroscopy/surgery										
26	45	62	82	**101**	125	158	209	**321**	365	131.32

Integrated Disability Durations, in days*

Median (mid-point) 23.0 Mean (average) 54.09
Mode (most frequent) 1 Calculated rec. 25

Percent of Cases
(3922 cases)

Range of Days (up to)	9	18	27	36	45	54	63	72	81	90	99	108	117	118+
Percent of Cases	21.0	7.9	4.4	3.5	4.9	1.7	3.2	3.0	1.0	1.1	1.3	2.8	0.9	6.8

*CDC NHIS cases with no lost workdays: 1430 (36.5%)

Impact on Total Absence: Prevalence 0.3984% of total lost workdays; Incidence 4.18 days per 100 workers

Occupational Disability Durations, in days

Median (mid-point) 14 - Benchmark Indemnity Costs $10,500

Percent of Cases
(4275 cases)

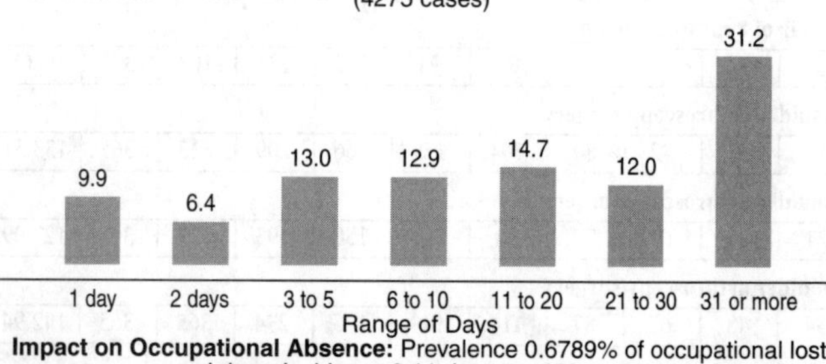

Impact on Occupational Absence: Prevalence 0.6789% of occupational lost workdays; Incidence 0.11 days per 100 workers

841 Sprains and strains of elbow and forearm

Return-To-Work Summary Guidelines		
Dataset	**Midrange**	**At-Risk**
Claims data	32 days	76 days
All absences	9 days	45 days

Return-To-Work "Best Practice" Guidelines
Moderate, clerical/modified work: 4 days
Moderate, manual work: 21 days
Severe, clerical/modified work: 7 days
Severe, manual work: 35-42 days

Capabilities & Activity Modifications:
Modified work: Repetitive motion activities not more than 4 times/hr; single upper extremity work if injured arm is non-dominant arm; lifting and carrying up to 3 lbs not more than 4 times/hr; pulling and pushing up to 5 lbs 3 times/hr; gripping using light tools (pens, scissors, etc) with 5-minute break at least every 20 min; avoid direct pressure on the elbow area; limit repetitive keying up to 15 keystrokes/min not more than 2 hrs/day; driving car up to 2 hrs/day; no full extension activities; possible immobilization by long arm splint or cast, tennis elbow splint, or wrist splint; no climbing ladders.
Regular manual work: Repetitive motion activities not more than 8 times/hr; use of injured dominant arm for moderate work; lifting and carrying up to 20 lbs not more than 15 times/hr; pulling and pushing up to 40 lbs 15 times/hr; gripping using moderate tools (pliers, screwdrivers, etc) full time; driving car or light truck up to 6 hrs/day or heavy truck up to 4 hrs/day; full extension activities up to 12 times/hr with up to 10 lbs of weight; possible immobilization by sling, wrist splint, or tennis elbow splint; climbing ladders up to 50 rungs/hr.
Description: Injury to the ligament (sprain) or to the muscle (strain) of the lower arm or elbow. Sprains and strains are usually accompanied by a tearing of the tissue as well as symptoms of pain, limited motion, swelling, bruising, and/or a change in sensation.
Other names: Sprained arm, Strained arm, Sprained elbow, Strained elbow
Procedure Summary (from ODG Treatment): Activity restrictions; Arthroplasty (elbow); Chiropractic; Cold packs; Deep transverse friction massage; Education; Electrical stimulation (E-STIM); Exercise; Fractures of humerus; Fractures of radius; Imaging; Iontophoresis; Laser doppler imaging (LDI); Manipulation; MRI's; Neural tension; Night splints; Nonprescription medications; Patient education; Phonophoresis; Physical therapy; Radiography; Return to work; Stretching; Surgery; Total elbow replacement (TER); Transcutaneous electrical neurostimulation (TENS); Ultrasound, diagnostic; Ultrasound, therapeutic; Work
Physical Therapy Guidelines:
Allow for fading of treatment frequency (from up to 3 visits per week to 1 or less), plus active self-directed home PT
Medical treatment: 9 visits over 8 weeks
Post-surgical treatment/ligament repair: 24 visits over 16 weeks
Chiropractic Guidelines:
Allow for fading of treatment frequency (from up to 3 visits per week to 1 or less), plus active self-directed home therapy
9 visits over 8 weeks

Workers' Comp Costs per Claim (based on 16,061 claims)					
Quartile	25%	50%	75%	Mean	% no cost
Indemnity	$1,134	$2,247	$4,956	$4,759	84%
Medical	$231	$441	$1,166	$1,366	4%
Total	$242	$462	$1,502	$2,162	4%

841 Sprains and strains of elbow and forearm

RTW Claims Data (Calendar-days away from work by decile)										
10%	20%	30%	40%	**50%**	60%	70%	80%	**90%**	100%	Mean
10	14	20	22	**32**	36	41	44	**76**	365	38.64

Integrated Disability Durations, in days*
Median (mid-point) 9.0 Mean (average) 22.20
Mode (most frequent) 4 Calculated rec. 11

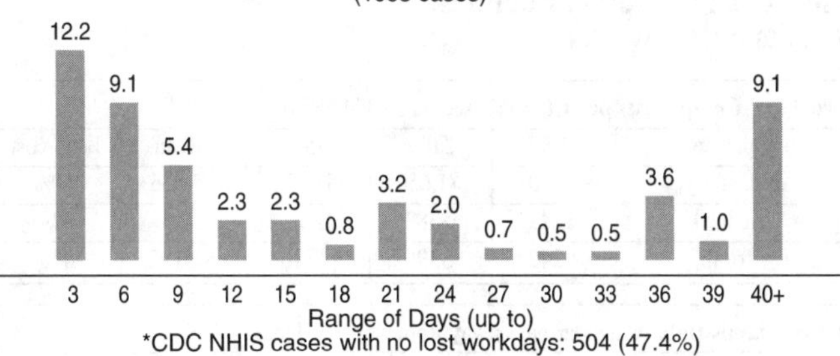

*CDC NHIS cases with no lost workdays: 504 (47.4%)

Impact on Total Absence: Prevalence 0.0366% of total lost workdays; Incidence 0.39 days per 100 workers

842 Sprains and strains of wrist and hand

Return-To-Work Summary Guidelines		
Dataset	**Midrange**	**At-Risk**
Claims data	21 days	51 days
All absences	7 days	35 days

Return-To-Work "Best Practice" Guidelines
Mild (grade I), clerical/modified work: 0 days
Mild, manual work: 5 days
Moderate (grade II), clerical/modified work: 7 days
Moderate, manual work: 21 days
Severe (grade III), clerical/modified work: 10 days
Severe, manual work: 35 days

Capabilities & Activity Modifications:
Modified work: Repetitive motion activities (w or w/o splint) not more than 4 times/hr; repetitive keying up to 15 keystrokes/min not more than 2 hrs/day; gripping and using light tools (pens, scissors, etc.) with 5-minute break at least every 20 min; no pinching; driving car up to 2 hrs/day; light work up to 5 lbs 3 times/hr; avoidance of prolonged periods in wrist flexion or extension.
Regular work (if not cause or aggravating to disability) : Repetitive motion activities not more than 25 times/hr; repetitive keying up to 45 keystrokes/min 8 hrs/day; gripping and using moderate tools (pliers, screwdrivers, etc.) fulltime; pinching up to 5 times/min; driving car or light truck up to 6 hrs/day or heavy truck up to 3 hrs/day; moderate to heavy work up to 35 lbs not more than 7 times/hr.
Description: Injury to the ligament (sprain) or to the muscle (strain) of the wrist or hand. Sprains and strains are usually accompanied by a tearing of the tissue as well as symptoms of pain, limited motion, swelling, bruising, and/or a change in sensation.
Other names: Sprained wrist, Strained wrist, Sprained hand, Strained hand
Procedure Summary (from ODG Treatment): Activity restrictions; Acupuncture; Arthrodesis (fusion); Arthroplasty (joint replacement); Casting versus splints; Chiropractic (manipulation); Cold packs; Computed tomography (CT); Continuous passive motion (CPM); de Quervain's tenosynovitis surgery; Dupuytren's release (fasciectomy); Ergonomic interventions; Exercises; Fasciotomy; Fusion; Imaging;

842 Sprains and strains of wrist and hand *(cont'd)*

Immobilization (treatment); Injection; Joint replacement; Mallet finger injuries (treatment); Manipulation; Modified duty; MRI's (magnetic resonance imaging); Nonprescription medications; Occupational therapy (OT); Physical therapy (PT); Plaster casting; Radiography (x-rays); Rest; Return to work; Splints; Surgery for broken wrist; TENS (transcutaneous electrical neurostimulation); Trapeziectomy; Triangular fibrocartilage complex (TFCC) reconstruction ; Trigger finger surgery; Vitamin C; Work; X-rays; Yoga

Physical Therapy Guidelines:
9 visits over 8 weeks

Workers' Comp Costs per Claim (based on 58,374 claims)					
Quartile	25%	50%	75%	Mean	% no cost
Indemnity	$830	$1,659	$3,171	$3,435	90%
Medical	$242	$389	$662	$821	4%
Total	$242	$399	$746	$1,192	4%

RTW Claims Data (Calendar-days away from work by decile)										
10%	20%	30%	40%	**50%**	60%	70%	80%	**90%**	100%	Mean
10	11	13	16	**21**	23	34	36	**51**	365	28.39

RTW Post Surgery (Calendar-days away from work by decile)										
10%	20%	30%	40%	**50%**	60%	70%	80%	**90%**	100%	Mean
Repair hand joint										
4	13	16	25	**40**	56	71	83	**201**	365	69.29
Wrist arthroscopy/surgery										
13	20	32	50	**71**	87	112	192	**341**	365	109.37

Integrated Disability Durations, in days*

Median (mid-point)	7.0	Mean (average)	14.47
Mode (most frequent)	1	Calculated rec.	7

Percent of Cases
(4372 cases)

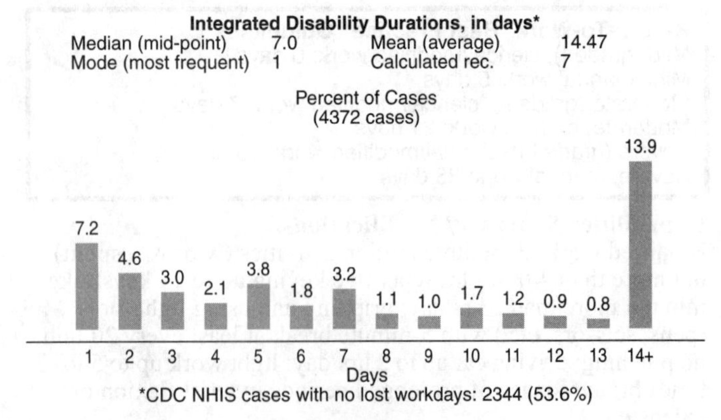

*CDC NHIS cases with no lost workdays: 2344 (53.6%)

Impact on Total Absence: Prevalence 0.0867% of total lost workdays; Incidence 0.91 days per 100 workers

Occupational Disability Durations, in days
Median (mid-point) 12 - Benchmark Indemnity Costs $9,000

Percent of Cases
(14155 cases)

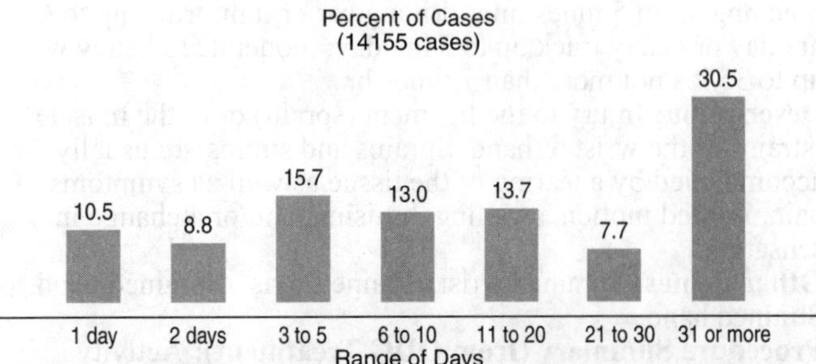

Impact on Occupational Absence: Prevalence 1.9269% of occupational lost workdays; Incidence 0.31 days per 100 workers

843 Sprains and strains of hip and thigh

Return-To-Work Summary Guidelines		
Dataset	**Midrange**	**At-Risk**
Claims data	21 days	51 days
All absences	8 days	36 days

Return-To-Work "Best Practice" Guidelines
Mild (grade I), clerical/modified work: 0 days
Mild, manual work: 7 days
Moderate (grade II), clerical/modified work: 5 days
Moderate, manual work: 21 days
Severe (grade III), clerical/modified work: 10 days
Severe, manual work: 35 days

Description: Injury to the ligament (sprain) or to the muscle (strain) of the hip or thigh. Sprains and strains are usually accompanied by a tearing of the tissue as well as symptoms of pain, limited motion, swelling, bruising, and/or a change in sensation.

Other names: Sprained hip, Strained hip, Sprained thigh, Strained thigh

Physical Therapy Guidelines:
9 visits over 8 weeks

Workers' Comp Costs per Claim (based on 10,752 claims)					
Quartile	25%	50%	75%	Mean	% no cost
Indemnity	$1,323	$2,709	$5,828	$5,783	78%
Medical	$231	$536	$1,722	$1,949	4%
Total	$242	$599	$2,489	$3,298	4%

RTW Claims Data (Calendar-days away from work by decile)										
10%	20%	30%	40%	**50%**	60%	70%	80%	**90%**	100%	Mean
9	11	13	17	**21**	24	34	36	**51**	365	28.85

Integrated Disability Durations, in days*

Median (mid-point)	8.0	Mean (average)	16.40
Mode (most frequent)	1	Calculated rec.	8

Percent of Cases
(1440 cases)

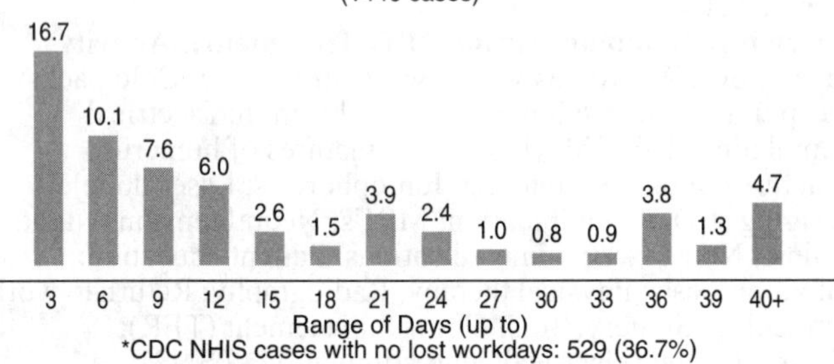

*CDC NHIS cases with no lost workdays: 529 (36.7%)

Impact on Total Absence: Prevalence 0.0441% of total lost workdays; Incidence 0.46 days per 100 workers

844 Sprains and strains of knee and leg

Return-To-Work Summary Guidelines		
Dataset	**Midrange**	**At-Risk**
Claims data	23 days	61 days
All absences	13 days	58 days

Return-To-Work "Best Practice" Guidelines
Mild (grade I), sedentary/modified work: 0 days
Mild, manual/standing work: 14 days
Moderate (grade II), sedentary/modified work: 5 days
Moderate, manual/standing work: 14-21 days
Severe (grade III - tear), sedentary/modified work: 14 days
Severe (tear), manual/standing work: 41-60 days

844 Sprains and strains of knee and leg *(cont'd)*

Capabilities & Activity Modifications:
Sedentary/modified work: Standing limited to 5-10 min/hr; walking only on a smooth surface using crutches with limited pressure on the foot; no walking on an irregular surface; no climbing stairs; no climbing ladders or hill climbing requiring frequent knee flexion; no activities requiring balance; no applying strength against bent knee (squatting, kneeling, crouching, stooping, pedaling, etc.); elevate leg half of time; may need immobilization; limited weight bearing.
Manual/standing work: Standing not more than 50 min/hr; walking on a smooth surface up to 1,200 ft/hr carrying up to 25 lbs; walking on an irregular surface up to 900 ft/hr carrying up to 25 lbs; climbing stairs up to 8 flights/hr carrying up to 40 lbs; climbing ladders up to 50 rungs/hr carrying up to 25 lbs; activities requiring balance up to 45 min/hr (if able to work with two hands without assistance for balance); applying strength against bent knee (pedaling, squatting, kneeling, etc.) up to 60 times/hr; may need brace for uneven ground or ladders.
Description: Injury to the ligament (sprain) or to the muscle (strain) of the knee or leg. Sprains and strains are usually accompanied by a tearing of the tissue as well as symptoms of pain, limited motion, swelling, bruising, and/or a change in sensation.
Other names: Sprained knee, Strained knee, Sprained leg, Strained leg

Excludes:
current tear of cartilage or meniscus of knee (836.0-836.2)
old tear of cartilage or meniscus of knee (717.0-717.5, 717.8-717.9)

Procedure Summary (from ODG Treatment): ACI; Activity restrictions; Anterior cruciate ligament (ACL) repair; ACL diagnostic tests; ACL injury rehabilitation; Acupuncture; Arthroplasty; Arthroscopy; Autologous cartilage implantation (ACI); Bone-growth stimulators; Braces; Canes; Cetylated fatty acids (CFA) topical cream; Chiropractic; Chondroplasty; Cold/heat packs; Cold lasers; Continuous-flow cryotherapy; Continuous passive motion (CPM); Corticosteroid injections; Crutches; Deep transverse friction massage (DTFM); Diagnostic arthroscopy; Education for knee replacement; Electromyographic biofeedback treatment; Exercise; Glucosamine; Hyaluronic acid injections; Imaging; Immobilization; Injections; Insoles; Interferential current therapy (IFC); Knee brace; Knee joint replacement; KT 1000 arthrometer; Lachman test; Lateral pull test and patellar tilt test; Lateral retinacular release; Low level laser therapy (LLLT); Magnet therapy; Manipulation; Meniscal allograft transplantation; Menisectomy; Microprocessor-controlled knee prostheses; Modified duty; Mosaicplasty; MRI's (magnetic resonance imaging); Non-surgical intervention for PFPS (patellofemoral pain syndrome); Occupational therapy; Orthoses; Osteochondral autograft transplant system (OATS); Osteotomy; Pharmacotherapy; Physical therapy; Pivot shift test (MacIntosh test) ; Posterior cruciate ligament (PCL) repair; Post-op ambulatory infusion pumps (local anesthetic); Prolotherapy; Prostheses (artificial limb); Pulsed magnetic field therapy (PMFT); Radiography; Return to work; SAMe (S-adenosylmethionine); Single photon emission computed tomography (SPECT); Static progressive stretch (SPS) therapy; Stretching and flexibility; Surgery; SynviscÒ; Therapeutic knee splint; Therapeutic ultrasound; Transcutaneous electrical neurostimulation (TENS); Ultrasound, diagnostic; Ultrasound, therapeutic; Ultrasound fracture healing (bone-growth stimulators); Viscosupplementation; Walkers; Walking aids (canes, crutches, braces, orthoses, & walkers); Work
Physical Therapy Guidelines:
Medical treatment: 12 visits over 8 weeks
Post-surgical treatment (ACL repair): 24 visits over 16 weeks
Chiropractic Guidelines:
12 visits over 8 weeks

Workers' Comp Costs per Claim (based on 47,874 claims)

Quartile	25%	50%	75%	Mean	% no cost
Indemnity	$1,281	$2,447	$5,355	$5,310	80%
Medical	$284	$557	$1,607	$1,979	4%
Total	$294	$609	$2,163	$3,083	4%

Disability Duration Adjustment Factors by Age

Age Group	18-24	25-34	35-44	45-54	55-64	65-74
Adjustment Factor	0.80	0.84	0.93	1.08	1.28	1.36

RTW Claims Data (Calendar-days away from work by decile)

10%	20%	30%	40%	**50%**	60%	70%	80%	**90%**	100%	Mean
12	14	15	19	**23**	33	42	51	**61**	365	33.40

RTW Post Surgery (Calendar-days away from work by decile)

	10%	20%	30%	40%	**50%**	60%	70%	80%	**90%**	100%	Mean
Knee arthroscopy, dx	16	27	37	46	**53**	64	81	116	**278**	365	87.67
Knee arthroscopy/surgery	17	27	34	41	**47**	60	88	124	**237**	365	86.12
Knee arthroscopy/surgery	16	28	38	45	**56**	65	95	135	**310**	365	95.51
Knee arthroscopy/surgery	17	29	38	47	**55**	73	94	144	**255**	365	95.78
Knee arthroscopy/surgery	18	31	41	55	**71**	89	116	142	**226**	365	102.21
Knee arthroscopy/surgery	18	27	38	47	**58**	77	104	152	**216**	365	95.26
Knee arthroscopy/surgery	15	25	33	41	**52**	65	87	130	**227**	365	86.97
Knee arthroscopy/surgery	24	41	57	69	**88**	109	132	169	**261**	365	114.83

Integrated Disability Durations, in days*

Median (mid-point)	13.0	Mean (average)	21.10
Mode (most frequent)	1	Calculated rec.	12

Percent of Cases
(5432 cases)

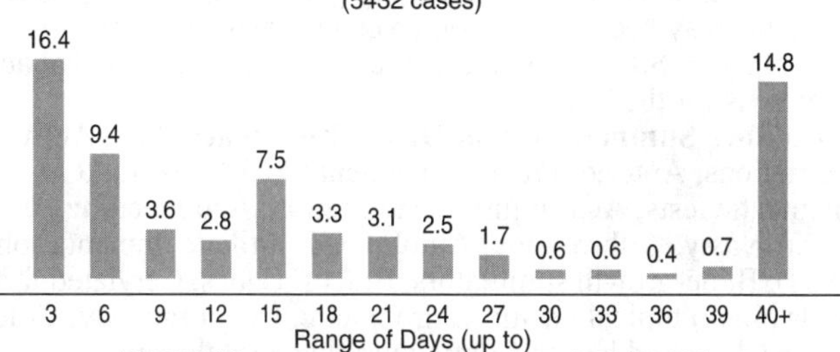

*CDC NHIS cases with no lost workdays: 1766 (32.5%)

Impact on Total Absence: Prevalence 0.2286% of total lost workdays; Incidence 2.40 days per 100 workers

844 Sprains and strains of knee and leg *(cont'd)*

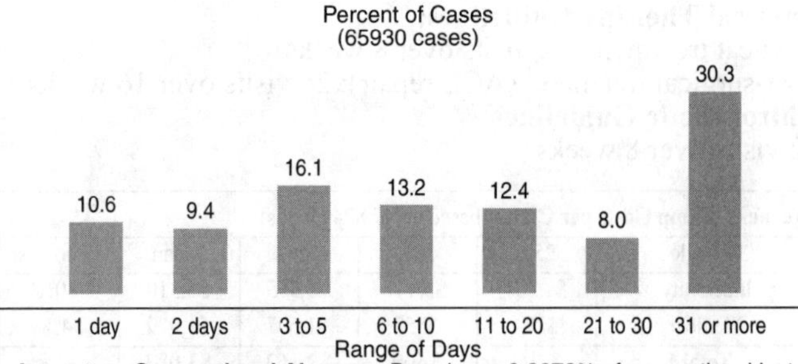

Impact on Occupational Absence: Prevalence 8.2272% of occupational lost workdays; Incidence 1.32 days per 100 workers

844.2 Cruciate ligament of knee

Return-To-Work Summary Guidelines		
Dataset	**Midrange**	**At-Risk**
Claims data	27 days	180 days
All absences	16 days	86 days

Return-To-Work "Best Practice" Guidelines
Mild (grade I), sedentary/modified work: 0 days
Mild, manual/standing work: 14 days
Moderate (grade II), sedentary/modified work: 5 days
Moderate, manual/standing work: 25 days
Severe (grade III - tear), ACL repair, sedentary/modified work: 35 days
Severe (tear), ACL repair, manual/standing work: 180 days
Tissue repair injection, sedentary/modified work: 14 days
Tissue repair injection, manual/standing work: 42 days

Capabilities & Activity Modifications:
Sedentary/modified work: Standing limited to 5-10 min/hr; walking only on a smooth surface using crutches with limited pressure on the foot; no walking on an irregular surface; no climbing stairs; no climbing ladders or hill climbing requiring frequent knee flexion; no activities requiring balance; no applying strength against bent knee (squatting, kneeling, crouching, stooping, pedaling, etc.); elevate leg half of time; may need immobilization; limited weight bearing.
Manual/standing work: Standing not more than 50 min/hr; walking on a smooth surface up to 1,200 ft/hr carrying up to 25 lbs; walking on an irregular surface up to 900 ft/hr carrying up to 25 lbs; climbing stairs up to 8 flights/hr carrying up to 40 lbs; climbing ladders up to 50 rungs/hr carrying up to 25 lbs; activities requiring balance up to 45 min/hr (if able to work with two hands without assistance for balance); applying strength against bent knee (pedaling, squatting, kneeling, etc.) up to 60 times/hr; may need brace for uneven ground or ladders.
Description: Sprain or strain of the cross-like ligament that acts as an axis for the knee.
Procedure Summary (from ODG Treatment): ACI; Activity restrictions; Anterior cruciate ligament (ACL) repair; ACL diagnostic tests; ACL injury rehabilitation; Acupuncture; Arthroplasty; Arthroscopy; Autologous cartilage implantation (ACI); Bone-growth stimulators; Braces; Canes; Cetylated fatty acids (CFA) topical cream; Chiropractic; Chondroplasty; Cold/heat packs; Cold lasers; Continuous-flow cryotherapy; Continuous passive motion (CPM); Corticosteroid injections; Crutches; Deep transverse friction massage (DTFM); Diagnostic arthroscopy; Education for knee replacement; Electromyographic biofeedback treatment; Exercise; Glucosamine; Hyaluronic acid injections; Imaging; Immobilization; Injections; Insoles; Interferential current

844.2 Cruciate ligament of knee *(cont'd)*

therapy (IFC); Knee brace; Knee joint replacement; KT 1000 arthrometer; Lachman test; Lateral pull test and patellar tilt test; Lateral retinacular release; Low level laser therapy (LLLT); Magnet therapy; Manipulation; Meniscal allograft transplantation; Meniscectomy; Microprocessor-controlled knee prostheses; Modified duty; Mosaicplasty; MRI's (magnetic resonance imaging); Non-surgical intervention for PFPS (patellofemoral pain syndrome); Occupational therapy; Orthoses; Osteochondral autograft transplant system (OATS); Osteotomy; Pharmacotherapy; Physical therapy; Pivot shift test (MacIntosh test) ; Posterior cruciate ligament (PCL) repair; Post-op ambulatory infusion pumps (local anesthetic); Prolotherapy; Prostheses (artificial limb); Pulsed magnetic field therapy (PMFT); Radiography; Return to work; SAMe (S-adenosylmethionine); Single photon emission computed tomography (SPECT); Static progressive stretch (SPS) therapy; Stretching and flexibility; Surgery; SynviscÒ; Therapeutic knee splint; Therapeutic ultrasound; Transcutaneous electrical neurostimulation (TENS); Ultrasound, diagnostic; Ultrasound, therapeutic; Ultrasound fracture healing (bone-growth stimulators); Viscosupplementation; Walkers; Walking aids (canes, crutches, braces, orthoses, & walkers); Work
Physical Therapy Guidelines:
Medical treatment: 12 visits over 8 weeks
Post-surgical: 24 visits over 16 weeks

Workers' Comp Costs per Claim (based on 2,366 claims)

Quartile	25%	50%	75%	Mean	% no cost
Indemnity	$3,560	$7,235	$15,792	$12,129	34%
Medical	$4,232	$11,398	$18,953	$13,948	0%
Total	$6,416	$15,981	$28,245	$21,941	0%

RTW Claims Data (Calendar-days away from work by decile)

10%	20%	30%	40%	**50%**	60%	70%	80%	**90%**	100%	Mean
12	14	16	22	**27**	37	45	53	**132**	365	47.20

RTW Post Surgery (Calendar-days away from work by decile)

10%	20%	30%	40%	**50%**	60%	70%	80%	**90%**	100%	Mean
Knee arthroscopy/surgery										
19	28	34	41	**57**	90	127	195	**365**	365	108.85
Knee arthroscopy/surgery										
20	35	48	59	**72**	96	129	169	**237**	365	105.66
Knee arthroscopy/surgery										
25	41	57	69	**89**	110	130	168	**255**	365	114.38

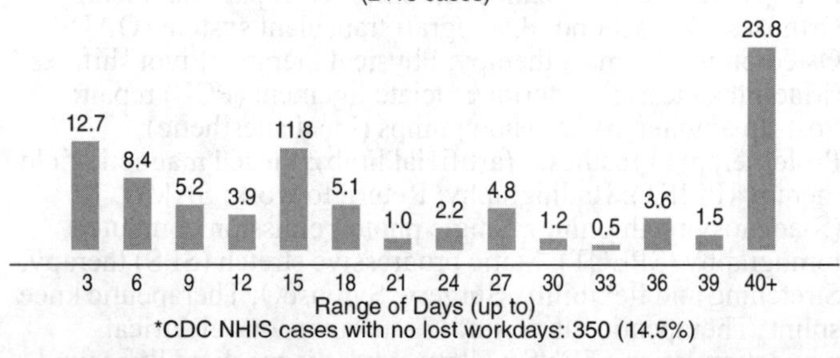

Impact on Total Absence: Prevalence 0.2148% of total lost workdays; Incidence 2.26 days per 100 workers

845 Sprains and strains of ankle and foot

Return-To-Work Summary Guidelines		
Dataset	Midrange	At-Risk
Claims data	20 days	46 days
All absences	9 days	41 days

Return-To-Work "Best Practice" Guidelines
Mild (grade I), sedentary/modified work: 0 days
Mild, manual/standing work: 5 days
Moderate (grade II), sedentary/modified work: 7 days
Moderate, manual/standing work: 14-21 days
Severe (grade III), sedentary/modified work: 10-20 days
Severe, manual/standing work, w/o cast: 42 days

Capabilities & Activity Modifications:
Sedentary/modified work: Standing limited to 5-10 min/hr; walking only on a smooth surface using crutches with limited pressure on the foot; no walking on an irregular surface; no climbing stairs; no climbing ladders or hill climbing requiring frequent knee flexion; no activities requiring balance; no applying strength against bent knee (squatting, kneeling, crouching, stooping, pedaling, etc.); elevate leg half of time; may need immobilization; limited weight bearing.
Manual/standing work: Standing not more than 50 min/hr; walking on a smooth surface up to 1,200 ft/hr carrying up to 25 lbs; walking on an irregular surface up to 900 ft/hr carrying up to 25 lbs; climbing stairs up to 8 flights/hr carrying up to 40 lbs; climbing ladders up to 50 rungs/hr carrying up to 25 lbs; activities requiring balance up to 45 min/hr (if able to work with two hands without assistance for balance); applying strength against bent knee (pedaling, squatting, kneeling, etc.) up to 60 times/hr; may need brace for uneven ground or ladders.
Description: Injury to the ligament (sprain) or to the muscle (strain) of the ankle or foot. Sprains and strains are usually accompanied by a tearing of the tissue as well as symptoms of pain, limited motion, swelling, bruising, and/or a change in sensation.
Other names: Sprained foot, Strained foot
Procedure Summary (from ODG Treatment):
Accommodative modalities; Achilles tendon ruptures (treatment); Activity restrictions; Actovegin; Ankle prostheses (total ankle replacement); Anterior drawer test; Anti-inflammatory medications (NSAIDs); Arthrodesis (fusion); Arthroplasty (total ankle replacement); Autologous conditioned serum (ACS); Bed rest; Biofeedback; Bone scan (imaging); Bracing (immobilization); Cast (immobilization); Causality; Chiropractic; Cold packs; Computed tomography (CT); Continuous-flow cryotherapy; Corticosteroids (topical); Diathermy; Dorsiflexion night splints; Education (patient); Elastic bandage (immobilization); Electron generating device; Exercise; Extracorporeal shock wave therapy (ESWT); Functional treatment; Fusion; Heat therapy (ice/heat); Heparin; Heel pads; Ice packs; Imaging; Immobilization; Ingrown toenail surgery; Injections; Insoles with magnetic foil; Inversion stress test; Iontophoresis; Lace-up ankle support; Laser therapy (LLLT); Lateral ligament ankle reconstruction (surgery); Lineal tomography; Low-intensity laser therapy (LLLT); Magnets; Magnetic resonance imaging (MRI); Manipulation; Massage; Mechanical treatment (taping/orthoses); Modified duty; Narcotics; Night splints; Nonprescription medications; Orthotic devices; Osteotomy; Ottawa ankle rules (OAR); Patient education; Phonophoresis; Physical therapy (PT); Prolotherapy (sclerotherapy); Radiography; Rest (RICE); Return to work; Sclerotherapy (prolotherapy); Semi-rigid ankle support; Shock wave therapy, extracorporeal (ESWT); Steroids (injection); Stretching (flexibility); Supports; Surgery; Surgery for achilles tendon ruptures; Surgery for ankle sprains; Surgery for

845 Sprains and strains of ankle and foot *(cont'd)*

calcaneal fractures; Surgery for hallux valgus; Surgery for plantar fasciitis; Surgery for tarsal tunnel syndrome; Talar tilt test; Tai Chi; Taping; Tension night splints (TNS); Therapeutic exercise; Thompson test; Total ankle replacement (arthroplasty); Transcutaneous electrical neurostimulation (TENS); Ultrasound, diagnostic; Ultrasound, therapeutic; Work

Workers' Comp Costs per Claim (based on 64,249 claims)					
Quartile	25%	50%	75%	Mean	% no cost
Indemnity	$798	$1,517	$2,804	$2,728	88%
Medical	$284	$441	$735	$801	4%
Total	$284	$462	$840	$1,154	4%

Disability Duration Adjustment Factors by Age						
Age Group	18-24	25-34	35-44	45-54	55-64	65-74
Adjustment Factor	0.80	0.84	0.93	1.08	1.28	1.36

RTW Claims Data (Calendar-days away from work by decile)										
10%	20%	30%	40%	**50%**	60%	70%	80%	**90%**	100%	Mean
10	12	14	15	**20**	21	25	41	**46**	365	26.98

RTW Post Surgery (Calendar-days away from work by decile)										
10%	20%	30%	40%	**50%**	60%	70%	80%	**90%**	100%	Mean
Repair achilles tendon										
7	18	38	59	**82**	95	100	125	**166**	365	90.27

Integrated Disability Durations, in days*
Median (mid-point) 9.0 Mean (average) 15.71
Mode (most frequent) 1 Calculated rec. 9

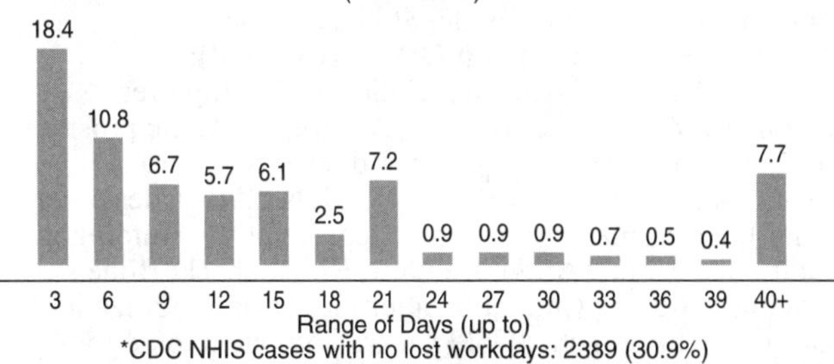

*CDC NHIS cases with no lost workdays: 2389 (30.9%)

Impact on Total Absence: Prevalence 0.2485% of total lost workdays; Incidence 2.61 days per 100 workers

Occupational Disability Durations, in days
Median (mid-point) 7 - Benchmark Indemnity Costs $5,250

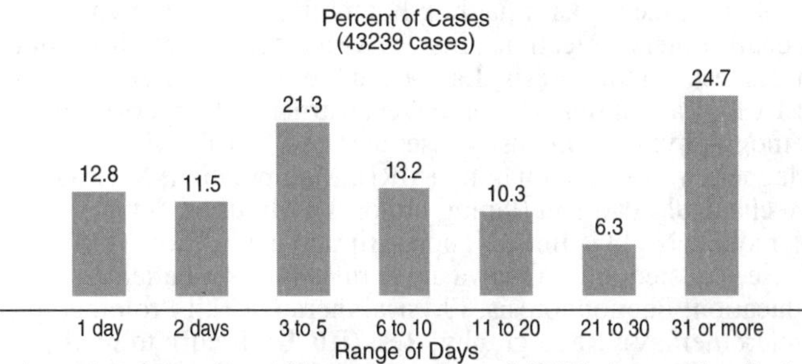

Impact on Occupational Absence: Prevalence 3.4336% of occupational lost workdays; Incidence 0.55 days per 100 workers

845.0 Ankle

Return-To-Work Summary Guidelines		
Dataset	Midrange	At-Risk
Claims data	21 days	63 days
All absences	6 days	50 days

845.0 Ankle *(cont'd)*

Return-To-Work "Best Practice" Guidelines
Ankle strapping/soft cast, mild sprain: 1 day
Ankle strapping/soft cast, severe sprain, sedentary/modified work (10 days crutches): 4-5 days
Ankle strapping/soft cast, severe sprain, manual/standing work: 21 days
With surgery, sedentary/modified work: 10 days
With surgery, manual/standing work, w/o cast: 49-63 days

Capabilities & Activity Modifications:
Sedentary/modified work: Standing limited to 5-10 min/hr; walking only on a smooth surface using crutches with limited pressure on the foot; no walking on an irregular surface; no climbing stairs; no climbing ladders or hill climbing requiring frequent knee flexion; no activities requiring balance; no applying strength against bent knee (squatting, kneeling, crouching, stooping, pedaling, etc.); elevate leg half of time; may need immobilization; limited weight bearing.
Manual/standing work: Standing not more than 50 min/hr; walking on a smooth surface up to 1,200 ft/hr carrying up to 25 lbs; walking on an irregular surface up to 900 ft/hr carrying up to 25 lbs; climbing stairs up to 8 flights/hr carrying up to 40 lbs; climbing ladders up to 50 rungs/hr carrying up to 25 lbs; activities requiring balance up to 45 min/hr (if able to work with two hands without assistance for balance); applying strength against bent knee (pedaling, squatting, kneeling, etc.) up to 60 times/hr; may need brace for uneven ground or ladders.
Description: Injury to the ligament (sprain) or to the muscle (strain) of the ankle. Sprains and strains are usually accompanied by a tearing of the tissue as well as symptoms of pain, limited motion, swelling, bruising, and/or a change in sensation.
Other names: Sprained ankle, Strained ankle
Procedure Summary (from ODG Treatment):
Accommodative modalities; Achilles tendon ruptures (treatment); Activity restrictions; Actovegin; Ankle prostheses (total ankle replacement); Anterior drawer test; Anti-inflammatory medications (NSAIDs); Arthrodesis (fusion); Arthroplasty (total ankle replacement); Autologous conditioned serum (ACS); Bed rest; Biofeedback; Bone scan (imaging); Bracing (immobilization); Cast (immobilization); Causality; Chiropractic; Cold packs; Computed tomography (CT); Continuous-flow cryotherapy; Corticosteroids (topical); Diathermy; Dorsiflexion night splints; Education (patient); Elastic bandage (immobilization); Electron generating device; Exercise; Extracorporeal shock wave therapy (ESWT); Functional treatment; Fusion; Heat therapy (ice/heat); Heparin; Heel pads; Ice packs; Imaging; Immobilization; Ingrown toenail surgery; Injections; Insoles with magnetic foil; Inversion stress test; Iontophoresis; Lace-up ankle support; Laser therapy (LLLT); Lateral ligament ankle reconstruction (surgery); Lineal tomography; Low-intensity laser therapy (LLLT); Magnets; Magnetic resonance imaging (MRI); Manipulation; Massage; Mechanical treatment (taping/orthoses); Modified duty; Narcotics; Night splints; Nonprescription medications; Orthotic devices; Osteotomy; Ottawa ankle rules (OAR); Patient education; Phonophoresis; Physical therapy (PT); Prolotherapy (sclerotherapy); Radiography; Rest (RICE); Return to work; Sclerotherapy (prolotherapy); Semi-rigid ankle support; Shock wave therapy, extracorporeal (ESWT); Steroids (injection); Stretching (flexibility); Supports; Surgery; Surgery for achilles tendon ruptures; Surgery for ankle sprains; Surgery for calcaneal fractures; Surgery for hallux valgus; Surgery for plantar fasciitis; Surgery for tarsal tunnel syndrome; Talar tilt test; Tai Chi; Taping; Tension night splints (TNS); Therapeutic exercise; Thompson test; Total ankle replacement (arthroplasty); Transcutaneous electrical neurostimulation (TENS); Ultrasound, diagnostic; Ultrasound, therapeutic; Work
Physical Therapy Guidelines:
Allow for fading of treatment frequency (from up to 3 visits per week to 1 or less), plus active self-directed home PT
Medical treatment: 9 visits over 8 weeks
Post-surgical treatment: 34 visits over 16 weeks
Chiropractic Guidelines:
Allow for fading of treatment frequency (from up to 3 visits per week to 1 or less), plus active self-directed home therapy
9 visits over 8 weeks

Workers' Comp Costs per Claim (based on 52,288 claims)

Quartile	25%	50%	75%	Mean	% no cost
Indemnity	$809	$1,554	$2,846	$2,773	87%
Medical	$294	$462	$756	$828	4%
Total	$294	$473	$861	$1,197	4%

RTW Claims Data (Calendar-days away from work by decile)

10%	20%	30%	40%	**50%**	60%	70%	80%	**90%**	100%	Mean
10	11	13	15	**21**	25	42	50	**63**	365	30.87

RTW Post Surgery (Calendar-days away from work by decile)

10%	20%	30%	40%	**50%**	60%	70%	80%	**90%**	100%	Mean
Repair achilles tendon										
7	18	38	59	**82**	95	100	125	**166**	365	90.27

Integrated Disability Durations, in days*
Median (mid-point) 6.0 Mean (average) 16.14
Mode (most frequent) 1 Calculated rec. 7

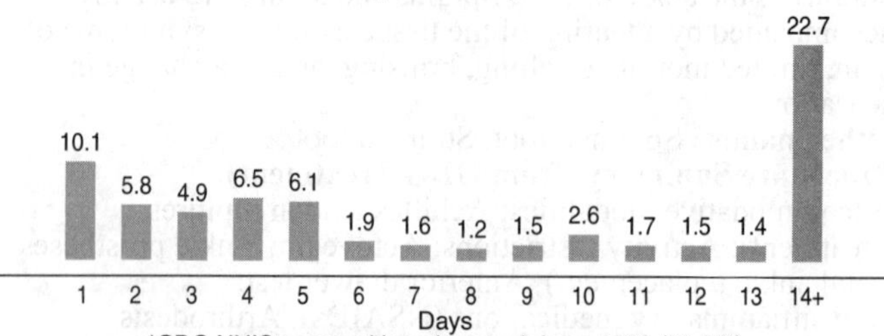

*CDC NHIS cases with no lost workdays: 1636 (30.5%)

Impact on Total Absence: Prevalence 0.1777% of total lost workdays; Incidence 1.87 days per 100 workers

846 Sprains and strains of sacroiliac region

Return-To-Work Summary Guidelines

Dataset	Midrange	At-Risk
Claims data	17 days	53 days
All absences	10 days	36 days

Return-To-Work "Best Practice" Guidelines
Mild (grade I), clerical/modified work: 0 days
Mild, manual work: 10 days
Severe (grade II-III), clerical/modified work: 0-3 days
Severe, manual work: 14-17 days
Severe, heavy manual work: 35 days

Capabilities & Activity Modifications:
Clerical/modified work: Lifting with knees (with a straight back, no stooping) not more than 5 lbs up to 3 times/hr; squatting up to 4 times/hr; standing or walking with a 5-minute break at least every 20 minutes; sitting with a 5-minute break

846 Sprains and strains of sacroiliac region *(cont'd)*

every 30 minutes; no extremes of extension or flexion; no extremes of twisting; no climbing ladders; driving car only up to 2 hrs/day.
Manual work: Lifting with knees (with a straight back) not more than 25 lbs up to 15 times/hr; squatting up to 16 times/hr; standing or walking with a 10-minute break at least every 1-2 hours; sitting with a 10-minute break every 1-2 hours; extremes of flexion or extension allowed up to 12 times/hr; extremes of twisting allowed up to 16 times/hr; climbing ladders allowed up to 25 rungs 6 times/hr; driving car or light truck up to a full work day; driving heavy truck up to 4 hrs/day.

Description: Injury to the ligament (sprain) or to the muscle (strain) of the groin. Sprains and strains are usually accompanied by a tearing of the tissue as well as symptoms of pain, limited motion, swelling, bruising, and/or a change in sensation.

Other names: Sprained groin, Strained groin

Procedure Summary (from ODG Treatment): Activity restrictions; Acupuncture; Adhesiolysis; Aerobic exercise; Age adjustment factors; Annuloplasty (IDET); Antidepressants; Anti-inflammatory medications; Aquatic therapy; Arthrodesis; Arthroplasty; Artificial disk; Back brace; Back schools; Bed rest; Behavioral treatment; Biofeedback; Bone-growth stimulators (BGS); Bone scan; Botulinum toxin (Botox); Chemonucleolysis (chymopapain); Chiropractic; Coblation nucleoplasty; Cognitive intervention; Colchicine; Cold/heat packs; Computerized range of motion (ROM); Corsets; CT & CT Myelography (computed tomography); Cutaneous laser treatment; Decompression; Diagnostic imaging; Diathermy; Differential Diagnosis; Disc prosthesis; Discectomy/ laminectomy; Discography; DRX (traction); Dynamic neutralization system (Dynesys); Education; Electrical stimulators (E-stim); Electromagnetic pulsed therapy; EMG's (electromyography); Epidural steroid injections (ESI's); Ergonomics interventions; Etanercept (Enbrel); Exercise; Facet-joint injections; Facet rhizotomy (radio frequency medial branch neurotomy); Feldenkrais; Flexibility; Fluoroscopy (for ESI's); Foraminotomy; Fusion (spinal); Fusion, endoscopic; Hardware; Heat therapy; Hemilaminectomy; H-wave stimulation (devices); IDD therapy (intervertebral disc decompression); IDET (intradiscal electrothermal anuloplasty); Imaging; Implantable pumps for narcotics; Implantable spinal cord stimulators; Implants; Infliximab (Remicade); Injections; Interferential therapy; Intradiscal electrothermal therapy (IDET); Intradiscal steroid injection; Intrathecal drug administration system; Kyphoplasty; Laminectomy/ laminotomy; Ligamentous injections; Lordex (traction); Low level laser therapy (LLLT); Lumbar supports; Magnet therapy; Manipulation; Manipulation under anesthesia (MUA) ; Massage; Mattress firmness; McKenzie method; Medications; MedX lumbar extension machine; Microcurrent electrical stimulation (MENS devices); Microdiscectomy; Modified duty; MR neurography; MRI's (magnetic resonance imaging); Muscle relaxants ; Myelography; Neuromodulation devices; Neuromuscular electrical stimulators (NMES); Neuroplasty; Neuroreflexotherapy; Nonprescription medications; Narcotics; Nucleoplasty; Occupational therapy (OT); Opioids; Oral corticosteroids; Percutaneous diskectomy (PCD); Percutaneous electrical nerve stimulation (PENS) ; Percutaneous endoscopic laser discectomy (PELD); Percutaneous epidural neuroplasty; Percutaneous intradiscal radiofrequency (thermocoagulation); Percutaneous neuromodulation therapy (PNT); Percutaneous vertebroplasty (PV); Physical therapy (PT); Pilates; Powered traction devices; Prolotherapy, also known as sclerotherapy; Psychological screening; Racz neurolysis; Radiofrequency neurotomy; Radiography (x-rays); Range of motion (ROM); Return to work; Sclerotherapy; Shoe insoles/shoe lifts; SPECT

846 Sprains and strains of sacroiliac region *(cont'd)*

(single photon emission computed tomography); Spinal cord stimulation (SCS); Standing MRI; Stimulators, electrical; Stretching; Supports & braces; Surface electromyography (SEMG); Surgery; Sympathetic therapy; Thermography (infrared stress thermography); Traction; Transcutaneous electrical neurostimulation (TENS) ; Trigger point injections; Tumor necrosis factor (TNF) modifiers; Ultrasound, diagnostic (imaging); Ultrasound, therapeutic; Vertebral axial decompression (VAX-D); Vertebroplasty; Videofluoroscopy (for range of motion); Work conditioning, work hardening; Work; X-rays; Yoga

Physical Therapy Guidelines:
Medical treatment: 10 visits over 8 weeks

Workers' Comp Costs per Claim (based on 70,315 claims)					
Quartile	25%	50%	75%	Mean	% no cost
Indemnity	$1,355	$2,825	$5,901	$5,774	77%
Medical	$284	$704	$2,142	$2,199	3%
Total	$294	$819	$3,098	$3,569	3%

RTW Claims Data (Calendar-days away from work by decile)										
10%	20%	30%	40%	**50%**	60%	70%	80%	**90%**	100%	Mean
10	12	14	15	**17**	21	29	36	**53**	365	28.97

Integrated Disability Durations, in days*

Median (mid-point) 10.0 Mean (average) 17.33
Mode (most frequent) 1 Calculated rec. 10

Percent of Cases
(4443 cases)

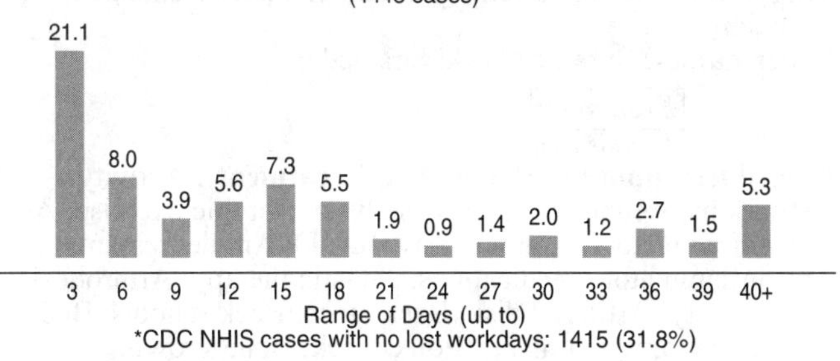

*CDC NHIS cases with no lost workdays: 1415 (31.8%)

Impact on Total Absence: Prevalence 0.1551% of total lost workdays; Incidence 1.63 days per 100 workers

Occupational Disability Durations, in days

Median (mid-point) 8 - Benchmark Indemnity Costs $6,000

Percent of Cases
(6745 cases)

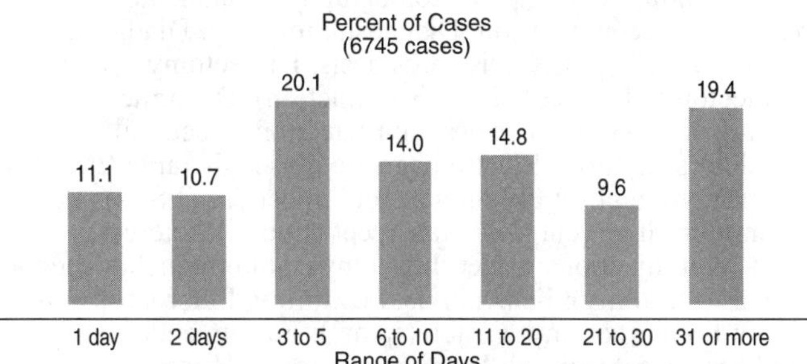

Impact on Occupational Absence: Prevalence 0.6121% of occupational lost workdays; Incidence 0.10 days per 100 workers

847 Sprains and strains of other and unspecified parts of back

Return-To-Work Summary Guidelines		
Dataset	**Midrange**	**At-Risk**
Claims data	17 days	61 days
All absences	11 days	39 days

847 Sprains and strains of other and unspecified parts of back *(cont'd)*

Return-To-Work "Best Practice" Guidelines
Mild (grade I), clerical/modified work: 0 days
Mild, manual work: 10 days
Severe (grade II-III), clerical/modified work: 0-3 days
Severe, manual work: 14-17 days
Severe, heavy manual work: 35 days
With radicular signs, see 722.1 (disc disorders)

Capabilities & Activity Modifications:
Clerical/modified work: Lifting with knees (with a straight back, no stooping) not more than 5 lbs up to 3 times/hr; squatting up to 4 times/hr; standing or walking with a 5-minute break at least every 20 minutes; sitting with a 5-minute break every 30 minutes; no extremes of extension or flexion; no extremes of twisting; no climbing ladders; driving car only up to 2 hrs/day.
Manual work: Lifting with knees (with a straight back) not more than 25 lbs up to 15 times/hr; squatting up to 16 times/hr; standing or walking with a 10-minute break at least every 1-2 hours; sitting with a 10-minute break every 1-2 hours; extremes of flexion or extension allowed up to 12 times/hr; extremes of twisting allowed up to 16 times/hr; climbing ladders allowed up to 25 rungs 6 times/hr; driving car or light truck up to a full work day; driving heavy truck up to 4 hrs/day.
Description: Injury to the ligament (sprain) or to the muscle (strain) of the back. Sprains and strains are usually accompanied by a tearing of the tissue as well as symptoms of pain, limited motion, swelling, bruising, and/or a change in sensation.
Other names: Sprained back, Strained back

Excludes:
lumbosacral (846.0)

Procedure Summary (from ODG Treatment): Activity restrictions; Acupuncture; Adhesiolysis; Aerobic exercise; Age adjustment factors; Annuloplasty (IDET); Antidepressants; Anti-inflammatory medications; Aquatic therapy; Arthrodesis; Arthroplasty; Artificial disk; Back brace; Back schools; Bed rest; Behavioral treatment; Biofeedback; Bone-growth stimulators (BGS); Bone scan; Botulinum toxin (Botox); Chemonucleolysis (chymopapain); Chiropractic; Coblation nucleoplasty; Cognitive intervention; Colchicine; Cold/heat packs; Computerized range of motion (ROM); Corsets; CT & CT Myelography (computed tomography); Cutaneous laser treatment; Decompression; Diagnostic imaging; Diathermy; Differential Diagnosis; Disc prosthesis; Discectomy/laminectomy; Discography; DRX (traction); Dynamic neutralization system (Dynesys); Education; Electrical stimulators (E-stim); Electromagnetic pulsed therapy; EMG's (electromyography); Epidural steroid injections (ESI's); Ergonomics interventions; Etanercept (Enbrel); Exercise; Facet-joint injections; Facet rhizotomy (radio frequency medial branch neurotomy); Feldenkrais; Flexibility; Fluoroscopy (for ESI's); Foraminotomy; Fusion (spinal); Fusion, endoscopic; Hardware; Heat therapy; Hemilaminectomy; H-wave stimulation (devices); IDD therapy (intervertebral disc decompression); IDET (intradiscal electrothermal anuloplasty); Imaging; Implantable pumps for narcotics; Implantable spinal cord stimulators; Implants; Infliximab (Remicade); Injections; Interferential therapy; Intradiscal electrothermal therapy (IDET); Intradiscal steroid injection; Intrathecal drug administration system; Kyphoplasty; Laminectomy/laminotomy; Ligamentous injections; Lordex (traction); Low level laser therapy (LLLT); Lumbar supports; Magnet therapy; Manipulation; Manipulation under anesthesia (MUA) ; Massage; Mattress firmness; McKenzie method; Medications; MedX lumbar extension machine; Microcurrent electrical stimulation (MENS devices); Microdiscectomy; Modified duty; MR neurography; MRI's (magnetic resonance imaging); Muscle relaxants ; Myelography; Neuromodulation devices; Neuromuscular electrical stimulators (NMES); Neuroplasty; Neuroreflexotherapy; Nonprescription medications; Narcotics; Nucleoplasty; Occupational therapy (OT); Opioids; Oral corticosteroids; Percutaneous diskectomy (PCD); Percutaneous electrical nerve stimulation (PENS) ; Percutaneous endoscopic laser discectomy (PELD); Percutaneous epidural neuroplasty; Percutaneous intradiscal radiofrequency (thermocoagulation); Percutaneous neuromodulation therapy (PNT); Percutaneous vertebroplasty (PV); Physical therapy (PT); Pilates; Powered traction devices; Prolotherapy, also known as sclerotherapy; Psychological screening; Racz neurolysis; Radiofrequency neurotomy; Radiography (x-rays); Range of motion (ROM); Return to work; Sclerotherapy; Shoe insoles/shoe lifts; SPECT (single photon emission computed tomography); Spinal cord stimulation (SCS); Standing MRI; Stimulators, electrical; Stretching; Supports & braces; Surface electromyography (SEMG); Surgery; Sympathetic therapy; Thermography (infrared stress thermography); Traction; Transcutaneous electrical neurostimulation (TENS) ; Trigger point injections; Tumor necrosis factor (TNF) modifiers; Ultrasound, diagnostic (imaging); Ultrasound, therapeutic; Vertebral axial decompression (VAX-D); Vertebroplasty; Videofluoroscopy (for range of motion); Work conditioning, work hardening; Work; X-rays; Yoga
Physical Therapy Guidelines:
Allow for fading of treatment frequency (from up to 3 visits per week to 1 or less), plus active self-directed home PT
10 visits over 5 weeks
Chiropractic Guidelines:
Therapeutic care --
Mild: up to 6 visits over 2 weeks
Severe: Trial of 6 visits over 2 weeks
Severe: With evidence of objective functional improvement, total of up to 18 visits over 6-8 weeks, avoid chronicity
Elective care -- not medically necessary

Workers' Comp Costs per Claim (based on 200,817 claims)

Quartile	25%	50%	75%	Mean	% no cost
Indemnity	$1,449	$2,919	$5,817	$5,576	78%
Medical	$263	$641	$1,974	$2,044	4%
Total	$273	$725	$2,856	$3,287	4%

Disability Duration Adjustment Factors by Age

Age Group	18-24	25-34	35-44	45-54	55-64	65-74
Adjustment Factor	0.66	0.74	1.07	1.10	1.35	1.64

RTW Claims Data (Calendar-days away from work by decile)

10%	20%	30%	40%	**50%**	60%	70%	80%	**90%**	100%	Mean
10	12	14	15	**17**	21	34	37	**61**	365	29.40

RTW Post Surgery (Calendar-days away from work by decile)

10%	20%	30%	40%	**50%**	60%	70%	80%	**90%**	100%	Mean
Neck spine fusion										
28	38	47	60	**75**	94	148	215	**304**	365	125.11
Low back disk surgery										
41	51	56	92	**142**	205	321	365	**365**	365	181.36
Neck spine disk surgery										
28	42	51	59	**76**	102	130	165	**304**	365	118.93

847 Sprains and strains of other and unspecified parts of back *(cont'd)*

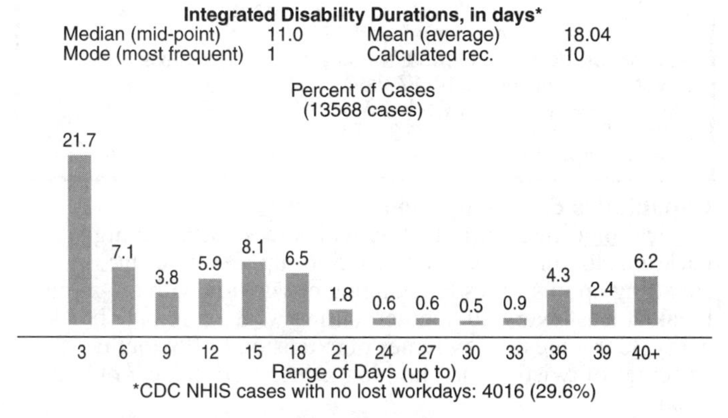

Impact on Total Absence: Prevalence 0.5094% of total lost workdays; Incidence 5.35 days per 100 workers

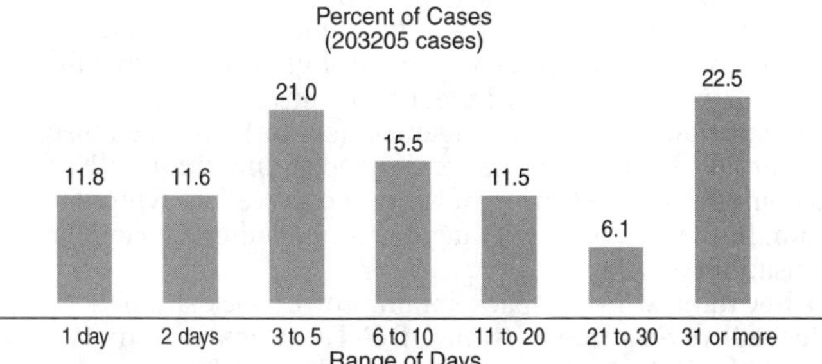

Impact on Occupational Absence: Prevalence 16.1365% of occupational lost workdays; Incidence 2.58 days per 100 workers

847.0 Neck

Return-To-Work Summary Guidelines		
Dataset	**Midrange**	**At-Risk**
Claims data	25 days	62 days
All absences	5 days	35 days

Return-To-Work "Best Practice" Guidelines
Whiplash grade 0 (Quebec Task Force grades): 0 days
Whiplash grade I-III, clerical/modified work: 5 days
Whiplash grade I-III, manual work: 21 days
Whiplash grade I-III, heavy manual work: 28 days
Whiplash grade IV: see 805 (fracture)

Capabilities & Activity Modifications:
Clerical/modified work: No lifting over shoulder; lifting to level of shoulder not more than 5 lbs up to 2 times/hr; standing or walking with a 5-minute break at least every 20 minutes; sitting with a 5-minute break every 30 minutes (using an operator head set if extended phone operations); no extremes of motion including extension or flexion; no extremes of twisting or lateral rotation; no climbing ladders; driving car only up to 2 hrs/day; possible use of cervical collar with change of position and stretching every 30 min; modify workstation or position to eliminate lifting away from body or using twisting motion.
Manual work: Lifting over shoulder not more than 25 lbs up to 15 times/hr; lifting to level of shoulder up to 30 lbs of weight not more than 15 times/hr; standing or walking with a 10-minute break at least every 1-2 hours; sitting with a 10-minute break every 1-2 hours; extremes of flexion or extension allowed up to 20 times/hr; extremes of twisting

847.0 Neck *(cont'd)*

allowed up to 16 times/hr; climbing ladders allowed up to 40 rungs 8 times/hr; driving car or light truck up to a full work day; driving heavy truck up to 4 hrs/day.
Description: Injury to the ligament (sprain) or to the muscle (strain) of the neck. Sprains and strains are usually accompanied by a tearing of the tissue as well as symptoms of pain, limited motion, swelling, bruising, and/or a change in sensation.
Other names: Sprained neck, Strained neck

Anterior longitudinal (ligament), cervical
Atlanto-axial (joints)
Atlanto-occipital (joints)
Whiplash injury

Excludes:
neck injury NOS (959.0)
thyroid region (848.2)

Procedure Summary (from ODG Treatment): Activity restrictions; Acupuncture; Arthrodesis (fusion); Arthroplasty; Back schools; Bed rest; Biofeedback; Bone scan; Botulinum toxin (injection); Cervical orthosis; Chiropractic care; Chymopapain (injection); Cognitive behavioral rehabilitation; Cold packs; Collars (cervical); Computed tomography (CT); Computerized range of motion (ROM); Corticosteroid injection; Decompression; Diathermy; Discography; Disc prosthesis; Discectomy/laminectomy; Education (patient); Electromyography (EMG); Electrotherapies; Electromagnetic therapy (PEMT); Epidural steroid injection (ESI); Ergonomics; Exercise; Facet-joint injections; Facet rhizotomy; Flexibility; Fluoroscopy (for ESI's); Fusion (spinal); H-Reflex tests; Heat/cold applications; High-dose methylprednisolone; Imaging; Immobilization (collars); Injections; Laminectomy; Laminoplasty; Laser therapy; Magnetic resonance imaging (MRI); Manipulation; Manipulation under anesthesia (MUA) ; Massage; Methylprednisolone; Multidisciplinary biopsychosocial (rehabilitation); Myelography; Nonprescription medications; Occupational therapy (OT); Opioids; Oral corticosteroids; Patient education; Percutaneous electrical nerve stimulation (PENS); Percutaneous neuromodulation therapy (PNT); Percutaneous radio-frequency neurotomy; Physical therapy (PT); Prolotherapy (also known as sclerotherapy); Pulsed electromagnetic therapy (PEMT); Radiofrequency neurotomy; Radiography (x-rays); Range of motion (ROM); Rest; Return to work; Sensory evoked potentials (SEPs); Soft collars; Steroids; Stretching; Surface EMG (electromyography); Surgery; Therapeutic exercises; Thermography (diagnostic); Traction; Transcutaneous electrical neurostimulation (TENS); Trigger point injections; Ultrasound, diagnostic (imaging); Ultrasound, therapeutic; Videofluoroscopy (for range of motion); Work
Physical Therapy Guidelines:
Allow for fading of treatment frequency (from up to 3 visits per week to 1 or less), plus active self-directed home PT
10 visits over 8 weeks
Chiropractic Guidelines:
(If not contraindicated by risk of stroke)
Mild (grade I): up to 6 visits over 2-3 weeks
Moderate (grade II): Trial of 6 visits over 2-3 weeks
Moderate (grade II): With evidence of objective functional improvement, total of up to 18 visits over 6-8 weeks, avoid chronicity
Severe (grade III & auto trauma): Trial of 10 visits over 4-6 weeks
Severe (grade III & auto trauma): With evidence of objective functional improvement, total of up to 25 visits over 26 weeks, avoid chronicity

847.0 Neck *(cont'd)*

Workers' Comp Costs per Claim (based on 67,106 claims)					
Quartile	25%	50%	75%	Mean	% no cost
Indemnity	$1,932	$3,612	$6,752	$6,259	74%
Medical	$378	$1,019	$2,919	$2,681	3%
Total	$399	$1,229	$4,494	$4,379	3%

RTW Claims Data (Calendar-days away from work by decile)										
10%	20%	30%	40%	**50%**	60%	70%	80%	**90%**	100%	Mean
11	14	19	21	**25**	28	31	41	**62**	104	30.30

RTW Post Surgery (Calendar-days away from work by decile)										
10%	20%	30%	40%	**50%**	60%	70%	80%	**90%**	100%	Mean
Neck spine fusion										
34	45	52	68	**76**	104	165	300	**365**	365	135.52
Neck spine disk surgery										
31	45	51	68	**76**	104	148	165	**304**	365	123.75

Integrated Disability Durations, in days*

Median (mid-point) 5.0 Mean (average) 14.33
Mode (most frequent) 1 Calculated rec. 6

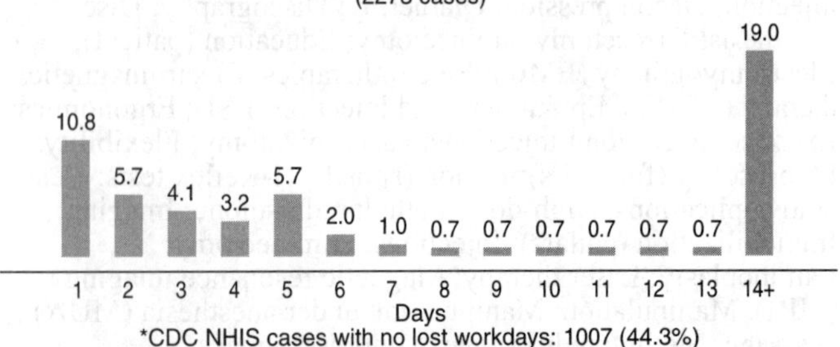

*CDC NHIS cases with no lost workdays: 1007 (44.3%)

Impact on Total Absence: Prevalence 0.0536% of total lost workdays; Incidence 0.56 days per 100 workers

Occupational Disability Durations, in days

Median (mid-point) 7 - Benchmark Indemnity Costs $5,250

Percent of Cases
(13598 cases)

14.1 | 12.1 | 17.9 | 12.8 | 10.6 | 5.7 | 27.0

1 day | 2 days | 3 to 5 | 6 to 10 | 11 to 20 | 21 to 30 | 31 or more

Range of Days

Impact on Occupational Absence: Prevalence 1.0798% of occupational lost workdays; Incidence 0.17 days per 100 workers

847.2 Lumbar sprains and strains

Return-To-Work Summary Guidelines		
Dataset	**Midrange**	**At-Risk**
Claims data	17 days	63 days
All absences	10 days	38 days

847.2 Lumbar sprains and strains *(cont'd)*

Return-To-Work "Best Practice" Guidelines
Mild (grade I), clerical/modified work: 0 days
Mild, manual/heavy manual work: 7-10 days
Severe (grade II-III), clerical/modified work: 0-3 days
Severe, manual work: 14-17 days
Severe, heavy manual work: 35 days
With radicular signs, see 722.1 (disc disorders)
Obesity comorbidity (BMI >= 30), multiply by: 1.31

Capabilities & Activity Modifications:
Clerical/modified work: Lifting with knees (with a straight back, no stooping) not more than 5 lbs up to 3 times/hr; squatting up to 4 times/hr; standing or walking with a 5-minute break at least every 20 minutes; sitting with a 5-minute break every 30 minutes; no extremes of extension or flexion; no extremes of twisting; no climbing ladders; driving car only up to 2 hrs/day.
Manual work: Lifting with knees (with a straight back) not more than 25 lbs up to 15 times/hr; squatting up to 16 times/hr; standing or walking with a 10-minute break at least every 1-2 hours; sitting with a 10-minute break every 1-2 hours; extremes of flexion or extension allowed up to 12 times/hr; extremes of twisting allowed up to 16 times/hr; climbing ladders allowed up to 25 rungs 6 times/hr; driving car or light truck up to a full work day; driving heavy truck up to 4 hrs/day.
Description: Injury to the ligament (sprain) or to the muscle (strain) of the lower back. Sprains and strains are usually accompanied by a tearing of the tissue as well as symptoms of pain, limited motion, swelling, bruising, and/or a change in sensation.
Other names: Lower back sprain, Lower back strain
Procedure Summary (from ODG Treatment): Activity restrictions; Acupuncture; Adhesiolysis; Aerobic exercise; Age adjustment factors; Annuloplasty (IDET); Antidepressants; Anti-inflammatory medications; Aquatic therapy; Arthrodesis; Arthroplasty; Artificial disk; Back brace; Back schools; Bed rest; Behavioral treatment; Biofeedback; Bone-growth stimulators (BGS); Bone scan; Botulinum toxin (Botox); Chemonucleolysis (chymopapain); Chiropractic; Coblation nucleoplasty; Cognitive intervention; Colchicine; Cold/heat packs; Computerized range of motion (ROM); Corsets; CT & CT Myelography (computed tomography); Cutaneous laser treatment; Decompression; Diagnostic imaging; Diathermy; Differential Diagnosis; Disc prosthesis; Discectomy/ laminectomy; Discography; DRX (traction); Dynamic neutralization system (Dynesys); Education; Electrical stimulators (E-stim); Electromagnetic pulsed therapy; EMG's (electromyography); Epidural steroid injections (ESI's); Ergonomics interventions; Etanercept (Enbrel); Exercise; Facet-joint injections; Facet rhizotomy (radio frequency medial branch neurotomy); Feldenkrais; Flexibility; Fluoroscopy (for ESI's); Foraminotomy; Fusion (spinal); Fusion, endoscopic; Hardware; Heat therapy; Hemilaminectomy; H-wave stimulation (devices); IDD therapy (intervertebral disc decompression); IDET (intradiscal electrothermal anuloplasty); Imaging; Implantable pumps for narcotics; Implantable spinal cord stimulators; Implants; Infliximab (Remicade); Injections; Interferential therapy; Intradiscal electrothermal therapy (IDET); Intradiscal steroid injection; Intrathecal drug administration system; Kyphoplasty; Laminectomy/ laminotomy; Ligamentous injections; Lordex (traction); Low level laser therapy (LLLT); Lumbar supports; Magnet therapy; Manipulation; Manipulation under anesthesia (MUA) ; Massage; Mattress firmness; McKenzie method; Medications; MedX lumbar extension machine; Microcurrent electrical stimulation (MENS devices); Microdiscectomy; Modified duty; MR neurography; MRI's (magnetic resonance imaging); Muscle relaxants ; Myelography; Neuromodulation devices;

847.2 Lumbar sprains and strains *(cont'd)*

Neuromuscular electrical stimulators (NMES); Neuroplasty; Neuroreflexotherapy; Nonprescription medications; Narcotics; Nucleoplasty; Occupational therapy (OT); Opioids; Oral corticosteroids; Percutaneous diskectomy (PCD); Percutaneous electrical nerve stimulation (PENS) ; Percutaneous endoscopic laser discectomy (PELD); Percutaneous epidural neuroplasty; Percutaneous intradiscal radiofrequency (thermocoagulation); Percutaneous neuromodulation therapy (PNT); Percutaneous vertebroplasty (PV); Physical therapy (PT); Pilates; Powered traction devices; Prolotherapy, also known as sclerotherapy; Psychological screening; Racz neurolysis; Radiofrequency neurotomy; Radiography (x-rays); Range of motion (ROM); Return to work; Sclerotherapy; Shoe insoles/shoe lifts; SPECT (single photon emission computed tomography); Spinal cord stimulation (SCS); Standing MRI; Stimulators, electrical; Stretching; Supports & braces; Surface electromyography (SEMG); Surgery; Sympathetic therapy; Thermography (infrared stress thermography); Traction; Transcutaneous electrical neurostimulation (TENS) ; Trigger point injections; Tumor necrosis factor (TNF) modifiers; Ultrasound, diagnostic (imaging); Ultrasound, therapeutic; Vertebral axial decompression (VAX-D); Vertebroplasty; Videofluoroscopy (for range of motion); Work conditioning, work hardening; Work; X-rays; Yoga

Physical Therapy Guidelines:

Allow for fading of treatment frequency (from up to 3 visits per week to 1 or less), plus active self-directed home PT
10 visits over 8 weeks

Chiropractic Guidelines:

Therapeutic care --
Mild: up to 6 visits over 2 weeks
Severe: Trial of 6 visits over 2 weeks
Severe: With evidence of objective functional improvement, total of up to 18 visits over 6-8 weeks, avoid chronicity
Elective care -- not medically necessary

Workers' Comp Costs per Claim (based on 95,654 claims)

Quartile	25%	50%	75%	Mean	% no cost
Indemnity	$1,281	$2,510	$5,103	$5,202	80%
Medical	$242	$546	$1,628	$1,780	4%
Total	$242	$609	$2,352	$2,862	4%

Disability Duration Adjustment Factors by Age

Age Group	18-24	25-34	35-44	45-54	55-64	65-74
Adjustment Factor	0.66	0.74	1.07	1.10	1.35	1.64

RTW Claims Data (Calendar-days away from work by decile)

10%	20%	30%	40%	**50%**	60%	70%	80%	**90%**	100%	Mean
10	12	14	15	**17**	21	34	37	**63**	365	30.27

RTW Post Surgery (Calendar-days away from work by decile)

	10%	20%	30%	40%	**50%**	60%	70%	80%	**90%**	100%	Mean
Low back disk surgery	41	51	58	92	**142**	205	321	365	**365**	365	182.98

847.2 Lumbar sprains and strains *(cont'd)*

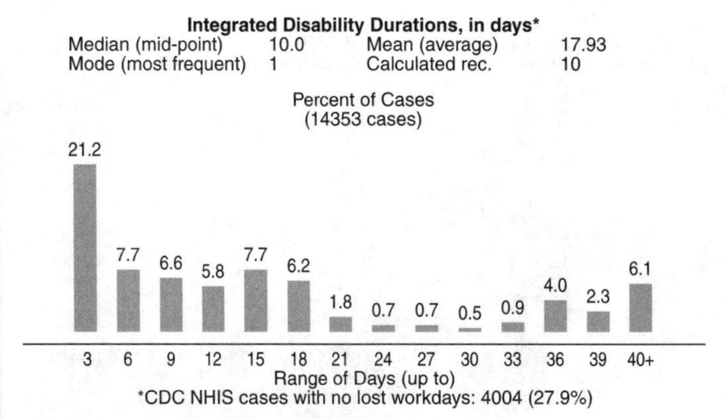

Impact on Total Absence: Prevalence 0.5485% of total lost workdays; Incidence 5.76 days per 100 workers

Occupational Disability Durations, in days
Median (mid-point) 7 - Benchmark Indemnity Costs $5,250

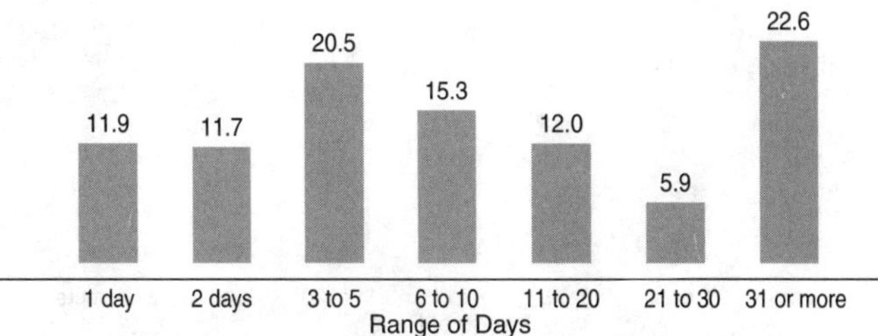

Impact on Occupational Absence: Prevalence 7.9982% of occupational lost workdays; Incidence 1.28 days per 100 workers

848 Other and ill-defined sprains and strains

Return-To-Work Summary Guidelines

Dataset	Midrange	At-Risk
Claims data	17 days	56 days
All absences	6 days	35 days

Workers' Comp Costs per Claim (based on 18,981 claims)

Quartile	25%	50%	75%	Mean	% no cost
Indemnity	$798	$1,512	$2,804	$3,143	89%
Medical	$158	$284	$525	$683	6%
Total	$168	$294	$630	$1,054	6%

RTW Claims Data (Calendar-days away from work by decile)

10%	20%	30%	40%	**50%**	60%	70%	80%	**90%**	100%	Mean
9	12	13	14	**17**	21	28	39	**56**	365	27.79

848 Other and ill-defined sprains and strains

Integrated Disability Durations, in days*

Median (mid-point) 6.0 Mean (average) 13.81
Mode (most frequent) 1 Calculated rec. 7

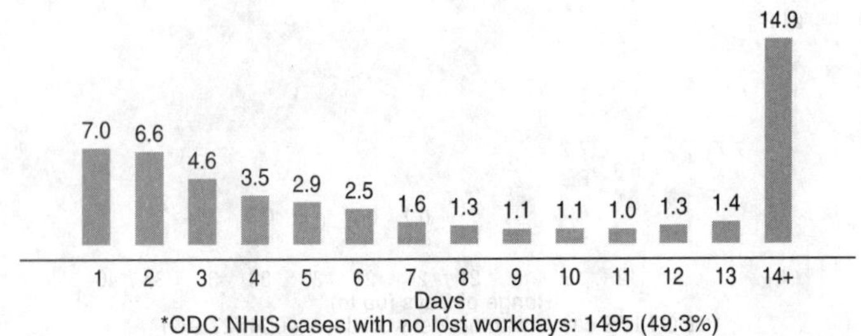

*CDC NHIS cases with no lost workdays: 1495 (49.3%)

Impact on Total Absence: Prevalence 0.0628% of total lost workdays; Incidence 0.66 days per 100 workers

Occupational Disability Durations, in days

Median (mid-point) 7 - Benchmark Indemnity Costs $5,250

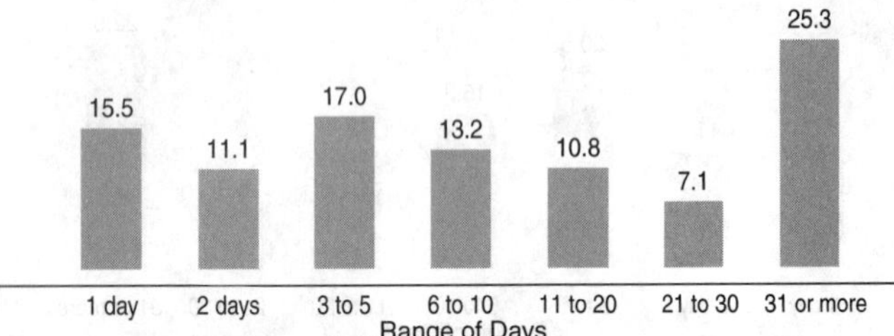

Impact on Occupational Absence: Prevalence 5.5364% of occupational lost workdays; Incidence 0.89 days per 100 workers

INTRACRANIAL INJURY, EXCLUDING THOSE WITH SKULL FRACTURE (850-854)

Excludes:

intracranial injury with skull fracture (800-801 and 803-804, except .0 and .5)
nerve injury (950.0-951.9)
open wound of head without intracranial injury (870.0-873.9)
skull fracture alone (800-801 and 803-804 with .0, .5)
The description "with open intracranial wound," used in the fourth-digit subdivisions, includes those specified as open or with mention of infection or foreign body.

The following fifth-digit subclassification is for use with categories 851-854:

0 unspecified state of consciousness
1 with no loss of consciousness
2 with brief [less than one hour] loss of consciousness
3 with moderate [1-24 hours] loss of consciousness
4 with prolonged [more than 24 hours] loss of consciousness and return to pre-existing conscious level
5 with prolonged [more than 24 hours] loss of consciousness, without return to pre-existing conscious level
6 with loss of consciousness of unspecified duration
9 with concussion, unspecified

INTRACRANIAL INJURY, EXCLUDING THOSE WITH SKULL FRACTURE (850-854) *(cont'd)*

RTW Claims Data (Calendar-days away from work by decile)										
10%	20%	30%	40%	**50%**	60%	70%	80%	**90%**	100%	Mean
11	13	14	16	**19**	27	29	35	**83**	365	41.60

Impact on Total Absence: Prevalence 0.3419% of total lost workdays; Incidence 3.59 days per 100 workers

Occupational Disability Durations, in days

Median (mid-point) 4 - Benchmark Indemnity Costs $3,000

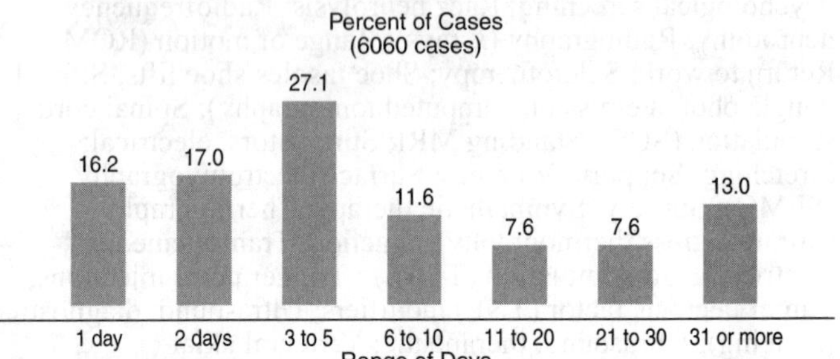

Impact on Occupational Absence: Prevalence 0.2749% of occupational lost workdays; Incidence 0.04 days per 100 workers

850 Concussion

Return-To-Work Summary Guidelines		
Dataset	**Midrange**	**At-Risk**
Claims data	16 days	32 days
All absences	6 days	29 days

Return-To-Work "Best Practice" Guidelines
Mild: 1 day
Severe, non-cognitive/modified work: 14 days
Severe, cognitive work: 28 days

Description: A brief loss of consciousness and sometimes memory after a head injury. Symptoms following a concussion usually include confusion, headache, sleepiness, dizziness, disorientation, and/or unconsciousness. These symptoms don't usually last more than 24 hours. More serious versions of those symptoms could develop days later depending on the extent of the injury.

Includes: commotio cerebri

Excludes:

Concussion with:
cerebral laceration or contusion (851.0-851.9)
cerebral hemorrhage (852-853)
head injury NOS (854)

Procedure Summary (from ODG Treatment): Activity restrictions; Acupuncture; Anticonvulsants; Antidepressants; Antiepilectics; Bed rest; Behavioral therapy; Botulinum toxin type A; Branched-chain amino acids (BCAAs); Cell transplantation therapy ; Complementary and alternative medicine (CAM); Corticosteroids (for acute traumatic brain injury); Cognitive therapy; Craniectomy; Craniotomy; CT (computed tomography); Decompressive surgery; EEG (Electroencephalography); Field of vision testing; Fluid resuscitation; Glasgow Coma Scale (GCS); Greater occipital nerve block (GONB); Hyperventilation; Hypothermia; Imaging; Interdisciplinary rehabilitation programs; Lumbar puncture; Mannitol; Melatonin; Methylphenidate; Modified Ashworth Scale (MAS); MRI (magnetic resonance imaging); Nutrition; Occupational therapy (OT); Oxygen therapy; PET (positron emission tomography); Physical therapy (PT); QEEG (Quantified Electroencephalography); Relaxation treatment (for

850 Concussion *(cont'd)*

migraines); Return to work; Sedation; Skull x-rays; Sleep aids; SPECT (single photon emission computed tomography); Steroids; Triptans; Vision evaluation; Wilsonii injecta; Work

Workers' Comp Costs per Claim (based on 5,312 claims)					
Quartile	25%	50%	75%	Mean	% no cost
Indemnity	$1,029	$2,809	$6,426	$6,136	84%
Medical	$567	$1,082	$2,048	$2,277	3%
Total	$588	$1,124	$2,415	$3,310	3%

RTW Claims Data (Calendar-days away from work by decile)										
10%	20%	30%	40%	**50%**	60%	70%	80%	**90%**	100%	Mean
12	13	14	15	**16**	19	27	29	**32**	365	22.67

Integrated Disability Durations, in days*

Median (mid-point) 6.0 Mean (average) 12.07
Mode (most frequent) 1 Calculated rec. 6

Percent of Cases
(2551 cases)

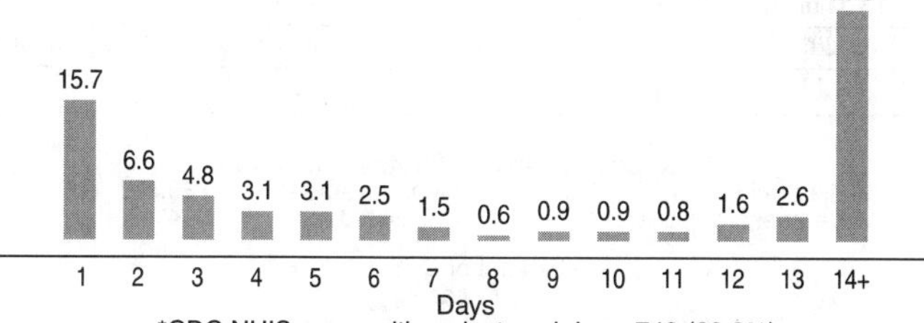

*CDC NHIS cases with no lost workdays: 748 (29.3%)

Impact on Total Absence: Prevalence 0.0643% of total lost workdays; Incidence 0.68 days per 100 workers

Occupational Disability Durations, in days

Median (mid-point) 4 - Benchmark Indemnity Costs $3,000

Percent of Cases
(5830 cases)

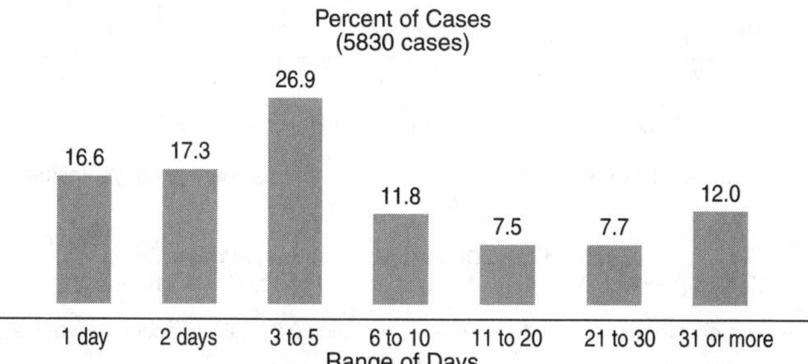

Impact on Occupational Absence: Prevalence 0.2645% of occupational lost workdays; Incidence 0.04 days per 100 workers

852 Subarachnoid, subdural, and extradural hemorrhage, following injury

Return-To-Work Summary Guidelines		
Dataset	**Midrange**	**At-Risk**
Claims data	61 days	365 days
All absences	60 days	365 days

Return-To-Work "Best Practice" Guidelines
Non-cognitive/modified work: 60-180 days
Cognitive work: 180 days to indefinite

Description: Bleeding from the lining of the brain following an injury.

Requires fifth digit. See beginning of section 850-854 for codes and definitions.

Excludes:

cerebral contusion or laceration (with hemorrhage) (851.0-851.9)

852 Subarachnoid, subdural, and extradural hemorrhage, following injury *(cont'd)*

Procedure Summary (from ODG Treatment): Activity restrictions; Acupuncture; Anticonvulsants; Antidepressants; Antiepilectics; Bed rest; Behavioral therapy; Botulinum toxin type A; Branched-chain amino acids (BCAAs); Cell transplantation therapy ; Complementary and alternative medicine (CAM); Corticosteroids (for acute traumatic brain injury); Cognitive therapy; Craniectomy; Craniotomy; CT (computed tomography); Decompressive surgery; EEG (Electroencephalography); Field of vision testing; Fluid resuscitation; Glasgow Coma Scale (GCS); Greater occipital nerve block (GONB); Hyperventilation; Hypothermia; Imaging; Interdisciplinary rehabilitation programs; Lumbar puncture; Mannitol; Melatonin; Methylphenidate; Modified Ashworth Scale (MAS); MRI (magnetic resonance imaging); Nutrition; Occupational therapy (OT); Oxygen therapy; PET (positron emission tomography); Physical therapy (PT); QEEG (Quantified Electroencephalography); Relaxation treatment (for migraines); Return to work; Sedation; Skull x-rays; Sleep aids; SPECT (single photon emission computed tomography); Steroids; Triptans; Vision evaluation; Wilsonii injecta; Work

Workers' Comp Costs per Claim (based on 137 claims)					
Quartile	25%	50%	75%	Mean	% no cost
Indemnity	$4,179	$11,177	$34,934	$23,932	31%
Medical	$10,227	$21,725	$45,371	$36,958	4%
Total	$13,146	$28,744	$77,931	$53,525	3%

RTW Claims Data (Calendar-days away from work by decile)										
10%	20%	30%	40%	**50%**	60%	70%	80%	**90%**	100%	Mean
16	27	39	58	**61**	99	145	183	**365**	365	119.65

Integrated Disability Durations, in days*

Median (mid-point) 60.0 Mean (average) 111.79
Mode (most frequent) 365 Calculated rec. 149

Percent of Cases
(83 cases)

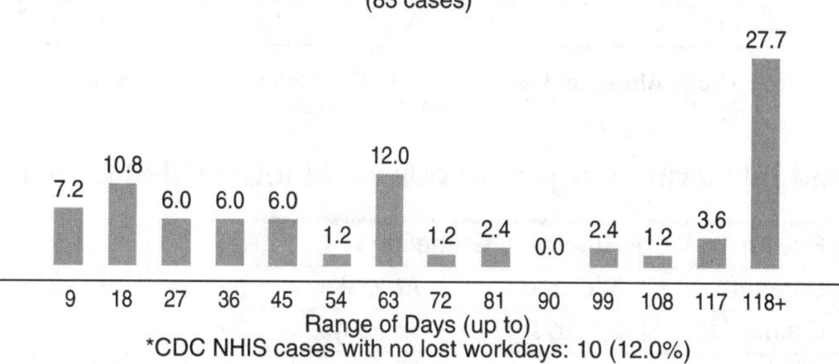

*CDC NHIS cases with no lost workdays: 10 (12.0%)

Impact on Total Absence: Prevalence 0.0241% of total lost workdays; Incidence 0.25 days per 100 workers

Occupational Disability Durations, in days

Median (mid-point) 7 - Benchmark Indemnity Costs $5,250
(40 cases)

Impact on Occupational Absence: Prevalence 0.0031% of occupational lost workdays

852.2 Subdural hemorrhage following injury without mention of open intracranial wound

Return-To-Work Summary Guidelines		
Dataset	**Midrange**	**At-Risk**
Claims data	31 days	58 days
All absences	17 days	58 days

Return-To-Work "Best Practice" Guidelines
Chronic: 21-42 days
Acute: 42 days to indefinite

852.2 Subdural hemorrhage following injury without mention of open intracranial wound

Description: Bleeding between the outer covering and the middle covering of the brain, usually as a result of head injury, causing brain cell destruction. Symptoms include severe headaches, vision problems, drowsiness, confusion, nausea, seizures, and/or weakness in one side of the body.
Other names: Intercranial hemorrhage
Procedure Summary (from ODG Treatment): Activity restrictions; Acupuncture; Anticonvulsants; Antidepressants; Antiepilectics; Bed rest; Behavioral therapy; Botulinum toxin type A; Branched-chain amino acids (BCAAs); Cell transplantation therapy ; Complementary and alternative medicine (CAM); Corticosteroids (for acute traumatic brain injury); Cognitive therapy; Craniectomy; Craniotomy; CT (computed tomography); Decompressive surgery; EEG (Electroencephalography); Field of vision testing; Fluid resuscitation; Glasgow Coma Scale (GCS); Greater occipital nerve block (GONB); Hyperventilation; Hypothermia; Imaging; Interdisciplinary rehabilitation programs; Lumbar puncture; Mannitol; Melatonin; Methylphenidate; Modified Ashworth Scale (MAS); MRI (magnetic resonance imaging); Nutrition; Occupational therapy (OT); Oxygen therapy; PET (positron emission tomography); Physical therapy (PT); QEEG (Quantified Electroencephalography); Relaxation treatment (for migraines); Return to work; Sedation; Skull x-rays; Sleep aids; SPECT (single photon emission computed tomography); Steroids; Triptans; Vision evaluation; Wilsonii injecta; Work

Workers' Comp Costs per Claim (based on 86 claims)

Quartile	25%	50%	75%	Mean	% no cost
Indemnity	$6,836	$15,377	$32,750	$20,202	33%
Medical	$8,988	$21,725	$57,215	$42,355	4%
Total	$12,905	$30,146	$77,931	$56,449	4%

RTW Claims Data (Calendar-days away from work by decile)

10%	20%	30%	40%	**50%**	60%	70%	80%	**90%**	100%	Mean
9	16	16	17	**31**	36	44	53	**58**	365	38.20

Impact on Total Absence: Prevalence 0.0011% of total lost workdays; Incidence 0.01 days per 100 workers

854 Intracranial injury of other and unspecified nature

Return-To-Work Summary Guidelines		
Dataset	**Midrange**	**At-Risk**
Claims data	23 days	364 days
All absences	7 days	85 days

Return-To-Work "Best Practice" Guidelines
Mild concussion: 3-7 days
Severe concussion, non-cognitive/modified work: 14 days to indefinite
Severe concussion, cognitive work: 84 days to indefinite

Requires fifth digit. See beginning of section 850-854 for codes and definitions.
Includes: brain injury NOS
head injury NOS

Procedure Summary (from ODG Treatment): Activity restrictions; Acupuncture; Anticonvulsants; Antidepressants; Antiepilectics; Bed rest; Behavioral therapy; Botulinum toxin type A; Branched-chain amino acids (BCAAs); Cell transplantation therapy ; Complementary and alternative medicine (CAM); Corticosteroids (for acute traumatic brain injury); Cognitive therapy; Craniectomy; Craniotomy; CT (computed tomography); Decompressive surgery; EEG (Electroencephalography); Field of vision testing; Fluid

854 Intracranial injury of other and unspecified nature *(cont'd)*

resuscitation; Glasgow Coma Scale (GCS); Greater occipital nerve block (GONB); Hyperventilation; Hypothermia; Imaging; Interdisciplinary rehabilitation programs; Lumbar puncture; Mannitol; Melatonin; Methylphenidate; Modified Ashworth Scale (MAS); MRI (magnetic resonance imaging); Nutrition; Occupational therapy (OT); Oxygen therapy; PET (positron emission tomography); Physical therapy (PT); QEEG (Quantified Electroencephalography); Relaxation treatment (for migraines); Return to work; Sedation; Skull x-rays; Sleep aids; SPECT (single photon emission computed tomography); Steroids; Triptans; Vision evaluation; Wilsonii injecta; Work

Workers' Comp Costs per Claim (based on 1,676 claims)

Quartile	25%	50%	75%	Mean	% no cost
Indemnity	$1,796	$5,786	$30,545	$27,326	69%
Medical	$431	$1,040	$2,940	$13,242	5%
Total	$483	$1,229	$5,450	$21,641	2%

RTW Claims Data (Calendar-days away from work by decile)

10%	20%	30%	40%	**50%**	60%	70%	80%	**90%**	100%	Mean
11	13	14	17	**23**	33	71	85	**364**	365	77.50

Integrated Disability Durations, in days*
Median (mid-point) 7.0 Mean (average) 39.83
Mode (most frequent) 1 Calculated rec. 14

Percent of Cases
(1317 cases)

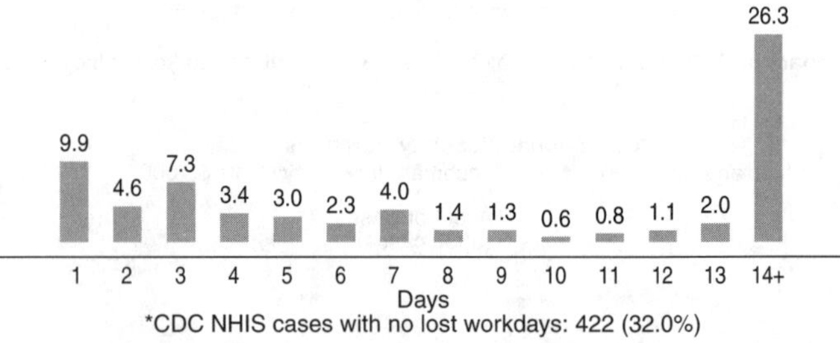

*CDC NHIS cases with no lost workdays: 422 (32.0%)

Impact on Total Absence: Prevalence 0.1053% of total lost workdays; Incidence 1.11 days per 100 workers

Occupational Disability Durations, in days
Median (mid-point) 14 - Benchmark Indemnity Costs $10,500
(170 cases)
Impact on Occupational Absence: Prevalence 0.0269% of occupational lost workdays

INTERNAL INJURY OF THORAX, ABDOMEN, AND PELVIS (860-869)

Includes: blast injuries of internal organs
blunt trauma of internal organs
bruise of internal organs
concussion injuries (except cerebral) of internal organs
crushing of internal organs
hematoma of internal organs
laceration of internal organs
puncture of internal organs
tear of internal organs
traumatic rupture of internal organs

Excludes:
concussion NOS (850.0-850.9)
flail chest (807.4)
foreign body entering through orifice (930.0-939.9)
injury to blood vessels (901.0-902.9)
The description "with open wound," used in the fourth-digit subdivisions, includes those with mention of infection or foreign body.

INTERNAL INJURY OF THORAX, ABDOMEN, AND PELVIS (860-869) *(cont'd)*

RTW Claims Data (Calendar-days away from work by decile)										
10%	20%	30%	40%	**50%**	60%	70%	80%	**90%**	100%	Mean
13	20	27	38	**45**	55	69	90	**131**	365	61.85

Impact on Total Absence: Prevalence 0.1553% of total lost workdays; Incidence 1.63 days per 100 workers

Occupational Disability Durations, in days
Median (mid-point) 24 - Benchmark Indemnity Costs $18,000
(70 cases)
Impact on Occupational Absence: Prevalence 0.0190% of occupational lost workdays

865 Injury to spleen

Return-To-Work Summary Guidelines		
Dataset	**Midrange**	**At-Risk**
Claims data	41 days	95 days
All absences	39 days	90 days

Return-To-Work "Best Practice" Guidelines
Without surgery, clerical/modified work: 0 days
Splenectomy, laparoscopic: 14 days
Splenectomy, open, clerical/modified work: 21 days
Splenectomy, open, manual work: 42 days

Description: A ruptured spleen is a common complication of car accidents, athletics, and beatings, causing large volumes of blood to pour into the abdomen. This could happen all at once or gradually. There will be tenderness and pain in the upper left abdominal area and there may be a broken rib on that side. There could also be pain in the left shoulder or neck.
Other names: Ruptured spleen

The following fifth-digit subclassification is for use with category 865:
- 0 unspecified injury
- 1 hematoma without rupture of capsule
- 2 capsular tears, without major disruption of parenchyma
- 3 laceration extending into parenchyma
- 4 massive parenchymal disruption
- 9 other

Workers' Comp Costs per Claim (based on 93 claims)					
Quartile	25%	50%	75%	Mean	% no cost
Indemnity	$1,901	$4,557	$11,214	$8,939	29%
Medical	$8,169	$14,669	$28,035	$23,659	0%
Total	$10,458	$18,638	$34,083	$30,044	0%

RTW Claims Data (Calendar-days away from work by decile)										
10%	20%	30%	40%	**50%**	60%	70%	80%	**90%**	100%	Mean
14	24	28	38	**41**	47	62	73	**95**	204	51.19

865 Injury to spleen *(cont'd)*

Integrated Disability Durations, in days*
Median (mid-point) 39.0 Mean (average) 46.21
Mode (most frequent) 1 Calculated rec. 31

Percent of Cases
(81 cases)

12.3 8.6 13.6 8.6 17.3 4.9 4.9 6.2 4.9 4.9 2.5 0.0 3.7 2.5

9 18 27 36 45 54 63 72 81 90 99 108 117 118+
Range of Days (up to)
*CDC NHIS cases with no lost workdays: 4 (4.9%)

Impact on Total Absence: Prevalence 0.0105% of total lost workdays; Incidence 0.11 days per 100 workers

OPEN WOUND (870-897)

Includes: animal bite
avulsion
cut
laceration
puncture wound
traumatic amputation

Excludes:
burn (940.0-949.5)
crushing (925-929.9)
puncture of internal organs (860.0-869.1)
superficial injury (910.0-919.9)
that incidental to:
dislocation (830.0-839.9)
fracture (800.0-829.1)
internal injury (860.0-869.1)
intracranial injury (851.0-854.1)
The description "complicated" used in the fourth-digit subdivisions includes those with mention of delayed healing, delayed treatment, foreign body, or major infection.

Occupational Disability Durations, in days
Median (mid-point) 4 - Benchmark Indemnity Costs $3,000

Percent of Cases
(130800 cases)

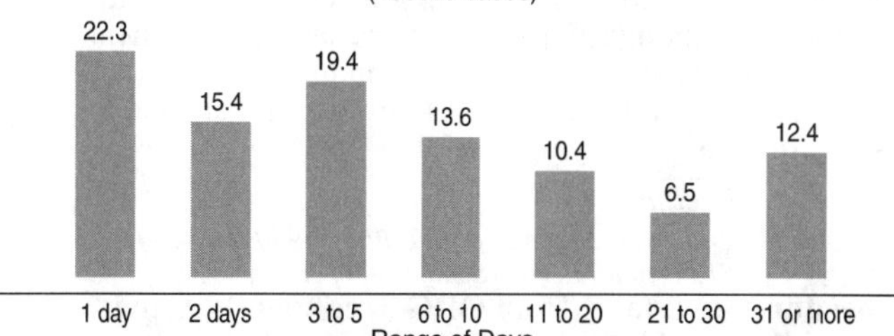

Range of Days
Impact on Occupational Absence: Prevalence 5.9353% of occupational lost workdays; Incidence 0.95 days per 100 workers

OPEN WOUND OF HEAD, NECK, AND TRUNK (870-879)

RTW Claims Data (Calendar-days away from work by decile)										
10%	20%	30%	40%	**50%**	60%	70%	80%	**90%**	100%	Mean
8	10	11	13	**14**	15	19	24	**38**	365	21.13

Impact on Total Absence: Prevalence 0.2272% of total lost workdays; Incidence 2.39 days per 100 workers

OPEN WOUND OF HEAD, NECK, AND TRUNK (870-879) *(cont'd)*

Occupational Disability Durations, in days
Median (mid-point) 3 - Benchmark Indemnity Costs $2,250

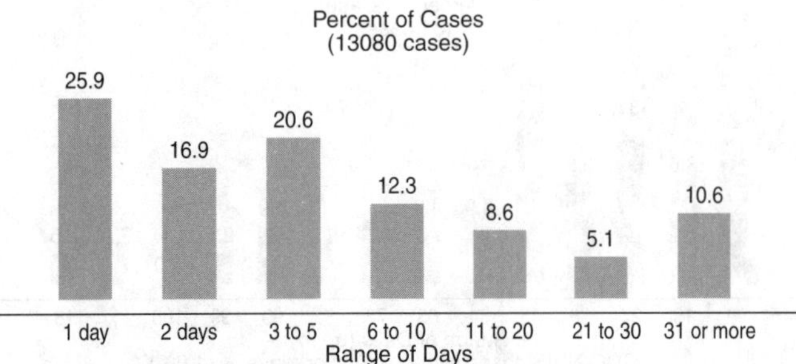

Impact on Occupational Absence: Prevalence 0.4451% of occupational lost workdays; Incidence 0.07 days per 100 workers

871 Open wound of eyeball

Return-To-Work Summary Guidelines		
Dataset	**Midrange**	**At-Risk**
Claims data	14 days	20 days
All absences	4 days	16 days

Return-To-Work "Best Practice" Guidelines
Modified work: 1 day
Regular work, loss of binocular-visual acuity, based on DOT rules: 14 days

Capabilities & Activity Modifications:
Modified work: In injuries occurring to one eye no binocular vision requirements, e.g., as required in the operation of high speed or mobile equipment (bilateral eye injuries such as welding flash burns, chemical burns, and allergic reactions, need to be off any work until the vision in one eye has returned to a functional level); limited stereopsis/fields of vision requirements; no exposure to significant vibration (e.g., affecting intra-ocular foreign bodies or retinal detachment); limit exposure to allergic substances (e.g., allergic conjuctivitis requiring removal of the substance from the workplace) and provision for hygiene to prevent spread of infection by direct contact or shared articles; wearing protective eyewear to prevent recurrent injury; possible workstation adjustment.
Description: An open cut or laceration in the eyeball, which may or may not cause internal hemorrhaging. Pain and loss of vision are among the symptoms.

Excludes:
2nd cranial nerve [optic] injury (950.0-950.9)
3rd cranial nerve [oculomotor] injury (951.0)

Procedure Summary (from ODG Treatment): Activity restrictions; Antibiotic therapy (for treatment of acute bacterial conjunctivitis); Bandage contact lens; Calf blood extract eye gel (vs. vitamin A and dexpanthenol); Computed tomography (CT); Contact lens after penetrating keratoplasty (PK); Diclofenac (ophthalmic solution); Emergency eye wash products; Erythromycin and sulfa compounds (for corneal abrasions involving contact lens use); Fibrin glue (versus N-butyl-2-cyanoacrylate in corneal perforations); Flurbiprofen (eye drops); Indomethacin (0.1%); Indomethacin/gentamicin eyedrops; Ophthalmic vasoconstrictor (drug products); Patching; Prophylactic intravitreal antibiotics; Protection methods (for eyes under general anaesthesia); Surgery for orbital floor fractures; Surgical treatment for hyphema; Surgery for optic neuropathy; Tetanus toxid; The management of optic neuropathy; Topical aminocaproic acid ; Topical corticosteroids

871 Open wound of eyeball *(cont'd)*

(for traumatic microhyphema); Topical nonsteroidal anti-inflammatory drops; Topical NSAIDs (especially Keterolac); Work

Workers' Comp Costs per Claim (based on 1,398 claims)					
Quartile	25%	50%	75%	Mean	% no cost
Indemnity	$830	$1,985	$7,077	$20,962	93%
Medical	$200	$357	$672	$1,203	7%
Total	$200	$357	$693	$2,888	7%

RTW Claims Data (Calendar-days away from work by decile)										
10%	20%	30%	40%	**50%**	60%	70%	80%	**90%**	100%	Mean
10	13	13	14	**14**	15	15	17	**20**	77	15.43

Integrated Disability Durations, in days*
Median (mid-point) 4.0 Mean (average) 7.12
Mode (most frequent) 1 Calculated rec. 4

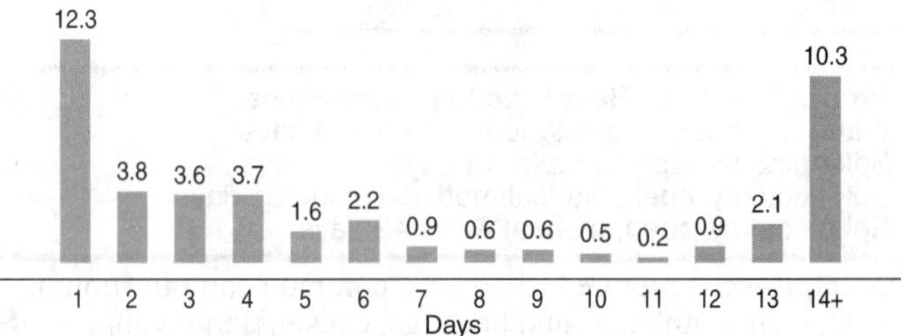

*CDC NHIS cases with no lost workdays: 542 (56.7%)

Impact on Total Absence: Prevalence 0.0087% of total lost workdays; Incidence 0.09 days per 100 workers

872 Open wound of ear

Return-To-Work Summary Guidelines		
Dataset	**Midrange**	**At-Risk**
Claims data	19 days	54 days
All absences	3 days	23 days

Return-To-Work "Best Practice" Guidelines
See 872.0

Workers' Comp Costs per Claim (based on 1,480 claims)					
Quartile	25%	50%	75%	Mean	% no cost
Indemnity	$294	$1,103	$2,069	$1,489	96%
Medical	$242	$462	$746	$716	6%
Total	$242	$467	$767	$777	6%

RTW Claims Data (Calendar-days away from work by decile)										
10%	20%	30%	40%	**50%**	60%	70%	80%	**90%**	100%	Mean
9	10	12	16	**19**	24	32	46	**54**	65	26.11

872 Open wound of ear *(cont'd)*

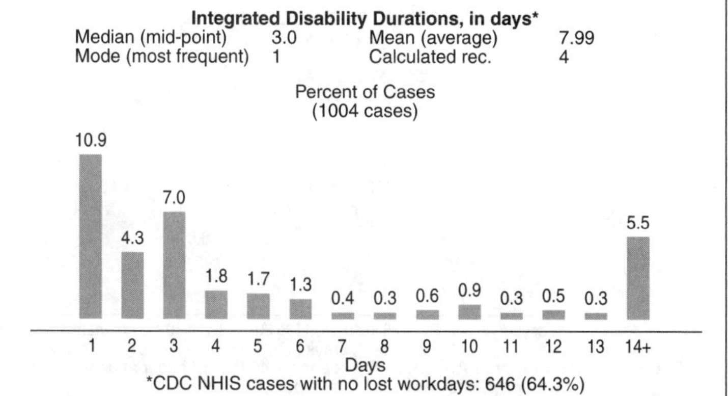

Impact on Total Absence: Prevalence 0.0084% of total lost workdays; Incidence 0.09 days per 100 workers

872.0 External ear, without mention of complication

Return-To-Work Summary Guidelines		
Dataset	**Midrange**	**At-Risk**
Claims data	17 days	52 days
All absences	3 days	20 days

Return-To-Work "Best Practice" Guidelines
Without hospitalization: 1 day
With hospitalization: 3 days

Workers' Comp Costs per Claim (based on 606 claims)					
Quartile	25%	50%	75%	Mean	% no cost
Medical	$284	$478	$767	$687	4%
Total	$294	$483	$809	$714	4%

RTW Claims Data (Calendar-days away from work by decile)										
10%	20%	30%	40%	**50%**	60%	70%	80%	**90%**	100%	Mean
9	11	12	13	**17**	25	32	47	**52**	64	26.04

Integrated Disability Durations, in days*
Median (mid-point) 3.0 Mean (average) 7.99
Mode (most frequent) 1 Calculated rec. 4

Percent of Cases
(378 cases)

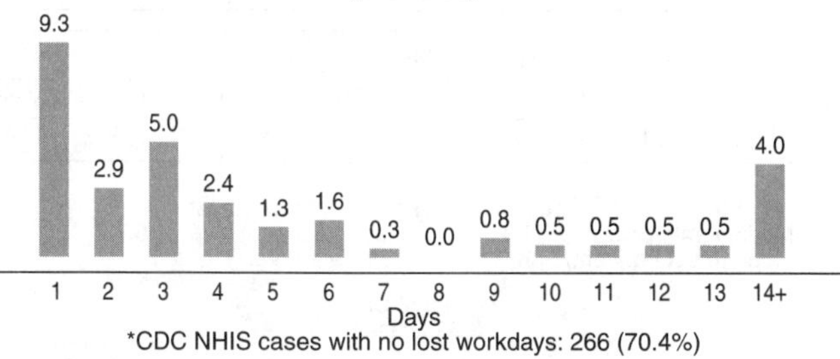

*CDC NHIS cases with no lost workdays: 266 (70.4%)

Impact on Total Absence: Prevalence 0.0026% of total lost workdays; Incidence 0.03 days per 100 workers

873 Other open wound of head

Return-To-Work Summary Guidelines		
Dataset	**Midrange**	**At-Risk**
Claims data	12 days	20 days
All absences	3 days	11 days

873 Other open wound of head *(cont'd)*

Return-To-Work "Best Practice" Guidelines
Minor: 0 days
Major, clerical/modified work: 3 days
Major, manual work: 7 days

Description: An open cut or laceration of the head, which may or may not cause internal hemorrhaging. Bleeding, pain, headache, and/or unconsciousness are among the symptoms.

Excludes:
that with mention of intracranial injury (851.0-854.1)

Procedure Summary (from ODG Treatment): Activity restrictions; Acupuncture; Anticonvulsants; Antidepressants; Antiepilectics; Bed rest; Behavioral therapy; Botulinum toxin type A; Branched-chain amino acids (BCAAs); Cell transplantation therapy ; Complementary and alternative medicine (CAM); Corticosteroids (for acute traumatic brain injury); Cognitive therapy; Craniectomy; Craniotomy; CT (computed tomography); Decompressive surgery; EEG (Electroencephalography); Field of vision testing; Fluid resuscitation; Glasgow Coma Scale (GCS); Greater occipital nerve block (GONB); Hyperventilation; Hypothermia; Imaging; Interdisciplinary rehabilitation programs; Lumbar puncture; Mannitol; Melatonin; Methylphenidate; Modified Ashworth Scale (MAS); MRI (magnetic resonance imaging); Nutrition; Occupational therapy (OT); Oxygen therapy; PET (positron emission tomography); Physical therapy (PT); QEEG (Quantified Electroencephalography); Relaxation treatment (for migraines); Return to work; Sedation; Skull x-rays; Sleep aids; SPECT (single photon emission computed tomography); Steroids; Triptans; Vision evaluation; Wilsonii injecta; Work

Workers' Comp Costs per Claim (based on 41,899 claims)					
Quartile	25%	50%	75%	Mean	% no cost
Indemnity	$441	$1,092	$2,205	$2,951	97%
Medical	$263	$441	$693	$716	7%
Total	$263	$452	$704	$800	7%

RTW Claims Data (Calendar-days away from work by decile)										
10%	20%	30%	40%	**50%**	60%	70%	80%	**90%**	100%	Mean
8	9	10	11	**12**	14	15	17	**20**	365	15.69

RTW Post Surgery (Calendar-days away from work by decile)										
10%	20%	30%	40%	**50%**	60%	70%	80%	**90%**	100%	Mean
Repair of wound or lesion										
2	3	4	6	**12**	15	19	39	**107**	365	38.67

Integrated Disability Durations, in days*
Median (mid-point) 3.0 Mean (average) 5.24
Mode (most frequent) 1 Calculated rec. 3

Percent of Cases
(5751 cases)

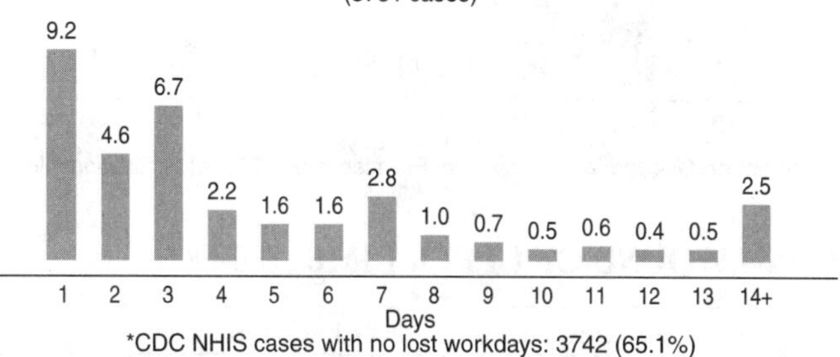

*CDC NHIS cases with no lost workdays: 3742 (65.1%)

Impact on Total Absence: Prevalence 0.0311% of total lost workdays; Incidence 0.33 days per 100 workers

879 Open wound of other and unspecified sites, except limbs

Return-To-Work Summary Guidelines		
Dataset	**Midrange**	**At-Risk**
Claims data	12 days	82 days
All absences	7 days	44 days

Return-To-Work "Best Practice" Guidelines
Minor: 0 days
Major, clerical/modified work: 3 days
Major, manual work: 8 days

Physical Therapy Guidelines:
24 visits over 8 weeks

Workers' Comp Costs per Claim (based on 961 claims)					
Quartile	25%	50%	75%	Mean	% no cost
Indemnity	$578	$1,559	$2,951	$3,058	94%
Medical	$179	$336	$609	$1,185	7%
Total	$179	$347	$662	$1,392	7%

RTW Claims Data (Calendar-days away from work by decile)										
10%	20%	30%	40%	**50%**	60%	70%	80%	**90%**	100%	Mean
8	9	9	10	**12**	15	29	44	**82**	365	34.09

Integrated Disability Durations, in days*
Median (mid-point) 7.0 Mean (average) 18.40
Mode (most frequent) 1 Calculated rec. 8

Percent of Cases
(882 cases)

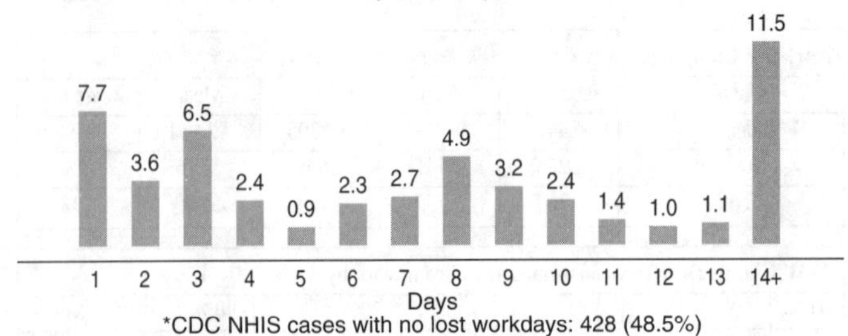

*CDC NHIS cases with no lost workdays: 428 (48.5%)

Impact on Total Absence: Prevalence 0.0246% of total lost workdays; Incidence 0.26 days per 100 workers

Occupational Disability Durations, in days
Median (mid-point) 2 - Benchmark Indemnity Costs $1,500

Percent of Cases
(780 cases)

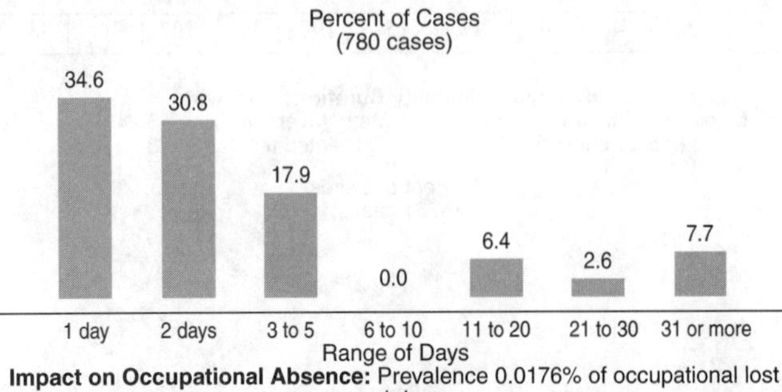

Impact on Occupational Absence: Prevalence 0.0176% of occupational lost workdays

OPEN WOUND OF UPPER LIMB (880-887)

RTW Claims Data (Calendar-days away from work by decile)										
10%	20%	30%	40%	**50%**	60%	70%	80%	**90%**	100%	Mean
9	11	13	15	**19**	25	39	56	**91**	365	34.26

Impact on Total Absence: Prevalence 0.4734% of total lost workdays; Incidence 4.97 days per 100 workers

OPEN WOUND OF UPPER LIMB (880-887)

Occupational Disability Durations, in days
Median (mid-point) 4 - Benchmark Indemnity Costs $3,000

Percent of Cases
(98100 cases)

21.7 15.1 19.2 13.5 10.6 6.6 13.3
1 day 2 days 3 to 5 6 to 10 11 to 20 21 to 30 31 or more
Range of Days

Impact on Occupational Absence: Prevalence 4.4515% of occupational lost workdays; Incidence 0.71 days per 100 workers

880 Open wound of shoulder and upper arm

Return-To-Work Summary Guidelines		
Dataset	**Midrange**	**At-Risk**
Claims data	18 days	91 days
All absences	5 days	54 days

Return-To-Work "Best Practice" Guidelines
Uncomplicated, clerical/modified work: 3 days
Uncomplicated, manual work: 7 days
Complicated, clerical/modified work: 7 days
Complicated, manual work: 14 days
Tendon repair, clerical/modified work: 14 days
Tendon repair, manual work: 91 days

The following fifth-digit subclassification is for use with category 880:
0 shoulder region
1 scapular region
2 axillary region
3 upper arm
9 multiple sites

Workers' Comp Costs per Claim (based on 2,561 claims)					
Quartile	25%	50%	75%	Mean	% no cost
Indemnity	$830	$1,990	$4,830	$3,658	95%
Medical	$189	$357	$578	$652	7%
Total	$189	$357	$578	$839	7%

RTW Claims Data (Calendar-days away from work by decile)										
10%	20%	30%	40%	**50%**	60%	70%	80%	**90%**	100%	Mean
9	12	14	15	**18**	25	39	84	**91**	122	35.47

Integrated Disability Durations, in days*
Median (mid-point) 5.0 Mean (average) 15.75
Mode (most frequent) 1 Calculated rec. 7

Percent of Cases
(1593 cases)

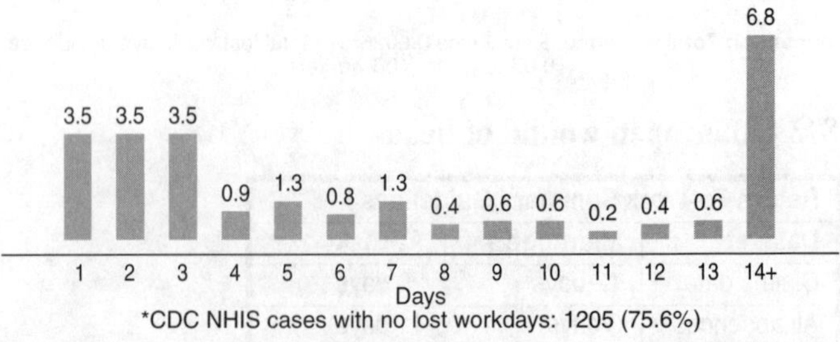

*CDC NHIS cases with no lost workdays: 1205 (75.6%)

Impact on Total Absence: Prevalence 0.0180% of total lost workdays; Incidence 0.19 days per 100 workers

880.1 Complicated

Return-To-Work Summary Guidelines		
Dataset	Midrange	At-Risk
Claims data	21 days	68 days
All absences	13 days	67 days

Return-To-Work "Best Practice" Guidelines
Clerical/modified work: 7 days
Manual work: 14 days

Description: Open wound of shoulder and upper arm with major infection, delayed treatment or healing, tissue loss, and/or foreign body.

Workers' Comp Costs per Claim (based on 124 claims)					
Quartile	25%	50%	75%	Mean	% no cost
Medical	$357	$541	$966	$1,638	2%
Total	$357	$557	$1,502	$1,998	2%

RTW Claims Data (Calendar-days away from work by decile)										
10%	20%	30%	40%	**50%**	60%	70%	80%	**90%**	100%	Mean
10	13	14	14	**21**	28	39	57	**68**	90	32.71

Integrated Disability Durations, in days*
Median (mid-point) 13.0 Mean (average) 20.55
Mode (most frequent) 2 Calculated rec. 12

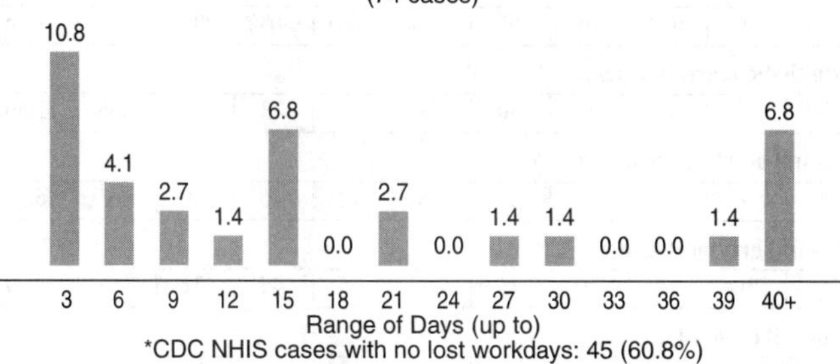

*CDC NHIS cases with no lost workdays: 45 (60.8%)

Impact on Total Absence: Prevalence 0.0017% of total lost workdays; Incidence 0.02 days per 100 workers

881 Open wound of elbow, forearm, and wrist

Return-To-Work Summary Guidelines		
Dataset	Midrange	At-Risk
Claims data	14 days	91 days
All absences	5 days	32 days

Return-To-Work "Best Practice" Guidelines
Minor: 0 days
Major, clerical/modified work: 3 days
Major, manual work: 8 days
Tendon repair, clerical/modified work: 14 days
Tendon repair, manual work: 91 days

Capabilities & Activity Modifications:
Modified work: Repetitive motion activities not more than 4 times/hr; single upper extremity work if injured arm is non-dominant arm; lifting and carrying up to 3 lbs not more than 4 times/hr; pulling and pushing up to 5 lbs 3 times/hr; gripping using light tools (pens, scissors, etc) with 5-minute break at least every 20 min; avoid direct pressure on the elbow area; limit repetitive keying up to 15 keystrokes/min not more than 2 hrs/day; driving car up to 2 hrs/day; no full extension activities; possible immobilization by long arm splint or cast, tennis elbow splint, or wrist splint; no climbing ladders.

881 Open wound of elbow, forearm, and wrist

Regular manual work: Repetitive motion activities not more than 8 times/hr; use of injured dominant arm for moderate work; lifting and carrying up to 20 lbs not more than 15 times/hr; pulling and pushing up to 40 lbs 15 times/hr; gripping using moderate tools (pliers, screwdrivers, etc) full time; driving car or light truck up to 6 hrs/day or heavy truck up to 4 hrs/day; full extension activities up to 12 times/hr with up to 10 lbs of weight; possible immobilization by sling, wrist splint, or tennis elbow splint; climbing ladders up to 50 rungs/hr.

Description: An open cut or laceration to the elbow, forearm, or wrist. Bleeding can be slight or severe, along with pain, and chance of infection.

The following fifth-digit subclassification is for use with category 881:
0 forearm
1 elbow
2 wrist

Procedure Summary (from ODG Treatment): Activity restrictions; Arthroplasty (elbow); Chiropractic; Cold packs; Deep transverse friction massage; Education; Electrical stimulation (E-STIM); Exercise; Fractures of humerus; Fractures of radius; Imaging; Iontophoresis; Laser doppler imaging (LDI); Manipulation; MRI's; Neural tension; Night splints; Nonprescription medications; Patient education; Phonophoresis; Physical therapy; Radiography; Return to work; Stretching; Surgery; Total elbow replacement (TER); Transcutaneous electrical neurostimulation (TENS); Ultrasound, diagnostic; Ultrasound, therapeutic; Work

Workers' Comp Costs per Claim (based on 34,572 claims)					
Quartile	25%	50%	75%	Mean	% no cost
Indemnity	$452	$1,134	$2,394	$2,274	96%
Medical	$242	$399	$599	$603	5%
Total	$252	$399	$609	$692	5%

RTW Claims Data (Calendar-days away from work by decile)										
10%	20%	30%	40%	**50%**	60%	70%	80%	**90%**	100%	Mean
8	9	10	12	**14**	15	23	49	**91**	106	28.39

RTW Post Surgery (Calendar-days away from work by decile)										
10%	20%	30%	40%	**50%**	60%	70%	80%	**90%**	100%	Mean
Repair forearm tendon/muscle										
4	10	15	22	**29**	38	49	81	**138**	365	60.38
Repair forearm tendon/muscle										
2	11	20	33	**49**	62	74	101	**261**	365	81.53

Integrated Disability Durations, in days*
Median (mid-point) 5.0 Mean (average) 13.24
Mode (most frequent) 1 Calculated rec. 6

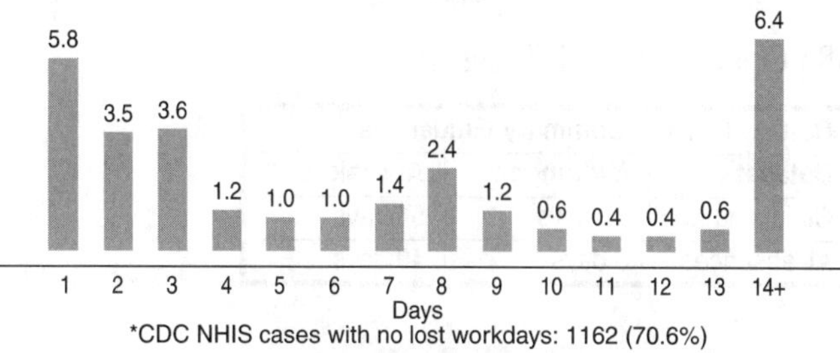

*CDC NHIS cases with no lost workdays: 1162 (70.6%)

Impact on Total Absence: Prevalence 0.0189% of total lost workdays; Incidence 0.20 days per 100 workers

882 Open wound of hand except finger(s) alone

Return-To-Work Summary Guidelines		
Dataset	**Midrange**	**At-Risk**
Claims data	15 days	92 days
All absences	5 days	46 days

Return-To-Work "Best Practice" Guidelines
Minor: 0 days
Major, clerical/modified work: 3 days
Major, manual work: 8 days
Tendon repair, clerical/modified work: 14 days
Tendon repair, manual work: 91 days

Description: An open cut or laceration of the hand (excluding the fingers). Bleeding can be slight or severe, along with pain, and chance of infection.

Workers' Comp Costs per Claim (based on 55,894 claims)					
Quartile	25%	50%	75%	Mean	% no cost
Indemnity	$431	$1,019	$2,237	$1,926	97%
Medical	$231	$378	$578	$536	6%
Total	$231	$378	$578	$605	6%

RTW Claims Data (Calendar-days away from work by decile)

10%	20%	30%	40%	**50%**	60%	70%	80%	**90%**	100%	Mean
8	9	11	13	**15**	17	27	69	**92**	365	33.58

RTW Post Surgery (Calendar-days away from work by decile)

10%	20%	30%	40%	**50%**	60%	70%	80%	**90%**	100%	Mean
Repair hand tendon										
3	4	10	16	**25**	32	48	60	**85**	365	39.27
Repair finger tendon										
2	7	13	19	**30**	38	47	62	**94**	346	47.15

Integrated Disability Durations, in days*
Median (mid-point) 5.0 Mean (average) 15.72
Mode (most frequent) 1 Calculated rec. 7

Percent of Cases
(3759 cases)

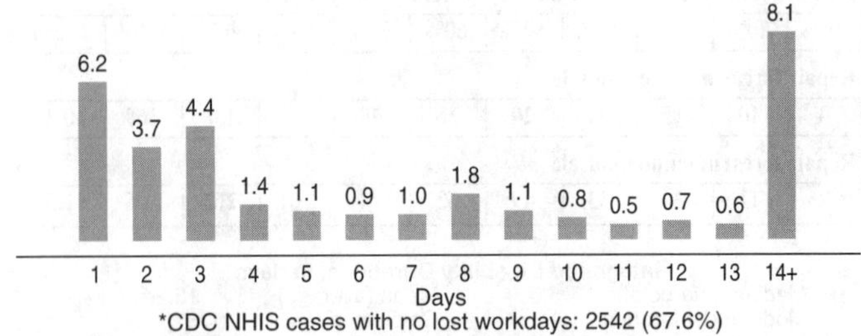

*CDC NHIS cases with no lost workdays: 2542 (67.6%)

Impact on Total Absence: Prevalence 0.0565% of total lost workdays; Incidence 0.59 days per 100 workers

883 Open wound of finger(s)

Return-To-Work Summary Guidelines		
Dataset	**Midrange**	**At-Risk**
Claims data	17 days	51 days
All absences	6 days	40 days

883 Open wound of finger(s) *(cont'd)*

Return-To-Work "Best Practice" Guidelines
Minor, clerical/modified work: 0 days
Minor, heavy manual work: 10 days
Major, clerical/modified work: 3 days
Major, heavy manual work: 21 days
With tendon involvement, clerical/modified work: 14 days
With tendon involvement, heavy manual work: 49 days

Description: An open cut or laceration of a finger, thumb, or nail. Bleeding can be slight or severe, along with pain, and chance of infection.

Includes: fingernail
thumb (nail)

Physical Therapy Guidelines:
9 visits over 8 weeks

Workers' Comp Costs per Claim (based on 199,401 claims)					
Quartile	25%	50%	75%	Mean	% no cost
Indemnity	$441	$1,155	$2,447	$2,133	96%
Medical	$221	$368	$567	$549	6%
Total	$221	$368	$567	$631	6%

RTW Claims Data (Calendar-days away from work by decile)

10%	20%	30%	40%	**50%**	60%	70%	80%	**90%**	100%	Mean
9	11	13	14	**17**	21	25	47	**51**	363	25.21

RTW Post Surgery (Calendar-days away from work by decile)

10%	20%	30%	40%	**50%**	60%	70%	80%	**90%**	100%	Mean
Skin tissue rearrangement										
3	9	15	23	**30**	41	58	73	**100**	365	52.50
Skn splt a-grft fac/nck/hf/g										
4	7	13	19	**24**	38	44	76	**103**	365	46.30
Skin full grft face/genit/hf										
5	10	12	20	**25**	29	36	45	**72**	153	32.09
Removal of foreign body										
1	2	3	3	**7**	11	26	34	**52**	365	23.30
Repair finger/hand tendon										
5	10	16	26	**41**	49	60	82	**109**	362	53.63
Repair finger/hand tendon										
4	12	19	29	**42**	55	72	87	**116**	365	59.52
Repair finger/hand tendon										
4	9	14	20	**34**	45	57	75	**110**	365	49.74
Repair hand tendon										
2	5	9	16	**26**	35	45	59	**79**	365	39.69
Repair finger tendon										
2	5	8	13	**19**	32	42	58	**85**	365	35.95
Release palm/finger tendon										
14	22	23	27	**36**	52	90	145	**248**	365	90.07
Treat finger fracture, each										
3	5	9	18	**23**	28	42	62	**79**	365	35.70
Amputation of finger/thumb										
6	10	24	30	**41**	46	56	88	**197**	365	64.55
Amputation of finger/thumb										
3	11	15	30	**36**	44	48	62	**117**	365	51.13
Repair of digit nerve										
4	6	13	20	**27**	36	51	69	**92**	365	45.00

883 Open wound of finger(s) *(cont'd)*

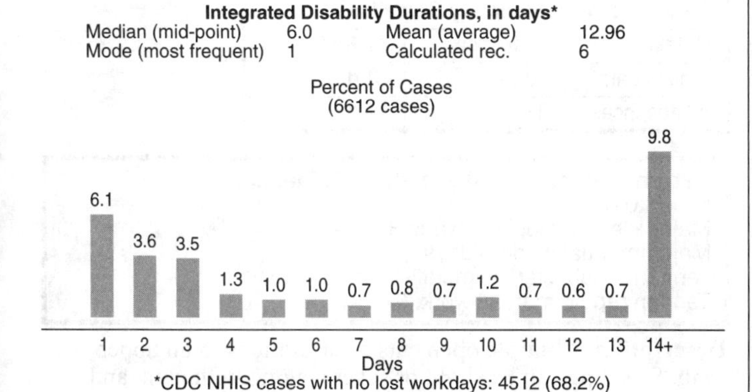

Impact on Total Absence: Prevalence 0.0804% of total lost workdays; Incidence 0.84 days per 100 workers

883.0 Without mention of complication

Return-To-Work Summary Guidelines		
Dataset	**Midrange**	**At-Risk**
Claims data	13 days	45 days
All absences	3 days	16 days

Return-To-Work "Best Practice" Guidelines
Clerical/modified work: 0 days
Manual work: 3 days
Heavy manual work: 10 days

Description: An open cut or laceration of a finger, thumb, or nail. Bleeding can be slight or severe, along with pain.

Workers' Comp Costs per Claim (based on 187,293 claims)					
Quartile	25%	50%	75%	Mean	% no cost
Indemnity	$336	$830	$1,544	$1,296	98%
Medical	$210	$357	$536	$435	6%
Total	$210	$357	$546	$467	6%

RTW Claims Data (Calendar-days away from work by decile)										
10%	20%	30%	40%	**50%**	60%	70%	80%	**90%**	100%	Mean
9	10	11	11	**13**	16	20	29	**45**	73	19.95

RTW Post Surgery (Calendar-days away from work by decile)										
10%	20%	30%	40%	**50%**	60%	70%	80%	**90%**	100%	Mean
Skin tissue rearrangement										
2	5	13	19	**27**	32	44	60	**77**	365	37.94
Skin full grft face/genit/hf										
5	10	12	21	**26**	29	33	41	**66**	145	30.11
Repair finger tendon										
2	4	6	10	**15**	20	34	47	**76**	220	27.70
Repair of digit nerve										
4	6	11	17	**20**	29	40	61	**97**	365	42.16

883.0 Without mention of complication *(cont'd)*

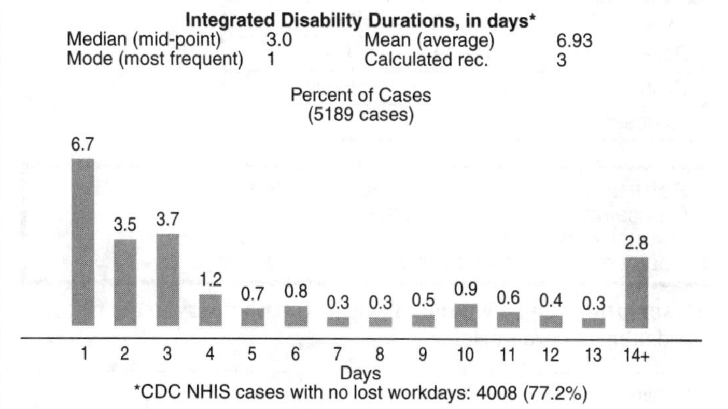

Impact on Total Absence: Prevalence 0.0242% of total lost workdays; Incidence 0.25 days per 100 workers

883.1 Complicated

Return-To-Work Summary Guidelines		
Dataset	**Midrange**	**At-Risk**
Claims data	22 days	60 days
All absences	8 days	46 days

Return-To-Work "Best Practice" Guidelines
Clerical/modified work: 3 days
Manual work: 7 days
Heavy manual work: 21 days

Description: Open wound of finger(s) with major infection, delayed treatment or healing, tissue loss, and/or foreign body.

Workers' Comp Costs per Claim (based on 6,692 claims)					
Quartile	25%	50%	75%	Mean	% no cost
Indemnity	$746	$1,575	$3,045	$2,650	87%
Medical	$273	$494	$977	$1,139	4%
Total	$273	$504	$1,103	$1,489	4%

RTW Claims Data (Calendar-days away from work by decile)										
10%	20%	30%	40%	**50%**	60%	70%	80%	**90%**	100%	Mean
10	14	17	20	**22**	27	35	46	**60**	72	29.10

Integrated Disability Durations, in days*
Median (mid-point) 8.0 Mean (average) 16.64
Mode (most frequent) 3 Calculated rec. 9

Percent of Cases
(215 cases)

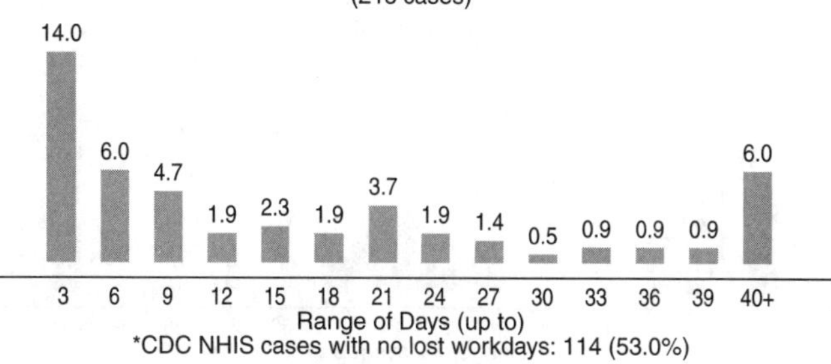

Impact on Total Absence: Prevalence 0.0049% of total lost workdays; Incidence 0.05 days per 100 workers

883.2 With tendon involvement

Return-To-Work Summary Guidelines		
Dataset	**Midrange**	**At-Risk**
Claims data	28 days	58 days
All absences	19 days	54 days

Return-To-Work "Best Practice" Guidelines
Clerical/modified work: 14 days
Manual work: 28 days
Heavy manual work: 49 days

Description: Open wound of finger(s) with injury to the fibrous cords that secure muscles.

Workers' Comp Costs per Claim (based on 5,417 claims)					
Quartile	25%	50%	75%	Mean	% no cost
Indemnity	$1,176	$2,478	$4,977	$3,910	66%
Medical	$851	$2,300	$4,883	$3,593	1%
Total	$945	$2,814	$6,279	$4,951	1%

RTW Claims Data (Calendar-days away from work by decile)

10%	20%	30%	40%	**50%**	60%	70%	80%	**90%**	100%	Mean
13	14	17	24	**28**	35	47	50	**58**	74	32.65

RTW Post Surgery (Calendar-days away from work by decile)

	10%	20%	30%	40%	**50%**	60%	70%	80%	**90%**	100%	Mean
Skin tissue rearrangement	4	13	16	24	**38**	54	73	82	**101**	322	53.10
Repair finger/hand tendon	4	9	14	24	**37**	48	59	81	**109**	362	51.29
Repair finger/hand tendon	4	12	19	30	**42**	54	69	85	**113**	365	57.94
Repair finger/hand tendon	5	10	14	24	**38**	47	59	75	**101**	365	50.59
Repair hand tendon	3	5	10	17	**26**	36	46	59	**78**	365	38.91
Repair finger tendon	2	4	8	13	**19**	32	41	57	**83**	365	35.09
Repair of digit nerve	5	9	15	27	**34**	47	58	72	**96**	365	49.03

Integrated Disability Durations, in days*
Median (mid-point) 19.0 Mean (average) 25.22
Mode (most frequent) 1 Calculated rec. 16

Percent of Cases
(163 cases)

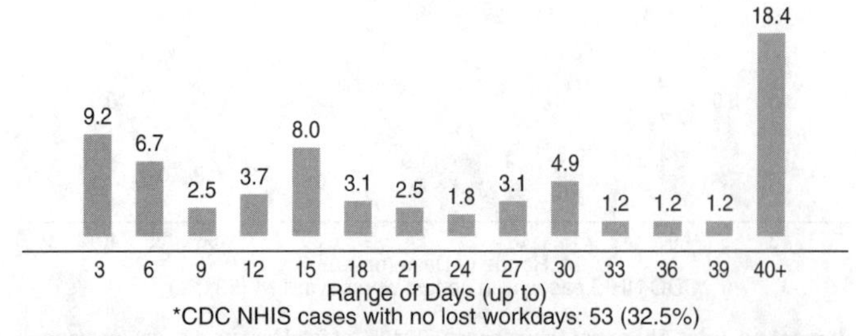

Range of Days (up to)
*CDC NHIS cases with no lost workdays: 53 (32.5%)

Impact on Total Absence: Prevalence 0.0081% of total lost workdays; Incidence 0.09 days per 100 workers

884 Multiple and unspecified open wound of upper limb

Return-To-Work Summary Guidelines		
Dataset	**Midrange**	**At-Risk**
Claims data	10 days	91 days
All absences	8 days	15 days

Return-To-Work "Best Practice" Guidelines
Minor: 0 days
Major, clerical/modified work: 3 days
Major, manual work: 8 days
Tendon repair, clerical/modified work: 14 days
Tendon repair, manual work: 91 days

Description: Multiple open cuts or lacerations to an upper limb. Bleeding can be slight or severe, along with pain, and chance of infection.

Includes: arm NOS
multiple sites of one upper limb
upper limb NOS

RTW Claims Data (Calendar-days away from work by decile)

10%	20%	30%	40%	**50%**	60%	70%	80%	**90%**	100%	Mean
8	8	9	9	**10**	12	14	15	**90**	93	21.61

Integrated Disability Durations, in days*
Median (mid-point) 8.0 Mean (average) 14.27
Mode (most frequent) 8 Calculated rec. 10

Percent of Cases
(146 cases)

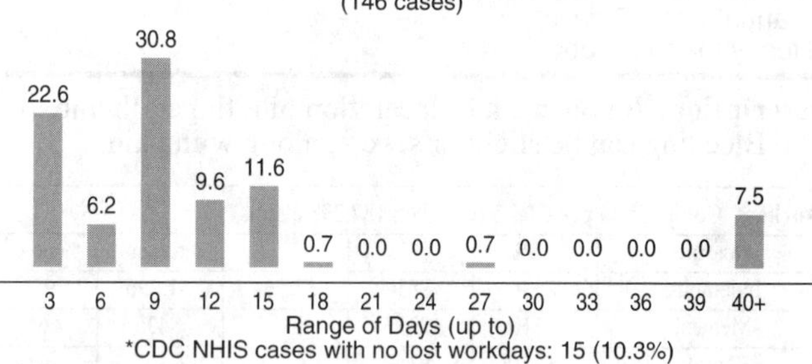

Range of Days (up to)
*CDC NHIS cases with no lost workdays: 15 (10.3%)

Impact on Total Absence: Prevalence 0.0055% of total lost workdays; Incidence 0.06 days per 100 workers

884.0 Without mention of complication

Return-To-Work Summary Guidelines		
Dataset	**Midrange**	**At-Risk**
Claims data	10 days	91 days
All absences	8 days	15 days

Return-To-Work "Best Practice" Guidelines
See 884

Occupational Disability Durations, in days
Median (mid-point) 3 - Benchmark Indemnity Costs $2,250

Percent of Cases
(15750 cases)

23.7 17.8 22.1 14.6 7.3 6.1 8.3
1 day 2 days 3 to 5 6 to 10 11 to 20 21 to 30 31 or more

Range of Days

Impact on Occupational Absence: Prevalence 0.5360% of occupational lost workdays; Incidence 0.09 days per 100 workers

884.1 Complicated

Return-To-Work Summary Guidelines		
Dataset	**Midrange**	**At-Risk**
Claims data	10 days	91 days
All absences	8 days	15 days

Return-To-Work "Best Practice" Guidelines
See 884

Occupational Disability Durations, in days
Median (mid-point) 4 - Benchmark Indemnity Costs $3,000

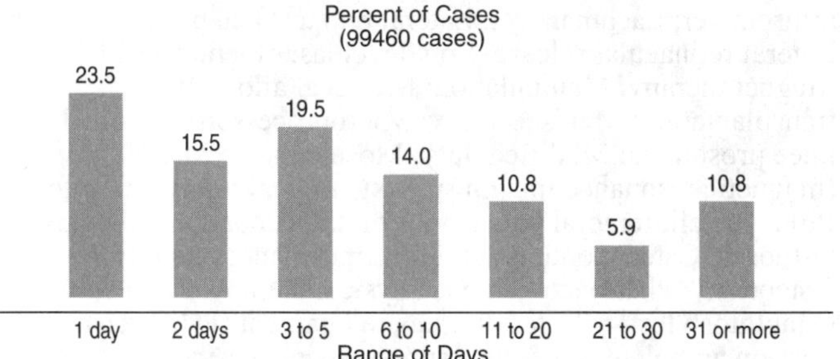

Impact on Occupational Absence: Prevalence 4.5132% of occupational lost workdays; Incidence 0.72 days per 100 workers

885 Traumatic amputation of thumb (complete) (partial)

Return-To-Work Summary Guidelines		
Dataset	**Midrange**	**At-Risk**
Claims data	35 days	113 days
All absences	28 days	112 days

Return-To-Work "Best Practice" Guidelines
Clerical/modified work: 21-28 days
Manual/regular work: 112 days

Description: Surgical removal of all or part of a limb that has been diseased or injured, in this case the thumb.

Includes: thumb(s) (with finger(s) of either hand)

Physical Therapy Guidelines:
Post-replantation surgery: 36 visits over 12 weeks

Workers' Comp Costs per Claim (based on 471 claims)					
Quartile	25%	50%	75%	Mean	% no cost
Indemnity	$4,736	$20,990	$25,200	$20,983	38%
Medical	$1,061	$2,620	$5,943	$5,389	1%
Total	$1,449	$9,450	$28,896	$18,610	1%

886 Traumatic amputation of other finger(s) (complete) (partial)

Return-To-Work Summary Guidelines		
Dataset	**Midrange**	**At-Risk**
Claims data	37 days	112 days
All absences	28 days	112 days

Return-To-Work "Best Practice" Guidelines
Clerical/modified work: 21-28 days
Manual/regular work: 112 days

Description: Surgical removal of all or part of a limb that has been diseased or injured, in this case one or more fingers.

Includes: finger(s) of one or both hands, without mention of thumb(s)

886 Traumatic amputation of other finger(s) (complete) (partial) *(cont'd)*

Physical Therapy Guidelines:
Medical treatment: 18 visits over 6 weeks
Post-replantation surgery: 36 visits over 12 weeks

Workers' Comp Costs per Claim (based on 3,770 claims)					
Quartile	25%	50%	75%	Mean	% no cost
Indemnity	$4,358	$8,600	$15,393	$12,826	30%
Medical	$1,460	$3,003	$5,964	$5,526	0%
Total	$2,636	$8,736	$17,997	$14,498	0%

Occupational Disability Durations, in days
Median (mid-point) 19 - Benchmark Indemnity Costs $14,250

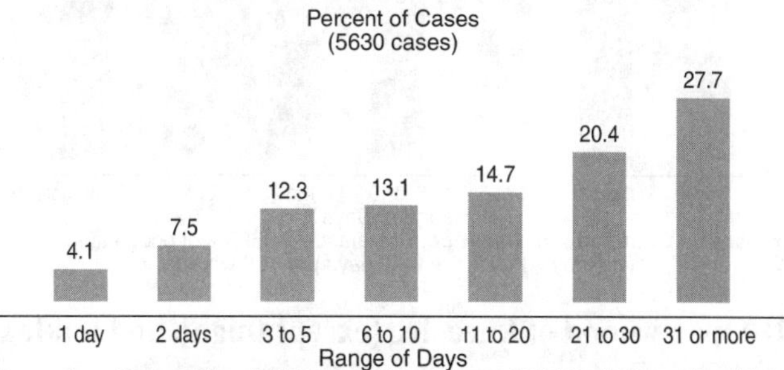

Impact on Occupational Absence: Prevalence 1.2134% of occupational lost workdays; Incidence 0.19 days per 100 workers

887 Traumatic amputation of arm and hand (complete) (partial)

Return-To-Work Summary Guidelines		
Dataset	**Midrange**	**At-Risk**
Claims data	153 days	224 days
All absences	153 days	196 days

Return-To-Work "Best Practice" Guidelines
Clerical/modified work: 56 days
Manual/regular work: 224 days

Description: Surgical removal of all or part of a limb that has been diseased or injured, in this case the arm or hand.

Physical Therapy Guidelines:
Post-replantation surgery: 48 visits over 26 weeks

Workers' Comp Costs per Claim (based on 68 claims)					
Quartile	25%	50%	75%	Mean	% no cost
Indemnity	$112,151	$138,941	$209,895	$171,629	0%
Medical	$60,732	$83,753	$162,761	$133,589	0%
Total	$172,778	$251,727	$371,312	$305,219	0%

Occupational Disability Durations, in days
Median (mid-point) 35 - Benchmark Indemnity Costs $26,250

Percent of Cases
(2360 cases)

2.5 3.8 8.9 11.0 9.3 11.9 52.5

1 day 2 days 3 to 5 6 to 10 11 to 20 21 to 30 31 or more
Range of Days

Impact on Occupational Absence: Prevalence 0.9370% of occupational lost workdays; Incidence 0.15 days per 100 workers

OPEN WOUND OF LOWER LIMB (890-897)

RTW Claims Data (Calendar-days away from work by decile)										
10%	20%	30%	40%	**50%**	60%	70%	80%	**90%**	100%	Mean
9	11	14	15	**19**	25	39	59	**91**	365	34.88

Impact on Total Absence: Prevalence 0.3741% of total lost workdays; Incidence 3.93 days per 100 workers

Occupational Disability Durations, in days
Median (mid-point) 6 - Benchmark Indemnity Costs $4,500

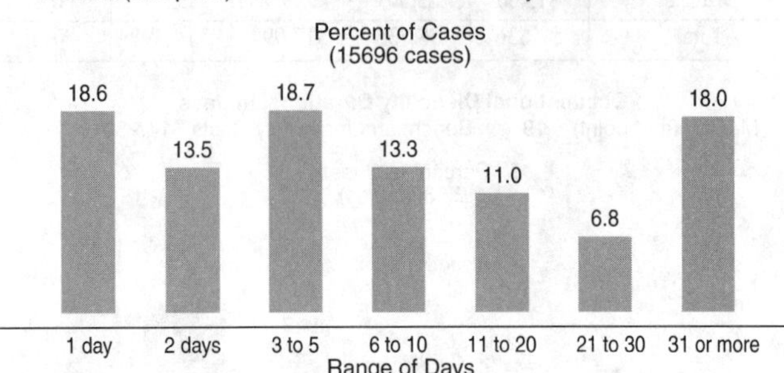

Impact on Occupational Absence: Prevalence 1.0683% of occupational lost workdays; Incidence 0.17 days per 100 workers

891 Open wound of knee, leg [except thigh], and ankle

Return-To-Work Summary Guidelines		
Dataset	**Midrange**	**At-Risk**
Claims data	14 days	92 days
All absences	6 days	54 days

Return-To-Work "Best Practice" Guidelines
Minor: 0 days
Major, clerical/modified work: 3 days
Major, manual work: 8 days
Major, heavy manual work: 14 days
Tendon repair, clerical/modified work: 14 days
Tendon repair, manual work: 91 days

Capabilities & Activity Modifications:
Sedentary/modified work: Standing limited to 5-10 min/hr; walking only on a smooth surface using crutches with limited pressure on the foot; no walking on an irregular surface; no climbing stairs; no climbing ladders or hill climbing requiring frequent knee flexion; no activities requiring balance; no applying strength against bent knee (squatting, kneeling, crouching, stooping, pedaling, etc.); elevate leg half of time; may need immobilization; limited weight bearing.
Manual/standing work: Standing not more than 50 min/hr; walking on a smooth surface up to 1,200 ft/hr carrying up to 25 lbs; walking on an irregular surface up to 900 ft/hr carrying up to 25 lbs; climbing stairs up to 8 flights/hr carrying up to 40 lbs; climbing ladders up to 50 rungs/hr carrying up to 25 lbs; activities requiring balance up to 45 min/hr (if able to work with two hands without assistance for balance); applying strength against bent knee (pedaling, squatting, kneeling, etc.) up to 60 times/hr; may need brace for uneven ground or ladders.
Description: Open cut or laceration to the knee, lower leg, or ankle. Bleeding can be slight or severe, along with pain, and chance of infection.

Includes: leg NOS
multiple sites of leg, except thigh

Excludes:
that of thigh (890.0-890.2)
with multiple sites of lower limb (894.0-894.2)

Procedure Summary (from ODG Treatment): ACI; Activity restrictions; Anterior cruciate ligament (ACL) repair; ACL diagnostic tests; ACL injury rehabilitation; Acupuncture;

891 Open wound of knee, leg [except thigh], and ankle *(cont'd)*

Arthroplasty; Arthroscopy; Autologous cartilage implantation (ACI); Bone-growth stimulators; Braces; Canes; Cetylated fatty acids (CFA) topical cream; Chiropractic; Chondroplasty; Cold/heat packs; Cold lasers; Continuous-flow cryotherapy; Continuous passive motion (CPM); Corticosteroid injections; Crutches; Deep transverse friction massage (DTFM); Diagnostic arthroscopy; Education for knee replacement; Electromyographic biofeedback treatment; Exercise; Glucosamine; Hyaluronic acid injections; Imaging; Immobilization; Injections; Insoles; Interferential current therapy (IFC); Knee brace; Knee joint replacement; KT 1000 arthrometer; Lachman test; Lateral pull test and patellar tilt test; Lateral retinacular release; Low level laser therapy (LLLT); Magnet therapy; Manipulation; Meniscal allograft transplantation; Meniscectomy; Microprocessor-controlled knee prostheses; Modified duty; Mosaicplasty; MRI's (magnetic resonance imaging); Non-surgical intervention for PFPS (patellofemoral pain syndrome); Occupational therapy; Orthoses; Osteochondral autograft transplant system (OATS); Osteotomy; Pharmacotherapy; Physical therapy; Pivot shift test (MacIntosh test) ; Posterior cruciate ligament (PCL) repair; Post-op ambulatory infusion pumps (local anesthetic); Prolotherapy; Prostheses (artificial limb); Pulsed magnetic field therapy (PMFT); Radiography; Return to work; SAMe (S-adenosylmethionine); Single photon emission computed tomography (SPECT); Static progressive stretch (SPS) therapy; Stretching and flexibility; Surgery; SynviscÒ; Therapeutic knee splint; Therapeutic ultrasound; Transcutaneous electrical neurostimulation (TENS); Ultrasound, diagnostic; Ultrasound, therapeutic; Ultrasound fracture healing (bone-growth stimulators); Viscosupplementation; Walkers; Walking aids (canes, crutches, braces, orthoses, & walkers); Work

Workers' Comp Costs per Claim (based on 15,438 claims)					
Quartile	25%	50%	75%	Mean	% no cost
Indemnity	$567	$1,339	$2,615	$2,624	95%
Medical	$231	$410	$651	$684	6%
Total	$231	$410	$672	$825	6%

RTW Claims Data (Calendar-days away from work by decile)										
10%	20%	30%	40%	**50%**	60%	70%	80%	**90%**	100%	Mean
8	9	11	13	**14**	17	30	68	**92**	365	33.20

Integrated Disability Durations, in days*

Median (mid-point)	6.0	Mean (average)	16.10
Mode (most frequent)	1	Calculated rec.	7

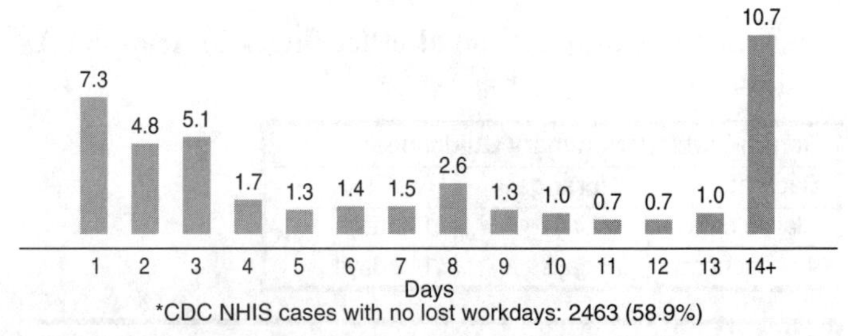

*CDC NHIS cases with no lost workdays: 2463 (58.9%)

Impact on Total Absence: Prevalence 0.0816% of total lost workdays; Incidence 0.86 days per 100 workers

892 Open wound of foot except toe(s) alone

Return-To-Work Summary Guidelines		
Dataset	Midrange	At-Risk
Claims data	21 days	92 days
All absences	4 days	52 days

Return-To-Work "Best Practice" Guidelines
Minor: 0 days
Major, clerical/modified work: 2 days
Major, manual/standing work: 14 days
Major, manual/standing work, also diabetic: 21 days
Tendon repair, clerical/modified work: 14 days
Tendon repair, manual/standing work: 91 days

Description: Open cut or laceration to the foot (excluding toes). Bleeding can be slight or severe, along with pain, and chance of infection.

Includes: heel

Workers' Comp Costs per Claim (based on 7,682 claims)					
Quartile	25%	50%	75%	Mean	% no cost
Indemnity	$326	$866	$1,596	$1,791	97%
Medical	$137	$231	$399	$424	7%
Total	$137	$231	$410	$490	7%

RTW Claims Data (Calendar-days away from work by decile)										
10%	20%	30%	40%	**50%**	60%	70%	80%	**90%**	100%	Mean
12	14	15	18	**21**	23	35	81	**92**	223	37.38

Integrated Disability Durations, in days*

Median (mid-point)	4.0	Mean (average)	16.51
Mode (most frequent)	1	Calculated rec.	6

Percent of Cases
(2764 cases)

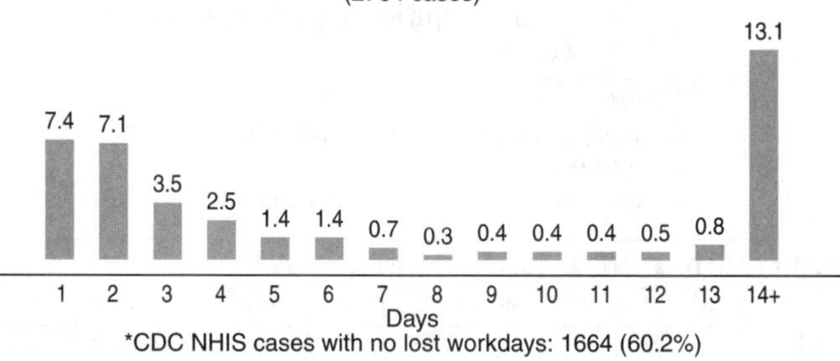

*CDC NHIS cases with no lost workdays: 1664 (60.2%)

Impact on Total Absence: Prevalence 0.0536% of total lost workdays; Incidence 0.56 days per 100 workers

893 Open wound of toe(s)

Return-To-Work Summary Guidelines		
Dataset	Midrange	At-Risk
Claims data	18 days	52 days
All absences	7 days	47 days

Return-To-Work "Best Practice" Guidelines
Minor: 0 days
Major, clerical/modified work: 3 days
Major, manual/standing work: 8 days
Major, manual/standing work, also diabetic: 14 days
With tendon involvement, clerical/modified work: 14 days
With tendon involvement, manual/standing work: 49 days

Description: Open cut or laceration to one or more toes. Bleeding can be slight or severe, along with pain, and chance of infection.

Includes: toenail

893 Open wound of toe(s) *(cont'd)*

Physical Therapy Guidelines:
24 visits over 8 weeks

Workers' Comp Costs per Claim (based on 1,644 claims)					
Quartile	25%	50%	75%	Mean	% no cost
Indemnity	$441	$856	$1,607	$1,219	94%
Medical	$189	$347	$599	$484	7%
Total	$189	$347	$620	$560	7%

RTW Claims Data (Calendar-days away from work by decile)										
10%	20%	30%	40%	**50%**	60%	70%	80%	**90%**	100%	Mean
9	11	13	14	**18**	23	32	47	**52**	70	25.71

Integrated Disability Durations, in days*

Median (mid-point)	7.0	Mean (average)	14.00
Mode (most frequent)	1	Calculated rec.	7

Percent of Cases
(1527 cases)

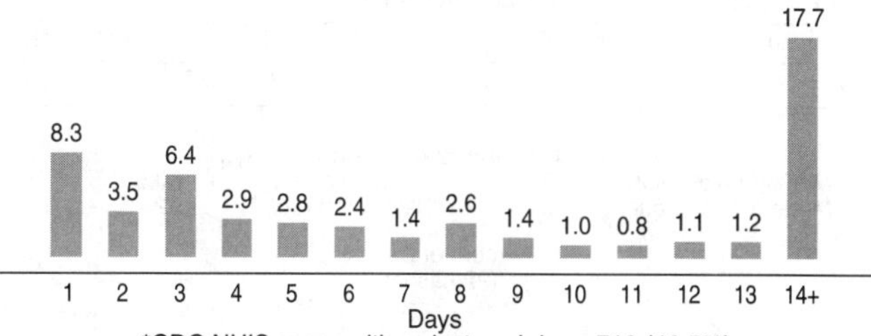

*CDC NHIS cases with no lost workdays: 710 (46.5%)

Impact on Total Absence: Prevalence 0.0338% of total lost workdays; Incidence 0.36 days per 100 workers

895 Traumatic amputation of toe(s) (complete) (partial)

Return-To-Work Summary Guidelines		
Dataset	Midrange	At-Risk
Claims data	54 days	111 days
All absences	50 days	100 days

Return-To-Work "Best Practice" Guidelines
Ordinary amputation & recision (stump disability): 14 days
Replantation surgery, sedentary/modified work: 24 days
Replantation surgery, manual/regular work: 48 days

Description: Surgical removal of all or part of a limb that has been diseased or injured, in this case one or more toes.

Includes: toe(s) of one or both feet

Physical Therapy Guidelines:
Post-replantation surgery: 20 visits over 12 weeks

Workers' Comp Costs per Claim (based on 177 claims)					
Quartile	25%	50%	75%	Mean	% no cost
Indemnity	$14,679	$26,460	$43,649	$35,402	3%
Medical	$6,710	$14,480	$34,241	$26,329	0%
Total	$19,950	$40,919	$80,304	$60,589	0%

896 Traumatic amputation of foot (complete) (partial)

Return-To-Work Summary Guidelines		
Dataset	Midrange	At-Risk
Claims data	67 days	222 days
All absences	51 days	180 days

896 Traumatic amputation of foot (complete) (partial) *(cont'd)*

Return-To-Work "Best Practice" Guidelines
Ordinary amputation & recision (stump disability): 21 days
Replantation surgery, sedentary/modified work: 35 days
Replantation surgery, manual/regular work: 112 days

Description: Surgical removal of all or part of a limb that has been diseased or injured, in this case the foot.
Physical Therapy Guidelines:
Post-replantation surgery: 48 visits over 26 weeks

Workers' Comp Costs per Claim (based on 48 claims)

Quartile	25%	50%	75%	Mean	% no cost
Indemnity	$101,336	$124,971	$168,084	$143,906	0%
Medical	$30,219	$65,720	$104,160	$83,114	0%
Total	$123,659	$193,316	$264,779	$227,019	0%

RTW Claims Data (Calendar-days away from work by decile)

10%	20%	30%	40%	**50%**	60%	70%	80%	**90%**	100%	Mean
14	42	43	63	**67**	115	148	156	**222**	257	99.69

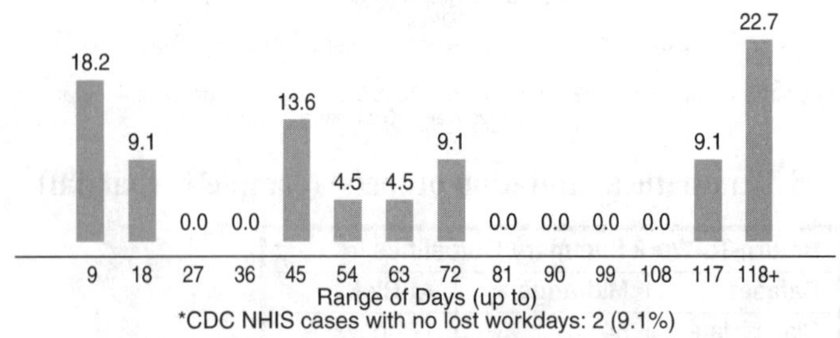

Impact on Total Absence: Prevalence 0.0047% of total lost workdays; Incidence 0.05 days per 100 workers

897 Traumatic amputation of leg(s) (complete) (partial)

Return-To-Work Summary Guidelines

Dataset	Midrange	At-Risk
Claims data	70 days	298 days
All absences	51 days	298 days

Return-To-Work "Best Practice" Guidelines
Ordinary amputation & revision (stump disability): 28 days
Replantation surgery, sedentary/modified work: 42 days
Replantation surgery, manual/regular work: 140 days

Description: Surgical removal of all or part of a limb that has been diseased or injured, in this case the leg.
Physical Therapy Guidelines:
Post-replantation surgery: 48 visits over 26 weeks

Workers' Comp Costs per Claim (based on 101 claims)

Quartile	25%	50%	75%	Mean	% no cost
Indemnity	$122,756	$168,641	$206,598	$172,355	0%
Medical	$102,375	$142,286	$198,996	$189,247	2%
Total	$243,548	$312,039	$375,134	$358,032	0%

RTW Claims Data (Calendar-days away from work by decile)

10%	20%	30%	40%	**50%**	60%	70%	80%	**90%**	100%	Mean
14	42	51	67	**70**	116	180	289	**298**	322	131.07

897 Traumatic amputation of leg(s) (complete) (partial) *(cont'd)*

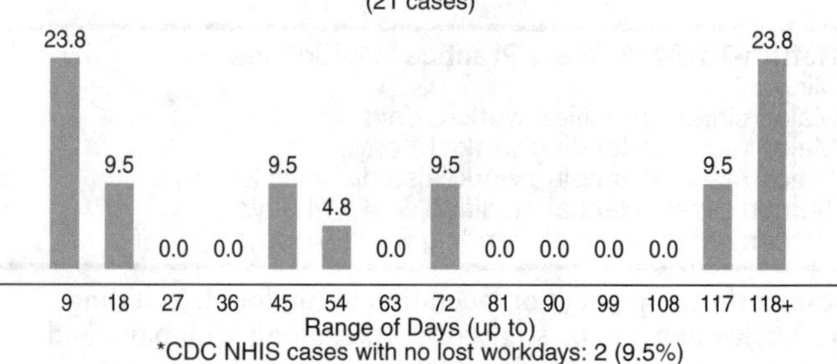

Impact on Total Absence: Prevalence 0.0054% of total lost workdays; Incidence 0.06 days per 100 workers

INJURY TO BLOOD VESSELS (900-904)

Includes: arterial hematoma of blood vessel, secondary to other injuries, e.g., fracture or open wound
avulsion of blood vessel, secondary to other injuries, e.g., fracture or open wound
cut of blood vessel, secondary to other injuries, e.g., fracture or open wound
laceration of blood vessel, secondary to other injuries, e.g., fracture or open wound
rupture of blood vessel, secondary to other injuries, e.g., fracture or open wound
traumatic aneurysm or fistula (arteriovenous) of blood vessel, secondary to other injuries, e.g., fracture or open wound

Excludes:
accidental puncture or laceration during medical procedure (998.2)
intracranial hemorrhage following injury (851.0-854.1)

RTW Claims Data (Calendar-days away from work by decile)

10%	20%	30%	40%	**50%**	60%	70%	80%	**90%**	100%	Mean
13	18	27	35	**36**	38	55	74	**89**	180	44.78

Impact on Total Absence: Prevalence 0.0226% of total lost workdays; Incidence 0.24 days per 100 workers

904 Injury to blood vessels of lower extremity and unspecified sites

Return-To-Work Summary Guidelines

Dataset	Midrange	At-Risk
Claims data	35 days	67 days
All absences	35 days	51 days

Return-To-Work "Best Practice" Guidelines
Mild: 7 days
Severe: 35 days

Workers' Comp Costs per Claim (based on 42 claims)

Quartile	25%	50%	75%	Mean	% no cost
Indemnity	$10,238	$27,253	$41,738	$36,264	27%
Medical	$13,104	$33,626	$142,947	$80,805	0%
Total	$13,104	$53,618	$194,544	$107,179	0%

904 Injury to blood vessels of lower extremity and unspecified sites *(cont'd)*

RTW Claims Data (Calendar-days away from work by decile)										
10%	20%	30%	40%	**50%**	60%	70%	80%	**90%**	100%	Mean
11	17	34	35	**35**	35	36	37	**67**	180	38.61

Integrated Disability Durations, in days*

Median (mid-point)	35.0	Mean (average)	33.65
Mode (most frequent)	35	Calculated rec.	35

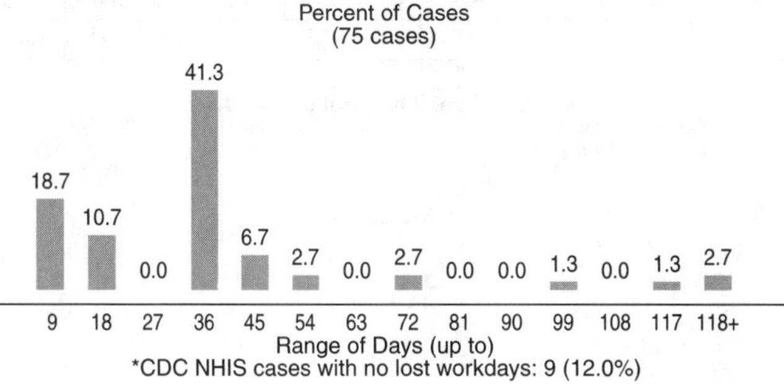

*CDC NHIS cases with no lost workdays: 9 (12.0%)

Impact on Total Absence: Prevalence 0.0065% of total lost workdays; Incidence 0.07 days per 100 workers

LATE EFFECTS OF INJURIES, POISONINGS, TOXIC EFFECTS, AND OTHER EXTERNAL CAUSES (905-909)

Note: These categories are to be used to indicate conditions classifiable to 800-999 as the cause of late effects, which are themselves classified elsewhere. The "late effects" include those specified as such, or as sequelae, which may occur at any time after the acute injury.

RTW Claims Data (Calendar-days away from work by decile)										
10%	20%	30%	40%	**50%**	60%	70%	80%	**90%**	100%	Mean
11	13	14	14	**15**	15	16	23	**54**	365	30.63

Impact on Total Absence: Prevalence 0.2955% of total lost workdays; Incidence 3.10 days per 100 workers

905 Late effects of musculoskeletal and connective tissue injuries

Return-To-Work Summary Guidelines		
Dataset	**Midrange**	**At-Risk**
Claims data	15 days	50 days
All absences	14 days	39 days

Procedure Summary (from ODG Treatment): Activity restrictions; Acupuncture; Anticonvulsants; Antidepressants; Antiepilectics; Bed rest; Behavioral therapy; Botulinum toxin type A; Branched-chain amino acids (BCAAs); Cell transplantation therapy ; Complementary and alternative medicine (CAM); Corticosteroids (for acute traumatic brain injury); Cognitive therapy; Craniectomy; Craniotomy; CT (computed tomography); Decompressive surgery; EEG (Electroencephalography); Field of vision testing; Fluid resuscitation; Glasgow Coma Scale (GCS); Greater occipital nerve block (GONB); Hyperventilation; Hypothermia; Imaging; Interdisciplinary rehabilitation programs; Lumbar puncture; Mannitol; Melatonin; Methylphenidate; Modified Ashworth Scale (MAS); MRI (magnetic resonance imaging); Nutrition; Occupational therapy (OT); Oxygen therapy; PET (positron emission tomography); Physical therapy (PT); QEEG (Quantified Electroencephalography); Relaxation treatment (for

905 Late effects of musculoskeletal and connective tissue injuries *(cont'd)*

migraines); Return to work; Sedation; Skull x-rays; Sleep aids; SPECT (single photon emission computed tomography); Steroids; Triptans; Vision evaluation; Wilsonii injecta; Work

RTW Claims Data (Calendar-days away from work by decile)										
10%	20%	30%	40%	**50%**	60%	70%	80%	**90%**	100%	Mean
11	13	14	14	**15**	16	17	30	**50**	365	30.18

Integrated Disability Durations, in days*

Median (mid-point)	14.0	Mean (average)	22.60
Mode (most frequent)	14	Calculated rec.	16

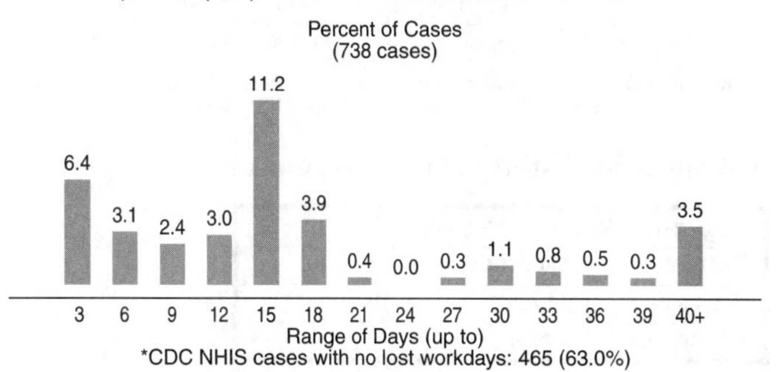

*CDC NHIS cases with no lost workdays: 465 (63.0%)

Impact on Total Absence: Prevalence 0.0182% of total lost workdays; Incidence 0.19 days per 100 workers

Occupational Disability Durations, in days

Median (mid-point) 14 - Benchmark Indemnity Costs $10,500

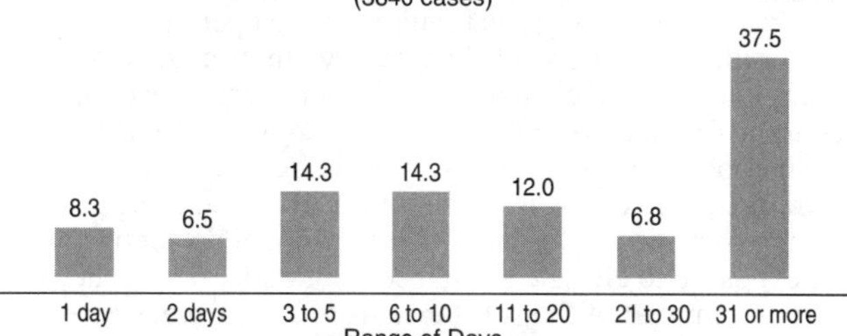

Impact on Occupational Absence: Prevalence 0.6098% of occupational lost workdays; Incidence 0.10 days per 100 workers

SUPERFICIAL INJURY (910-919)

Excludes:

burn (blisters) (940.0-949.5)
contusion (920-924.9)
foreign body:
granuloma (728.82)
inadvertently left in operative wound (998.4)
residual, in soft tissue (729.6)
insect bite, venomous (989.5)
open wound with incidental foreign body (870.0-897.7)

RTW Claims Data (Calendar-days away from work by decile)										
10%	20%	30%	40%	**50%**	60%	70%	80%	**90%**	100%	Mean
9	10	11	12	**13**	16	18	20	**24**	365	15.53

Impact on Total Absence: Prevalence 0.3181% of total lost workdays; Incidence 3.34 days per 100 workers

SUPERFICIAL INJURY (910-919) *(cont'd)*

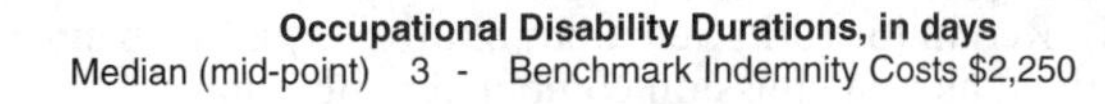

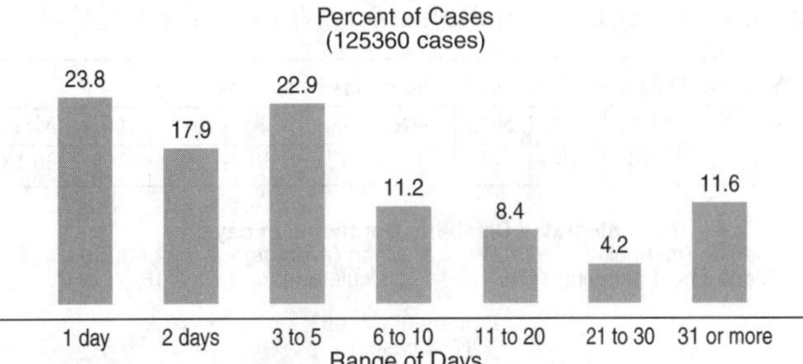

Impact on Occupational Absence: Prevalence 4.2663% of occupational lost workdays; Incidence 0.68 days per 100 workers

918 Superficial injury of eye and adnexa

Return-To-Work Summary Guidelines		
Dataset	**Midrange**	**At-Risk**
Claims data	11 days	16 days
All absences	1 days	7 days

Return-To-Work "Best Practice" Guidelines
Medical treatment not required: 0 days
With eye patch: 1 day

Capabilities & Activity Modifications:
Modified work: In injuries occurring to one eye no binocular vision requirements, e.g., as required in the operation of high speed or mobile equipment (bilateral eye injuries such as welding flash burns, chemical burns, and allergic reactions, need to be off any work until the vision in one eye has returned to a functional level); limited stereopsis/fields of vision requirements; no exposure to significant vibration (e.g., affecting intra-ocular foreign bodies or retinal detachment); limit exposure to allergic substances (e.g., allergic conjuctivitis requiring removal of the substance from the workplace) and provision for hygiene to prevent spread of infection by direct contact or shared articles; wearing protective eyewear to prevent recurrent injury; possible workstation adjustment.
Description: A surface injury/scratch to the eye. Symptoms include light sensitivity, blurry vision, and pain that is made worse by eyelid movement.

Excludes:
burn (940.0-940.9)
foreign body on external eye (930.0-930.9)

Procedure Summary (from ODG Treatment): Activity restrictions; Antibiotic therapy (for treatment of acute bacterial conjunctivitis); Bandage contact lens; Calf blood extract eye gel (vs. vitamin A and dexpanthenol); Computed tomography (CT); Contact lens after penetrating keratoplasty (PK); Diclofenac (ophthalmic solution); Emergency eye wash products; Erythromycin and sulfa compounds (for corneal abrasions involving contact lens use); Fibrin glue (versus N-butyl-2-cyanoacrylate in corneal perforations); Flurbiprofen (eye drops); Indomethacin (0.1%); Indomethacin/gentamicin eyedrops; Ophthalmic vasoconstrictor (drug products); Patching; Prophylactic intravitreal antibiotics; Protection methods (for eyes under general anaesthesia); Surgery for orbital floor fractures; Surgical treatment for hyphema; Surgery for optic neuropathy; Tetanus toxid; The management of optic neuropathy; Topical aminocaproic acid ; Topical corticosteroids (for traumatic microhyphema); Topical nonsteroidal anti-inflammatory drops; Topical NSAIDs (especially Keterolac); Work

918 Superficial injury of eye and adnexa *(cont'd)*

Workers' Comp Costs per Claim (based on 42,425 claims)					
Quartile	25%	50%	75%	Mean	% no cost
Indemnity	$158	$441	$1,082	$1,258	99%
Medical	$147	$242	$368	$285	6%
Total	$147	$242	$368	$300	6%

RTW Claims Data (Calendar-days away from work by decile)										
10%	20%	30%	40%	**50%**	60%	70%	80%	**90%**	100%	Mean
8	9	9	10	**11**	12	13	14	**16**	91	13.28

Integrated Disability Durations, in days*
Median (mid-point) 1.0 Mean (average) 3.04
Mode (most frequent) 1 Calculated rec. 2

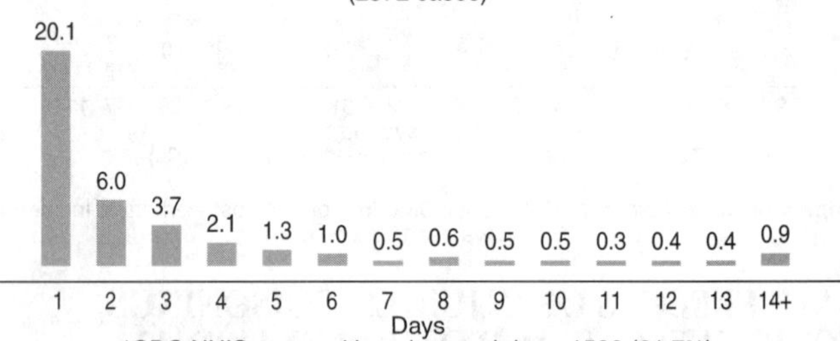

*CDC NHIS cases with no lost workdays: 1586 (61.7%)

Impact on Total Absence: Prevalence 0.0088% of total lost workdays; Incidence 0.09 days per 100 workers

918.1 Cornea

Return-To-Work Summary Guidelines		
Dataset	**Midrange**	**At-Risk**
Claims data	11 days	17 days
All absences	1 days	4 days

Return-To-Work "Best Practice" Guidelines
Medical treatment not required: 0 days
With eye patch, modified work: 0 days
With eye patch, regular work: 1 day

Capabilities & Activity Modifications:
Modified work: In injuries occurring to one eye no binocular vision requirements, e.g., as required in the operation of high speed or mobile equipment (bilateral eye injuries such as welding flash burns, chemical burns, and allergic reactions, need to be off any work until the vision in one eye has returned to a functional level); limited stereopsis/fields of vision requirements; no exposure to significant vibration (e.g., affecting intra-ocular foreign bodies or retinal detachment); limit exposure to allergic substances (e.g., allergic conjuctivitis requiring removal of the substance from the workplace) and provision for hygiene to prevent spread of infection by direct contact or shared articles; wearing protective eyewear to prevent recurrent injury; possible workstation adjustment.
Description: Damage to the top layer of cells on the front of the eye caused by injury or debris/dust that scratch the eye. Symptoms include light sensitivity, blurry vision, and pain that is made worse by eyelid movement.

Corneal abrasion
Superficial laceration

Excludes:
corneal injury due to contact lens (371.82)

Procedure Summary (from ODG Treatment): Activity restrictions; Antibiotic therapy (for treatment of acute bacterial conjunctivitis); Bandage contact lens; Calf blood extract eye gel

918.1 Cornea *(cont'd)*

(vs. vitamin A and dexpanthenol); Computed tomography (CT); Contact lens after penetrating keratoplasty (PK); Diclofenac (ophthalmic solution); Emergency eye wash products; Erythromycin and sulfa compounds (for corneal abrasions involving contact lens use); Fibrin glue (versus N-butyl-2-cyanoacrylate in corneal perforations); Flurbiprofen (eye drops); Indomethacin (0.1%); Indomethacin/gentamicin eyedrops; Ophthalmic vasoconstrictor (drug products); Patching; Prophylactic intravitreal antibiotics; Protection methods (for eyes under general anaesthesia); Surgery for orbital floor fractures; Surgical treatment for hyphema; Surgery for optic neuropathy; Tetanus toxid; The management of optic neuropathy; Topical aminocaproic acid ; Topical corticosteroids (for traumatic microhyphema); Topical nonsteroidal anti-inflammatory drops; Topical NSAIDs (especially Keterolac); Work

Workers' Comp Costs per Claim (based on 38,032 claims)

Quartile	25%	50%	75%	Mean	% no cost
Indemnity	$147	$441	$1,124	$1,234	99%
Medical	$158	$242	$378	$286	6%
Total	$158	$242	$378	$300	6%

RTW Claims Data (Calendar-days away from work by decile)

10%	20%	30%	40%	**50%**	60%	70%	80%	**90%**	100%	Mean
8	9	9	10	**11**	12	13	14	**17**	20	11.90

Integrated Disability Durations, in days*

Median (mid-point)	1.0	Mean (average)	2.24
Mode (most frequent)	1	Calculated rec.	1

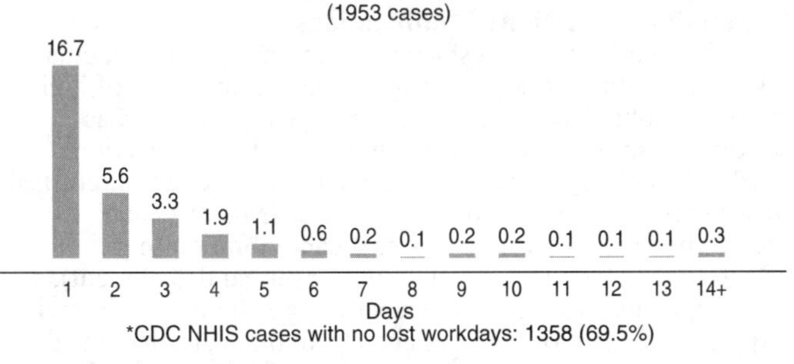

*CDC NHIS cases with no lost workdays: 1358 (69.5%)

Impact on Total Absence: Prevalence 0.0039% of total lost workdays; Incidence 0.04 days per 100 workers

919 Superficial injury of other, multiple, and unspecified sites

Return-To-Work Summary Guidelines

Dataset	Midrange	At-Risk
Claims data	10 days	25 days
All absences	5 days	13 days

Return-To-Work "Best Practice" Guidelines
See 919.0

Excludes:
multiple sites classifiable to the same three-digit category (910.0-918.9)

RTW Claims Data (Calendar-days away from work by decile)

10%	20%	30%	40%	**50%**	60%	70%	80%	**90%**	100%	Mean
8	8	9	10	**10**	13	14	16	**25**	50	14.23

919 Superficial injury of other, multiple, and unspecified sites *(cont'd)*

Integrated Disability Durations, in days*

Median (mid-point)	5.0	Mean (average)	6.65
Mode (most frequent)	1	Calculated rec.	4

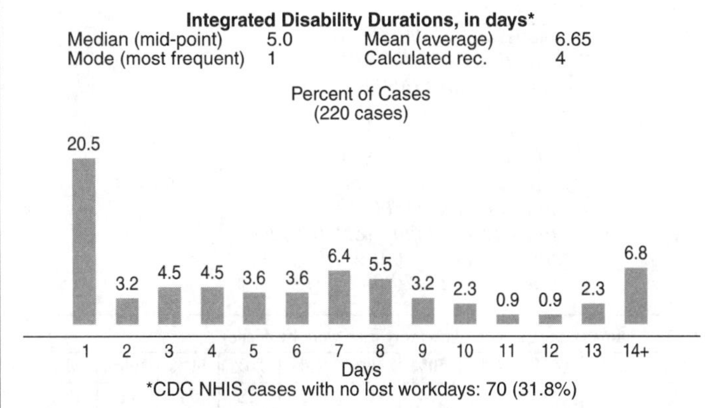

*CDC NHIS cases with no lost workdays: 70 (31.8%)

Impact on Total Absence: Prevalence 0.0029% of total lost workdays; Incidence 0.03 days per 100 workers

Occupational Disability Durations, in days
Median (mid-point) 5 - Benchmark Indemnity Costs $3,750

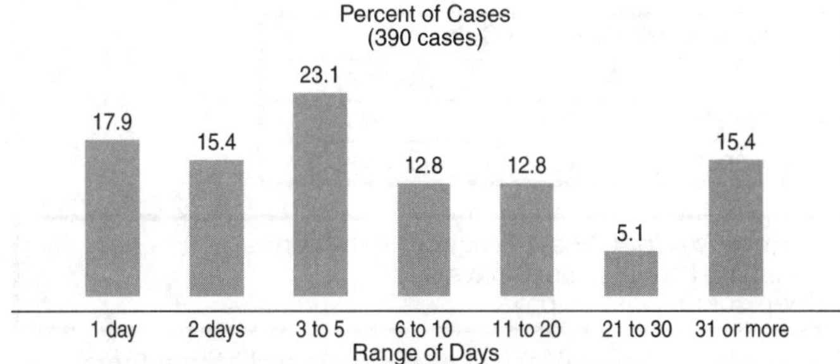

Impact on Occupational Absence: Prevalence 0.0221% of occupational lost workdays

919.0 Abrasion or friction burn without mention of infection

Return-To-Work Summary Guidelines

Dataset	Midrange	At-Risk
Claims data	10 days	25 days
All absences	5 days	13 days

Return-To-Work "Best Practice" Guidelines
Without surgery: 0-1 days
With surgery: 7 days

Description: Surface damage to the skin without infection. Bleeding is often of the oozing type. Although they are usually not serious, reconstructive surgery may be needed if deeper tissue layers are damaged.

CONTUSION WITH INTACT SKIN SURFACE (920-924)

Includes: bruise without fracture or open wound
hematoma without fracture or open wound

CONTUSION WITH INTACT SKIN SURFACE (920-924) *(cont'd)*

Excludes:
concussion (850.0-850.9)
hemarthrosis (840.0-848.9)
internal organs (860.0-869.1)
that incidental to:
crushing injury (925-929.9)
dislocation (830.0-839.9)
fracture (800.0-829.1)
internal injury (860.0-869.1)
intracranial injury (850.0-854.1)
nerve injury (950.0-957.9)
open wound (870.0-897.7)

RTW Claims Data (Calendar-days away from work by decile)										
10%	20%	30%	40%	**50%**	60%	70%	80%	**90%**	100%	Mean
9	10	11	13	**14**	16	19	22	**31**	365	18.72

Impact on Total Absence: Prevalence 0.5910% of total lost workdays; Incidence 6.21 days per 100 workers

920 Contusion of face, scalp, and neck except eye(s)

Return-To-Work Summary Guidelines		
Dataset	**Midrange**	**At-Risk**
Claims data	11 days	22 days
All absences	3 days	13 days

Return-To-Work "Best Practice" Guidelines
Superficial contusions: 0 days
Deep contusions: 10 days

Description: Bruise of the face, scalp, or neck. Symptoms include localized tenderness, pain, swelling, and blue/purple color where the bruise forms.

Cheek
Ear (auricle)
Gum
Lip
Mandibular joint area
Nose
Throat

Workers' Comp Costs per Claim (based on 25,278 claims)					
Quartile	25%	50%	75%	Mean	% no cost
Indemnity	$431	$872	$1,397	$1,287	98%
Medical	$158	$315	$693	$549	11%
Total	$158	$315	$725	$585	11%

RTW Claims Data (Calendar-days away from work by decile)										
10%	20%	30%	40%	**50%**	60%	70%	80%	**90%**	100%	Mean
9	10	10	10	**11**	12	13	14	**22**	289	14.57

920 Contusion of face, scalp, and neck except eye(s) *(cont'd)*

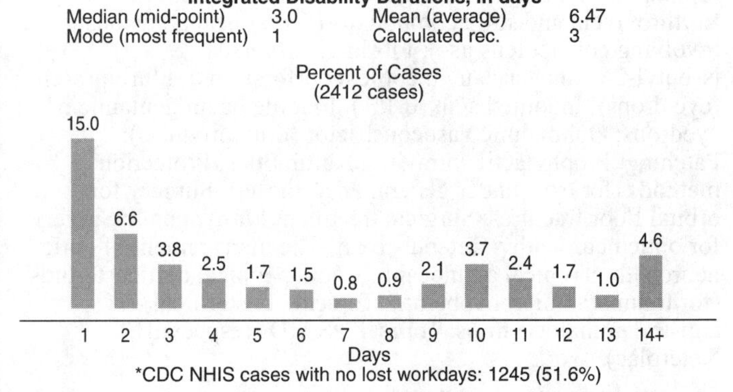

Impact on Total Absence: Prevalence 0.0223% of total lost workdays; Incidence 0.23 days per 100 workers

921 Contusion of eye and adnexa

Return-To-Work Summary Guidelines		
Dataset	**Midrange**	**At-Risk**
Claims data	11 days	15 days
All absences	3 days	12 days

Return-To-Work "Best Practice" Guidelines
Superficial contusions: 0 days
Injury to eyeball, without associated intraocular injury: 10 days

Capabilities & Activity Modifications:
Modified work: In injuries occurring to one eye no binocular vision requirements, e.g., as required in the operation of high speed or mobile equipment (bilateral eye injuries such as welding flash burns, chemical burns, and allergic reactions, need to be off any work until the vision in one eye has returned to a functional level); limited stereopsis/fields of vision requirements; no exposure to significant vibration (e.g., affecting intra-ocular foreign bodies or retinal detachment); limit exposure to allergic substances (e.g., allergic conjuctivitis requiring removal of the substance from the workplace) and provision for hygiene to prevent spread of infection by direct contact or shared articles; wearing protective eyewear to prevent recurrent injury; possible workstation adjustment.
Description: Bruise of the eye or area around the eye. Symptoms include localized tenderness, pain, swelling, and blue/purple color where the bruise forms. Eye may be swollen shut.
Procedure Summary (from ODG Treatment): Activity restrictions; Antibiotic therapy (for treatment of acute bacterial conjunctivitis); Bandage contact lens; Calf blood extract eye gel (vs. vitamin A and dexpanthenol); Computed tomography (CT); Contact lens after penetrating keratoplasty (PK); Diclofenac (ophthalmic solution); Emergency eye wash products; Erythromycin and sulfa compounds (for corneal abrasions involving contact lens use); Fibrin glue (versus N-butyl-2-cyanoacrylate in corneal perforations); Flurbiprofen (eye drops); Indomethacin (0.1%); Indomethacin/gentamicin eyedrops; Ophthalmic vasoconstrictor (drug products); Patching; Prophylactic intravitreal antibiotics; Protection methods (for eyes under general anaesthesia); Surgery for orbital floor fractures; Surgical treatment for hyphema; Surgery for optic neuropathy; Tetanus toxid; The management of optic neuropathy; Topical aminocaproic acid ; Topical corticosteroids

921 Contusion of eye and adnexa *(cont'd)*

(for traumatic microhyphema); Topical nonsteroidal anti-inflammatory drops; Topical NSAIDs (especially Keterolac); Work

Workers' Comp Costs per Claim (based on 4,435 claims)					
Quartile	25%	50%	75%	Mean	% no cost
Indemnity	$420	$840	$1,586	$1,865	97%
Medical	$147	$252	$431	$387	9%
Total	$147	$252	$441	$452	9%

RTW Claims Data (Calendar-days away from work by decile)										
10%	20%	30%	40%	**50%**	60%	70%	80%	**90%**	100%	Mean
9	10	10	10	**11**	11	12	13	**15**	69	12.12

Integrated Disability Durations, in days*

Median (mid-point) 3.0 Mean (average) 5.36
Mode (most frequent) 1 Calculated rec. 3

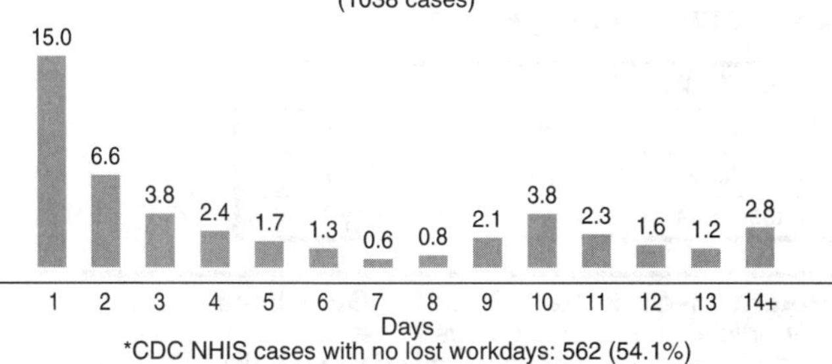

*CDC NHIS cases with no lost workdays: 562 (54.1%)

Impact on Total Absence: Prevalence 0.0075% of total lost workdays; Incidence 0.08 days per 100 workers

922 Contusion of trunk

Return-To-Work Summary Guidelines		
Dataset	**Midrange**	**At-Risk**
Claims data	12 days	28 days
All absences	5 days	16 days

Return-To-Work "Best Practice" Guidelines
Superficial contusions: 0 days
Deep contusions: 10 days

Capabilities & Activity Modifications:
Clerical/modified work: Lifting with knees (with a straight back, no stooping) not more than 5 lbs up to 3 times/hr; squatting up to 4 times/hr; standing or walking with a 5-minute break at least every 20 minutes; sitting with a 5-minute break every 30 minutes; no extremes of extension or flexion; no extremes of twisting; no climbing ladders; driving car only up to 2 hrs/day.
Manual work: Lifting with knees (with a straight back) not more than 25 lbs up to 15 times/hr; squatting up to 16 times/hr; standing or walking with a 10-minute break at least every 1-2 hours; sitting with a 10-minute break every 1-2 hours; extremes of flexion or extension allowed up to 12 times/hr; extremes of twisting allowed up to 16 times/hr; climbing ladders allowed up to 25 rungs 6 times/hr; driving car or light truck up to a full work day; driving heavy truck up to 4 hrs/day.
Description: Bruise of the breast, back, abdominal wall, or chest wall. Symptoms include localized tenderness, swelling, pain, and blue/purple color where the bruise forms.
Procedure Summary (from ODG Treatment): Activity restrictions; Acupuncture; Adhesiolysis; Aerobic exercise; Age adjustment factors; Annuloplasty (IDET); Antidepressants; Anti-inflammatory medications; Aquatic therapy; Arthrodesis;

922 Contusion of trunk *(cont'd)*

Arthroplasty; Artificial disk; Back brace; Back schools; Bed rest; Behavioral treatment; Biofeedback; Bone-growth stimulators (BGS); Bone scan; Botulinum toxin (Botox); Chemonucleolysis (chymopapain); Chiropractic; Coblation nucleoplasty; Cognitive intervention; Colchicine; Cold/heat packs; Computerized range of motion (ROM); Corsets; CT & CT Myelography (computed tomography); Cutaneous laser treatment; Decompression; Diagnostic imaging; Diathermy; Differential Diagnosis; Disc prosthesis; Discectomy/laminectomy; Discography; DRX (traction); Dynamic neutralization system (Dynesys); Education; Electrical stimulators (E-stim); Electromagnetic pulsed therapy; EMG's (electromyography); Epidural steroid injections (ESI's); Ergonomics interventions; Etanercept (Enbrel); Exercise; Facet-joint injections; Facet rhizotomy (radio frequency medial branch neurotomy); Feldenkrais; Flexibility; Fluoroscopy (for ESI's); Foraminotomy; Fusion (spinal); Fusion, endoscopic; Hardware; Heat therapy; Hemilaminectomy; H-wave stimulation (devices); IDD therapy (intervertebral disc decompression); IDET (intradiscal electrothermal anuloplasty); Imaging; Implantable pumps for narcotics; Implantable spinal cord stimulators; Implants; Infliximab (Remicade); Injections; Interferential therapy; Intradiscal electrothermal therapy (IDET); Intradiscal steroid injection; Intrathecal drug administration system; Kyphoplasty; Laminectomy/laminotomy; Ligamentous injections; Lordex (traction); Low level laser therapy (LLLT); Lumbar supports; Magnet therapy; Manipulation; Manipulation under anesthesia (MUA) ; Massage; Mattress firmness; McKenzie method; Medications; MedX lumbar extension machine; Microcurrent electrical stimulation (MENS devices); Microdiscectomy; Modified duty; MR neurography; MRI's (magnetic resonance imaging); Muscle relaxants ; Myelography; Neuromodulation devices; Neuromuscular electrical stimulators (NMES); Neuroplasty; Neuroreflexotherapy; Nonprescription medications; Narcotics; Nucleoplasty; Occupational therapy (OT); Opioids; Oral corticosteroids; Percutaneous diskectomy (PCD); Percutaneous electrical nerve stimulation (PENS) ; Percutaneous endoscopic laser discectomy (PELD); Percutaneous epidural neuroplasty; Percutaneous intradiscal radiofrequency (thermocoagulation); Percutaneous neuromodulation therapy (PNT); Percutaneous vertebroplasty (PV); Physical therapy (PT); Pilates; Powered traction devices; Prolotherapy, also known as sclerotherapy; Psychological screening; Racz neurolysis; Radiofrequency neurotomy; Radiography (x-rays); Range of motion (ROM); Return to work; Sclerotherapy; Shoe insoles/shoe lifts; SPECT (single photon emission computed tomography); Spinal cord stimulation (SCS); Standing MRI; Stimulators, electrical; Stretching; Supports & braces; Surface electromyography (SEMG); Surgery; Sympathetic therapy; Thermography (infrared stress thermography); Traction; Transcutaneous electrical neurostimulation (TENS) ; Trigger point injections; Tumor necrosis factor (TNF) modifiers; Ultrasound, diagnostic (imaging); Ultrasound, therapeutic; Vertebral axial decompression (VAX-D); Vertebroplasty; Videofluoroscopy (for range of motion); Work conditioning, work hardening; Work; X-rays; Yoga

Workers' Comp Costs per Claim (based on 37,913 claims)					
Quartile	25%	50%	75%	Mean	% no cost
Indemnity	$746	$1,491	$2,783	$2,684	92%
Medical	$221	$389	$725	$795	9%
Total	$221	$399	$788	$1,035	8%

RTW Claims Data (Calendar-days away from work by decile)										
10%	20%	30%	40%	**50%**	60%	70%	80%	**90%**	100%	Mean
9	10	10	11	**12**	13	14	18	**28**	365	16.24

922 Contusion of trunk *(cont'd)*

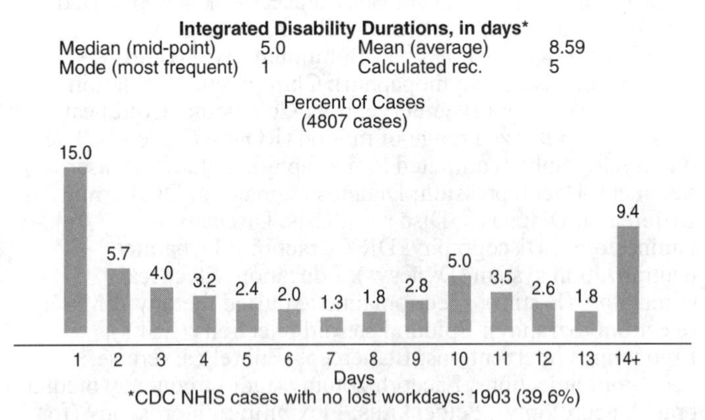

Impact on Total Absence: Prevalence 0.0737% of total lost workdays; Incidence 0.77 days per 100 workers

Occupational Disability Durations, in days
Median (mid-point) 7 - Benchmark Indemnity Costs $5,250

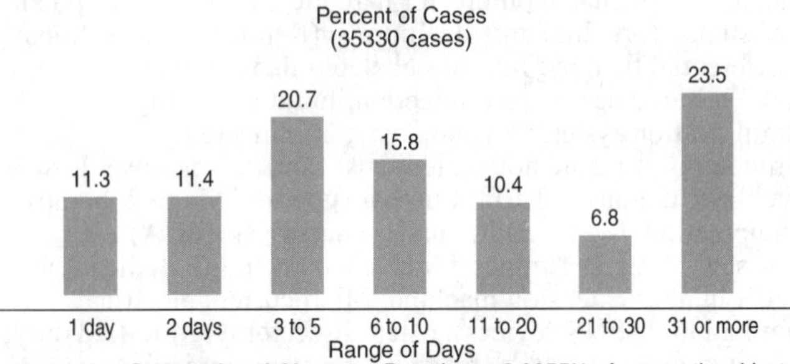

Impact on Occupational Absence: Prevalence 2.8055% of occupational lost workdays; Incidence 0.45 days per 100 workers

922.4 Genital organs

Return-To-Work Summary Guidelines		
Dataset	**Midrange**	**At-Risk**
Claims data	22 days	30 days
All absences	4 days	27 days

Return-To-Work "Best Practice" Guidelines
Superficial contusions: 0 days
Deep contusions: 7 days
Testicle, surgical repair: 28 days

Description: Bruise of the genitals. Symptoms include localized tenderness, pain, swelling, and blue/purple color where the bruise forms.

Labium (majus) (minus)
Penis
Perineum
Scrotum
Testis
Vagina
Vulva

Workers' Comp Costs per Claim (based on 690 claims)					
Quartile	25%	50%	75%	Mean	% no cost
Indemnity	$315	$872	$1,890	$1,593	92%
Medical	$158	$284	$536	$508	5%
Total	$158	$284	$536	$642	5%

RTW Claims Data (Calendar-days away from work by decile)										
10%	20%	30%	40%	**50%**	60%	70%	80%	**90%**	100%	Mean
9	11	12	13	**22**	27	28	29	**30**	40	20.36

922.4 Genital organs *(cont'd)*

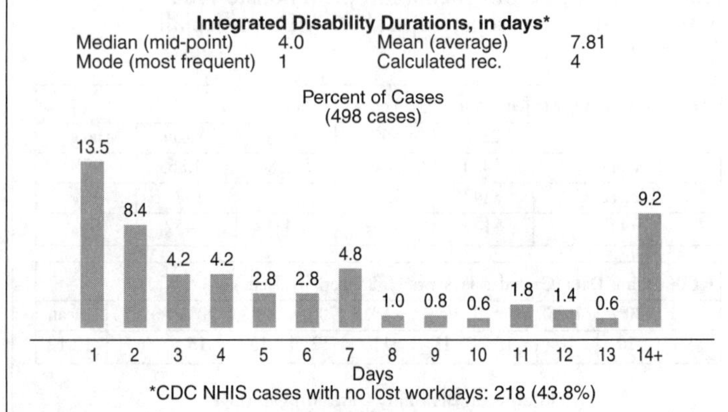

Impact on Total Absence: Prevalence 0.0064% of total lost workdays; Incidence 0.07 days per 100 workers

923 Contusion of upper limb

Return-To-Work Summary Guidelines		
Dataset	**Midrange**	**At-Risk**
Claims data	21 days	44 days
All absences	5 days	24 days

Return-To-Work "Best Practice" Guidelines
Superficial contusions: 0 days
Deep contusions, clerical/modified work: 5 days
Deep contusions, manual work: 21 days

Capabilities & Activity Modifications:
Modified work: Repetitive motion activities not more than 4 times/hr; single upper extremity work if injured arm is non-dominant arm; lifting and carrying up to 3 lbs not more than 4 times/hr; pulling and pushing up to 5 lbs 3 times/hr; gripping using light tools (pens, scissors, etc) with 5-minute break at least every 20 min; avoid direct pressure on the elbow area; limit repetitive keying up to 15 keystrokes/min not more than 2 hrs/day; driving car up to 2 hrs/day; no full extension activities; possible immobilization by long arm splint or cast, tennis elbow splint, or wrist splint; no climbing ladders.
Regular manual work: Repetitive motion activities not more than 8 times/hr; use of injured dominant arm for moderate work; lifting and carrying up to 20 lbs not more than 15 times/hr; pulling and pushing up to 40 lbs 15 times/hr; gripping using moderate tools (pliers, screwdrivers, etc) full time; driving car or light truck up to 6 hrs/day or heavy truck up to 4 hrs/day; full extension activities up to 12 times/hr with up to 10 lbs of weight; possible immobilization by sling, wrist splint, or tennis elbow splint; climbing ladders up to 50 rungs/hr.
Description: Bruise of an upper limb. Symptoms include localized tenderness, pain, swelling, and blue/purple color where the bruise forms.
Procedure Summary (from ODG Treatment): Activity restrictions; Arthroplasty (elbow); Chiropractic; Cold packs; Deep transverse friction massage; Education; Electrical stimulation (E-STIM); Exercise; Fractures of humerus; Fractures of radius; Imaging; Iontophoresis; Laser doppler imaging (LDI); Manipulation; MRI's; Neural tension; Night splints; Nonprescription medications; Patient education; Phonophoresis; Physical therapy; Radiography; Return to work; Stretching; Surgery; Total elbow replacement (TER); Transcutaneous electrical neurostimulation (TENS); Ultrasound, diagnostic; Ultrasound, therapeutic; Work

923 Contusion of upper limb *(cont'd)*

Workers' Comp Costs per Claim (based on 114,181 claims)					
Quartile	25%	50%	75%	Mean	% no cost
Indemnity	$536	$1,239	$2,205	$1,960	95%
Medical	$210	$315	$494	$467	7%
Total	$210	$315	$504	$569	7%

RTW Claims Data (Calendar-days away from work by decile)										
10%	20%	30%	40%	**50%**	60%	70%	80%	**90%**	100%	Mean
10	13	17	20	**21**	22	23	25	**44**	365	25.58

Integrated Disability Durations, in days*

Median (mid-point) 5.0 Mean (average) 10.96
Mode (most frequent) 1 Calculated rec. 5

Percent of Cases
(5758 cases)

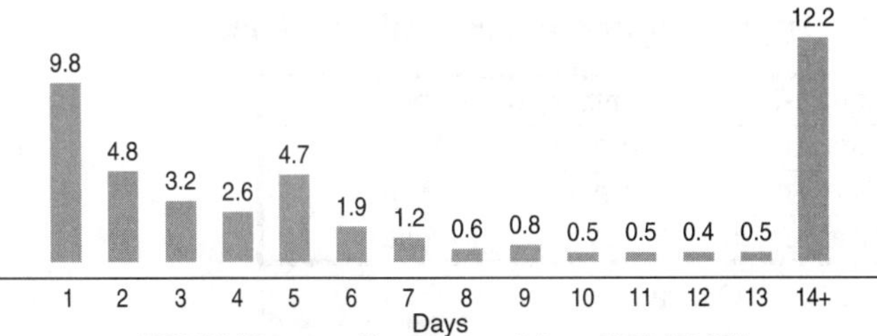

*CDC NHIS cases with no lost workdays: 3239 (56.3%)

Impact on Total Absence: Prevalence 0.0816% of total lost workdays; Incidence 0.86 days per 100 workers

923.2 Wrist and hand(s), except finger(s) alone

Return-To-Work Summary Guidelines		
Dataset	**Midrange**	**At-Risk**
Claims data	21 days	44 days
All absences	3 days	22 days

Return-To-Work "Best Practice" Guidelines
See 923

Workers' Comp Costs per Claim (based on 43,428 claims)					
Quartile	25%	50%	75%	Mean	% no cost
Indemnity	$557	$1,239	$2,174	$1,870	95%
Medical	$221	$326	$494	$466	6%
Total	$221	$326	$504	$570	6%

RTW Claims Data (Calendar-days away from work by decile)										
10%	20%	30%	40%	**50%**	60%	70%	80%	**90%**	100%	Mean
10	13	16	20	**21**	22	24	29	**44**	68	23.50

923.2 Wrist and hand(s), except finger(s) alone

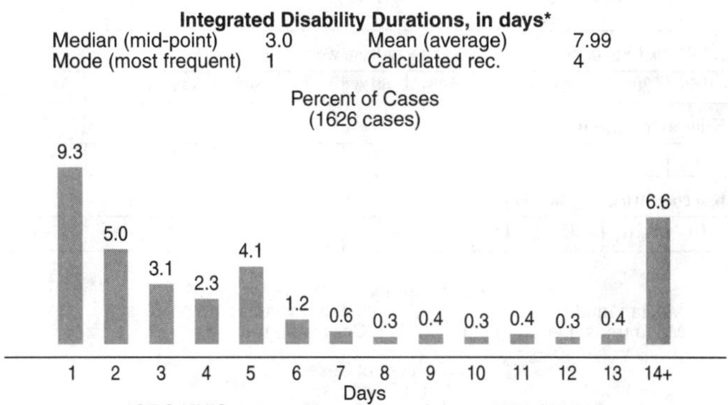

*CDC NHIS cases with no lost workdays: 1070 (65.8%)

Impact on Total Absence: Prevalence 0.0131% of total lost workdays; Incidence 0.14 days per 100 workers

Occupational Disability Durations, in days

Median (mid-point) 4 - Benchmark Indemnity Costs $3,000

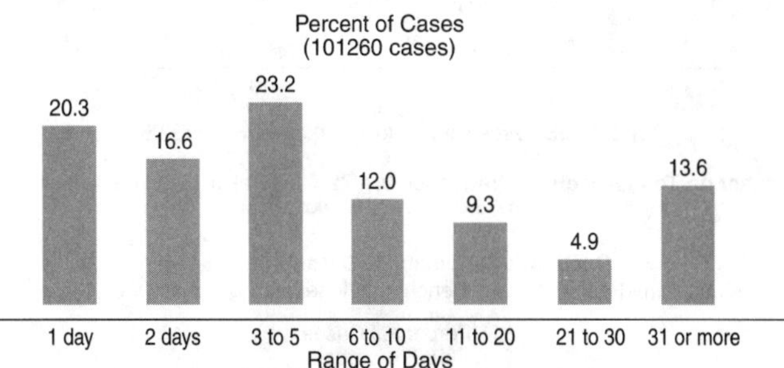

Impact on Occupational Absence: Prevalence 4.5948% of occupational lost workdays; Incidence 0.74 days per 100 workers

924 Contusion of lower limb and of other and unspecified sites

Return-To-Work Summary Guidelines		
Dataset	**Midrange**	**At-Risk**
Claims data	14 days	27 days
All absences	7 days	17 days

Return-To-Work "Best Practice" Guidelines
Superficial contusions: 0 days
Deep contusions, clerical/sedentary work: 7 days
Deep contusions, manual/standing work: 14 days

Description: Bruise of a lower limb or unspecified site. Symptoms include localized tenderness, pain, swelling, and blue/purple color where the bruise forms.

Workers' Comp Costs per Claim (based on 90,436 claims)					
Quartile	25%	50%	75%	Mean	% no cost
Indemnity	$651	$1,323	$2,552	$2,399	92%
Medical	$210	$336	$567	$604	9%
Total	$210	$347	$599	$810	9%

RTW Claims Data (Calendar-days away from work by decile)										
10%	20%	30%	40%	**50%**	60%	70%	80%	**90%**	100%	Mean
9	11	13	14	**14**	15	16	18	**27**	365	19.36

924 Contusion of lower limb and of other and unspecified sites *(cont'd)*

RTW Post Surgery (Calendar-days away from work by decile)										
10%	20%	30%	40%	**50%**	60%	70%	80%	**90%**	100%	Mean
Knee arthroscopy/surgery										
24	27	39	46	**55**	65	93	144	**279**	365	95.99
Knee arthroscopy/surgery										
16	26	35	41	**48**	57	73	93	**131**	365	71.54

Integrated Disability Durations, in days*

Median (mid-point)	7.0	Mean (average)	10.42
Mode (most frequent)	1	Calculated rec.	6

Percent of Cases
(7899 cases)

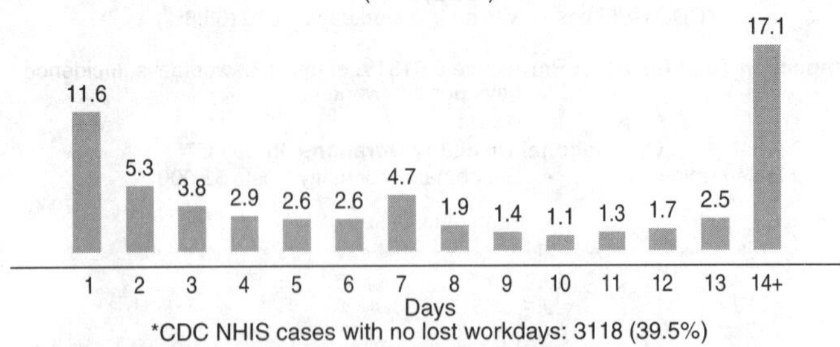

*CDC NHIS cases with no lost workdays: 3118 (39.5%)

Impact on Total Absence: Prevalence 0.1472% of total lost workdays; Incidence 1.55 days per 100 workers

Occupational Disability Durations, in days
Median (mid-point) 8 - Benchmark Indemnity Costs $6,000

Percent of Cases
(18020 cases)

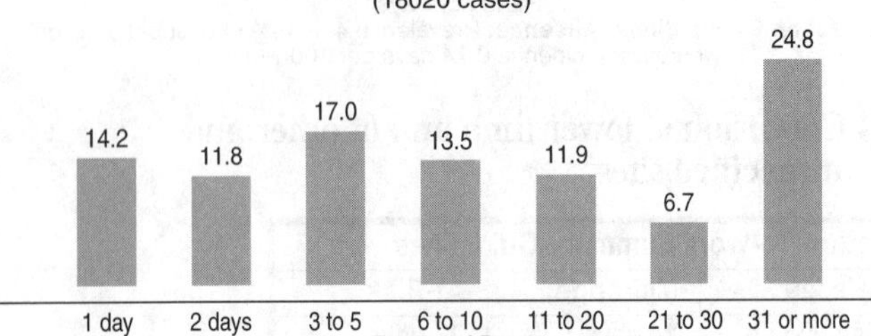

Impact on Occupational Absence: Prevalence 1.6353% of occupational lost workdays; Incidence 0.26 days per 100 workers

CRUSHING INJURY (925-929)

Excludes:
concussion (850.0-850.9)
fractures (800-829)
internal organs (860.0-869.1)
that incidental to:
internal injury (860.0-869.1)
intracranial injury (850.0-854.1)

RTW Claims Data (Calendar-days away from work by decile)										
10%	20%	30%	40%	**50%**	60%	70%	80%	**90%**	100%	Mean
11	14	19	25	**30**	41	55	74	**110**	365	55.73

Impact on Total Absence: Prevalence 1.1272% of total lost workdays; Incidence 11.84 days per 100 workers

CRUSHING INJURY (925-929) *(cont'd)*

Occupational Disability Durations, in days
Median (mid-point) 10 - Benchmark Indemnity Costs $7,500

Percent of Cases
(15410 cases)

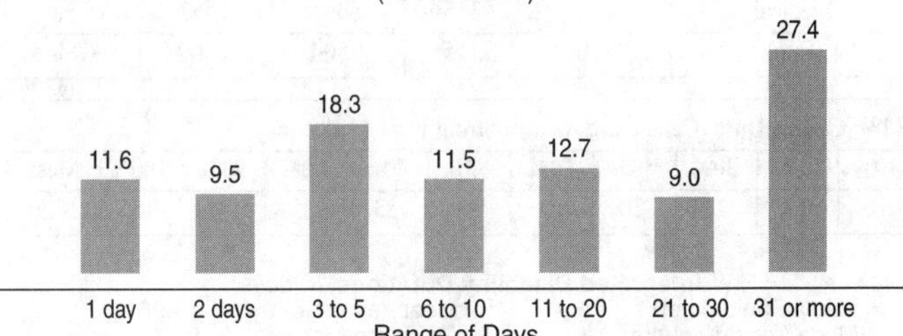

Range of Days

Impact on Occupational Absence: Prevalence 1.7481% of occupational lost workdays; Incidence 0.28 days per 100 workers

925 Crushing injury of face, scalp, and neck

Return-To-Work Summary Guidelines		
Dataset	**Midrange**	**At-Risk**
Claims data	13 days	42 days
All absences	13 days	42 days

Cheek
Ear
Larynx
Pharynx
Throat

RTW Claims Data (Calendar-days away from work by decile)										
10%	20%	30%	40%	**50%**	60%	70%	80%	**90%**	100%	Mean
12	12	12	13	**13**	14	28	28	**42**	42	20.17

Impact on Total Absence: Prevalence 0.0003% of total lost workdays

925.1 Crushing injury of face and scalp

Return-To-Work Summary Guidelines		
Dataset	**Midrange**	**At-Risk**
Claims data	13 days	42 days
All absences	13 days	42 days

Return-To-Work "Best Practice" Guidelines
Minor: 7-21 days
Severe, extensive: 28 days to indefinite

Cheek
Ear

926 Crushing injury of trunk

Return-To-Work Summary Guidelines		
Dataset	**Midrange**	**At-Risk**
Claims data	42 days	364 days
All absences	31 days	364 days

Return-To-Work "Best Practice" Guidelines
Minor: 7-21 days
Severe, extensive: 28 days to indefinite

Excludes:
crush injury of internal organs (860.0-869.1)

926 Crushing injury of trunk *(cont'd)*

Workers' Comp Costs per Claim (based on 86 claims)					
Quartile	25%	50%	75%	Mean	% no cost
Indemnity	$3,308	$6,872	$51,251	$31,491	42%
Medical	$546	$5,287	$10,742	$7,748	2%
Total	$2,258	$10,332	$38,073	$25,770	0%

RTW Claims Data (Calendar-days away from work by decile)

10%	20%	30%	40%	**50%**	60%	70%	80%	**90%**	100%	Mean
14	21	28	32	**42**	61	88	145	**364**	365	102.54

Integrated Disability Durations, in days*
Median (mid-point) 31.0 Mean (average) 83.39
Mode (most frequent) 2 Calculated rec. 37

Percent of Cases
(72 cases)

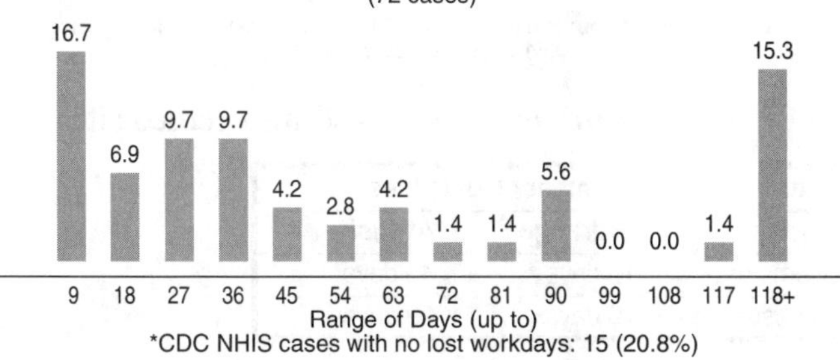

*CDC NHIS cases with no lost workdays: 15 (20.8%)

Impact on Total Absence: Prevalence 0.0140% of total lost workdays; Incidence 0.15 days per 100 workers

927 Crushing injury of upper limb

Return-To-Work Summary Guidelines		
Dataset	**Midrange**	**At-Risk**
Claims data	27 days	73 days
All absences	6 days	55 days

Workers' Comp Costs per Claim (based on 12,861 claims)					
Quartile	25%	50%	75%	Mean	% no cost
Indemnity	$830	$1,659	$3,507	$3,270	88%
Medical	$263	$431	$756	$840	5%
Total	$263	$441	$840	$1,237	5%

RTW Claims Data (Calendar-days away from work by decile)

10%	20%	30%	40%	**50%**	60%	70%	80%	**90%**	100%	Mean
11	13	17	20	**27**	34	45	57	**73**	220	34.72

RTW Post Surgery (Calendar-days away from work by decile)

10%	20%	30%	40%	**50%**	60%	70%	80%	**90%**	100%	Mean
Skin tissue rearrangement										
6	15	23	31	**40**	50	109	158	**310**	365	91.40

927 Crushing injury of upper limb *(cont'd)*

Integrated Disability Durations, in days*
Median (mid-point) 6.0 Mean (average) 17.88
Mode (most frequent) 1 Calculated rec. 8

Percent of Cases
(8890 cases)

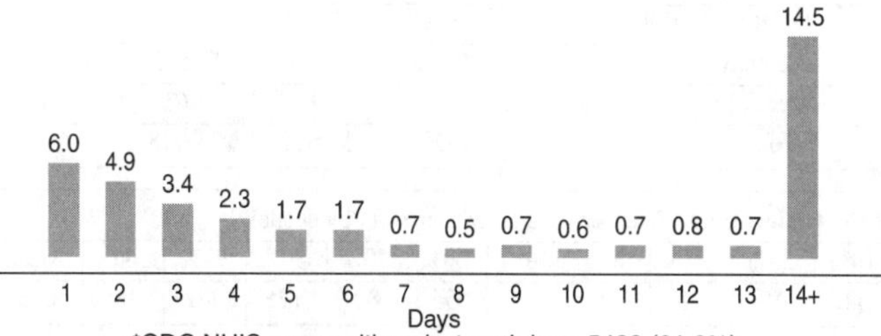

*CDC NHIS cases with no lost workdays: 5422 (61.0%)

Impact on Total Absence: Prevalence 0.1832% of total lost workdays; Incidence 1.92 days per 100 workers

927.1 Elbow and forearm

Return-To-Work Summary Guidelines		
Dataset	**Midrange**	**At-Risk**
Claims data	30 days	95 days
All absences	12 days	67 days

Return-To-Work "Best Practice" Guidelines
Minor: 7-14 days
Amputation, clerical/modified work: 28-56 days
Amputation, manual work: 56 days to indefinite

Workers' Comp Costs per Claim (based on 390 claims)					
Quartile	25%	50%	75%	Mean	% no cost
Indemnity	$840	$1,638	$4,967	$4,457	77%
Medical	$294	$515	$1,103	$1,457	4%
Total	$305	$567	$1,596	$2,544	4%

RTW Claims Data (Calendar-days away from work by decile)

10%	20%	30%	40%	**50%**	60%	70%	80%	**90%**	100%	Mean
13	14	17	26	**30**	40	55	59	**95**	365	60.84

Integrated Disability Durations, in days*
Median (mid-point) 12.0 Mean (average) 34.90
Mode (most frequent) 1 Calculated rec. 15

Percent of Cases
(274 cases)

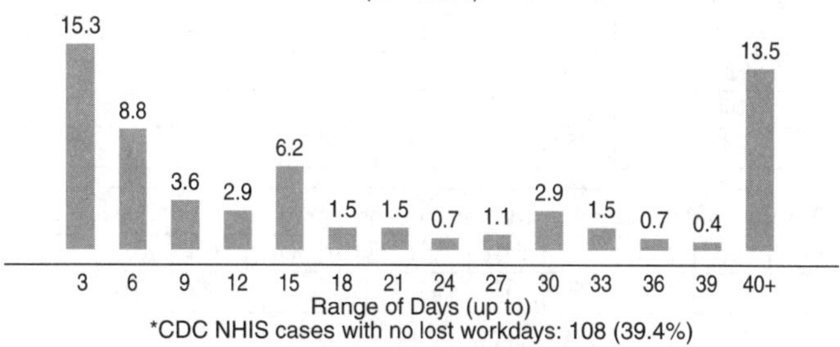

*CDC NHIS cases with no lost workdays: 108 (39.4%)

Impact on Total Absence: Prevalence 0.0171% of total lost workdays; Incidence 0.18 days per 100 workers

928 Crushing injury of lower limb

Return-To-Work Summary Guidelines		
Dataset	**Midrange**	**At-Risk**
Claims data	33 days	242 days
All absences	22 days	178 days

928 Crushing injury of lower limb *(cont'd)*

Return-To-Work "Best Practice" Guidelines
See 928.0

Workers' Comp Costs per Claim (based on 2,565 claims)					
Quartile	25%	50%	75%	Mean	% no cost
Indemnity	$903	$2,237	$5,156	$5,572	76%
Medical	$305	$525	$1,145	$1,637	4%
Total	$305	$557	$1,827	$3,045	4%

RTW Claims Data (Calendar-days away from work by decile)										
10%	20%	30%	40%	**50%**	60%	70%	80%	**90%**	100%	Mean
11	19	23	28	**33**	54	82	125	**242**	365	83.37

Integrated Disability Durations, in days*

Median (mid-point)	22.0	Mean (average)	59.06
Mode (most frequent)	1	Calculated rec.	26

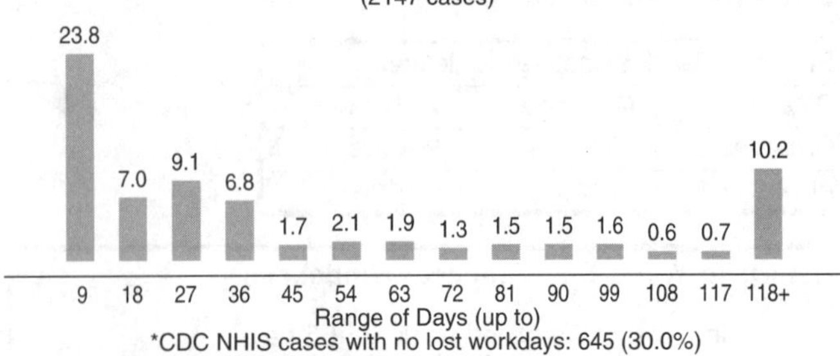

*CDC NHIS cases with no lost workdays: 645 (30.0%)

Impact on Total Absence: Prevalence 0.2622% of total lost workdays; Incidence 2.75 days per 100 workers

928.3 Toe(s)

Return-To-Work Summary Guidelines		
Dataset	**Midrange**	**At-Risk**
Claims data	32 days	140 days
All absences	14 days	100 days

Return-To-Work "Best Practice" Guidelines
Minor: 0-7 days
Amputation, clerical/sedentary work: 14-28 days
Amputation, manual/standing work: 28-140 days

Workers' Comp Costs per Claim (based on 671 claims)					
Quartile	25%	50%	75%	Mean	% no cost
Indemnity	$441	$1,160	$2,426	$1,715	83%
Medical	$231	$399	$662	$599	5%
Total	$242	$425	$851	$905	5%

RTW Claims Data (Calendar-days away from work by decile)										
10%	20%	30%	40%	**50%**	60%	70%	80%	**90%**	100%	Mean
13	14	19	28	**32**	54	80	95	**140**	205	55.34

928.3 Toe(s) *(cont'd)*

Integrated Disability Durations, in days*

Median (mid-point)	14.0	Mean (average)	34.66
Mode (most frequent)	1	Calculated rec.	16

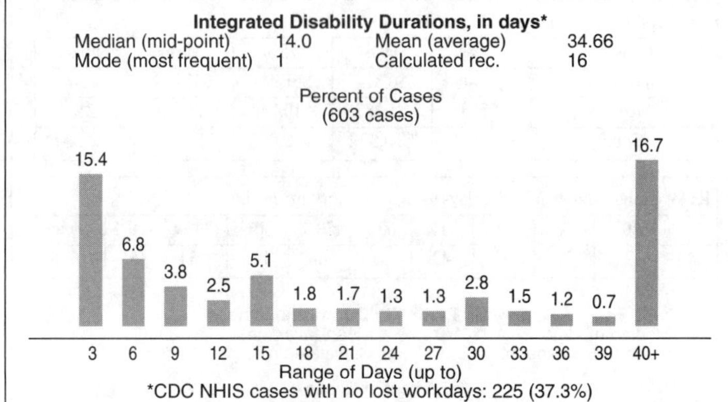

*CDC NHIS cases with no lost workdays: 225 (37.3%)

Impact on Total Absence: Prevalence 0.0387% of total lost workdays; Incidence 0.41 days per 100 workers

929 Crushing injury of multiple and unspecified sites

Return-To-Work Summary Guidelines		
Dataset	**Midrange**	**At-Risk**
Claims data	15 days	48 days
All absences	13 days	39 days

Excludes:
multiple internal injury NOS (869.0-869.1)

RTW Claims Data (Calendar-days away from work by decile)										
10%	20%	30%	40%	**50%**	60%	70%	80%	**90%**	100%	Mean
10	13	14	14	**15**	30	30	39	**48**	48	24.14

Impact on Total Absence: Prevalence 0.0005% of total lost workdays; Incidence 0.01 days per 100 workers

Occupational Disability Durations, in days
Median (mid-point) 5 - Benchmark Indemnity Costs $3,750

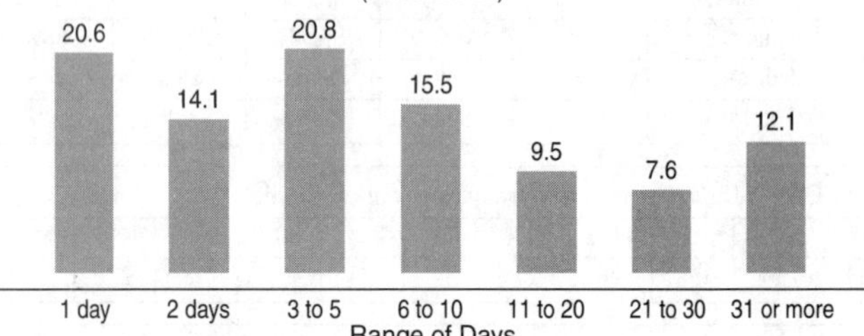

Impact on Occupational Absence: Prevalence 0.4498% of occupational lost workdays; Incidence 0.07 days per 100 workers

EFFECTS OF FOREIGN BODY ENTERING THROUGH ORIFICE (930-939)

Excludes:
foreign body:
granuloma (728.82)
inadvertently left in operative wound (998.4, 998.7)
in open wound (800-839, 851-897)
residual, in soft tissues (729.6)
superficial without major open wound (910-919 with .6 or .7)

RTW Claims Data (Calendar-days away from work by decile)										
10%	20%	30%	40%	**50%**	60%	70%	80%	**90%**	100%	Mean
8	9	10	10	**11**	12	13	14	**18**	57	12.70

Impact on Total Absence: Prevalence 0.0132% of total lost workdays; Incidence 0.14 days per 100 workers

934 Foreign body in trachea, bronchus, and lung

Return-To-Work Summary Guidelines		
Dataset	**Midrange**	**At-Risk**
Claims data	11 days	18 days
All absences	2 days	6 days

Return-To-Work "Best Practice" Guidelines
Medical treatment, without hospitalization: 0 days
Medical treatment, with hospitalization: 7 days
Bronchoscopy, local anesthesia: 0 days
Bronchoscopy, general anesthesia: 1 day

Description: A foreign body in the respiratory system could cause minor or serious breathing problems.

BURNS (940-949)

Includes: burns from:
electrical heating appliance
electricity
flame
hot object
lightning
radiation
chemical burns (external) (internal)
scalds

Excludes:
friction burns (910-919 with .0, .1)
sunburn (692.71)

RTW Claims Data (Calendar-days away from work by decile)										
10%	20%	30%	40%	**50%**	60%	70%	80%	**90%**	100%	Mean
10	13	15	19	**23**	28	33	55	**69**	365	30.59

Impact on Total Absence: Prevalence 1.4514% of total lost workdays; Incidence 15.24 days per 100 workers

Occupational Disability Durations, in days
Median (mid-point) 4 - Benchmark Indemnity Costs $3,000

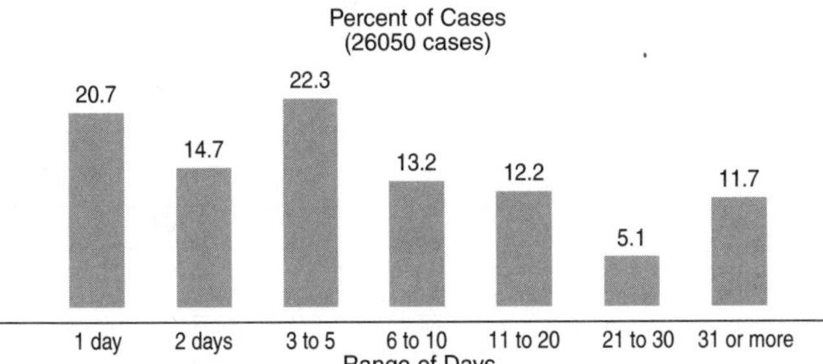

Impact on Occupational Absence: Prevalence 1.1820% of occupational lost workdays; Incidence 0.19 days per 100 workers

941 Burn of face, head, and neck

Return-To-Work Summary Guidelines		
Dataset	**Midrange**	**At-Risk**
Claims data	22 days	70 days
All absences	8 days	53 days

941 Burn of face, head, and neck *(cont'd)*

Return-To-Work "Best Practice" Guidelines
First degree: 0 days
Second degree, < 3 square inches: 0 days
Second degree, >= 3 square inches: 10 days
Third degree, < 3 square inches: 21 days
Third degree, >= 3 square inches: 28 days
Third degree, > 30 square inches (1% BSA), modified work: 56 days
Third degree, > 30 square inches (1% BSA), regular work: 70 days

Capabilities & Activity Modifications:
Modified work: Mild heat exposure (under 80 degrees Fahrenheit); limit
exposure to liquids (dressing over burn must be dry); limit exposure to dirty or dusty environment.
Description: Tissue of the face, head or neck that has been damaged by heat, electricity, radiation, or chemicals. First-degree burns involve only the surface layer of skin and cause redness, pain, and swelling. Second degree burns are deeper into the epidermis and top layer of the dermis causing pain, redness, blisters, swelling, and hypersensitivity. Third degree burns affect the entire thickness of the skin causing the skin to become white and soft, or black, charred, and leathery with no feeling when touched because of nerve ending destruction.

Excludes:
mouth (947.0)

The following fifth-digit subclassification is for use with category 941:
0 face and head, unspecified site
1 ear [any part]
2 eye (with other parts of face, head, and neck)
3 lip(s)
4 chin
5 nose (septum)
6 scalp [any part]
Temple (region)
7 forehead and cheek
8 neck
9 multiple sites [except with eye] of face, head, and neck

Procedure Summary (from ODG Treatment): 2400 mOsm solutions; Acticoat; Activity restrictions; Apligraf®; Benzodiazepines; Burn size calculations; Citalopram; Cooling (with ice or cold water); Dexamethasone; Early tangential excision (and skin grafting); Early tracheostomy (ET); Enteral feeding ; Euglycemic hyperinsu-linemia; Flucloxacillin; Growth hormone; High frequency percussive ventilation (HFPV); Honey dressing; Human allogeneic epidermal sheets; Hyperbaric oxygen therapy; Immune-enhancing diets (IEDs); Insulin; Insulin and glucose; Interferon-gamma-1b (IFN-gamma); Itch control ; Lignocaine-prilocaine (EMLA) cream; Massage therapy; Moist exposed burn ointment (MEBO); Music therapy; Occupational therapy; Oxandrolone; Physical therapy (PT); Potato peel; Propranolol; Psychological debriefing (PD); Recombinant bovine fibroblast growth factor (rbFGF); Silver sulfadiazine (SSD); Skin grafts; Sucralfate cream; Teicoplanin; Therapeutic touch (TT); Therapeutic ultrasound; Topical corticosteroid (treatment of sunburn); Topical local anesthesia; Tourniquet use; TransCyte; Trimethoprim-sulfamethoxazole (TMP-SMX); Work

941 Burn of face, head, and neck *(cont'd)*

Workers' Comp Costs per Claim (based on 6,063 claims)					
Quartile	25%	50%	75%	Mean	% no cost
Indemnity	$651	$1,460	$2,709	$4,936	92%
Medical	$168	$263	$452	$1,469	6%
Total	$168	$263	$494	$1,905	6%

RTW Claims Data (Calendar-days away from work by decile)										
10%	20%	30%	40%	**50%**	60%	70%	80%	**90%**	100%	Mean
10	12	15	19	**22**	26	30	52	**63**	365	29.24

Integrated Disability Durations, in days*

Median (mid-point) 8.0 Mean (average) 16.03
Mode (most frequent) 1 Calculated rec. 8

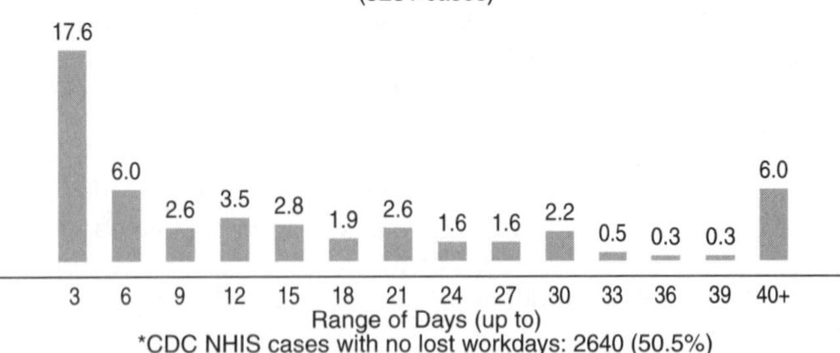

*CDC NHIS cases with no lost workdays: 2640 (50.5%)

Impact on Total Absence: Prevalence 0.1227% of total lost workdays; Incidence 1.29 days per 100 workers

942 Burn of trunk

Return-To-Work Summary Guidelines		
Dataset	**Midrange**	**At-Risk**
Claims data	27 days	70 days
All absences	10 days	55 days

Return-To-Work "Best Practice" Guidelines
First degree: 0 days
Second degree, < 3 square inches: 0 days
Second degree, >= 3 square inches: 10 days
Third degree, < 3 square inches, clerical/modified work: 21 days
Third degree, >= 3 square inches, clerical/modified work: 28 days
Third degree, > 30 square inches, clerical/modified work: 56 days
Third degree, < 3 square inches, manual work: 21 days
Third degree, >= 3 square inches, manual work: 35 days
Third degree, > 30 square inches, manual work: 70 days

Capabilities & Activity Modifications:
Modified work: Mild heat exposure (under 80 degrees Fahrenheit); limit
exposure to liquids (dressing over burn must be dry); limit exposure to dirty or dusty environment.
Description: Body tissue that has been damaged by heat, electricity, radiation, or chemicals. See 941 for symptoms.

Excludes:
scapular region (943.0-943.5 with fifth-digit 6)

942 Burn of trunk *(cont'd)*

The following fifth-digit subclassification is for use with category 942:
0 trunk, unspecified site
1 breast
2 chest wall, excluding breast and nipple
3 abdominal wall
Flank
Groin
4 back [any part]
Buttock
Interscapular region
5 genitalia
Labium (majus) (minus)
Penis
Perineum
Scrotum
Testis
Vulva
9 other and multiple sites of trunk

Procedure Summary (from ODG Treatment): 2400 mOsm solutions; Acticoat; Activity restrictions; Apligraf®; Benzodiazepines; Burn size calculations; Citalopram; Cooling (with ice or cold water); Dexamethasone; Early tangential excision (and skin grafting); Early tracheostomy (ET); Enteral feeding ; Euglycemic hyperinsu-linemia; Flucloxacillin; Growth hormone; High frequency percussive ventilation (HFPV); Honey dressing; Human allogeneic epidermal sheets; Hyperbaric oxygen therapy; Immune-enhancing diets (IEDs); Insulin; Insulin and glucose; Interferon-gamma-1b (IFN-gamma); Itch control ; Lignocaine-prilocaine (EMLA) cream; Massage therapy; Moist exposed burn ointment (MEBO); Music therapy; Occupational therapy; Oxandrolone; Physical therapy (PT); Potato peel; Propranolol; Psychological debriefing (PD); Recombinant bovine fibroblast growth factor (rbFGF); Silver sulfadiazine (SSD); Skin grafts; Sucralfate cream; Teicoplanin; Therapeutic touch (TT); Therapeutic ultrasound; Topical corticosteroid (treatment of sunburn); Topical local anesthesia; Tourniquet use; TransCyte; Trimethoprim-sulfamethoxazole (TMP-SMX); Work

Workers' Comp Costs per Claim (based on 2,626 claims)					
Quartile	25%	50%	75%	Mean	% no cost
Indemnity	$767	$1,712	$3,434	$5,039	87%
Medical	$189	$326	$609	$2,676	6%
Total	$189	$336	$693	$3,369	6%

RTW Claims Data (Calendar-days away from work by decile)										
10%	20%	30%	40%	**50%**	60%	70%	80%	**90%**	100%	Mean
10	13	17	21	**27**	31	36	51	**68**	180	32.09

Integrated Disability Durations, in days*

Median (mid-point) 10.0 Mean (average) 18.58
Mode (most frequent) 1 Calculated rec. 10

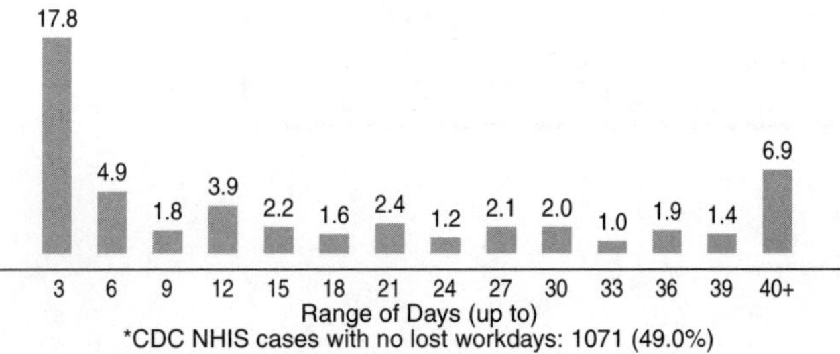

*CDC NHIS cases with no lost workdays: 1071 (49.0%)

Impact on Total Absence: Prevalence 0.0611% of total lost workdays; Incidence 0.64 days per 100 workers

943 Burn of upper limb, except wrist and hand

Return-To-Work Summary Guidelines		
Dataset	Midrange	At-Risk
Claims data	21 days	70 days
All absences	5 days	51 days

Return-To-Work "Best Practice" Guidelines
First degree: 0 days
Second degree, < 3 square inches: 0 days
Second degree, >= 3 square inches: 10 days
Third degree, < 3 square inches: 14 days
Third degree, >= 3 square inches: 28 days
Third degree, > 30 square inches, modified work: 56 days
Third degree, > 30 square inches, regular work: 70 days

Capabilities & Activity Modifications:
Modified work: Mild heat exposure (under 80 degrees Fahrenheit); limit
exposure to liquids (dressing over burn must be dry); limit exposure to dirty or dusty environment.
Description: Tissue of an upper limb except the wrist or hand that has been damaged by heat, electricity, radiation, or chemicals. See 941 for symptoms.

The following fifth-digit subclassification is for use with category 943:
0 upper limb, unspecified site
1 forearm
2 elbow
3 upper arm
4 axilla
5 shoulder
6 scapular region
9 multiple sites of upper limb, except wrist and hand

Procedure Summary (from ODG Treatment): 2400 mOsm solutions; Acticoat; Activity restrictions; Apligraf®; Benzodiazepines; Burn size calculations; Citalopram; Cooling (with ice or cold water); Dexamethasone; Early tangential excision (and skin grafting); Early tracheostomy (ET); Enteral feeding ; Euglycemic hyperinsu-linemia; Flucloxacillin; Growth hormone; High frequency percussive ventilation (HFPV); Honey dressing; Human allogeneic epidermal sheets; Hyperbaric oxygen therapy; Immune-enhancing diets (IEDs); Insulin; Insulin and glucose; Interferon-gamma-1b (IFN-gamma); Itch control ; Lignocaine-prilocaine (EMLA) cream; Massage therapy; Moist exposed burn ointment (MEBO); Music therapy; Occupational therapy; Oxandrolone; Physical therapy (PT); Potato peel; Propranolol; Psychological debriefing (PD); Recombinant bovine fibroblast growth factor (rbFGF); Silver sulfadiazine (SSD); Skin grafts; Sucralfate cream; Teicoplanin; Therapeutic touch (TT); Therapeutic ultrasound; Topical corticosteroid (treatment of sunburn); Topical local anesthesia; Tourniquet use; TransCyte; Trimethoprim-sulfamethoxazole (TMP-SMX); Work

Workers' Comp Costs per Claim (based on 10,798 claims)					
Quartile	25%	50%	75%	Mean	% no cost
Indemnity	$494	$1,292	$2,552	$3,010	93%
Medical	$158	$263	$441	$800	9%
Total	$158	$263	$452	$1,025	9%

RTW Claims Data (Calendar-days away from work by decile)										
10%	20%	30%	40%	**50%**	60%	70%	80%	**90%**	100%	Mean
10	12	14	16	**21**	28	32	55	**68**	131	29.45

943 Burn of upper limb, except wrist and hand

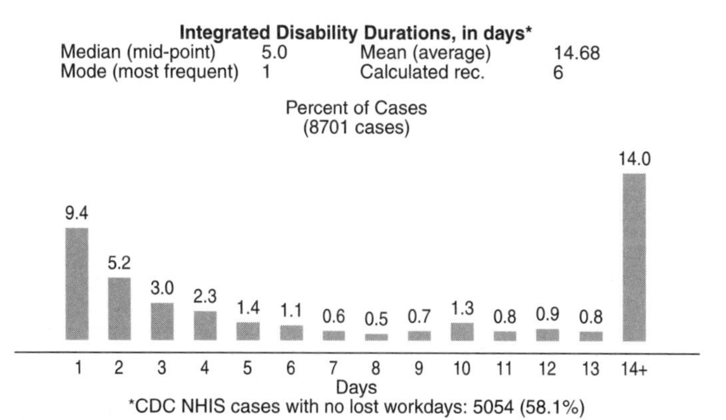

Impact on Total Absence: Prevalence 0.1583% of total lost workdays; Incidence 1.66 days per 100 workers

944 Burn of wrist(s) and hand(s)

Return-To-Work Summary Guidelines		
Dataset	Midrange	At-Risk
Claims data	23 days	70 days
All absences	5 days	52 days

Return-To-Work "Best Practice" Guidelines
First degree: 0 days
Second degree, < 3 square inches: 0 days
Second degree, >= 3 square inches: 14 days
Third degree, < 3 square inches: 21 days
Third degree, >= 3 square inches: 28 days
Third degree, > 30 square inches, modified work: 56 days
Third degree, > 30 square inches, regular work: 70 days

Capabilities & Activity Modifications:
Modified work: Mild heat exposure (under 80 degrees Fahrenheit); limit
exposure to liquids (dressing over burn must be dry); limit exposure to dirty or dusty environment.
Description: Hand or wrist tissue that has been damaged by heat, electricity, radiation, or chemicals. See 941 for symptoms.

The following fifth-digit subclassification is for use with category 944:
0 hand, unspecified site
1 single digit [finger (nail)] other than thumb
2 thumb (nail)
3 two or more digits, not including thumb
4 two or more digits including thumb
5 palm
6 back of hand
7 wrist
8 multiple sites of wrist(s) and hand(s)

Procedure Summary (from ODG Treatment): 2400 mOsm solutions; Acticoat; Activity restrictions; Apligraf®; Benzodiazepines; Burn size calculations; Citalopram; Cooling (with ice or cold water); Dexamethasone; Early tangential excision (and skin grafting); Early tracheostomy (ET); Enteral feeding ; Euglycemic hyperinsu-linemia; Flucloxacillin; Growth hormone; High frequency percussive ventilation (HFPV); Honey dressing; Human allogeneic epidermal sheets; Hyperbaric oxygen therapy; Immune-enhancing diets (IEDs); Insulin; Insulin and glucose; Interferon-gamma-1b (IFN-gamma); Itch control ; Lignocaine-prilocaine (EMLA) cream; Massage therapy; Moist exposed burn ointment (MEBO); Music therapy; Occupational therapy; Oxandrolone; Physical therapy (PT); Potato peel; Propranolol; Psychological debriefing (PD); Recombinant bovine fibroblast growth factor

944 Burn of wrist(s) and hand(s) *(cont'd)*

(rbFGF); Silver sulfadiazine (SSD); Skin grafts; Sucralfate cream; Teicoplanin; Therapeutic touch (TT); Therapeutic ultrasound; Topical corticosteroid (treatment of sunburn); Topical local anesthesia; Tourniquet use; TransCyte; Trimethoprim-sulfamethoxazole (TMP-SMX); Work

Workers' Comp Costs per Claim (based on 17,757 claims)

Quartile	25%	50%	75%	Mean	% no cost
Indemnity	$420	$924	$2,121	$2,190	94%
Medical	$168	$252	$420	$527	8%
Total	$168	$263	$431	$669	8%

RTW Claims Data (Calendar-days away from work by decile)

10%	20%	30%	40%	**50%**	60%	70%	80%	**90%**	100%	Mean
11	14	16	20	**23**	28	32	56	**69**	163	30.94

Integrated Disability Durations, in days*

Median (mid-point) 5.0 Mean (average) 14.57
Mode (most frequent) 1 Calculated rec. 6

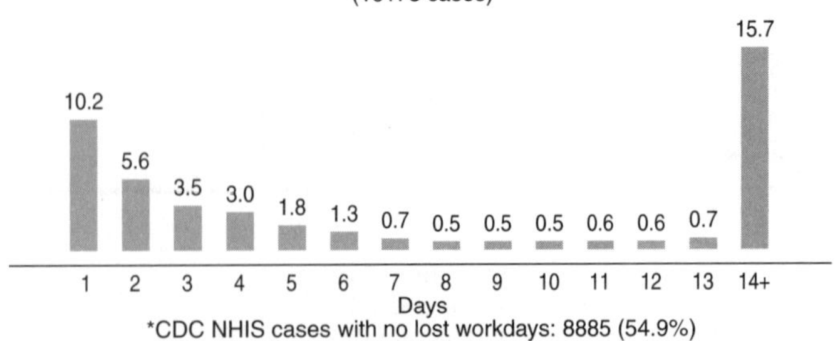

*CDC NHIS cases with no lost workdays: 8885 (54.9%)

Impact on Total Absence: Prevalence 0.3139% of total lost workdays; Incidence 3.30 days per 100 workers

944.2 Blisters, epidermal loss [second degree]

Return-To-Work Summary Guidelines		
Dataset	**Midrange**	**At-Risk**
Claims data	22 days	70 days
All absences	5 days	50 days

Return-To-Work "Best Practice" Guidelines
See 944

Workers' Comp Costs per Claim (based on 11,470 claims)

Quartile	25%	50%	75%	Mean	% no cost
Indemnity	$357	$840	$1,712	$1,490	93%
Medical	$179	$284	$452	$416	5%
Total	$179	$284	$473	$519	5%

RTW Claims Data (Calendar-days away from work by decile)

10%	20%	30%	40%	**50%**	60%	70%	80%	**90%**	100%	Mean
11	14	16	19	**22**	27	31	55	**68**	115	29.90

944.2 Blisters, epidermal loss [second degree]

Integrated Disability Durations, in days*

Median (mid-point) 5.0 Mean (average) 14.86
Mode (most frequent) 1 Calculated rec. 6

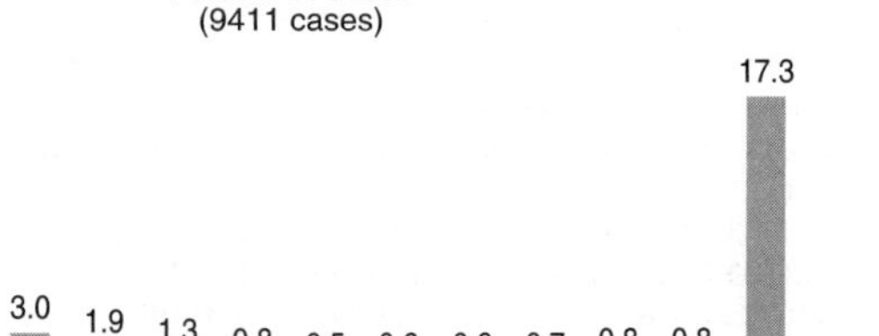

*CDC NHIS cases with no lost workdays: 4941 (52.5%)

Impact on Total Absence: Prevalence 0.1963% of total lost workdays; Incidence 2.06 days per 100 workers

Occupational Disability Durations, in days

Median (mid-point) 5 - Benchmark Indemnity Costs $3,750

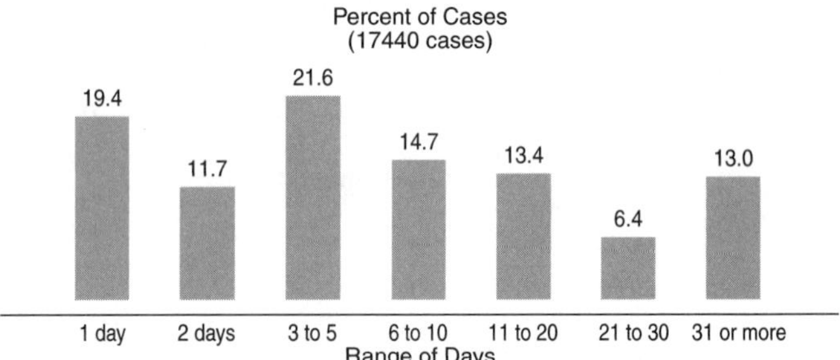

Impact on Occupational Absence: Prevalence 0.9892% of occupational lost workdays; Incidence 0.16 days per 100 workers

INJURY TO NERVES AND SPINAL CORD (950-957)

Includes: division of nerve
lesion in continuity (with open wound)
traumatic neuroma (with open wound)
traumatic transient paralysis (with open wound)

Excludes:
accidental puncture or laceration during medical procedure (998.2)

RTW Claims Data (Calendar-days away from work by decile)

10%	20%	30%	40%	**50%**	60%	70%	80%	**90%**	100%	Mean
13	18	24	32	**43**	57	72	90	**120**	365	57.36

Impact on Total Absence: Prevalence 0.2615% of total lost workdays; Incidence 2.75 days per 100 workers

953 Injury to nerve roots and spinal plexus

Return-To-Work Summary Guidelines		
Dataset	**Midrange**	**At-Risk**
Claims data	48 days	126 days
All absences	23 days	119 days

Return-To-Work "Best Practice" Guidelines
Clerical/modified work: 7 days
Manual work: 21 days
Heavy manual work: 49 days

Description: Damage to the nerve roots and spinal nerves, which could cause pain, loss of sensation, muscle weakness, and lack of coordination or movement.

953 Injury to nerve roots and spinal plexus *(cont'd)*

Workers' Comp Costs per Claim (based on 108 claims)					
Quartile	25%	50%	75%	Mean	% no cost
Indemnity	$6,563	$12,537	$29,012	$32,474	14%
Medical	$4,746	$10,584	$28,917	$24,408	0%
Total	$11,603	$22,943	$60,827	$52,326	0%

RTW Claims Data (Calendar-days away from work by decile)										
10%	20%	30%	40%	**50%**	60%	70%	80%	**90%**	100%	Mean
13	19	21	22	**48**	50	58	89	**126**	180	55.31

Integrated Disability Durations, in days*

Median (mid-point)	23.0	Mean (average)	47.64
Mode (most frequent)	21	Calculated rec.	29

Percent of Cases
(85 cases)

16.5 9.4 20.0 0.0 0.0 15.3 3.5 4.7 0.0 2.4 1.2 1.2 1.2 10.6

9 18 27 36 45 54 63 72 81 90 99 108 117 118+

Range of Days (up to)

*CDC NHIS cases with no lost workdays: 12 (14.1%)

Impact on Total Absence: Prevalence 0.0102% of total lost workdays; Incidence 0.11 days per 100 workers

953.4 Brachial plexus

Return-To-Work Summary Guidelines		
Dataset	**Midrange**	**At-Risk**
Claims data	66 days	173 days
All absences	57 days	157 days

Return-To-Work "Best Practice" Guidelines
Diagnostic testing: 0 days
Treatment, clerical/modified work: 14 days
Treatment, manual work: 42 days

Description: Damage to the brachial nerves in the shoulder area causing a sudden shoulder ache (it could be in the arms and neck as well), changes in sensation, muscle weakness even after the pain subsides, and lack of coordination.

Workers' Comp Costs per Claim (based on 70 claims)					
Quartile	25%	50%	75%	Mean	% no cost
Indemnity	$6,636	$11,408	$20,864	$28,168	14%
Medical	$4,400	$10,584	$25,295	$22,956	0%
Total	$11,603	$22,743	$59,073	$47,318	0%

RTW Claims Data (Calendar-days away from work by decile)										
10%	20%	30%	40%	**50%**	60%	70%	80%	**90%**	100%	Mean
19	20	26	57	**66**	89	126	131	**173**	178	81.75

953.4 Brachial plexus *(cont'd)*

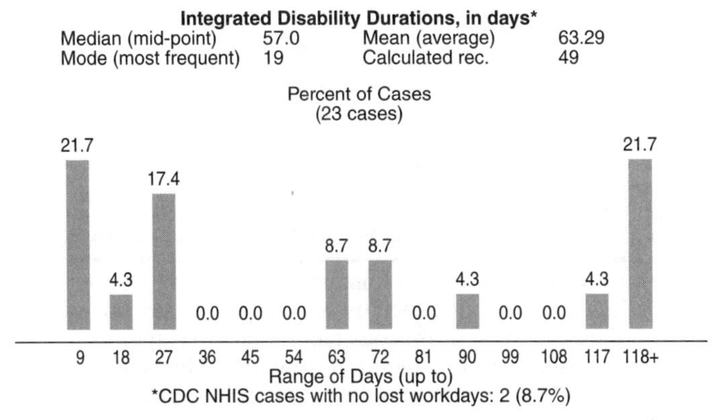

Impact on Total Absence: Prevalence 0.0039% of total lost workdays; Incidence 0.04 days per 100 workers

POISONING BY DRUGS, MEDICINAL AND BIOLOGICAL SUBSTANCES (960-979)

Includes: overdose of these substances
wrong substance given or taken in error

Excludes:
adverse effects ["hypersensitivity," "reaction," etc.] of correct substance properly administered. Such cases are to be classified according to the nature of the adverse effect, such as:
- *adverse effect NOS (995.2)*
- *allergic lymphadenitis (289.3)*
- *aspirin gastritis (535.4)*
- *blood disorders (280.0-289.9)*
- *dermatitis:*
  - *contact (692.0-692.9)*
  - *due to ingestion (693.0-693.9)*
- *nephropathy (583.9)*
- *[The drug giving rise to the adverse effect may be identified by use of categories E930-E949.]*

drug dependence (304.0-304.9)
drug reaction and poisoning affecting the newborn (760.0-779.9)
nondependent abuse of drugs (305.0-305.9)
pathological drug intoxication (292.2)
Use additional code to specify the effects of the poisoning

RTW Claims Data (Calendar-days away from work by decile)										
10%	20%	30%	40%	**50%**	60%	70%	80%	**90%**	100%	Mean
8	8	8	12	**13**	14	15	16	**21**	365	35.93

Impact on Total Absence: Prevalence 0.0021% of total lost workdays; Incidence 0.02 days per 100 workers

977 Poisoning by other and unspecified drugs and medicinal substances

Return-To-Work Summary Guidelines		
Dataset	**Midrange**	**At-Risk**
Claims data	13 days	21 days
All absences	5 days	14 days

Return-To-Work "Best Practice" Guidelines
See 977.9

977.9 Unspecified drug or medicinal substance

Return-To-Work Summary Guidelines		
Dataset	Midrange	At-Risk
Claims data	13 days	21 days
All absences	5 days	14 days

Return-To-Work "Best Practice" Guidelines
Without hospitalization: 2 days
With hospitalization (not involving suicide): 7 days to by report

Description: Injury, death, or impairment of organ function as a result of a toxic substance swallowed, inhaled, or absorption through the skin, eyes, or mucous membranes. Symptoms include malaise, vomiting, blood in stool, pale blue skin, diarrhea, difficulty breath, weakness, irritability, and/or dizziness.
Other names: Poisoning, Overdose, Intoxication

RTW Claims Data (Calendar-days away from work by decile)										
10%	20%	30%	40%	**50%**	60%	70%	80%	**90%**	100%	Mean
8	8	8	12	**13**	14	15	16	**21**	365	35.93

Integrated Disability Durations, in days*
Median (mid-point) 5.0 Mean (average) 11.50
Mode (most frequent) 2 Calculated rec. 6

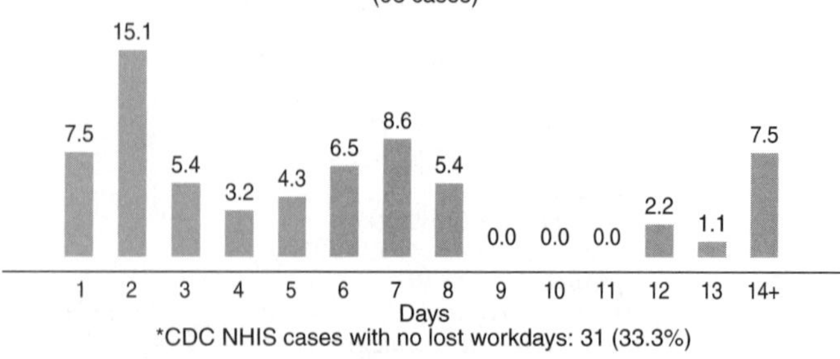

*CDC NHIS cases with no lost workdays: 31 (33.3%)

Impact on Total Absence: Prevalence 0.0021% of total lost workdays; Incidence 0.02 days per 100 workers

TOXIC EFFECTS OF SUBSTANCES CHIEFLY NONMEDICINAL AS TO SOURCE (980-989)

Excludes:
burns from chemical agents (ingested) (947.0-947.9)
localized toxic effects indexed elsewhere (001.0-799.9)
respiratory conditions due to external agents (506.0-508.9)
Use additional code to specify the nature of the toxic effect

RTW Claims Data (Calendar-days away from work by decile)										
10%	20%	30%	40%	**50%**	60%	70%	80%	**90%**	100%	Mean
8	9	11	14	**16**	20	21	25	**45**	365	24.47

Impact on Total Absence: Prevalence 0.0489% of total lost workdays; Incidence 0.51 days per 100 workers

TOXIC EFFECTS OF SUBSTANCES CHIEFLY NONMEDICINAL AS TO SOURCE (980-989) *(cont'd)*

Occupational Disability Durations, in days
Median (mid-point) 2 - Benchmark Indemnity Costs $1,500

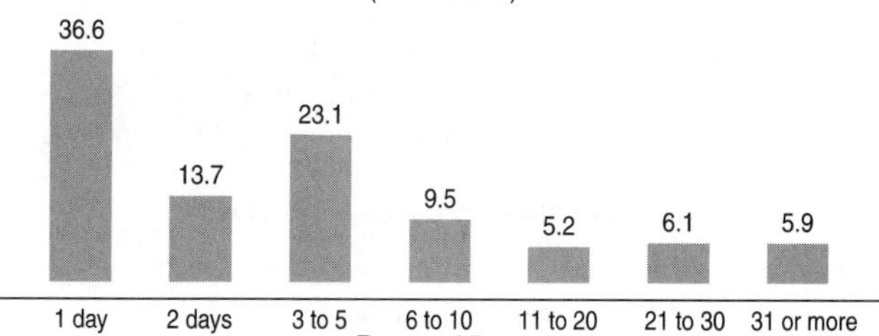

Impact on Occupational Absence: Prevalence 0.1604% of occupational lost workdays; Incidence 0.03 days per 100 workers

984 Toxic effect of lead and its compounds (including fumes)

Return-To-Work Summary Guidelines		
Dataset	Midrange	At-Risk
Claims data	16 days	56 days
All absences	2 days	13 days

Return-To-Work "Best Practice" Guidelines
Chemical absorption, without convulsions (evaluate occupational exposure): 0-2 days
Without convulsions, with encephalopathy: 21-56 days
With convulsions: 42 days to indefinite

Description: Lead poisoning usually occurring from inhalation of dust and fumes, although sometimes from oral ingestion and skin absorption. The poison gathers mostly in the bones, with 10 to 20 percent found in the soft tissues (mainly the brain and kidney). Symptoms include headache, memory loss, weakness, loss of appetite and coordination, abdominal pain and/or other gastrointestinal problems.
Other names: Lead poisoning

Includes: that from all sources except medicinal substances

Workers' Comp Costs per Claim (based on 63 claims)					
Quartile	25%	50%	75%	Mean	% no cost
Indemnity	$1,901	$5,518	$10,185	$7,625	45%
Medical	$210	$604	$1,512	$2,101	9%
Total	$504	$2,258	$6,038	$6,069	0%

987 Toxic effect of other gases, fumes, or vapors

Return-To-Work Summary Guidelines		
Dataset	Midrange	At-Risk
Claims data	21 days	35 days
All absences	2 days	20 days

Return-To-Work "Best Practice" Guidelines
Chemical exposure, no symptoms: 0 days
Chemical exposure, mild, irritant symptoms: 1 day
Chemical exposure, bronchoconstriction only: 7 days
Chemical exposure, pulmonary, laryngeal edema: 21 days

Description: Vapors or gases of corrosive chemicals (acids, caustics) cause acute inflamation of the respiratory tract when inhaled. Short lived exposures to low air levels result in mild mucosal irritation usually without sequelae. Inhalation of

987 Toxic effect of other gases, fumes, or vapors

exceptionally high air concentrations may cause bronchoconstriction, and/or pulmonary edema and rarely fibrosis.

Other names: Irritant vapors and gases

Workers' Comp Costs per Claim (based on 6,156 claims)					
Quartile	25%	50%	75%	Mean	% no cost
Indemnity	$683	$1,764	$4,515	$4,183	97%
Medical	$200	$368	$641	$627	5%
Total	$210	$368	$672	$775	5%

989 Toxic effect of other substances, chiefly nonmedicinal as to source

Return-To-Work Summary Guidelines		
Dataset	**Midrange**	**At-Risk**
Claims data	14 days	72 days
All absences	2 days	10 days

Workers' Comp Costs per Claim (based on 9,890 claims)					
Quartile	25%	50%	75%	Mean	% no cost
Indemnity	$84	$536	$2,426	$4,817	99%
Medical	$116	$189	$336	$308	9%
Total	$116	$189	$336	$348	9%

RTW Claims Data (Calendar-days away from work by decile)										
10%	20%	30%	40%	**50%**	60%	70%	80%	**90%**	100%	Mean
9	10	13	14	**14**	16	18	30	**72**	365	31.78

Integrated Disability Durations, in days*

Median (mid-point) 2.0 Mean (average) 5.97

Mode (most frequent) 1 Calculated rec. 3

Percent of Cases
(3107 cases)

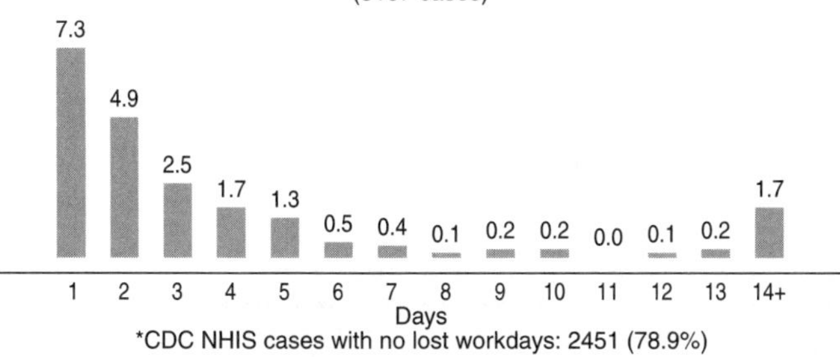

*CDC NHIS cases with no lost workdays: 2451 (78.9%)

Impact on Total Absence: Prevalence 0.0115% of total lost workdays; Incidence 0.12 days per 100 workers

989.5 Venom

Return-To-Work Summary Guidelines		
Dataset	**Midrange**	**At-Risk**
Claims data	9 days	29 days
All absences	2 days	7 days

Return-To-Work "Best Practice" Guidelines
Without hospitalization: 1 day
With hospitalization, depending on specific venom: 7 days

Description: Toxic venom injected into the body by a poisonous insect, spider, snake, or lizard. Reactions to the toxicity can be immediate or can happen several hours after the bite. Specific symptoms depend on the type of venom injected. General symptoms include pain, swelling, itching, or burning, with more serious cases having symptoms of vomiting, diarrhea, cramps, fever, chills, rapid heartbeat, sweating,

989.5 Venom *(cont'd)*

faintness, headache, blood in the stools, dizziness, loss of coordination, and/or breathing problems. Extremely serious cases require hospitalization and can sometimes lead to death.

Bites of venomous snakes, lizards, and spiders
Tick paralysis

Workers' Comp Costs per Claim (based on 9,371 claims)					
Quartile	25%	50%	75%	Mean	% no cost
Indemnity	$74	$247	$830	$1,242	99%
Medical	$116	$189	$326	$298	9%
Total	$116	$189	$326	$306	9%

RTW Claims Data (Calendar-days away from work by decile)										
10%	20%	30%	40%	**50%**	60%	70%	80%	**90%**	100%	Mean
8	8	9	9	**9**	10	11	18	**29**	95	15.85

Integrated Disability Durations, in days*

Median (mid-point) 2.0 Mean (average) 3.61

Mode (most frequent) 1 Calculated rec. 2

Percent of Cases
(2564 cases)

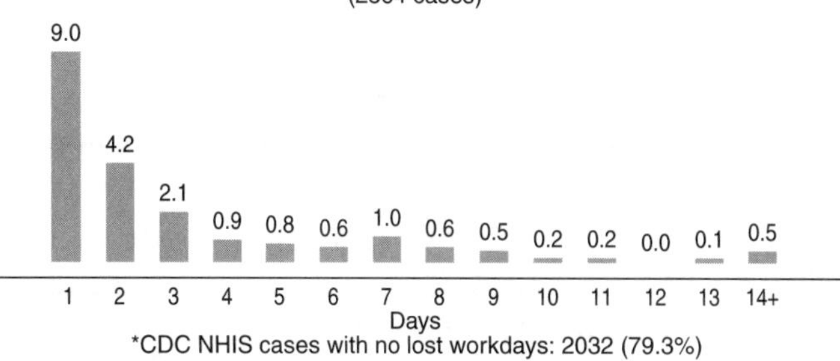

*CDC NHIS cases with no lost workdays: 2032 (79.3%)

Impact on Total Absence: Prevalence 0.0056% of total lost workdays; Incidence 0.06 days per 100 workers

Occupational Disability Durations, in days

Median (mid-point) 3 - Benchmark Indemnity Costs $2,250

Percent of Cases
(4420 cases)

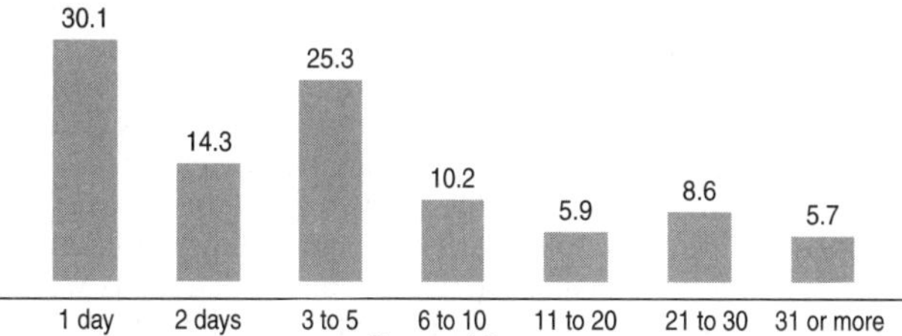

Impact on Occupational Absence: Prevalence 0.1504% of occupational lost workdays; Incidence 0.02 days per 100 workers

OTHER AND UNSPECIFIED EFFECTS OF EXTERNAL CAUSES (990-995)

RTW Claims Data (Calendar-days away from work by decile)										
10%	20%	30%	40%	**50%**	60%	70%	80%	**90%**	100%	Mean
10	12	13	14	**14**	15	16	18	**44**	365	27.28

Impact on Total Absence: Prevalence 0.3136% of total lost workdays; Incidence 3.29 days per 100 workers

OTHER AND UNSPECIFIED EFFECTS OF EXTERNAL CAUSES (990-995) *(cont'd)*

Occupational Disability Durations, in days
Median (mid-point) 3 - Benchmark Indemnity Costs $2,250

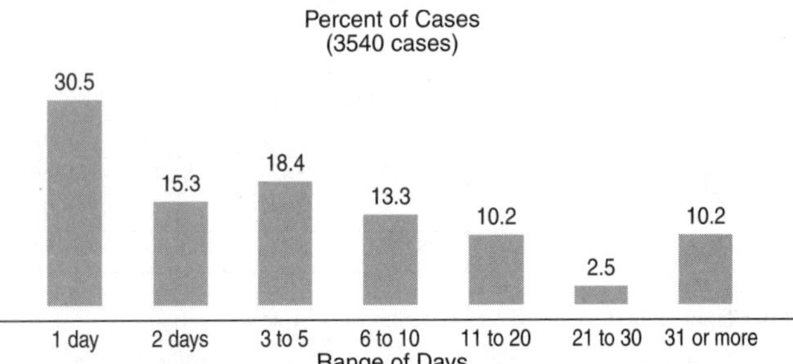

Impact on Occupational Absence: Prevalence 0.1204% of occupational lost workdays; Incidence 0.02 days per 100 workers

990 Effects of radiation, unspecified

Return-To-Work Summary Guidelines		
Dataset	**Midrange**	**At-Risk**
Claims data	15 days	115 days
All absences	13 days	66 days

Return-To-Work "Best Practice" Guidelines
Vision loss due to UV radiation, modified work: 1 day
Vision loss due to UV radiation, regular work (evaluate occupational exposure): 7 days

Capabilities & Activity Modifications:
Modified work: In injuries occurring to one eye no binocular vision requirements, e.g., as required in the operation of high speed or mobile equipment (bilateral eye injuries such as welding flash burns, chemical burns, and allergic reactions, need to be off any work until the vision in one eye has returned to a functional level); limited stereopsis/fields of vision requirements; no exposure to significant vibration (e.g., affecting intra-ocular foreign bodies or retinal detachment); limit exposure to allergic substances (e.g., allergic conjuctivitis requiring removal of the substance from the workplace) and provision for hygiene to prevent spread of infection by direct contact or shared articles; wearing protective eyewear to prevent recurrent injury; possible workstation adjustment.
Description: Exposure to radiation because of a complication of radiation therapy causing temporary loss of vision, as well as nausea, headache, malaise, loss of appetite, and/or increased heartbeat.

Complication of:
  phototherapy
  radiation therapy
Radiation sickness

Excludes:
specified adverse effects of radiation. Such conditions are to be classified according to the nature of the adverse effect, as:
  burns (940.0-949.5)
  dermatitis (692.7-692.8)
  leukemia (204.0-208.9)
  pneumonia (508.0)
  sunburn (692.71)
[The type of radiation giving rise to the adverse effect may be identified by use of the E codes.]

RTW Claims Data (Calendar-days away from work by decile)

10%	20%	30%	40%	**50%**	60%	70%	80%	**90%**	100%	Mean
10	13	14	14	**15**	16	42	50	**115**	180	37.48

990 Effects of radiation, unspecified *(cont'd)*

Integrated Disability Durations, in days*
Median (mid-point) 13.0 Mean (average) 25.15
Mode (most frequent) 1 Calculated rec. 13

Percent of Cases
(69 cases)

Range of Days (up to)	3	6	9	12	15	18	21	24	27	30	33	36	39	40+
Percent	11.6	5.8	5.8	2.9	13.0	4.3	0.0	0.0	0.0	0.0	0.0	0.0	0.0	13.0

*CDC NHIS cases with no lost workdays: 30 (43.5%)

Impact on Total Absence: Prevalence 0.0028% of total lost workdays; Incidence 0.03 days per 100 workers

991 Effects of reduced temperature

Return-To-Work Summary Guidelines		
Dataset	**Midrange**	**At-Risk**
Claims data	14 days	44 days
All absences	4 days	16 days

Workers' Comp Costs per Claim (based on 285 claims)

Quartile	25%	50%	75%	Mean	% no cost
Medical	$126	$231	$410	$495	7%
Total	$126	$231	$431	$707	7%

Occupational Disability Durations, in days
Median (mid-point) 39 - Benchmark Indemnity Costs $29,250
(290 cases)
Impact on Occupational Absence: Prevalence 0.1283% of occupational lost workdays; Incidence 0.02 days per 100 workers

991.1 Frostbite of hand

Return-To-Work Summary Guidelines		
Dataset	**Midrange**	**At-Risk**
Claims data	28 days	72 days
All absences	5 days	71 days

Return-To-Work "Best Practice" Guidelines
Medical treatment, clerical/modified work: 0 days
Medical treatment, manual work: 5 days
Sympathectomy, localized: 7 days
Sympathectomy/ganglionectomy, clerical/modified work: 21 days
Sympathectomy/ganglionectomy, manual work: 28 days
With gangrene, amputation, sedentary work: 24 days
With gangrene, amputation of finger, manual work: 35 days
With gangrene, amputation, manual work: 48 days

Description: See 991.3

Workers' Comp Costs per Claim (based on 127 claims)

Quartile	25%	50%	75%	Mean	% no cost
Medical	$147	$231	$420	$569	6%
Total	$147	$263	$525	$877	6%

RTW Claims Data (Calendar-days away from work by decile)

10%	20%	30%	40%	**50%**	60%	70%	80%	**90%**	100%	Mean
12	14	15	24	**28**	42	70	71	**72**	73	39.75

991.1 Frostbite of hand *(cont'd)*

Integrated Disability Durations, in days*

Median (mid-point)	5.0	Mean (average)	20.45
Mode (most frequent)	1	Calculated rec.	8

Percent of Cases
(70 cases)

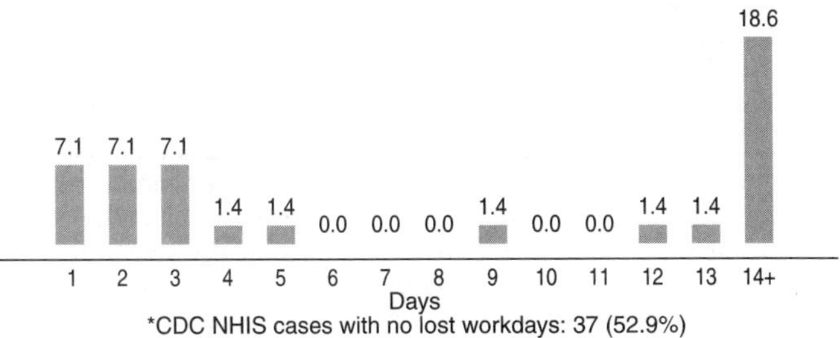

Days
*CDC NHIS cases with no lost workdays: 37 (52.9%)

Impact on Total Absence: Prevalence 0.0019% of total lost workdays; Incidence 0.02 days per 100 workers

991.3 Frostbite of other and unspecified sites

Return-To-Work Summary Guidelines		
Dataset	**Midrange**	**At-Risk**
Claims data	14 days	48 days
All absences	4 days	16 days

Return-To-Work "Best Practice" Guidelines
Medical treatment: 0 days
Sympathectomy, localized: 7 days
Sympathectomy/ganglionectomy, clerical/modified work: 21 days
Sympathectomy/ganglionectomy, manual work: 28 days
With gangrene, amputation, sedentary work: 24 days
With gangrene, amputation, manual work: 48 days

Description: Injury to the skin caused by prolonged exposure to extreme cold in which one or more parts of the body are permanently damaged. Initial symptoms include pain, prickling, itching, white waxy skin and pins and needles followed by numbness. Eventually the skin becomes red and swollen, and then black. Thawing brings burning pain and tenderness. The tissue could eventually recover or gangrene could develop.

Workers' Comp Costs per Claim (based on 55 claims)					
Quartile	25%	50%	75%	Mean	% no cost
Medical	$116	$236	$378	$296	3%
Total	$116	$236	$378	$381	3%

Occupational Disability Durations, in days
Median (mid-point) 9 - Benchmark Indemnity Costs $6,750
(110 cases)
Impact on Occupational Absence: Prevalence 0.0112% of occupational lost workdays

992 Effects of heat and light

Return-To-Work Summary Guidelines		
Dataset	**Midrange**	**At-Risk**
Claims data	11 days	14 days
All absences	2 days	10 days

Return-To-Work "Best Practice" Guidelines
See 992.0

992 Effects of heat and light *(cont'd)*

Excludes:
burns (940.0-949.5)
diseases of sweat glands due to heat (705.0-705.9)
malignant hyperpyrexia following anesthesia (995.89)
sunburn (692.71)

Workers' Comp Costs per Claim (based on 1,701 claims)					
Quartile	25%	50%	75%	Mean	% no cost
Medical	$305	$536	$914	$772	5%
Total	$305	$536	$924	$785	5%

RTW Claims Data (Calendar-days away from work by decile)										
10%	20%	30%	40%	**50%**	60%	70%	80%	**90%**	100%	Mean
9	9	10	10	**11**	11	11	13	**14**	254	13.58

Integrated Disability Durations, in days*

Median (mid-point)	2.0	Mean (average)	4.30
Mode (most frequent)	1	Calculated rec.	2

Percent of Cases
(1204 cases)

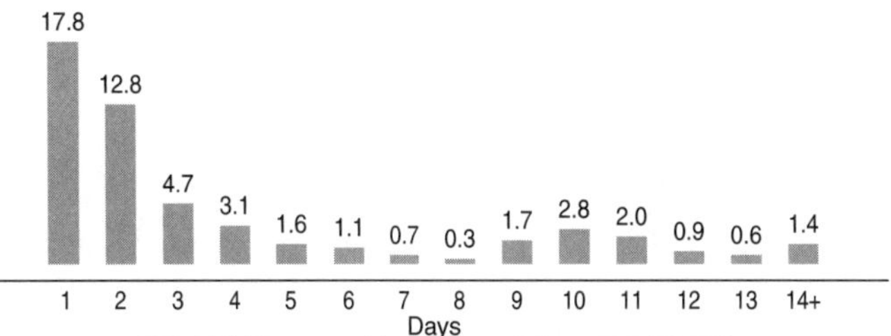

Days
*CDC NHIS cases with no lost workdays: 584 (48.5%)

Impact on Total Absence: Prevalence 0.0078% of total lost workdays; Incidence 0.08 days per 100 workers

Occupational Disability Durations, in days
Median (mid-point) 2 - Benchmark Indemnity Costs $1,500

Percent of Cases
(3020 cases)

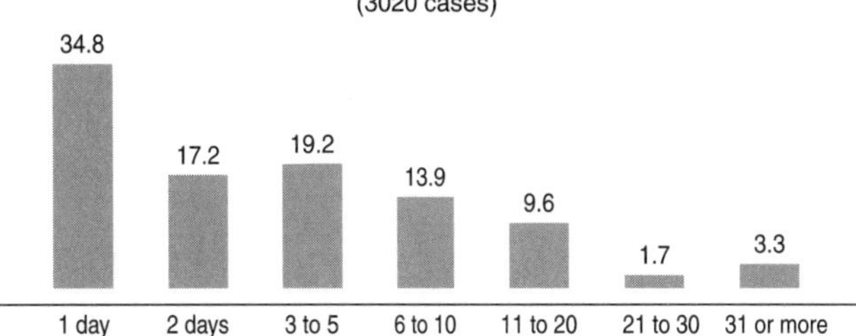

Range of Days
Impact on Occupational Absence: Prevalence 0.0685% of occupational lost workdays; Incidence 0.01 days per 100 workers

992.0 Heat stroke and sunstroke

Return-To-Work Summary Guidelines		
Dataset	**Midrange**	**At-Risk**
Claims data	10 days	14 days
All absences	9 days	13 days

Return-To-Work "Best Practice" Guidelines
Without hospitalization (depending on occupational evaluation): 1-2 days
With hospitalization: 10 days

Description: A life threatening condition resulting from prolonged exposure to extreme heat in which a person cannot sweat enough to lower body temperature. Warning symptoms include headache, dizziness, weakness, confusion, or fatigue, as well as hot, flushed, dry skin. Heart rate increases, body temperature rises, and there could be convulsions, collapse or damage to the brain, heart, liver, kidneys, or blood system.

992.0 Heat stroke and sunstroke *(cont'd)*

Heat apoplexy
Heat pyrexia
Ictus solaris
Siriasis
Thermoplegia

Workers' Comp Costs per Claim (based on 38 claims)					
Quartile	25%	50%	75%	Mean	% no cost
Medical	$525	$1,019	$1,911	$3,797	15%
Total	$620	$1,071	$4,064	$4,351	15%

RTW Claims Data (Calendar-days away from work by decile)										
10%	20%	30%	40%	**50%**	60%	70%	80%	**90%**	100%	Mean
9	10	10	10	**10**	11	12	13	**14**	29	11.56

Integrated Disability Durations, in days*
Median (mid-point) 9.0 Mean (average) 7.63
Mode (most frequent) 10 Calculated rec. 9

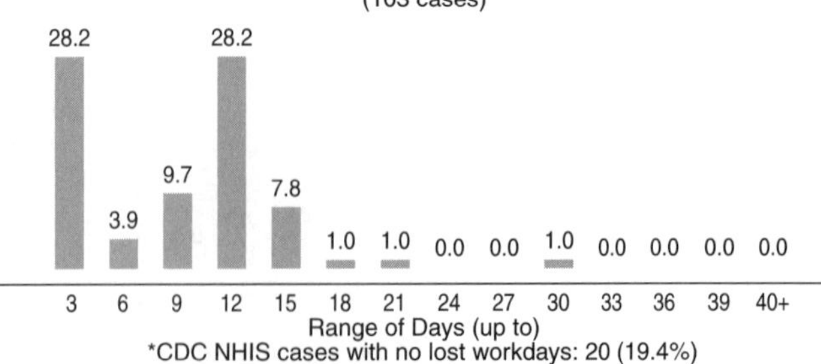

*CDC NHIS cases with no lost workdays: 20 (19.4%)

Impact on Total Absence: Prevalence 0.0018% of total lost workdays; Incidence 0.02 days per 100 workers

Occupational Disability Durations, in days
Median (mid-point) 3 - Benchmark Indemnity Costs $2,250

Percent of Cases
(300 cases)

10.0 40.0 30.0 6.7 6.7 0.0 6.7

1 day 2 days 3 to 5 6 to 10 11 to 20 21 to 30 31 or more
Range of Days

Impact on Occupational Absence: Prevalence 0.0102% of occupational lost workdays

992.2 Heat cramps

Return-To-Work Summary Guidelines		
Dataset	**Midrange**	**At-Risk**
Claims data	11 days	14 days
All absences	2 days	10 days

Return-To-Work "Best Practice" Guidelines
Without hospitalization: 1 day
With hospitalization: 3 days

Description: Muscle contractions as a result of high environmental temperatures.

992.5 Heat exhaustion, unspecified

Return-To-Work Summary Guidelines		
Dataset	**Midrange**	**At-Risk**
Claims data	11 days	17 days
All absences	3 days	11 days

Return-To-Work "Best Practice" Guidelines
Without hospitalization (day of presentation only): 0-1 days
With hospitalization: 1-5 days

Description: Condition caused by excessive exposure to heat, causing fatigue, low blood pressure, and sometimes collapse. Symptoms are a result of loss of fluids from heavy sweating and can also include weakness, anxiety, faintness, slow heartbeat, clammy cold skin, and/or confusion.
Other names: Heat collapse, Heat prostration
Heat prostration NOS

Workers' Comp Costs per Claim (based on 1,564 claims)					
Quartile	25%	50%	75%	Mean	% no cost
Medical	$305	$536	$914	$722	4%
Total	$305	$536	$924	$726	4%

RTW Claims Data (Calendar-days away from work by decile)										
10%	20%	30%	40%	**50%**	60%	70%	80%	**90%**	100%	Mean
8	9	10	10	**11**	12	13	14	**17**	365	24.33

Integrated Disability Durations, in days*
Median (mid-point) 3.0 Mean (average) 7.03
Mode (most frequent) 1 Calculated rec. 4

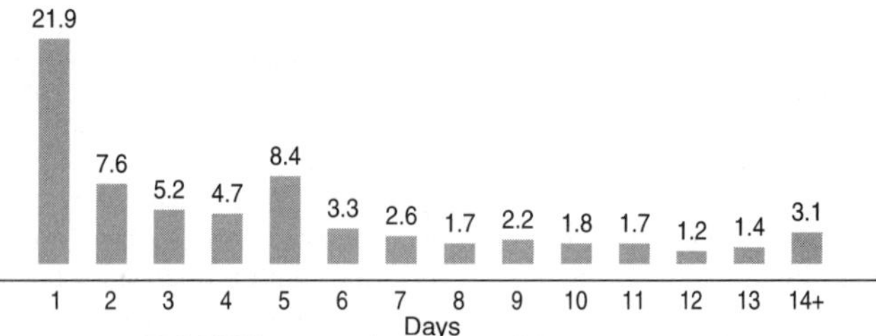

*CDC NHIS cases with no lost workdays: 543 (33.4%)

Impact on Total Absence: Prevalence 0.0224% of total lost workdays; Incidence 0.24 days per 100 workers

993 Effects of air pressure

Return-To-Work Summary Guidelines		
Dataset	**Midrange**	**At-Risk**
Claims data	15 days	16 days
All absences	4 days	16 days

Return-To-Work "Best Practice" Guidelines
Medical treatment, modified work (no diving or flying): 0-1 days
Medical treatment, regular work: 7 days
Tympanostomy/myringotomy, modified work: 2 days
Tympanostomy/myringotomy, regular work: 10 days

Workers' Comp Costs per Claim (based on 198 claims)					
Quartile	25%	50%	75%	Mean	% no cost
Medical	$137	$210	$378	$335	7%
Total	$137	$210	$399	$381	5%

993 Effects of air pressure *(cont'd)*

Occupational Disability Durations, in days
Median (mid-point) 11 - Benchmark Indemnity Costs $8,250

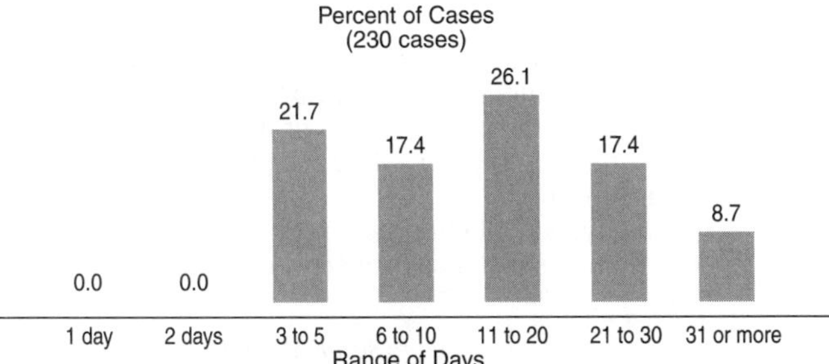

Impact on Occupational Absence: Prevalence 0.0287% of occupational lost workdays

994 Effects of other external causes

Return-To-Work Summary Guidelines		
Dataset	**Midrange**	**At-Risk**
Claims data	24 days	112 days
All absences	2 days	26 days

Excludes:
certain adverse effects not elsewhere classified (995.0-995.8)

Workers' Comp Costs per Claim (based on 4,494 claims)

Quartile	25%	50%	75%	Mean	% no cost
Indemnity	$830	$2,315	$6,867	$15,572	95%
Medical	$179	$368	$725	$760	7%
Total	$189	$378	$756	$1,544	6%

RTW Claims Data (Calendar-days away from work by decile)

10%	20%	30%	40%	**50%**	60%	70%	80%	**90%**	100%	Mean
9	11	15	19	**24**	35	42	59	**112**	171	41.57

Integrated Disability Durations, in days*
Median (mid-point) 2.0 Mean (average) 10.52
Mode (most frequent) 1 Calculated rec. 4

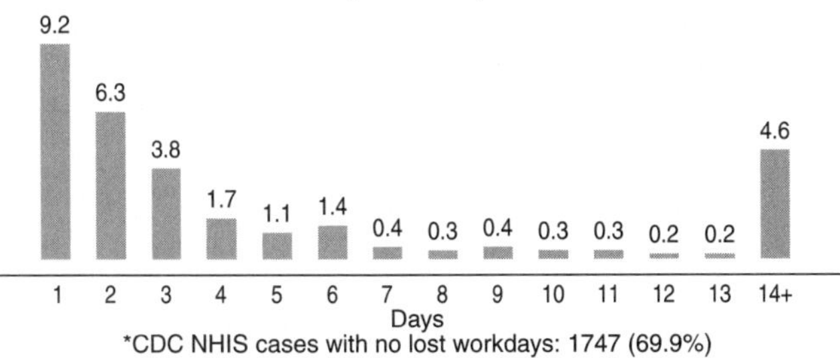

*CDC NHIS cases with no lost workdays: 1747 (69.9%)

Impact on Total Absence: Prevalence 0.0234% of total lost workdays; Incidence 0.25 days per 100 workers

994.6 Motion sickness

Return-To-Work Summary Guidelines		
Dataset	**Midrange**	**At-Risk**
Claims data	24 days	112 days
All absences	2 days	26 days

Return-To-Work "Best Practice" Guidelines
Avoid motion-induced jobs: 0 days

994.6 Motion sickness *(cont'd)*

Air sickness
Seasickness
Travel sickness

994.8 Electrocution and nonfatal effects of electric current

Return-To-Work Summary Guidelines		
Dataset	**Midrange**	**At-Risk**
Claims data	37 days	364 days
All absences	4 days	64 days

Return-To-Work "Best Practice" Guidelines
Moderate: 7-14 days
Severe, cardiac arrest, clerical/modified work: 21-42 days
Severe, cardiac arrest, manual work: 64 days to indefinite

Shock from electric current

Excludes:
electric burns (940.0-949.5)

Workers' Comp Costs per Claim (based on 2,476 claims)

Quartile	25%	50%	75%	Mean	% no cost
Indemnity	$1,218	$2,111	$5,985	$12,739	94%
Medical	$242	$483	$935	$943	6%
Total	$242	$504	$998	$1,779	5%

RTW Claims Data (Calendar-days away from work by decile)

10%	20%	30%	40%	**50%**	60%	70%	80%	**90%**	100%	Mean
12	15	20	22	**37**	42	63	67	**364**	365	73.50

Integrated Disability Durations, in days*
Median (mid-point) 4.0 Mean (average) 30.23
Mode (most frequent) 1 Calculated rec. 10

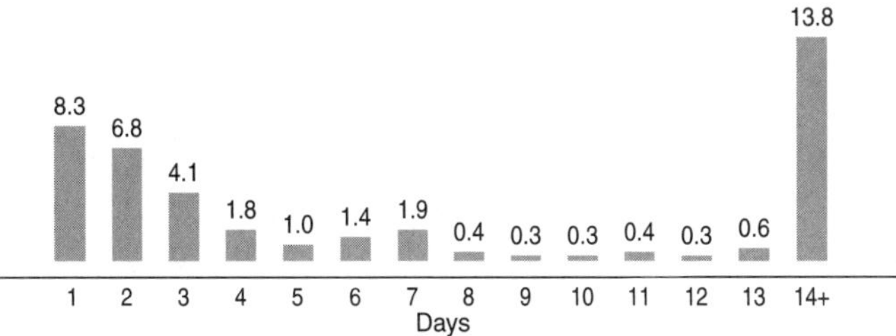

*CDC NHIS cases with no lost workdays: 917 (58.6%)

Impact on Total Absence: Prevalence 0.0579% of total lost workdays; Incidence 0.61 days per 100 workers

Occupational Disability Durations, in days
Median (mid-point) 5 - Benchmark Indemnity Costs $3,750

Percent of Cases
(1600 cases)

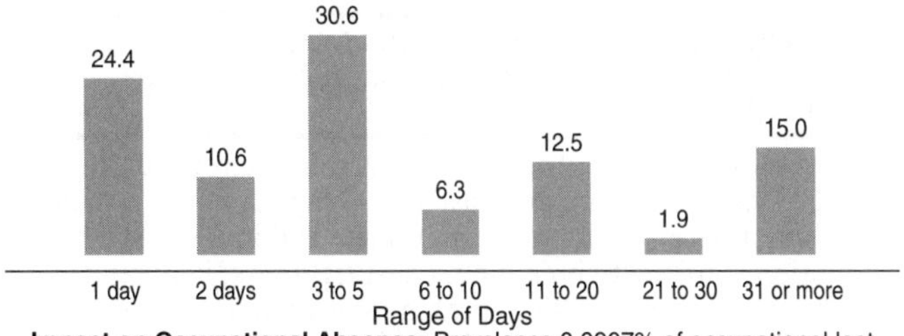

1 day	2 days	3 to 5	6 to 10	11 to 20	21 to 30	31 or more
24.4	10.6	30.6	6.3	12.5	1.9	15.0

Range of Days

Impact on Occupational Absence: Prevalence 0.0907% of occupational lost workdays; Incidence 0.01 days per 100 workers

995 Certain adverse effects not elsewhere classified

Return-To-Work Summary Guidelines		
Dataset	Midrange	At-Risk
Claims data	14 days	36 days
All absences	4 days	14 days

Return-To-Work "Best Practice" Guidelines
See 995.0

Note: This category is to be used to identify the effects not elsewhere classifiable of unknown, undetermined, or ill-defined causes. This category may also be used to provide an additional code to identify the effects of conditions classified elsewhere.

Excludes:
complications of surgical and medical care (996.0-999.9)

Workers' Comp Costs per Claim (based on 695 claims)					
Quartile	25%	50%	75%	Mean	% no cost
Indemnity	$452	$2,636	$4,547	$6,766	96%
Medical	$137	$221	$462	$455	11%
Total	$137	$221	$473	$768	11%

RTW Claims Data (Calendar-days away from work by decile)										
10%	20%	30%	40%	**50%**	60%	70%	80%	**90%**	100%	Mean
9	9	11	13	**14**	15	15	17	**36**	365	29.58

Integrated Disability Durations, in days*
Median (mid-point) 4.0 Mean (average) 8.42
Mode (most frequent) 1 Calculated rec. 4

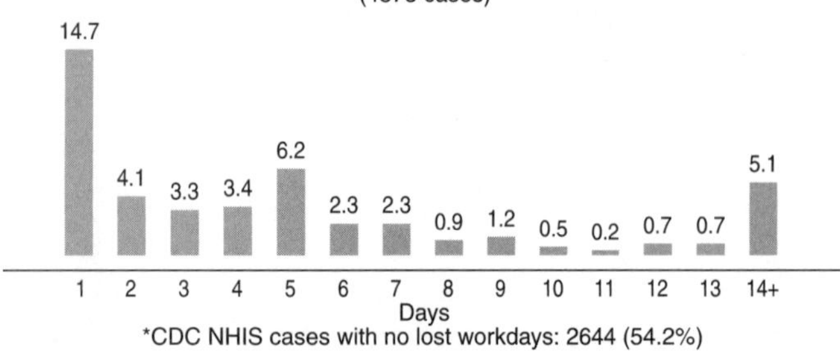

*CDC NHIS cases with no lost workdays: 2644 (54.2%)

Impact on Total Absence: Prevalence 0.0555% of total lost workdays; Incidence 0.58 days per 100 workers

995.0 Other anaphylactic shock

Return-To-Work Summary Guidelines		
Dataset	Midrange	At-Risk
Claims data	14 days	36 days
All absences	4 days	14 days

Return-To-Work "Best Practice" Guidelines
Medical treatment (consider occupational allergy): 1 day
With hospitalization: 5 days

Description: An acute, life-threatening allergic reaction of the immune system to a foreign substance. Symptoms begin with in two hours after exposure to the substance and include agitation, palpitations, difficulty breathing, chest tightness, itchy and flushed skin, hives, swelling, profuse sweating, coughing, and/or sneezing. Serious cases can result in total obstruction of the respiratory system and circulatory collapse, causing convulsions, loss of consciousness and bladder control, and/or stroke.

Other names: Anaphylaxis

Allergic shock NOS or due to adverse effect of correct medicinal substance properly administered
Anaphylactic reaction NOS or due to adverse effect of correct medicinal substance properly administered
Anaphylaxis NOS or due to adverse effect of correct medicinal substance properly administered

Excludes:
anaphylactic reaction to serum (999.4)
anaphylactic shock due to adverse food reaction (995.60-995.69)
Code also any underlying condition such as:
poisoning by drugs, medicinals and biologic substances (960-979)
toxic effects of substances chiefly nonmedical as to source (980-989)
Use additional E code to identify external cause, such as:
adverse effects of correct medicinal substance properly administered [E930-E949]

Impact on Total Absence: Prevalence 0.0002% of total lost workdays

995.2 Other and unspecified adverse effect of drug, medicinal and biological substance (due) to correct medicinal substance properly administered

Return-To-Work Summary Guidelines		
Dataset	Midrange	At-Risk
Claims data	15 days	18 days
All absences	13 days	17 days

Return-To-Work "Best Practice" Guidelines
Moderate: 3 days
Severe: 14 days

Adverse effect to correct medicinal substance properly administered
Allergic reaction to correct medicinal substance properly administered
Hypersensitivity to correct medicinal substance properly administered
Idiosyncrasy due to correct medicinal substance properly administered
Drug:
hypersensitivity NOS
reaction NOS

Excludes:
pathological drug intoxication (292.2)

Workers' Comp Costs per Claim (based on 63 claims)					
Quartile	25%	50%	75%	Mean	% no cost
Medical	$147	$242	$473	$969	15%
Total	$158	$268	$599	$1,089	15%

RTW Claims Data (Calendar-days away from work by decile)										
10%	20%	30%	40%	**50%**	60%	70%	80%	**90%**	100%	Mean
12	13	14	14	**15**	15	16	16	**18**	365	18.97

995.2 Other and unspecified adverse effect of drug, medicinal and biological substance (due) to correct medicinal substance properly

Integrated Disability Durations, in days*

Median (mid-point) 13.0 Mean (average) 12.25
Mode (most frequent) 14 Calculated rec. 13

Percent of Cases
(4925 cases)

15.8 8.0 3.5 3.2 19.8 9.7 0.2 0.0 0.1 0.1 0.1 0.1 0.0 0.8

3 6 9 12 15 18 21 24 27 30 33 36 39 40+
Range of Days (up to)
*CDC NHIS cases with no lost workdays: 1901 (38.6%)

Impact on Total Absence: Prevalence 0.1094% of total lost workdays; Incidence 1.15 days per 100 workers

995.3 Allergy, unspecified

Return-To-Work Summary Guidelines		
Dataset	**Midrange**	**At-Risk**
Claims data	16 days	58 days
All absences	3 days	56 days

Return-To-Work "Best Practice" Guidelines
Medical treatment (unless occupational): 0 days
Medical treatment, regular work (if work related): 14-56 days

Description: Hypersensitivity of the immune system to a foreign substance causing symptoms of rash, swelling, congestion, sneezing, tearing, earache, cough, breathing problems, sore throat, and/or gastrointestinal symptoms.

Allergic reaction NOS
Hypersensitivity NOS
Idiosyncrasy NOS

Excludes:
allergic reaction NOS to correct medicinal substance properly administered (995.2)
specific types of allergic reaction, such as:
allergic diarrhea (558.9)
dermatitis (691.0-693.9)
hayfever (477.0-477.9)

Workers' Comp Costs per Claim (based on 562 claims)					
Quartile	25%	50%	75%	Mean	% no cost
Medical	$137	$210	$378	$345	11%
Total	$137	$210	$389	$445	11%

Disability Duration Adjustment Factors by Age						
Age Group	18-24	25-34	35-44	45-54	55-64	65-74
Adjustment Factor	0.88	0.80	0.75	1.12	1.82	1.92

RTW Claims Data (Calendar-days away from work by decile)										
10%	20%	30%	40%	**50%**	60%	70%	80%	**90%**	100%	Mean
12	14	14	15	**16**	27	56	57	**58**	365	35.25

995.3 Allergy, unspecified *(cont'd)*

Integrated Disability Durations, in days*

Median (mid-point) 3.0 Mean (average) 14.51
Mode (most frequent) 1 Calculated rec. 5

Percent of Cases
(1132 cases)

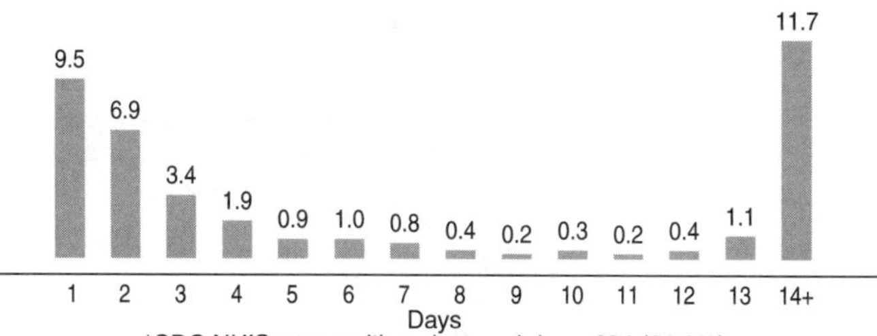

Days
*CDC NHIS cases with no lost workdays: 694 (61.3%)

Impact on Total Absence: Prevalence 0.0187% of total lost workdays; Incidence 0.20 days per 100 workers

Occupational Disability Durations, in days

Median (mid-point) 2 - Benchmark Indemnity Costs $1,500

Percent of Cases
(560 cases)

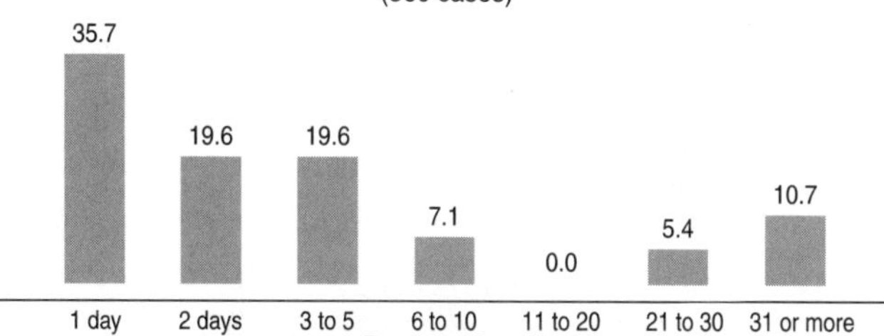

Range of Days

Impact on Occupational Absence: Prevalence 0.0127% of occupational lost workdays

COMPLICATIONS OF SURGICAL AND MEDICAL CARE, NOT ELSEWHERE CLASSIFIED (996-999)

Excludes:
adverse effects of medicinal agents (001.0-799.9, 995.0-995.8)
burns from local applications and irradiation (940.0-949.5)
complications of:
conditions for which the procedure was performed
surgical procedures during abortion, labor, and delivery (630-676.9)
poisoning and toxic effects of drugs and chemicals (960.0-989.9)
postoperative conditions in which no complications are present, such as:
artificial opening status (V44.0-V44.9)
closure of external stoma (V55.0-V55.9)
fitting of prosthetic device (V52.0-V52.9)
specified complications classified elsewhere
anesthetic shock (995.4)
electrolyte imbalance (276.0-276.9)
postlaminectomy syndrome (722.80-722.83)
postmastectomy lymphedema syndrome (457.0)
postoperative psychosis (293.0-293.9)
any other condition classified elsewhere in the Alphabetic Index when described as due to a procedure

RTW Claims Data (Calendar-days away from work by decile)										
10%	20%	30%	40%	**50%**	60%	70%	80%	**90%**	100%	Mean
11	13	14	15	**15**	17	29	50	**100**	365	41.00

Impact on Total Absence: Prevalence 0.1749% of total lost workdays; Incidence 1.84 days per 100 workers

996 Complications peculiar to certain specified procedures

Return-To-Work Summary Guidelines		
Dataset	**Midrange**	**At-Risk**
Claims data	14 days	20 days
All absences	10 days	20 days

Includes: complications, not elsewhere classified, in the use of artificial substitutes [e.g., Dacron, metal, Silastic, Teflon] or natural sources [e.g., bone] involving:
anastomosis (internal)
graft (bypass) (patch)
implant
internal device:
catheter
electronic
fixation
prosthetic
reimplant
transplant

Excludes:
accidental puncture or laceration during procedure (998.2)
complications of internal anastomosis of:
gastrointestinal tract (997.4)
urinary tract (997.5)
other specified complications classified elsewhere, such as:
hemolytic anemia (283.1)
functional cardiac disturbances (429.4)
serum hepatitis (070.2-070.3)

Workers' Comp Costs per Claim (based on 403 claims)					
Quartile	25%	50%	75%	Mean	% no cost
Indemnity	$7,382	$16,002	$45,056	$29,018	18%
Medical	$12,726	$25,431	$59,346	$40,585	1%
Total	$18,459	$42,488	$95,393	$64,296	1%

996.3 Mechanical complication of genitourinary device, implant, and graft

Return-To-Work Summary Guidelines		
Dataset	**Midrange**	**At-Risk**
Claims data	14 days	20 days
All absences	10 days	20 days

Impact on Total Absence: Prevalence 0.0002% of total lost workdays

996.32 Due to intrauterine contraceptive device

Return-To-Work Summary Guidelines		
Dataset	**Midrange**	**At-Risk**
Claims data	14 days	42 days
All absences	10 days	20 days

Return-To-Work "Best Practice" Guidelines
Medical treatment: 0 days
Laparoscopy: 7 days
Laparotomy, clerical/modified work: 28 days
Laparotomy, manual work: 42 days

Description: Tearing of the muscular wall of the uterus during the insertion of an intrauterine contraceptive device that may pierce through the uterine wall into the abdominal cavity. This is more likely to happen if the uterus is soft, such as after a birth

or abortion, or if the individual moves during the insertion. Symptoms include vaginal bleeding, pelvic or abdominal pain, and/or failure to find and IUD string.
Other names: Perforation of uterus

ICD9 KEYWORD INDEX